Advanced
Urologic
Surgery

Advanced Urologic Surgery

EDITED BY

Rudolf Hohenfellner

Department of Urology,
University of Mainz, Mainz, Germany

John Fitzpatrick

Department of Surgery, Mater Misericordiae Hospital,
University College Dublin,
Dublin, Ireland

Jack McAninch

Department of Urology, San Francisco General Hospital,
San Francisco, USA

THIRD EDITION

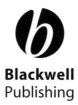

Blackwell
Publishing

© 2005 by Blackwell Publishing Ltd

Blackwell Publishing, Inc., 350 Main Street, Malden, Massachusetts 02148-5020, USA
Blackwell Publishing Ltd, 9600 Garsington Road, Oxford OX4 2DQ, UK
Blackwell Publishing Asia Pty Ltd, 550 Swanston Street, Carlton, Victoria 3053,
Australia

Library of Congress Cataloging-in-Publication Data

Advanced urologic surgery / [edited by] Rudolf Hohenfellner, John Fitzpatrick, Jack
McAninch. — 3rd ed.
    p.   ;   cm.
  Rev. ed. of: Innovations in urologic surgery, 1997.
  Includes bibliographical references.
  1. Genitourinary organs — Surgery.
  [DNLM: 1. Urogenital System — surgery.   2. Urogenital Diseases — surgery.   3.
Urogenital Surgical Procedures — methods.]
I. Hohenfellner, Rudolf.   II. Fitzpatrick, John M.   III. McAninch, Jack W.   IV.
Innovations in urologic surgery.   V. Title.

  RD571.A35 2005   2005002630
  617.4′6 — dc22

A catalogue record for this title is available from the British Library

ISBN-13: 978-1-4051-2213-9
ISBN-10: 1-4051-2213-7

Set in 10 on 12pt Minion by SNP Best-set Typesetter Ltd., Hong Kong
Printed and bound in India by Replika Press Pvt. Ltd

Commissioning Editor: Stuart Taylor
Development Editor: Rebecca Huxley
Production Controller: Kate Charman

For further information on Blackwell Publishing, visit our website:
http://www.blackwellpublishing.com

The publisher's policy is to use permanent paper from mills that operate a sustainable
forestry policy, and which has been manufactured from pulp processed using acid-free and
elementary chlorine-free practices. Furthermore, the publisher ensures that the text paper
and cover board used have met acceptable environmental accreditation standards.

Contents

Preface to Third Edition

The aim of the editors in producing this textbook, the third edition of *Advanced Urologic Surgery*, remains the same as that declared in the preface to the second edition: we wish to produce a stimulating and up-to-date operative textbook that will supply the reader with a mainly pictorial interpretation of technical advancements and innovations, with a number of interesting modifications and suggested improvements, based on the large experience of a stellar group of well-known international urologists. The amount of text is kept to a minimum, and is structured into a series of concise bullet points that provide step-by-step information. We believe that this methodology will be of greater value to the reader than page after page of prose, however purple that might have been!

The first edition was reasonably limited and published exclusively in German. It was so instantly well received that further reprints were required within the first year of its appearance in print, as well as translation becoming standardized and with a further emphasis on pictorial representation of the various surgical techniques. This third edition, now entitled *Advanced Urologic Surgery*, has further developed the artistic format, but each author has been asked to supply, in bullet points, a number of different aspects about the surgical technique they discuss. Each author outlines the indications for the procedure in question, the limitations and contraindications, any specific preoperative management or instruments required, and then a brief description of the surgical technique, if possible overlaying their technique on any important anatomical principles. Potential complications are also described. Finally, the authors of each chapter draw on their own extensive experience and provide tips to the reader, which should be of help when performing the surgery.

At this point, we must express our considerable gratitude to Gottfried Müller, whose outstanding artwork has been a feature of the book, adding significantly to its readability and attractiveness as a product.

It has not been our intention to relentlessly work our way through all of the surgical procedures known in urology. In the preface to the second edition, it was pointed out that there were, for example, over 300 surgical procedures described in the treatment of hypospadias, and that it would clearly be impossible to cover even a fraction of these, and this is still the case with the third edition. However, all of the currently recommended techniques for the full range of urologic conditions are included in this textbook. Some of the traditionally employed standard techniques may not appear in these pages, as the emphasis in many places is on the description of newly introduced but already accepted urologic procedures. We believe that the reader will find value and enjoyment when reading this textbook, either as a 'cover-to-cover' read, or if the reader wishes to dip into the particular section that applies to their area of interest.

It has been a feature of the previous editions that readers felt free to communicate their views about the book to the editors and to the publishers. Once again, we would encourage this. The interaction between reader and editor/publisher is a help to both, from our point of view helping us to produce an excellent product which will be of continuing value to our readers.

We very much hope that you will enjoy reading this book.

R. Hohenfellner
J. M. Fitzpatrick
J. McAninch

Preface to Second Edition

Surgical atlases and operative textbooks which are often produced with a great deal of effort seldom elude an all too rapid ageing process. The more dilatory the co-authors participating, the longer the period of time it takes from planning and production to the finished product. From this sorrowful realization was born the concept of *Innovations in Urologic Surgery*. The aim was to produce a stimulating operative textbook with an animated interpretation of technical advancements and innovations or supplements, modifications and improvement proposals for standardized and new procedures.

The first edition, published in 1994, was limited and published only in the German language. The huge national and international interest which followed, led to two further German reprints in the same year and translations into Italian, Japanese, Portuguese, Spanish and now English.

For the purpose of limiting and systematizing the text, we completely revised the first German publication into categories according to indication, contraindication, instruments, approach, step by step technique, operative tricks, postoperative care and special features.

Reviews from surgeons familiar with the specific problems of each procedure provide an objective approach and at the same time contributed towards the evaluation of each respective technique. Three stars (***) represent standardized, proven over many years, recommended procedures; two stars: technically largely standardized, details could be improved upon, proven regarding reproducibility and long-term results with guaranteed data; one star: a new procedure, possibly useful and reproducible although without conclusive results.

In accordance with the concept described in the introduction, we re-evaluated the already published procedures. Analysis of information from congresses and operation seminars proved particularly helpful in this respect. The interest and demand for a particular technique can be calculated from the number of lectures, poster and video contributions. Additionally, the published complications demonstrated the reproducibility as well as possible technical shortcomings. For example, an analysis of 'neuralgic ureter implantation sites' in continent urinary reservoirs showed the occurrence of a predominantly short-term postoperative obstruction rate of up to 8%. Accordingly there was considerable interest in the antirefluxive 'Hassan implantation' with a minimal complication rate including also dilated, thick-walled ureters. Despite the comparative short follow-up of only 2 years, this alternative procedure was included.

The reader will undoubtedly search in vain for some of the more traditionally employed 'gold standard' techniques, which have proved their worth and from which there is no reason to deviate. Consequently, the reader will most probably not miss these all too familiar techniques. Nevertheless the editors are particularly grateful for comments and correspondence on these subjects. It is only through continuous dialogue with operating surgeons that these animated operative techniques can fulfil the original intentions.

Many authors who participated in the first German edition will miss their contributions in this English language version. The prevailing reasons were either high published complication rates or technical improvements developed in alternative procedures. The emphasis lies deliberately on a 'selection' of operative techniques; an undoubtedly problematic undertaking. On the other hand the reader may feel spoiled for choice in view of, for example, the 300 surgical procedures for hypospadias correction published up until 1995. If only 20 from this number were reproduced, as is the case in the average surgical atlas, the situation would not be any better. Should the reader not systematically follow for example, 'hypospadiology', he or she may not realize that a procedure perhaps favored by an institution for over 10 years and published in various national and international surgical textbooks has been abandoned due to a high late complication rate. *Innovations in Urologic Surgery* seeks to do justice to such a situation.

At this point we would like to express our gratitude to Mr Brammer who, apart from his artistic skills, possesses the necessary capacity and composure to produce high quality illustrations under the exacting demands of deadline pressure. Furthermore, we thank the reviewer for their critical and time-consuming work. Last but not least, our thanks go to Mrs Hug who ran the entire scientific secretariat superbly.

R. Hohenfellner
A. Novick
J. Fichtner

Contributors

Abbou, C.-C.
Service d'Urologie
Centre Hospitalier Universitaire Henri Mondor
Paris
France

Albers, P.
Klinik und Poliklinik für Urologie
Rheinische Friedrich-Wilhelms Universität
Bonn
Germany

Alken, P.
Department of Urology
University Hospital Mannheim
Mannheim
Germany

Alsikafi, N. F.
Department of Urology
University of Chicago Hospitals
Mount Sinai Hospital
Chicago
Illinois
USA

Assenmacher, Chr.
Service D'Urologie
Hôpital St. Elisabeth
Uccle
Belgium

Austen, M.
Klinik für Urologie und Kinderurologie
Klinikum Fulda
Fulda
Germany

Bastian, P. J.
Klinik und Poliklinik für Urologie
Rheinische Friedrich-Wilhelms Universität
Bonn
Germany

Black, P. C.
Department of Urology
Harborview Medical Center
Seattle
Washington
USA

Bollens, R.
Service D'Urologie
Hôpital Erasme
Bruxelles
Belgium

Bracka, A.
Department for Plastic Surgery
Wordsley Hospital
Stourbridge
UK

Braun, M.
Klinik für Urologie und Kinderurologie
Städtisches Klinikum
Fulda
Germany

Braun, P.-M.
Klinik für Urologie und Kinderurologie
Universitätsklinikum Schleswig-Holstein
Campus Kiel
Kiel
Germany

Bräutigam, B.
Waldstrasse 49
64569 Nauheim
Germany

Bürger, R. A.
Urologische Klinik und Poliklinik
St. Katharinen Krankenhaus
Frankfurt
Germany

D'Elia, G.
77 Viale Parioli
Rome

Dekuyper, P.
Dienst Urologie
Maria Middelaresziekenhius
Gent
Belgium

Dénes, F. T.
Urologic Clinic
Uropediatric Unit
São Paulo University Medical School Hospital
São Paulo
Brazil

Eicke, M.
Neurologische Universitätsklinik
Mainz
Germany

Elliott, S. P.
Department of Urology
University of California
San Francisco
California
USA

Engelmann, U.
Urologische Klink und Poliklinik
Medizinische Einrichtungen der Universität
  zu Köln
Köln
Germany

Engrav, L. H.
Division of Plastic Surgery
Department of Surgery
Harborview Medical Center and University of
  Washington
Seattle
Washington
USA

Fichtner, J.
Department of Urology
Johanniter Hospital
Steinbrinkstr. 96
Oberhausen
Germany

Filipas, D.
Department of Urology
University of Vienna
Vienna
Austria

Fillet, M.
Service D'Urologie
CHU Liège
Liège
Belgium

Fisch, M.
Allgemeines Krankenhaus Harburg
Urologisches Zentrum Hamburg
Hamburg
Germany

Fischer, A.
Abt. für Gynäkologie und Geburtshilfe
SCIVIAS-Krankenhaus St Josef
Rüdesheim am Rhein
Germany

Fitzpatrick, J. M.
Department of Surgery
Mater Misericordiae Hospital
University College Dublin
Dublin
Ireland

Fornara, P.
Department of Urology
Martin Luther University Halle-Wittenberg
Halle
Germany

Franc-Guimond, J.
Hôpital Sainte-Justine
University of Montreal
Montreal
Quebec
Canada

Gill, I. S.
Section of Laparoscopic and Minimally Invasive
   Surgery
Glickman Urological Institute
Cleveland Clinic Foundation
Cleveland
Ohio
USA

González, R.
A. I. duPont Hospital for Children
Wilmington Delaware and Thomas Jefferson
   University
Philadelphia
Pennsylvania
USA

Grady, R. W.
Department of Urology
Harborview Medical Center
Seattle
Washington
USA

Hiller, W. F. A.
Department of Surgery
Klinikum Lippe-Detmold
Detmold
Germany

Höckel, M.
Department of Obstetrics/Gynecology
University of Leipzig Medical Center
Leipzig
Germany

Hohenfellner, R.
Department of Urology
University of Mainz
Mainz
Germany

Homberg, R.
Department of Urology and Paediatric Urology
Ammerlandklinik
Westerstede
Germany

Howaldt, H.-P.
Department of Maxillo-Facial and Facial Plastic
   Surgery
Medical School
Justus Liebig University of Giessen
Giessen
Germany

Hoznek, A.
Service d'Urologie
Centre Hospitalier Universitaire Henri Mondor
Paris
France

Humke, U.
Department of Urology
Katharinenhospital
Stuttgart
Germany

Jünemann, K.-P.
Klinik für Urologie und Kinderurologie
Universitätsklinikum Schleswig-Holstein
Campus Kiel
Kiel
Germany

Jünger, T. H.
Department of Maxillo-Facial and Facial Plastic
   Surgery
Medical School
Justus Liebig University of Giessen
Giessen
Germany

Kälble, T.
Klinik für Urologie und Kinderurologie
Klinikum Fulda
Fulda
Germany

Kerschbaumer, F.
Department of Orthopedics
Johann Wolfgang Goethe University
Frankfurt
Germany

Kollias, A.
Department of Urology and Paediatric Urology
Ammerlandklinik
Westerstede
Germany

Langen, P. H.
Afdeling Urologie
Vie Curi Medisch
Centrum voor Noord Limburg
Venlo
The Netherlands

Latal, D.†
Department of Urology
Medical School Vienna
Vienna
Austria

Lau, H.
Department of Urology
Westmead Hospital
Darcy Road
Westmead
Australia

Leissner, J.
Department of Urology
Bonn University
Bonn
Germany

Libertino, J.
Department of Urology
Lahey Clinic Medical Center
Burlington
Massachusetts
USA

Lindenmeir, T.
Department of Urology
Otto von Guericke University
Magdeburg
Germany

Lodde, M.
Department of Urology
General Hospital of Bolzano/Bozen
Bolzano/Bozen
Italy

Macedo, Jr, A.
Division of Urology
Federal University of São Paulo
São Paulo
Brazil

Managadze, L.
Clinical and Experimental Development
    Foundation for Adult and Pediatric Urology
Tiblissi
Georgia
USA

Martens, P.
Dienst Urologie
Virga Jesseziekenhuis
Wasselt
Belgium

McAninch, J, W.
Department of Urology
University of California
and
San Francisco General Hospital
San Francisco
California
USA

Melchior, S. W.
Department of Urology
University of Mainz
Mainz
Germany

Michel, M. S.
Department of Urology
University Hospital Mannheim
Mannheim
Germany

Mitchell, M. E.
Children's Hospital
Seattle
Washington
USA

Mottrie, A.
Dienst Urologie
OLV Zienkenhuis
Aalst
Belgium

Müller, S. C.
Department of Urology
Bonn University
Bonn
Germany

Nicolas, H.
Service D'Urologie
Hôpital Le Citadelle
Liège
Belgium

Nitti, V. W.
Department of Urology
New York University School of Medicine
New York
USA

Olianas, R.
Allgemeines Krankenhaus Harburg
Urologisches Zentrum Hamburg
Hamburg
Germany

Pansadoro, V.
559 via Aurelia
Rome

Perovic, S. V.
Department of Urology
University Children's Hospital
Belgrade
Serbia and Montenegro

Pycha, A.
Department of Urology
General Hospital of Bolzano/Bozen
Bolzano/Bozen
Italy

Salomon, L.
Service d'Urologie
Centre Hospitalier Universitaire Henri Mondor
Paris
France

Scarpero, H. M.
Department of Urology
New York University School of Medicine
New York
USA

Schmiedt, W.
Klinik und Poliklinik für Herz-, Thorax- und
    Gefäßchirurgie
Universitätsklinik Mainz
Mainz
Germany

Schönberger, B.
Urological Clinic
Humboldt University
Berlin
Germany

Schreiter, F.
Urological Clinic Hamburg-Harburg
University of Witten/Herdecke
Hamburg
Germany

Seif, C.
Klinik für Urologie und Kinderurologie
Universitätsklinikum Schleswig-Holstein
Campus Kiel
Kiel
Germany

Sorcini, A.
Department of Urology
Lahey Clinic

Srougi, E. M.
Division of Urology
Federal State of São Paulo
São Paulo
Brazil

Stackl, W.
Urologische Abteilung Krankenstalten
    Rudolfstiftung
Wien
Juchgasse
Austria

Steffens, J.
Department of Urology and Pediatric Urology
St Antonius Hospital
Eschweiler
Germany

Stein, R.
Department of Urology
Medical School
Johannes Gutenberg University of Mainz
Mainz
Germany

Steinberg, A. P.
Department of Urology
McGill University
Montreal
Quebec
Canada

Stief, C. G.
Department of Urology
Ludwigs-Maximilians Universität München
Munich
Germany

Stolzenburg, J.-U.
Department of Urology
University of Leipzig
Leipzig
Germany

Svensson, L.
Department of Cardiothoracic Surgery
Lahey Clinic

Tal, Raanan
Institute of Urology
Rabin Medical Center
Golda-Hasharon Campus
Petah Tikva
Israel

Van Velthoven, R.
Service D'Urologie
Institut Bordet
Bruxelles
Belgium

Varol, C.
Department of Urology
Nepean Hospital
Sydney
Australia

Wammack, R.
Katholische Kliniken Essen-Nord gGmbH
Klinik für Urologie und Neurourologie
Essen
Germany

Wessells, H.
Department of Urology
Harborview Medical Center and University of
    Washington
Seattle
Washington
USA

Witzsch, U. H. Fr.
Krankenhaus Nordwest
Klinik für Urologie und Kinderurologie
Frankfurt
Germany

Zacharias, M.
Department of Urology
Martin Luther University Halle-Wittenberg
Halle
Germany

Ziegler, M,
Department of General and Pediatric Urology
University Hospital of Saarland
Homburg/Saar
Germany

Zumbé, J.
Klinik für Urologie
Klinikum Leverkusen
Leverkusen
Germany

Section 1
Kidney and Ureter

Part 1.1
Kidney and Upper Ureter

Chapter 1
Posterior Lumbotomy

V. Pansadoro

Introduction

This technique was first published by H. Lurz in 1956 and is the author's method of choice for pyeloplasty whenever the laparoscopic approach is not possible. It is relatively easy to perform, demonstrate, and teach, with a short learning curve. There is limited exposure but it is good enough for the planned procedure.

Patient counseling and consent

As for a routine surgical procedure.

Indications

This procedure is indicated in surgical pyeloplasty and in approaches to the lumbar ureter.

Limitation and risks

- Very high kidney.
- Very short patient.

Contraindications

The technique is contraindicated in patients with previous cancer surgery, a horseshoe kidney, an anteriorly placed renal pelvis, and a history of previous surgery.

Preoperative management

As routine for kidney surgery.

Anesthesia

Blended, general, and peridural anesthesia.

Special instruments/suture material

- Bookwalter self-retaining retractor.

Operative technique

Anatomy

The lumbodorsal region is delineated by three bony structures: the iliac crest, the 12th rib, and the spinal processes. Between these three structures are the sacrospinalis muscle and the quadratus lumborum muscle. Two factors contribute to the originality of the Lurz approach: the incision is exactly on the quadratus lumborum muscle, which is situated in the center of the dorsolumbar region, and the operating field is widened by mobilization of the 12th rib after the costovertebral ligament is severed.

Patient's position

The position of the patient on the operating table is important and needs emphasis. It is characterized by three main features. The laterolateral axis makes a 45° angle with the operating table. It is not necessary for the table to be bent too much because the muscles do not need to be stretched; on the contrary, it is better if they are relaxed to allow easier retraction. The thorax is turned ventrally and the pelvis dorsally to allow a better opening of the dorsolumbar space. The legs and the upper arm are positioned as usual for a flank incision (Fig. 1.1).

Skin incision

Once the iliac crest, the 12th rib, and the spinal processes have been localized, the sacrospinalis muscle can be identified easily and the surgeon is able to localize the quadratus lumborum. This muscle goes from the medial part of the 12th rib to the mid third of the iliac crest; its upper third is under the sacrospinalis muscle. The skin incision is made over the quadratus lumborum muscle and begins at the costovertebral angle, over the lateral part of the sacrospinalis muscle, and with a slightly oblique course extends down to the iliac crest,

3–5 cm in front of the anterior margin of the sacrospinalis muscle (Fig. 1.2).

Approach to the kidney

The incision of the muscular plane has the shape of a 'Y', with the sacrospinalis muscle contained between the two arms of the Y (Fig. 1.3). The incision of the muscular layers is a step-by-step procedure that should open the flank safely and exactly, and avoid any injury to the muscle and nerves present in this region. After the incision of the subcutaneous fat, the last fibers of the latissimus dorsi and the serratus dorsalis caudalis muscles are cut.

As the incision is deepened in its cranial portion, the posterior aspect of the lumbodorsal fascia is opened and the fibers of the sacrospinalis muscle are uncovered (Fig. 1.4). These fibers are easily identified by their craniocaudal direction. By cutting through the posterior lumbodorsal fascia around the sacrospinalis muscle, the surgeon completes the incision of the superficial arm of the Y. The sacrospinalis muscle is then prepared in its lateral and deep aspect and is retracted medially, uncovering the anterior aspect of the lumbodorsal fascia and, under this, the quadratus lumborum muscle (Fig. 1.5). When the fascia between these two muscles is incised, the deep arm of the Y is completed and the lumbodorsal fascia is severed caudally over the quadratus lumborum. Following strictly the direction of the fibers of this muscle, the surgeon completes the limb of the Y (Fig. 1.6). Retracting this muscle medially, we uncover the posterior aspect of the perirenal (Gerota's) fascia and identify the iliohypogastric and ilioinguinal nerves. This fascia must be incised between these nerves, which are retracted to each side by two Richardson retractors, reaching the perirenal area (Fig. 1.7).

Ureterolithotomy

In the event a ureterolithotomy must be performed, a deeper retractor should be inserted in the anterior aspect of the wound, so the inferior pole of the kidney can be lifted and moved cranially. Usually the ureter can be identified by simple inspection of the posterior aspect of the retroperitoneal space (Fig. 1.8). An oblique ureterotomy is preferred, and a 5/0 extramucosal running suture is used for closure. Of course the posterior approach is not indicated for stones lying lower than the iliac crest.

Ureteropyeloplasty

When the need for a ureteropyeloplasty arises, the pelvis lies directly in the center of the incision, and the operation can be done without any further dissection. It is helpful to expose the renal sinus with the aid of a small peanut. The kidney can then be moved anteriorly and superficially with two Gil-Vernet retractors. Usually after this maneuver a self-retaining retractor can be inserted and the pyeloplasty can be done with great ease (Fig. 1.9).

Wound closure

The wound closure is accomplished with interrupted 1/0 absorbable sutures, in one layer, on the lumbodorsal fascia. The quadratus lumborum and sacrospinalis muscles will regain their normal positions. Patients will usually experience an almost painless recovery.

Tips

Before surgery obtain a KUB in a supine and standing position to evaluate the kidney's mobility. Avoid fixed kidneys. By incising the costovertebral ligament the 12th rib can be retracted easily obtaining a wider exposure.

The surgeon who uses posterior lumbotomy must learn how to get the best exposure with this relatively small incision. During the opening phase, two Richardson retractors are used, and after the renal sinus has been prepared, two Gil-Vernet sinus retractors are essential to bring the kidney into the best position. Only then is a self-retaining retractor used to provide the best exposure, with the kidney lifted and positioned in the center of the incision.

Postoperative care

As routine for kidney surgery.

Complications

Care must be taken not to injure the ileoinguinal and ileohypogastric nerves to avoid secondary anesthesia of the corresponding region. Temporary hypotonus of muscles of the anterolateral abdominal wall, caused by stretching of the corresponding nerves, may happen.

Troubleshooting

The patient's positioning is of the utmost importance to get the best from the incision. The posterior lumbotomy is a fast, easy, relatively painless, and minimally traumatic approach to the kidney and upper ureter but the working space is more limited than usual. The surgeon who uses the posterior lumbotomy technique should avoid using it for the wrong indications.

Results

The muscle-sparing incision, lack of postoperative pain, absence of postoperative laparocele, and short hospitalization are the rewards of this approach.

To do

It is the perfect incision for a skinny patient, with a mobile kidney and a posteriorly placed dilated pelvis.

Not to do

The surgeon who uses this approach should know the limits of the incision and use it for the right indications.

References

1 Bergmann EV. Über Nierenextirpation. Berl Klin Wochenschr 1885;39:46–8.
2 Gil-Vernet J. New surgical concept in removing renal calculi. Urol Int 1965;20:255–88.
3 Guyon F. Leçons cliniques sur les Maladies des Voies Urinaires. J.B. Ballière, Paris, 1881.
4 Israel J. Ein Fall von Nierenextirpation. Berl Klin Wochenschr 1883;37:689.
5 Lury H. Ein muskelschonender Lumbalschnitt zur Freilegung der Niere. Chirurg 1956;27:125–8.
6 Lurz L, Lurz H. Die Eingriffe an den Harnorganen, Nebennieren und männlichen Geschlechtsorganen. In: Allgemeine und spezielle chirurgische Operationslehre, 2nd edn (Guleke N, Zenker R, eds). Springer Verlag, Berlin, 1961.
7 Lutzeyer Wl, Lymberoupoulos S. Der Lumbodorsale Zugang zur Niere (Lurz): Indikation, klinische Erfahrung, und kritische Beurteilung. Urologe A 1970;9:324–9.
8 Pansadoro V. La via posteriore nella Chirurgia del Rene e dell'Uretere. Atti Soc Ital Urol 1977:414–20.
9 Rosenstein P. Ein funktioneller Lumbalschnitt zur Freilegung der Niere. Z Urol Chir 1925;7:119–26.
10 Sigel A, Held L. Die Zugangswege der Nierenchirurgie. Urologe A 1963;2:144–53.
11 Simon G. Extirpation einer Niere am Menschen. Dtsch Klin 1870;22:137–9.

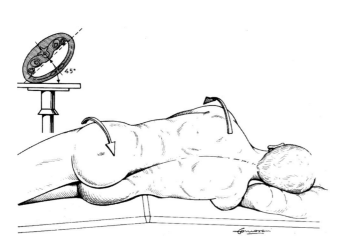

Figure 1.1 Position of the patient on the operating table.

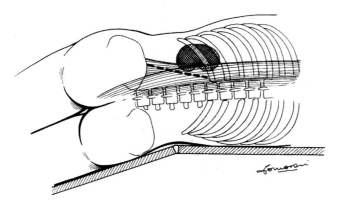

Figure 1.2 Skin incision.

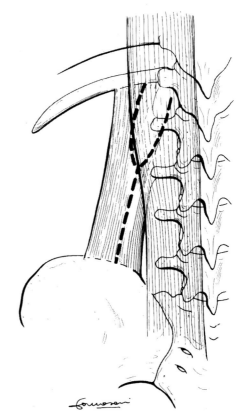

Figure 1.3 The approach to the kidney has the shape of a 'Y'.

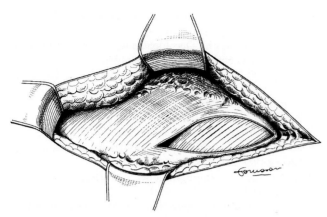

Figure 1.4 By incising the superficial arm of the 'Y', the fibers of the sacrospinalis muscle are uncovered.

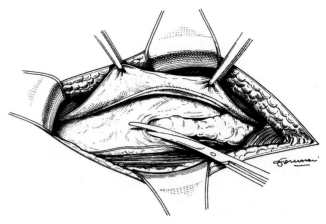

Figure 1.7 The iliohypogastric and ilioinguinal nerves are exposed, and the perineal space is entered between the two.

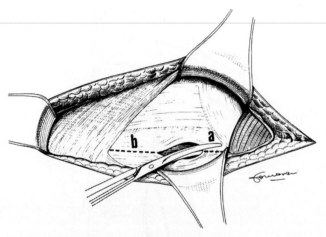

Figure 1.5 When the sacrospinalis muscle is retracted medially, the quadratus lumborum muscle is exposed under the deep aspect of the lumbodorsal fascia (a–b, the costovertebral ligament).

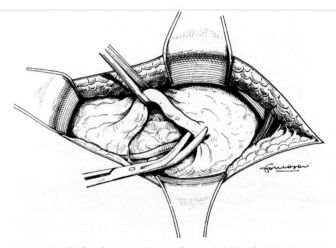

Figure 1.8 The lumbar ureter is usually easy to identify with proper anterior retraction.

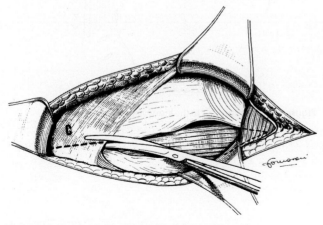

Figure 1.6 Incision of the limb of the 'Y' over the quadratus lumborum (c, the lumbodorsal fascia).

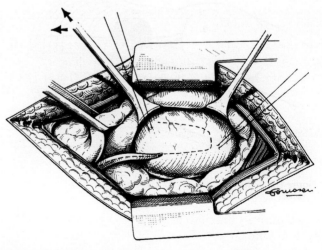

Figure 1.9 The proper use of two sinus retractors allows visualization of the entire renal pelvis.

Chapter 2
Laparoscopic Pyeloplasty

J.-U. Stolzenburg

Introduction

The Anderson–Hynes pyeloplasty is the most commonly performed surgical procedure for the correction of congenital or acquired pyeloureteric junction (PUJ) obstruction. It is widely recognized as the gold standard technique. Global interest in the procedure was initiated with the first laparoscopic pyeloplasty performed in 1993 [5]. With constant improvements in laparoscopic instruments over the past decade, many centers have progressed from the classic open operation to an entirely laparoscopic technique.

An evaluation of the laparoscopic versus open technique reveals comparable results. Success rates of over 90% have been reported following the laparoscopic procedure in adults as well as in children [1–3,6]. Additionally, the results of the laparoscopic Anderson–Hynes pyeloplasty have been 10–25% more successful when compared to other minimally invasive techniques (percutaneous antegrade or retrograde endopyelotomy). With endoluminal techniques, there is an ever present risk of injuring a crossing vessel, resulting in hemorrhage and potential renal loss. The magnification of the telescope allows for accurate dissection of the renal hilum with easy identification of any aberrant vessels that can be safely preserved [4]. Further advantages of the laparoscopic technique include its minimal invasiveness, lesser postoperative analgesia requirement, quicker recovery time, and improved cosmetic results.

Indications

These are identical to the open Anderson–Hynes pyeloplasty.

Contraindications

- Active urinary tract infection.
- Renal malrotations.
- Large renal calculi.
- Abdominal aortic aneurysm or prior abdominal surgery (here a retroperitoneal approach is recommended).
- Cardiorespiratory limitation (such a patient is unable to tolerate a capnoperitoneum).
- Previous attempt at PUJ obstruction repair (depending on the surgeon's experience).

Preoperative management

This is identical to the open Anderson–Hynes pyeloplasty. Note that the preoperative placement of a ureteric stent/catheter is not recommended.

Special instruments/suture material

- Standard laparoscopic tower/monitor.
- 10 mm, 0° telescope (optional 30° telescope).
- Veress cannula.
- 1 × 12 mm trocar (for optic).
- 3 × 5 mm trocars.
- Bipolar forceps: 5 mm.
- Atraumatic dissectors: 5 mm.
- Metzenbaum scissors.
- Hook scissors.
- Irrigation sucker: 5 mm.
- Needle holder: 5 mm.

Surgical approach

Transperitoneal access is an easier approach for the beginner and the overview is better with more space for instrument placement and handling. Aberrant vessels can be readily identified and dissected free without mobilizing the kidney. A disadvantage of this approach is the potential injury to the intraperitoneal organs.

Operative technique

- Insert an indwelling catheter, with the patient in a lateral position without hyperextension.
- Peritoneal access is gained initially with a Veress cannula.

Insufflate the peritoneal cavity with CO_2 at 12 mmHg pressure and insert a 10/12 mm safety trocar (Versaport).

• In obese patients the optical trocar should be placed into the pararectal line for optimal visualization of the retroperitoneal ureter and kidney. An optional minilaparotomy is an alternative for safe trocar placement.

• Insert the telescope and place the other three trocars under vision.

• Divide any adhesions.

• The Toldt's line is incised and the colon is mobilized medially. For a left-sided operation, mobilization needs to include the splenic flexure, and for a right side the hepatic flexure. The mobilization needs to continue 4 cm below the lower pole of the kidney.

• Identify the ureter, which lies medial and caudal to the lower pole of the kidney. Dissect and isolate the ureter up to the renal pelvis.

• A large dilated renal pelvis can be easily dissected free including the PUJ and the proximal ureter.

• To guarantee a tension-free anastomosis, 5 cm of proximal ureter needs to be mobilized, ensuring that the periureteric adventitia is maintained around the ureter to prevent ischemia. Only bipolar cautery should be used for hemostasis at the renal pelvis.

• A transperitoneal approach allows excellent visualization of any aberrant vessels that can be dissected free without injury and without compromise to the renal blood supply.

• Division of the ureter is made obliquely in a cranial medial to a caudal lateral direction below the stenosis. If an aberrant lower pole vessel is present, anterior transposition of the divided ureter is required prior to its repair.

• Spatulate the lateral aspect of the ureter for 1.5 cm.

• Rhomboid resection of the renal pelvis: care must be taken not to resect too much tissue and enter the renal calyces, which may result in scaring and narrowing.

• Any associated calculi can be retrieved and placed into an Endobag® to be removed at the end of the operation.

• The reconstruction of the pyeloureteral anastomosis follows the exact principles of the open Anderson–Hynes operation.

Tips

• Before cutting the PUJ, a 'stay' suture is placed on the medial margin of the ureter and caudally of the stricture to avoid malpositioning (rotation) of the ureter. The stay suture is removed after the first anastomotic suture.

• Once the posterior wall anastomosis has been completed, a 0.038 inch Terumo® guidewire (Terumo Corporation, Tokyo)

is inserted via the cranial trocar through the ureter into the bladder. A 6 or 7 Fr double-J catheter is placed over this wire into the renal pelvis. No other internal drain is required (e.g. nephrostomy tube).

• If the angle of the cranial trocar does not allow for easy guidewire placement into the ureter, a two-part puncture needle (diameter 1.3 mm/17.5; Bard-Angiomed, Germany) can be inserted into a more appropriate site. The guidewire and double-J catheter can be introduced through this following minor dilatation of the tract. Alternatively, the wire is totally inserted into the abdominal cavity and removed through a 5 mm port for double-J stent insertion.

• Drain placement can be achieved by introducing a laparoscopic grasper through the cranial trocar and out from the caudal trocar site. The caudal trocar is removed and a 20 Fr Robinson drain grasped and placed into the operative site.

• A stay suture may be needed to assist with the operation. A straight needle (KS needle, 2/0 Vicryl) is inserted through the lateral abdominal wall and placed through the renal pelvis and out where it is fixed on the skin.

• Renal calculi that are difficult to find can be retrieved with the aid of a flexible cystoscope and a Dormia basket. A 5 mm trocar will need to be exchanged for a 10/12 mm trocar for passage of the cystoscope. Alternatively a 5 mm telescope is placed through one of the other trocars and the (umbilical) 10/12 mm trocar site is used for the flexible cystoscope.

Postoperative care

The urethral catheter is removed 2–3 days after the procedure. The urethral stent is removed 3–4 weeks later.

References

1 Chen RN, Moore RG, Kavoussi LR. Laparoscopic pyeloplasty. Indications, technique, and long-term outcome. Urol Clin North Am 1998;25(2):323–30.

2 Janetschek G, Peschel R, Frauscher F, Franscher F. Laparoscopic pyeloplasty. Urol Clin North Am 2000;27(4):695–704.

3 Pattaras JG, Moore RG. Laparoscopic pyeloplasty. J Endourol 2000;14(10):895–904.

4 Rehman J, Landman J, Sundaram C, Clayman RV. Missed anterior crossing vessels during open retroperitoneal pyeloplasty: laparoscopic transperitoneal discovery and repair. J Urol 2001;166(2): 593–6.

5 Schuessler WW, Grune MT, Tecuanhuey LV, Preminger GM. Laparoscopic dismembered pyeloplasty. J Urol 1993;150:1795–9.

6 Tan HL. Laparoscopic Anderson–Hynes dismembered pyeloplasty in children. J Urol 1999;162:1045–8.

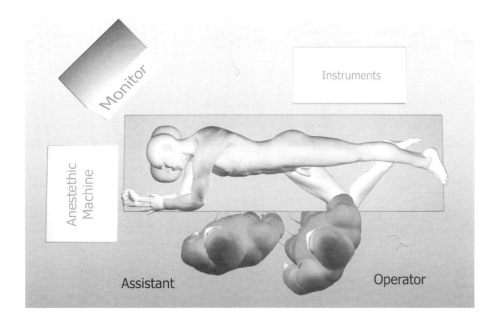

Figure 2.1 Room set-up for a laparoscopic pyeloplasty.

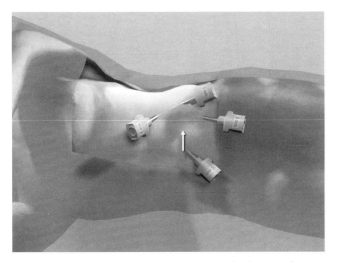

Figure 2.2 Trocar positions for laparoscopic pyeloplasty. In obese patients the optical trocar should be placed in the pararectal line (arrow).

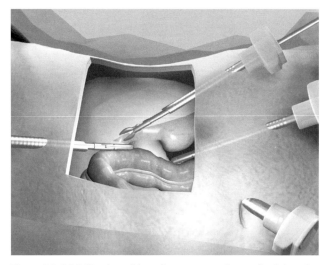

Figure 2.3 Mobilization of the colon to expose the renal pelvis and the upper ureter.

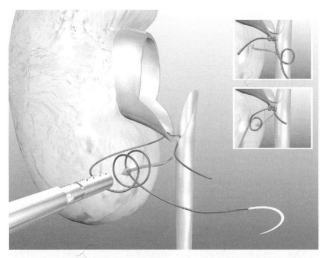

Figure 2.4 The technique of laparoscopic suturing. The first stitch is placed at the distal tip of the transected renal pelvis and the medial part of the spatulated ureter.

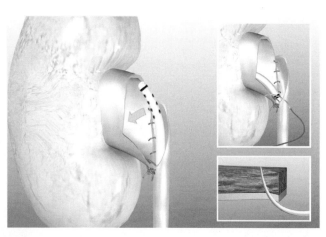

Figure 2.6 After the dorsal pyeloureteral anastomosis is completed, the ventral defect is closed by running suture. The detail shows the technique of stitching, which involves taking more muscularis and less urothelium.

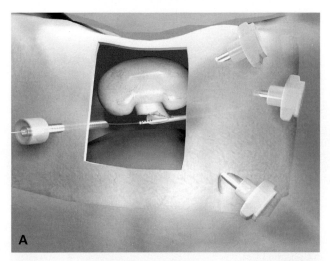

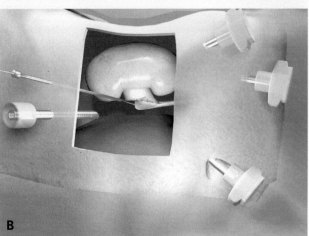

Figure 2.5 Double-J catheter placement in an antegrade fashion using a Terumo® guidewire: (A) via the cranial trocar, and (B) using a two-part puncture needle (see Tips).

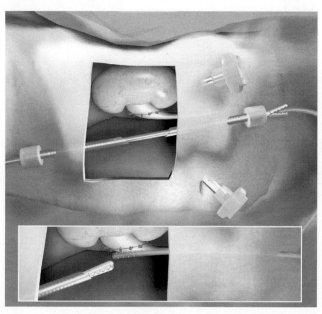

Figure 2.7 Drain placement (20 Fr Robinson drainage).

Chapter 3
Division of the Horseshoe Kidney and Pyeloplasty

J. Fichtner and S. W. Melchior

Introduction

There is an ongoing discussion about the necessity of bridge resection in horseshoe kidney versus pyeloplasty only. However, in the authors' experience, recurrent obstruction and stone recurrence were observed in patients treated previously by percutaneous litholapaxy ESWL, as well as in open renal stone surgery with or without Anderson–Hynes pyeloplasty but with the bridge untouched.

Indications

This approach is indicated in primary or recurrent symptomatic ureteropelvic obstruction with or without kidney stone formation.

Limitations and risks

• Primary stone formation without ureteropelvic obstruction treated by ESWL or litholapaxy runs a risk of stone recurrence.
• Borderline split renal function in recurrent ureteropelvic junction obstruction and/or staghorn stone formation.

Contraindications

The chance detection of a symptomatic normal kidney that is found to be dilated.

Special instruments/suture material

• Standard suture material (4/0, 5/0 Macon, PDS, and Monocryl).
• 8 Fr pyelostomy splint.
• 6 Fr ureter splint.

Operative technique

• Make a supracostal incision (above the 12th rib) extended medially.

• The dilated renal pelvis will be found immediately in front of the kidney. Take particular care when the lesion crosses vessels.
• Explore the ureter crossing the bridge ventrally and medially, and place a vessel loop.
• Explore the bridge dorsally and observe the broad variety of vessels arising from the iliac artery and lumbar arteries.
• Using careful blunt dissection, the thin isthmus is freed and lifted up.
• Use bulldog clamps to first identify the extension of ischemia before you ligate it.
• Use deep parenchyma sutures on both sides of the isthmus before it is divided by electrocautery.
• Cover the contralateral margin of the bridge with a running, watertight, capsulated fibrosa, 5/0 Maxon suture, and fatty tissue.
• Resect the ipsilateral stump of the ischemia bridge, which is fixed to the psoas later on (transversopexy).
• An Anderson–Hynes plastic side-to-side anastomosis is performed; by lifting up the crossing vessels, it should be made as long as possible.

Tips

• Take care when there is a ureter lesion of the contracted contralateral side.
• Keep the isthmus sutures long otherwise it will slip on the contracted side when the isthmus is divided.
• Isthmus urinomas can be avoided by a watertight suture line.
• Using ipsilateral bridge resection, the lower calyx can be opened and used for the Anderson–Hynes plastic anastomosis.
• In cases of recurrent operations, the fatty capsule can be substituted by the greater omentum. It is important to prevent scar formation around the ureter (secondary obstruction).

Postoperative care

• Remove the pararenal drain on day 2 or 3 and the splint on day 7.

• Lift up the pyelostomy 15 cm on day 10 and clamp it for 1 h.
• Remove the pyelostomy if the patient is without pain.

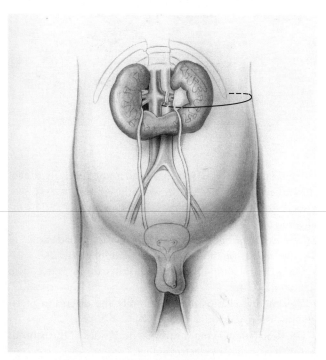

Figure 3.1 Flank incision above the 12th rib.

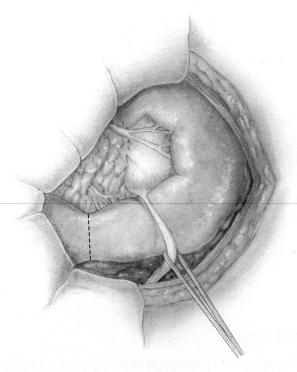

Figure 3.3 Vessel loop on the ipsilateral ureter.

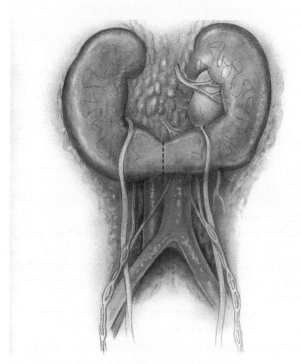

Figure 3.2 Division of the isthmus at the thinnest part.

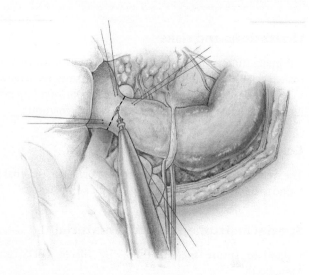

Figure 3.4 Division of the isthmus with electrocautery and the placement of stay sutures.

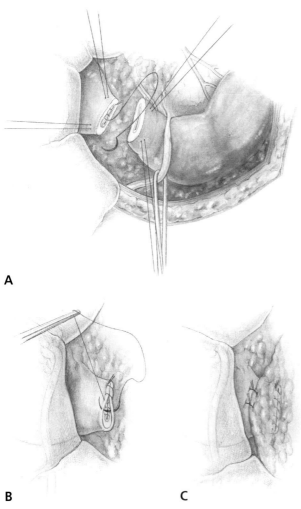

A

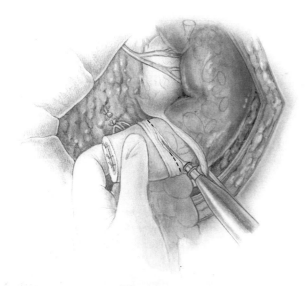

B

C

Figure 3.5 Running capsular stuture and covering with perirenal fat.

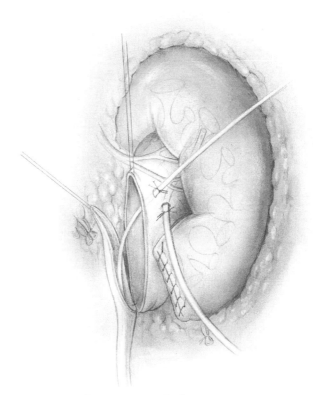

Figure 3.7 Anderson–Hynes pyeloplasty.

Figure 3.6 Resection of the bridge.

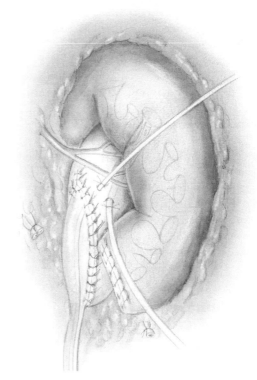

Figure 3.8 Completed pyeloplasty.

Chapter 4
Double Systems

M. Fisch and J. Leissner

Introduction

There are still controversies concerning the best strategy, but consensus has been reached concerning the following strategies:
- Place a percutaneous tube in case of a high febrile upper tract infection (UTI).
- Wait and see in small orthotopic ureteroceles.
- In symptomatic babies, first incise endoscopically vesically located ureteroceles for decompression.
- Use the Lich–Gregoir procedure in nondilated refluxive double systems.
- In a case of renal function demonstrated in MAG 3 (region of interest) of >20%, resection of the ureterocele with trigonal support and 'butterfly' implantation of both ureters using the psoas hitch technique should be done.
- Partial kidney and ureter resection in nonfunctioning upper systems with a psoas hitch for the lower ureter in order to preserve the lower segment from reflux, which occurs quite often if the dilated ureter is removed.
- Unilateral ectopic ureteroceles: carefully resect the roof endoscopically, step by step in several sessions to avoid incontinence later on.
- Children with solitary kidneys or bilateral ectopic ureteroceles that are incontinent, require urinary diversion.
- Young women with partial incontinence or recurrent intermittent vaginal discharge are highly suspect for a vaginal ectopic partially obstructed megaureter filled with pus. Perform an MRI.

Patient counseling and consent

See Chapter 13.

Indications

In primary implantation of both ureters with borderline split renal function of the lower or upper part, heminephrectomy is indicated later on in persistent UTI or if hypertension occurs. (See Chapter 13.)

Preoperative management

See Chapter 13.

Anesthesia

See Chapter 13.

Operative technique

Implantation of both ureters (psoas hitch)
- Use the parainguinal standard incision. Identify, ligate, and dissect the vasa epigastrica and the round ligament. Identify and arm the spermatic chord by vessel loop. Identify, cut, and ligate the lateral umbilical cord crossing both ureters just underneath.
- Both ureters, identified in the common sheath, should be separated above the common sheath, carefully.
- In 'butterfly' implantation of both ureters, ligate and dissect both ureters, usually 3 cm above the ureter–bladder junction in order to preserve the blood supply and the branches of the plexus pelvicus.
- Shorten the ureter stumps until capillary bleeding occurs. Spatulate each at 12 o'clock for 1 cm.
- Side-to-side anastomosis is performed using 5/0 Monocryl with interrupted sutures (Fig. 4.1).
- The standard psoas hitch procedure is performed and both ureters are commonly implanted antirefluxive in a tunnel wide enough to ensure sufficient blood supply.
- Splints are inserted and a cystostomy is placed through stab incisions and is fixed separately.

Heminephrectomy; ureterectomy; resection of the ureterocele–ureter implantation
• This is the gold standard procedure in nonfunctioning upper or lower parts of the double kidney.
• Use a standard supracostal 12 or 11 flank incision.
• For surgical details, see Figs 4.2–4.20.
• The wound is closed and the patient turned for a parainguinal incision.

Tips

• During preparation the mobile kidney may become 'blue' due to compression of the renal vessels. This is a temporary effect if it is turned back immediately.
• Initially clamp the isolated segmental vessels before ligation (irreversible!).
• Argon gas is effective in parenchymal superficial coagulation and facilitates adaptation of the harness parenchyma.
• Dissect the ureter through the supracostal incision as far down (distally) as possible; this facilitates further dissection later on, performed via the second parainguinal incision.

Postoperative care

See Chapter 13.

Complications

• Prolonged urine secretion out of the pararenal drain will stop spontaneously in the majority of cases. Open revision should not be before 3 weeks: parenchyma resection.
• Nonfunctioning kidney: thromboses of renal vein; nephrectomy.
• See also Chapter 13.

Results

The rate of reoperation in a total of 413 patients with double systems was 3.5% in primary antirefluxive operations and 7% if heminephrectomy was carried out in the same session. In contrast, primary incision of the ureterocele alone was effective in only 42%, and heminephrectomy in only 36% if performed without an antirefluxive procedure. The strategy described above represents our learning curve since 1968 and has been the gold standard for the last 20 years.

References

1 Jelloul L, Berger D, Frey P. Endoscopic management of ureteroceles in children. Eur Urol 1997;32:321–7.
2 von Wallenberg-Pachaly H, Voges G, Riedmiller H, Hohenfellner R. Therapiekonzept bei kindlichen Doppelnieren. Verhandlungsbericht der Deutschen Gesellschaft für Urologie, No. 40. Meeting 28 September to 1 October 1988. Springer Verlag, Saarbrücken.

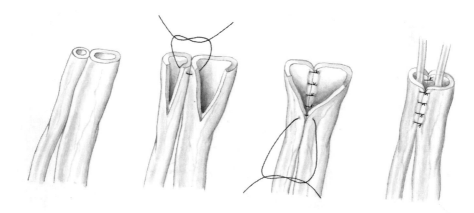

Figure 4.1 Butterfly ureteroanastomosis (see Chapter 13).

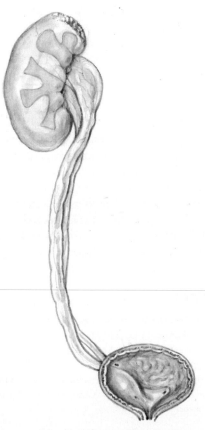

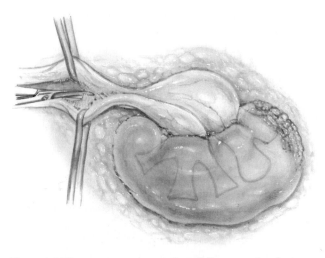

Figure 4.4 The ureters are separated carefully, preserving the longitudinal vessels under the adventitia.

Figure 4.2 Duplex system: refluxive ureteral orifice of the lower moiety; upper part with ureterocele.

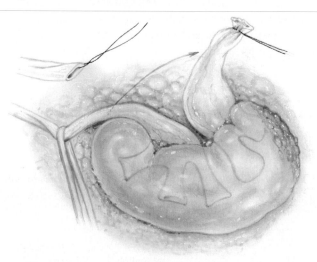

Figure 4.5 The dilated ureter is ligated and dissected. Preparation is continued from the dorsal side first.

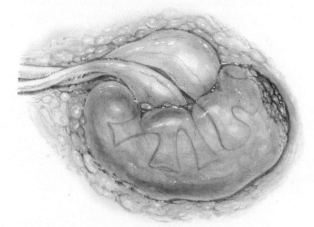

Figure 4.3 The kidney should be first explored dorsally.

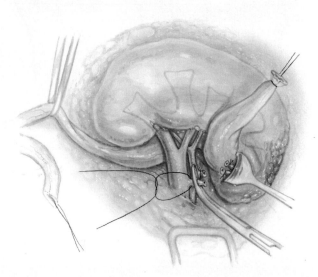

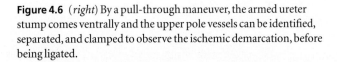

Figure 4.6 (*right*) By a pull-through maneuver, the armed ureter stump comes ventrally and the upper pole vessels can be identified, separated, and clamped to observe the ischemic demarcation, before being ligated.

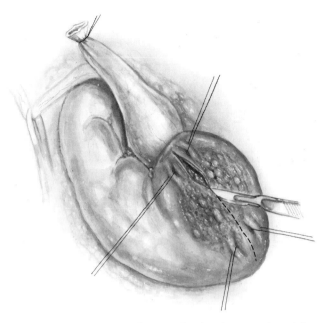

Figure 4.7 The fibrous capsule is spatulated and separated carefully from the parenchyma. If preserved, it will cover the parenchyma defect to prevent fistula formation.

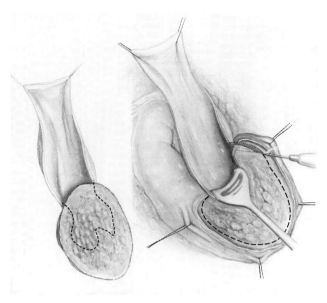

Figure 4.9 With an eyelid retractor inserted in the sinus renalis, the ischemic pole is lifted upwards.

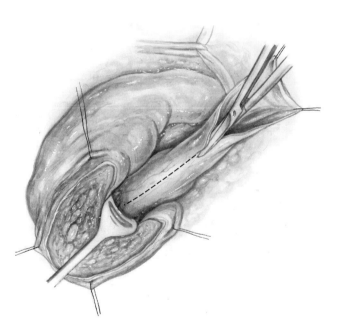

Figure 4.8 The ureter is opened longitudinally.

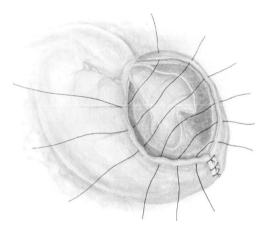

Figure 4.10 Parenchyma resection is performed with the backside of the calyx untouched and is coagulated using argon gas. The renal capsular is closed watertight with a running 5/0 Monocryl suture.

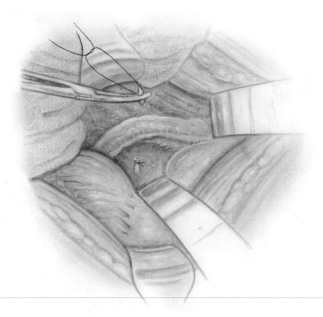

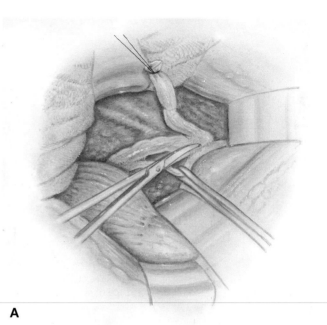

A

Figure 4.11 The lateral umbilical cord is dissected. Both ureters in the common sheet are identified.

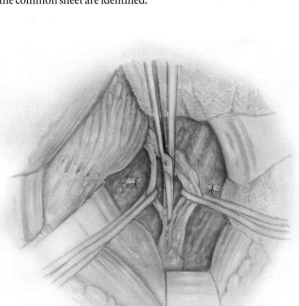

B

Figure 4.13 The separated and ligated ureter is dissected.

Figure 4.12 The ureters are dissected carefully.

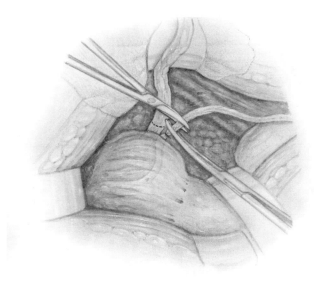

Figure 4.14 The lower ureter is dissected and cut 3 cm above the bladder entrance.

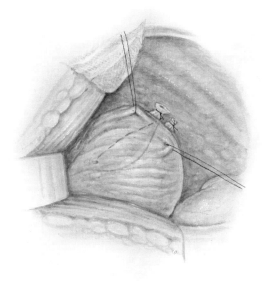

Figure 4.16 The bladder is opened between the stay sutures.

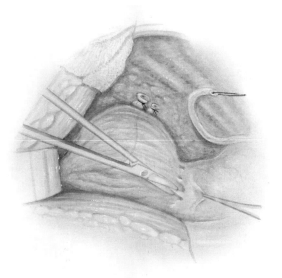

Figure 4.15 The bladder is freed.

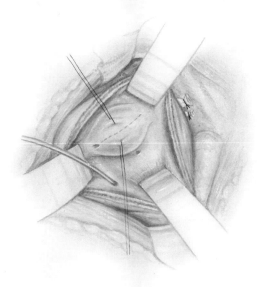

Figure 4.17 The ureterocele is opened longitudinally. The contralateral orifice is identified and a 6 Fr splint is inserted and fixed by a 5/0 Vicryl rapid suture.

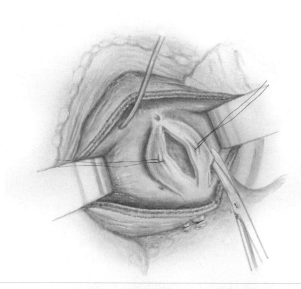

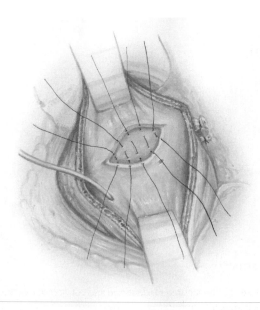

Figure 4.18 The ureterocele is resected.

Figure 4.19 The trigonal support is performed with deep interrupted detrusor sutures of 4/0 Monocryl. The ureter of the lower moiety is reimplanted using the classic psoas hitch technique (see Chapter 13).

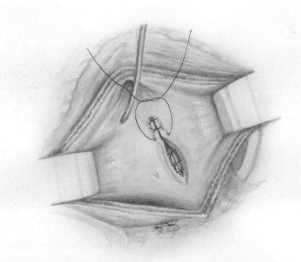

Figure 4.20 The mucosa is closed.

Chapter 5
Crossed Pyelopyelostomy

R. Stein

Introduction

When using the transuretero-ureterostomy, one of the difficulties is the different caliber of the ureters. The advantage of the crossed pyelopyelostomy is the wide anastomosis between the renal pelvises. The indications for this operation are quite rare [1].

Indications

• A contralateral hypoplastic or shrunken kidney (<30% split renal function in the MAG 3 clearance) with a normal kidney and a nonrefluxing ureter on the other site (VCUG preoperative).

Anesthesia

General anesthesia.

Special instruments/suture material

As for pyeloplasty; 6/0 and 7/0 Vicryl or Monocryl are needed for suturing.

Operative technique

• Make a vertical midline incision extending about 5 cm above and below the umbilicus and opening of the peritoneum.
• Incise the peritoneum lateral to the descending colon and the sigmoid or the cecum and ascending colon, depending on the side of the scarred/stenotic ureter with a normal functioning kidney.
• Explore the scarred ureter, which is usually fixed in scar tissue after previous surgery. The ureter is sharply transected from the lateral abdominal wall. Ligation of the ureter should be as distal as possible, in case of persistent reflux close to the bladder. Prepare the ureter up to the kidney.
• Resect an oval part of the renal pelvis.

• Explore the contralateral kidney (hypoplastic kidney) after mobilization of the cecum and ascending colon or the descending colon.
• Mobilize the kidney and ligate the kidney vessels without disturbing the adrenal gland. Careful preparation of the proximal ureter should be made without compromising the blood supply.
• The ureter is mobilized distally to its crossing with the iliac vessels. Care is taken not to damage the blood supply of the ureter in the fibroareolar tissue along its medial side.
• The renal parenchyma is detached from the renal pelvis. There is oval excision of the renal pelvis near the calices.
• In cases with a right hypoplastic kidney, the right ureter is pulled through a wide window in the mesenterium above the mesenterica inferior artery. In cases with a hypoplastic left kidney, pull through the left ureter. Care should be taken to avoid any kinking of the ureter.
• Anastomosis of both renal pelvises is made with interrupted watertight sutures (6/0 or 7/0 Vicryl, or 6/0 Monocryl). The suture size depends on the thickness of the pelvic wall. A pyelostomy is inserted.

Tips

• To guarantee a wide anastomosis the renal pelvis of the hypoplastic kidney is resected near the calices.
• To relieve any tension from the anastomosis, the upper renal suspension apparatus can be separated and the kidney lowered for up to 3 cm.

Postoperative care

• At the 10th postoperative day, a water manometer is connected to the pyelostomy tube and the intrapelvic pressure is measured. It should be between 12 and 15 cmH$_2$O. In doubt, the patency of the anastomosis can be checked fluoroscopically. If the findings are normal, the tube is removed.
• Follow up using sonography.

Reference

1 Hohenfellner R, Jonas U. Trans-Kaliko-Ureterostomie. Akt Urol 1971;2:43–6.

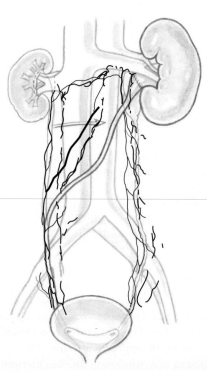

Figure 5.1 Schematic drawing of the blood supply of the ureters, as well as the operative technique for the crossed pyelopyelostomy from the right to the left side.

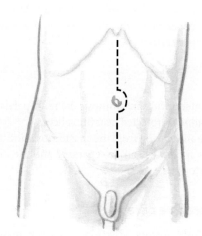

Figure 5.2 The vertical medial incision.

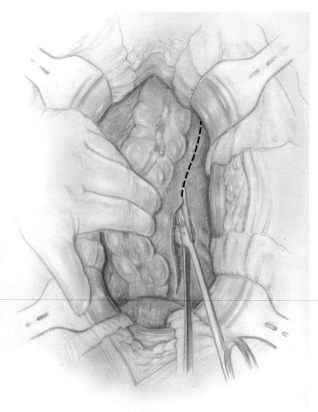

Figure 5.3 Incision of the posterior peritoneum lateral to the sigmoid colon up to the descending colon.

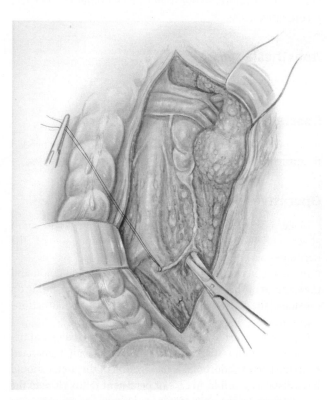

Figure 5.4 Ligation of the stenotic ureter should be as distal as possible and the scarred ureter should be dissected up to the renal pelvis.

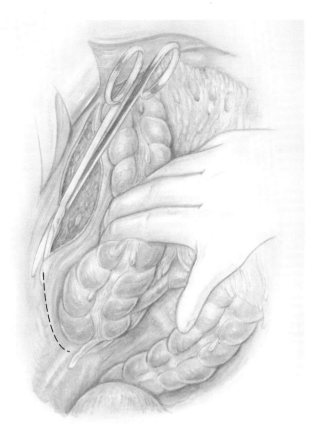

Figure 5.5 Mobilization of the cecum and ascending colon to expose the contralateral kidney.

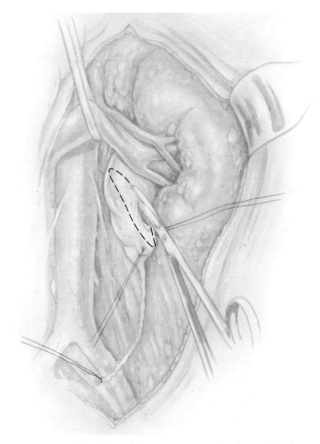

Figure 5.6 Oval excision of the ureter proximal and cranial to the ureteropelvic junction.

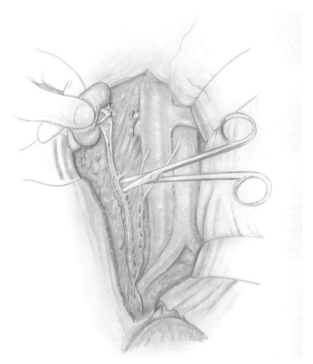

Figure 5.7 Exploration of the contralateral kidney, ligation of the renal artery and vein, and careful preparation of the ureter caudal to the crossing of the iliac vessels. The blood supply comes medially.

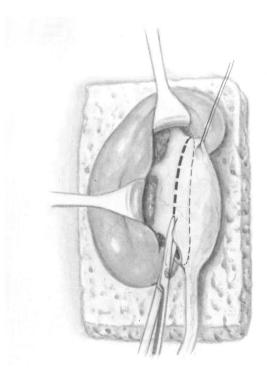

Figure 5.8 Oval resection of the renal pelvis near the calices.

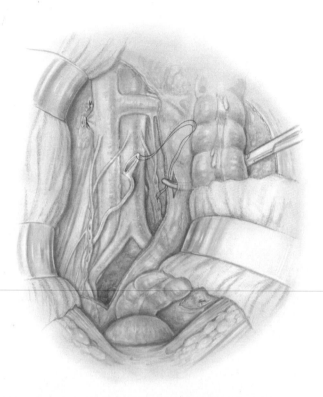

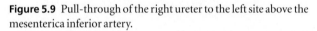

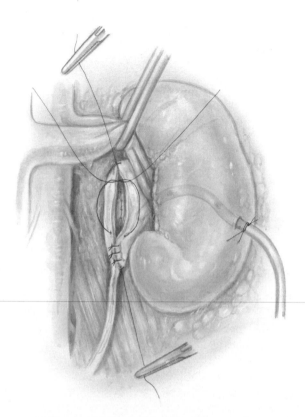

Figure 5.9 Pull-through of the right ureter to the left site above the mesenterica inferior artery.

Figure 5.10 Side-to-side anastomosis of the two renal pelvises with single sutures (6/0 or 7/0 Vicryl or 6/0 Monocryl, depending on the size of the wall of the pelvis) and placement of the pyelostomy.

Chapter 6
Surgical Therapy for Retrocaval Ureter

G. D'Elia

Introduction

This is a congenital anomaly arising from the inferior vena cava. The right ureter becomes trapped behind the vena cava when the infrarenal vena cava derives from either the persistent right subcardinal or postcardinal vein rather than, as normal, from the supracardinal vein. Despite its congenital origin, symptoms are usually absent in childhood. It presents clinically with pain from ureteral obstruction in the third or fourth decade of life.

Patient counseling and consent

There is a risk of ureteral stenosis, renal deterioration, and kidney loss.

Indications

- Recurrent renal colic.
- Symptomatic upper tract dilatation with renal function deterioration.
- Pyelonephritis.
- Stone disease.

Limitations and risks

If ipsilateral renal function is <15% on scintigraphy and the patient is symptomatic, perform a nephrectomy.

Contraindications

Contraindicated in asymptomatic patients with upper tract dilatation but a normal outwash pattern.

Preoperative management

- Intravenous pyelography or antegrade descending pyelography through a percutaneous nephrostomy.

- Retrograde ureterography and renal dynamic scintigraphy if needed.

Anesthesia

General anesthesia.

Special instruments/suture material

Have ready a ureteral stent and pyelostomy tube.

Operative technique

See Figs 6.1–6.5.

Tips

Taking down the adhesions between the ureter and the vena cava is the most delicate and time-consuming part of the procedure. After that, the procedure is the same as a dismembered pyeloplasty. During dissection of the adhesions between the ureter and the vena cava, take care not to damage the longitudinal vessels that feed the ureteral adventitia.

Postoperative care

- Remove the drain on day 3–5.
- Remove the ureteral stent on day 8.
- If a pyelostomy was placed, measure the renal pelvic pressure and descending pyelography before removing the pyelostomy.
- If the renal pelvis pressure is <15 cmH$_2$O and there is free passage of the contrast media, remove the pyelostomy tube.

Complications

In rare cases a Satinsky clamp on the inferior vena cava is required if adhesions between the ureter and vena cava itself are difficult to dissect.

Troubleshooting

The extrarenal renal pelvis might be extremely dilated. After opening it, you can use a flap of it to bridge a long ureteral defect. If the dismembered pyeloplasty anastomosis is under tension perform renal mobilization and nephropexy.

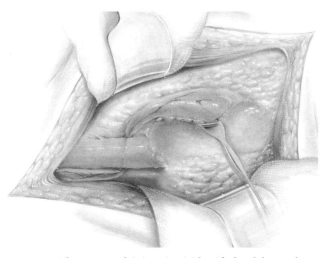

Figure 6.2 The ureteropelvic junction is identified and the renal sinus dissected to expose the dilated renal pelvis.

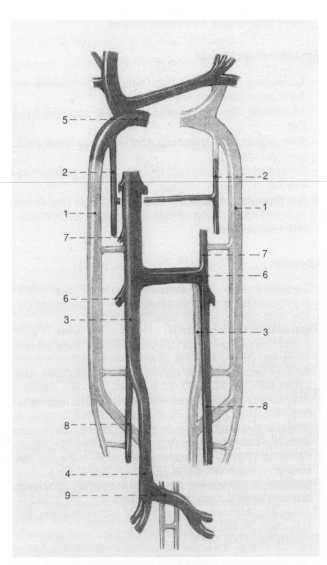

Figure 6.1 Development of the vena caval system (vessels in regression are in light gray): 1, vena cardinalis caudalis; 2, supracardinal vein (on the right it gives rise to the azygos vein, on the left to the hemiazygos vein); 3, subcardinal vein (on the right it gives rise to the inferior vena cava, on the left to the gonadal vein); 4, vena sacrocardinalis; 5, superior vena cava; 6, renal veins; 7, adrenal veins; 8, gonadal vein; 9, common iliac veins.

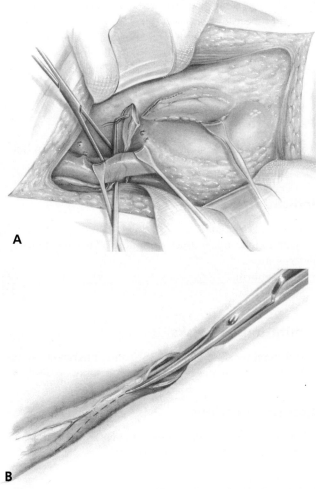

Figure 6.3 (A) The ureter is exposed and divided just caudal to the ureteropelvic junction, the adhesions between the vena cava and ureter are dissected, and the distal ureteric stump is placed ventral to the vena cava. (B) Longitudinal opening of the ureter.

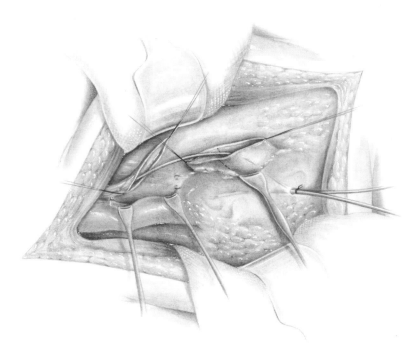

Figure 6.4 After positioning a ureteral stent, the spatulated ureter is anastomosed to the renal pelvis.

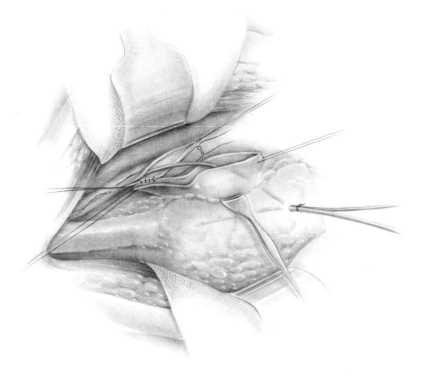

Figure 6.5 Anderson–Hynes pyeloplasty.

Chapter 7

Extraperitoneal Laparoscopic Radical Nephrectomy and Nephroureterectomy

A. Hoznek, L. Salomon, and C.-C. Abbou

Introduction

Radical nephrectomy represents the gold standard treatment of kidney cancer. Its principles were described by Robson in 1963: primary ligature of the renal artery and vein, removal of the kidney together with its envelopes including Gerota's fascia and the adrenal gland, and regional lymphadenectomy. These principles are still considered valid, although during the last decade the operative approach has been modernized. Since the first laparoscopic radical nephrectomy reported by Clayman in 1991, this minimally invasive technology has gained much popularity. Three variants are currently used worldwide: the transperitoneal laparoscopic, the extraperitoneal laparoscopic, and the hand-assisted approach for radical nephrectomy.

All these techniques have their specific advantages and drawbacks [1]. The transperitoneal laparoscopic approach is preferred by many surgeons because it offers a large working space. Hand-assisted laparoscopic renal surgery is a hybrid procedure, during which the surgeon places his nondominant hand into the abdominal cavity. This helps to overcome some inherent obstacles associated with conventional laparoscopy, such as loss of tactile feedback and special orientation, thereby lessening the learning curve. In our department, we decided to develop the extraperitoneal laparoscopic approach because access to the renal pedicle is quicker, safer, and easier. Post-operative morbidity is diminished because of the absence of intraperitoneal complications—patients have less pain and there is no ileus.

Nephroureterectomy is indicated for upper tract urothelial cancer. The first step of this procedure is identical to radical nephrectomy, but the procedure is completed by the excision of a bladder cuff and removal of the operative specimen through an iliac incision.

Indications

- Renal cell cancer: the main indication is represented by tumors of less than 7 cm in diameter (T1 tumors). With larger tumors, laparoscopy loses its advantages somewhat because of the large parietal opening required to extract the specimen.
- Upper tract urothelial cancer: the gold standard is represented by radical ureteronephrectomy.

Contraindications

Local spread to the perirenal fat or to the renal vein is an absolute contraindication. A past history of retroperitoneal lumbar surgery is a relative contraindication as it makes the dissection difficult. In this case, traditional open surgery may be considered.

Preoperative management

The patient must fast starting at midnight on the night before surgery. Determination of blood type and cross-match are carried out. When inducing anesthesia, prophylactic antibiotic therapy with a second generation cephalosporin is administered. Prophylactic treatment with low molecular weight heparin is begun on the day of surgery.

Special instruments/suture material

- Video unit: preferably two monitors; insufflation system; suction device; monopolar and bipolar cautery energy source.
- Trocars: 12 mm blunt port trocar; two 12 mm trocars; two 5 mm trocars.
- Laparoscope: 0° lens.
- Primary surgeon: rotating tip coagulating scissors; bipolar coagulator; suction irrigation; clip applier with medium to large (9 mm) metallic clips; linear stapler (Endo-GIA); entrapment sac (Endo-Catch); and needle holder (required only exceptionally).
- Assistant: two 5 mm fenestrated graspers.

In addition, for nephroureterectomy, standard open surgical instruments are required.

Operative technique

• A nasogastric tube and a Foley catheter are inserted prior to surgery.

• The patient is positioned in lateral decubitus, with the lumbar support raised to its maximum height. The legs are flexed slightly forward and paced on the anterior leg rest. The posterior leg rest is removed to leave room for the assistant who holds the laparoscope and camera.

• A mini-lumbotomy (2 cm incision) is done in the posterior axillary line 1–2 cm below the 12th rib (Fig. 7.2A, a). The abdominal wall and the transversalis fascia are incised. The posterior pararenal space is dissected with the finger, and the peritoneal reflection is pushed forward. Two 5 mm trocars are inserted under digital guidance in the anterior axillary line, one in the upper part and one in the lower part of the abdomen (Fig. 7.2A, d and e). A 12 mm trocar is placed 2 cm above the iliac crest, in the mid axillary line (Fig. 7.2A, c). A 12 mm trocar is placed in the posterior axillary line above the iliac crest (Fig. 7.2A, b). The blunt port trocar is placed and anchored with sutures to the initial mini-lumbotomy.

• After insufflation and insertion of the laparoscope, the psoas muscle is identified and the posterior pararenal space dissected. The surgeon uses trocars 'a' and 'b' (Fig. 7.2A), dissects with rotating tip coagulating scissors, and holds the suction irrigation in the other hand. Suction irrigation allows him to maintain a permanently clean operative field, by removing blood and smoke. In addition, together with the scissors, it allows tissue dissection. The camera is inserted through trocar 'c' and the assistant helps in retracting the kidney and puts the renal pedicle under tension with two forceps.

• Gerota's fascia is incised giving access to the perirenal space.

• On the left side, the ureter and/or the genital vein are identified.

• On the right side, the inferior vena cava, the genital vein, and the ureter are exposed.

• Dissection continues upward along these structures, leading to the renal pedicle.

• The renal vein and the renal artery are dissected. On the left side, the reno-azygo-lumbar vein and the genital vein, which drain directly into the renal vein, are also dissected.

• The renal artery is secured with 9 mm metallic clips. The renal artery is sectioned. On the left side this makes the adrenal vein appear, which is anterior to the renal artery.

• The dissection of the renal vein is completed. This allows safe placement of the linear stapler on the vein. The renal vein is section ligatured.

• The mobilization of the kidney surrounded by perirenal fat and Gerota's fascia begins at its posterior surface and is extended cephalad. At this point the anterior and lateral attachments are left intact. They keep the kidney suspended and, along with the retraction effect of the pneumoretroperitoneum, facilitate the posterior cleavage. The surgeon reaches the diaphragm and can free the superior pole entirely.

• The operative specimen should not include the adrenal gland in case of a small tumor situated at the lower pole of the kidney. In such circumstances, the adrenal vein is not sectioned. The adrenal is dissected by cleaving the plane between the renal capsule and the surrounding fatty tissue at the anterior face of the kidney at its upper pole. If an adrenelectomy is necessary, the adrenal vein is first clipped and sectioned, and the adrenal gland is included in the operative specimen.

• The dissection continues at the anterior aspect of the kidney, in the anterior pararenal space.

• The lower pole of the kidney is freed.

• In case of radical nephrectomy, the ureter is clip ligated and sectioned.

• During nephroureterectomy, the ureter should not be opened. The dissection is continued as far as possible caudally. Then, the patient is placed in the dorsal decubitus position. An oblique iliac incision allows the surgeon to expose the bladder. The ureter is dissected in its whole length and is excised together with a bladder cuff. The bladder is closed with 4/0 PDS Vicryl.

• In the case of both radical nephrectomy and nephroureterectomy, the operative specimen is removed through an iliac incision. Prior to removal, in the case of radical nephrectomy, the specimen is placed into an Endo-Catch in order to avoid direct parietal contact with the tumor.

• The site of the extraction is closed in two layers. A suction drain is left for 24 h. Trocar sites are closed with intracutaneous absorbable running sutures.

Tips

• *Access creation*: when doing the mini-lumbotomy, the surgeon has to be sure that he entered the posterior pararenal space. This cleavage plan is easily identified by the possibility of palpating the posterior surface of the 12th rib.

• *Dissection of the renal pedicles*: to identify the zone where the dissection of the renal pedicle should start, simply place the instrument in trocar 'a' perpendicular to the abdominal wall (Fig. 7.2A). The tip of the instrument points toward the zone where the renal pedicle would be expected. On the right side, simply follow the inferior vena cava cephalad. Be careful with the right gonadic vein, it can easily tear off the inferior vena cava.

• *Ligature of the renal artery*: the more proximal clip on the renal artery has to be placed at a safe distance from the aorta (at least 5–10 mm). This is because if the clip accidentally cuts or injures a calcified artery, one should be able to clamp more proximally, near the aorta.

• *Ligature of the renal vein*: the Endo-GIA has to be placed sufficiently near the kidney to allow putting a forceps on the distal portion of the vein in case of malfunctioning of the Endo-GIA.

• *Dissection of the upper pole*: optimal triangulation of instruments can be obtained if the surgeon uses trocars 'a' and 'e' (Fig. 7.2).

• *Dissection of the anterior pararenal space*: this is an avascular plane, and usually no hemostasis is required. However, if bleeding occurs, do not use monopolar electrocautery.

• *Specimen entrapment*: be sure to open the endobag respecting the inscription 'this side up'. Otherwise it is impossible to open the sac correctly.

Postoperative care

Radical nephrectomy

The day after surgery, the Foley catheter and suction drain are usually removed and the patient returns to a full diet. The patient leaves the hospital on the third or fourth postoperative day.

Nephroureterectomy

The Foley catheter is maintained for 4 days. The patient leaves the hospital on day 5 or 6.

Troubleshooting

• *Injury to the vena cava* results in limited bleeding because of the absence of a pressure gradient between the blood in the venous system and the pneumoretroperitoneum. A surgeon performing laparoscopic nephrectomy should be sufficiently skilled and trained in reconstructive laparoscopic surgery. In this case, suturing the injury is not a major challenge.

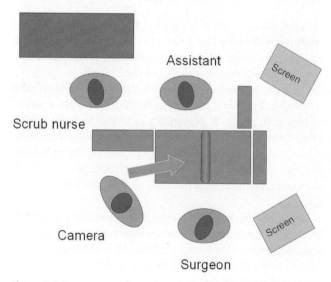

Figure 7.1 Room set-up for extraperitoneal laparoscopic radical nephrectomy. The primary surgeon stands behind the patient, with his assistant and the scrub nurse in front of him. A second assistant or the scrub nurse holds the camera. The optimum is to have two video screens.

• *Injury of the peritoneum* sometimes occurs accidentally but interferes only mildly with the rest of the surgery.

Reference

1 Hoznek A, Salomon L, Gettman M, Stolzenburg JU, Abbou CC. Justification of extraperitoneal laparoscopic access for surgery of the upper urinary tract. Curr Urol Rep 2004;5:93–9.

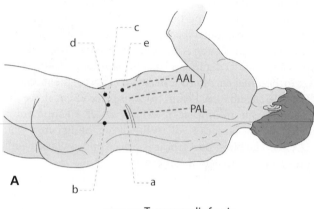

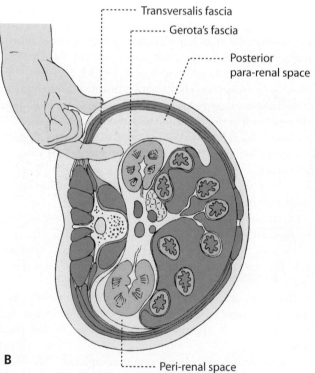

Figure 7.2 (A) Trocar placement showing the mini-lumbotomy and finger dissection of the retroperitoneal space, placement of two 5 mm trocars in the anterior axillary line (AAL) (d, e), one 12 mm trocar in the mid axillary line (MAL) (c), one 12 mm trocar in the posterior axillary line (PAL) (b), and one blunt port trocar into the initial mini-lumbotomy (a). (B) The mini-lumbotomy in the PAL 1–2 cm below the 12th rib and finger dissection of the posterior pararenal space.

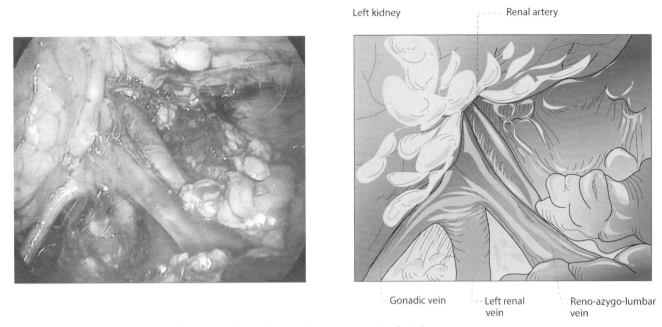

Figure 7.3 View of the left renal pedicle. (For color, see Plate 7.3, between pp. 112 and 113.)

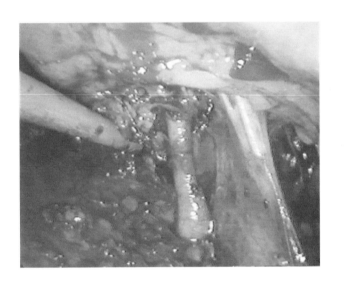
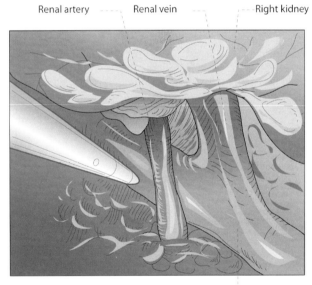

Figure 7.4 View of the right renal pedicle. (For color, see Plate 7.4.)

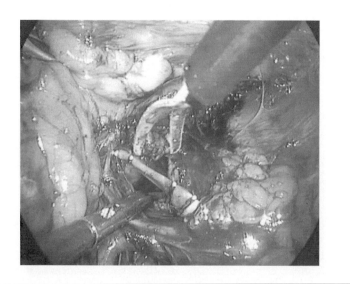
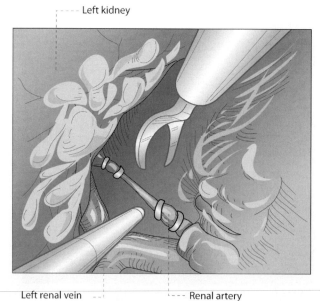

Left kidney

Left renal vein   Renal artery

Figure 7.5 Clipping (9 mm metallic clips, three clips proximally and two clips distally) and sectioning of the renal artery. (For color, see Plate 7.5, between pp. 112 and 113.)

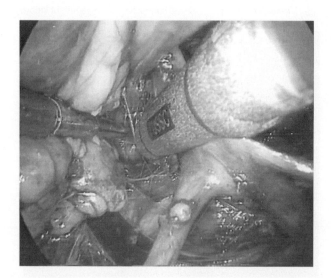
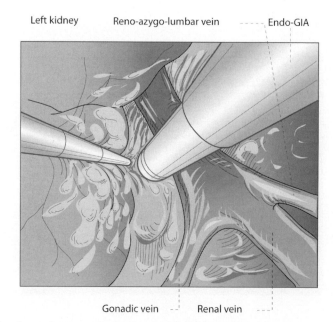

Left kidney   Reno-azygo-lumbar vein   Endo-GIA

Gonadic vein   Renal vein

Figure 7.6 Sectioning of the renal vein with a linear stapler. Make sure that the stapler is completely closed around the vein. (For color, see Plate 7.6.)

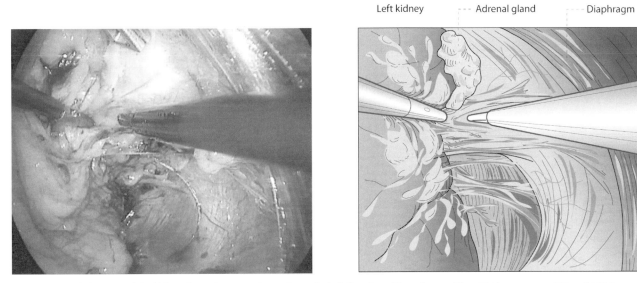

Left kidney --- Adrenal gland --- Diaphragm

Figure 7.7 Mobilization of the kidney from the posterior to the cephalad direction. (For color, see Plate 7.7, between pp. 112 and 113.)

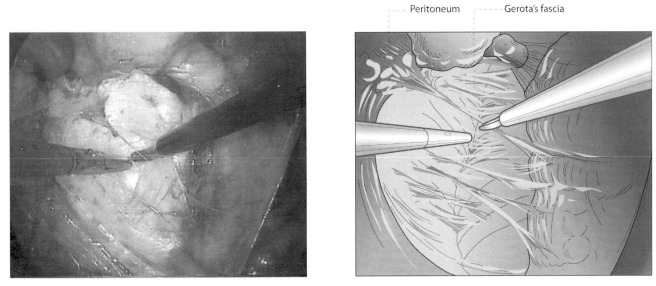

Peritoneum --- Gerota's fascia

Figure 7.8 Mobilization of the kidney is continued anteriorly between the peritoneum and Gerota's fascia. (For color, see Plate 7.8.)

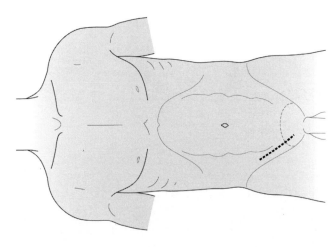

Figure 7.9 For nephroureterectomy the patient is placed in the dorsal decubitus position. An inguinal incision is performed to free the whole ureter including a bladder cuff.

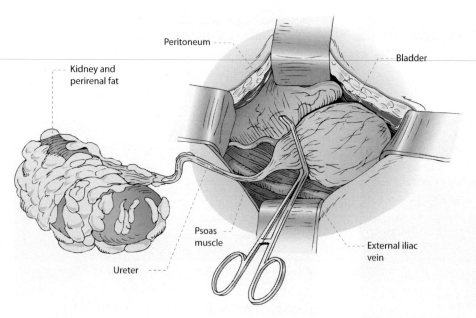

Figure 7.10 Removing the specimen (kidney, ureter, bladder cuff).

Chapter 8
Laparoscopic Transperitoneal Radical Nephrectomy and Laparoscopic Live Donor Nephrectomy

C. Varol, H. Lau and J.-U. Stolzenburg

Introduction

The reduction of pain and recovery time associated with laparoscopic transperitoneal radical nephrectomy (LTN) and live donor nephrectomy (LLDN) has made these techniques increasingly popular worldwide. The transperitoneal approach is recommended for its clear and early identification of anatomical landmarks and generous working space. The technical issues, however, in LLDN of vascular length, ischemia time, and limited access has prevented its universal adaptation. Surgeons should become familiar with ablative nephrectomy before taking up LLDN.

Prior to embarking on laparoscopic surgery, a good understanding of laparoscopic principles and capnoperitoneum physiology is required. The surgeon must be aware of the various energy sources available for dissection, hemostatic clips, and staples for vascular control.

Laparoscopic transperitoneal radical nephrectomy

Patient counseling and consent

The patient must be informed of the potential risks of laparoscopy and the possibility of converting to an open approach if deemed necessary.

Contraindications

Relative contraindications
- Grossly obese patient where the instrument length may not be adequate.
- Severe intraperitoneal or retroperitoneal adhesions.
- Abdominal aortic aneurysm.
- Xanthogranulomatous pyelonephritis.

Definite contraindications
- Renal cell carcinoma stage >T2 or >10 cm in diameter.
- Tumor with renal hilar enlarged lymph nodes.
- Tumor with vena cava involvement.

Preoperative management

- Deep venous thrombosis prophylaxis: compression stockings, subcutaneous anticoagulation, and intraoperative calf compressors.
- A light bowel preop may facilitate handling of the colon.
- A good CT scan demonstrating the tumor and the renal vessels is essential.

Anesthesia

A general anesthetic is required to enable peritoneal insufflation and distension. An indwelling catheter and nasogastric tube are required for gastric decompression.

Special instruments/suture material

- A laparoscopic tower with a high flow CO_2 insufflator and a 30° laparoscope (0° optional).
- One 12 mm Hasson trochar.
- One 12 mm and two 5 mm ports.
- 5 mm bipolar forceps and 5 mm monopolar scissors.
- 10 mm right-angle forceps.
- 5 mm Maryland and Duckbill dissectors.
- 5 mm sharp grasping forceps with locking handle.
- 5 mm laparoscopic sucker.
- Endo-GIA® for ligation of the renal vein and large renal artery.
- Large and medium laparoscopic clip applicator.
- Endo-Catch® 15 mm with a 15 mm port.
- Ribbon gauze 5 cm wide, 30 cm long.
- An ultrasonic dissector.
- A laparoscopic needle holder, open retractor, and scalpel must always be ready.

Operative technique

Patient position

• Insert an indwelling catheter, compression stockings, and nasogastric tube.
• Place the patient in a lateral decubitus and slightly flexed position. The pressure points must be protected.
• The abdomen is aligned to the edge of the operating table and the elbow is placed as cranial as possible to allow unrestricted movements for the laparoscopic instruments (Fig. 8.1).

Port placement

• The placement of ports can change depending on the surgeon's preference. The authors use an inverted triangle (Fig. 8.2) with the apex (camera port) at the mid-clavicular line 2–4 cm below the surface marking of the renal hilum (transpyloric plane).
• A Hasson technique is used to gain intraperitoneal access.
• All subsequent ports are placed following the establishment of a capnoperitoneum and under vision. The two operating ports are along the anterior axillary line, one just below the costal margin and the other superior and medial to the anterior superior iliac spine.
• For a right-sided nephrectomy, insert an additional port for liver retraction (5 mm) below the xiphoid process. A 5 mm locking forceps is used to lift the liver with the forceps tip secured to the posterior diaphragm avoiding manual traction.
• Position a lateral port (5 mm) for lateral renal traction (right or left nephrectomy). Place this just medial to the tip of the 12th rib (Fig. 8.1).

Right laparoscopic transperitoneal nephrectomy
Colon reflection

• Gallbladder adhesions are divided before retracting the right liver lobe cephalad.
• To assist with the liver retraction, a 5 mm port is introduced into the epigastrium.
• A toothed forceps is positioned below the liver and is used to lift it up prior to being fixed to the posterior diaphragm.
• The ascending colon is mobilized on the white line of Toldt (Fig. 8.2). The plane between the mesocolon and Gerota's fascia is developed. The dissection extends 3–5 cm caudal to the lower pole of the kidney and just below the liver cranially.
• The Kocher maneuver is performed on the duodenum exposing the inferior vena cava. The lateral Gerota's fascia attachment should not be dissected until the renal vessels are divided.

Hilar dissection

• The location of the renal vessels will be cranial to the camera port site, in the transpyloric plane. In slim patients with minimal perinephric fat, the renal vein will be immediately visible. To assist in localizing the renal vein, the gonadal vein is identi-

fied and traced cranially on its lateral surface to the inferior vena cava insertion. The renal vein is located cranial to this insertion site.
• With difficult dissections, a 5 mm lateral port is placed at the tip of the 12th rib, in line with the camera port, to lift the kidney laterally (Fig. 8.1).
• Isolate the renal vein with the Maryland or right-angle dissector. The renal artery is posterior to the vein and may be difficult to find and ligate. The renal vein can be retracted superiorly or inferiorly with the Maryland dissector or alternatively a 0/0 polyglycolic acid tie can be slung around the vein to retract it. This can also be used guide the Endo-GIA® onto the vein (Fig. 8.3).
• First, the renal artery(s) is ligated with a large laparoscopic clip. Excess clipping is avoided on the artery, to minimize its interference with the renal vein stapling.
• The renal vein is ligated with an Endo-GIA® device (Fig. 8.3). Further clips are applied to the renal artery(s) (three proximal and one distal) before its division.

Lower pole dissection

• The hilar dissection continues posteriorly and inferiorly on the psoas muscle to the ureter.
• The ureter is double clipped and divided.
• The gonadal vein retracted medially is preserved or alternatively ligated with clips if damaged.

Upper pole dissection

• The hilar dissection continues up along the vena cava for a short distance before entering the plane between the upper pole of the kidney and the adrenal gland.
• Capsular veins present need to be clipped or bipolarized. An ultrasonic dissector device is ideal here.
• Complete the dissection by freeing the lateral attachment of Gerota's fascia.

Kidney removal

• Place the kidney into an Endo-Catch® bag and remove it via the caudal port site. This will need to be slightly enlarged to accommodate the kidney.
• If morcellation of the kidney is to be performed, a Lap-Sac® bag is required to prevent spillage. The authors do not practice this, for risk of tumor spillage and port site metastases.

Left laparoscopic transperitoneal nephrectomy

• The epigastric port for liver retraction is not required for a left-sided nephrectomy.
• The descending colon is mobilized up to the splenic flexure and 3 cm below the lower pole of the kidney. Divide the lienorenal and phrenicocolic ligaments if necessary. Alternatively, the line of dissection remains lateral to the spleen. Mobilizing the spleen with the left colon instead of separating the spleen from the splenic flexure reduces risk of spleen injury risk.

- The dissection is continued until the colon is displaced medially, exposing the renal hilum.
- When identification of the renal vein is difficult, mobilize the left gonadal vein at the lower pole of the kidney on its medial aspect to its renal vein insertion.
- The remainder of the procedure is similar to that of a right-sided LTN.

Tips

- Set goals. In the early learning phase set a time limit. It is important to realize that an open conversion is not a failure but a serious complication is.
- Obese patients need to have their port placement more lateral to allow easier access to the renal hilum. This will also overcome problems of instrument length reaching the upper and lower renal poles.
- A good quality 5 mm, 30° telescope can be used.
- Following the Hasson trocar, insert the working trocars under vision with the intra-abdominal pressure temporarily raised to 20 mmHg. This allows safe and easier port placement.
- A 5 cm wide, 30 cm strip of ribbon gauze can be inserted via the 12 mm port for removing any blood or sucker filtration, minimizing losses of the capnoperitoneum. Use the gauze also for protected retraction on the colon, spleen, or duodenum. The authors recommend this for minor bleeding over irrigation.
- Nonurgent open conversion: complete the dissection in the upper and lower pole before conversion to reduce the size of incision. This is usually from the tip of the 12th rib to the camera port.
- Urgent open conversion: if the ribbon gauze is already present, use it for compression to control the bleeding.

Laparoscopic live donor nephrectomy

Contraindications

Candidate selection is the same as for open live donor nephrectomy. Age, comorbidity—particularly conditions that may impair the donor's renal function—and malignancy are the important issues.

Relative contraindications include obesity, previous surgery, vascular anomalies, and rarely inflammatory disease in the retroperitoneum. The procedure is contraindicated if, on the right, the renal artery bifurcates before the lateral border of the inferior vena cava (IVC).

Preoperative management

A 3D CT angiogram or MR angiogram allows for clarification of the renal vascular anatomy. The position, numbers, and presence of the accessory vessels is required. Adequate hydration is needed to ensure diuresis after transplantation.

Anesthesia

General anesthesia with 3–5 L of intravenous fluid hydration. Mannitol, Lasix, and intravenous heparin have been advocated without documented improvement of graft function, and are not used by the author.

Special instruments/suture material

These are the same as for LTN plus:
- Endo-TA® (instead of the Endo-GIA®).
- Hemolok® clips plus a laparoscopic applicator (13 and 16 mm).
- Kidney dissection table: intravenous giving set, cold Ross solution, crushed frozen saline, and a fine artery dissection tray.

Operative technique

Patient position and port insertion
The patient is prepared and positioned as in LTN. Premark the mid-line and extraction site in the lower abdomen. A 6 cm Pfannenstiel incision is used to extract the kidney.

Colon reflection
Lateral colon adhesions are divided to expose the anterior Gerota's fascia. An important landmark is the gonadal vein which can be followed superiorly to the renal vein.

Ureteric mobilization
The ureter is deep to the gonadal vein. It needs to be mobilized to the level of the iliac bifurcation with careful attention to preserve the periureteric microcirculation. Monopolar diathermy should not be used around the ureter.

Hilar dissection
- The renal vein is carefully freed, looking out for lumber veins. The renal vein is usually freed just medial to the adrenal vein on the left with the junction of the IVC on the right.
- The renal artery is dissected to its origin on the left and to just behind the lateral border of the IVC on the right.
- A Veseloop® (8 cm), blue for veins and yellow for arteries, is helpful in manipulating the vessels.

Kidney mobilization
The kidney is then completely mobilized. Gerota's fascia is entered near the upper pole kidney preserving the adrenal gland. The upper pole is freed, followed by division of any posterior attachments. The renal artery is clearly seen from behind; make sure not to kink it as the kidney is very mobile now.

Ureteric division
The ureter is clipped (with a large laparoscopic clip) and divided at the level of the iliac bifurcation. The clip will prevent urine leak into the operation field, which would worsen vision.

Kidney removal

• Make a 6 cm Pfannenstiel incision as previously marked. Take care not to split the rectus in the mid-line in order to minimize gas leakage. A 15 mm port is inserted under vision followed by the 15 mm Endo-Catch® bag.

• The Endo-Catch® bag is deployed over the kidney and around the renal vessels, pre-bagging it ready for removal.

• Ensure a large laparoscopic clip, scissors, Endo-TA® and a laparoscopic sucker are all ready for use. Clip the artery at least three times near its origin (and start recording ischemia time). Divide it at least 2 mm lateral to the last clip. Expect minimal back bleeding (Fig. 8.4).

• Apply the Endo-TA® as proximal as possible on the collapsed renal vein. (A Hemolok® clip can be used instead of an Endo-TA® for the renal vein.)

• Release the Endo-TA® and inspect the staple line. If complete, cut the renal vein lateral to it. The back bleeding should be brisk but very brief. Remove the veseloops. Pull the string of the Endo-Catch® bag, which is hanging out through the extraction incision (Fig. 8.5). Dilate the extraction site by inserting the two index fingers into the wound and retract. The kidney should be perfused immediately after extraction.

Tips

In addition to the tips for LTN (given above), the following may be used for LLDN:

• Surgeons may prefer hand assistance for either the entire operation or just the division of the artery and vein.

• An Endo-TA® allows for a longer vein by applying staples only on the patient side and allows inspection of the staple line before cutting. An extra large Hemolok® can give similar advantages. This also reduces hemocongestion of the kidney and minimizes renal rupture during extraction.

• Avoid excessive clips around the renal vein. Suture tie the adrenal vein to facilitate rapid staple application onto the renal vein.

• Beware the inferior mesenteric vein, which runs parallel and anterior to the gonadal vein.

• A hand inserted via the lower abdominal Pfannenstiel incision without a 'hand assist device' can be used instead of the Endo-Catch®. The author uses a hand for kidney extraction in larger kidneys that can be difficult to fit into the Endo-Catch® quickly.

• An oblique incision in the iliac fossa just lateral to the rectus is an excellent alternative to a Pfannenstiel incision in obese patients.

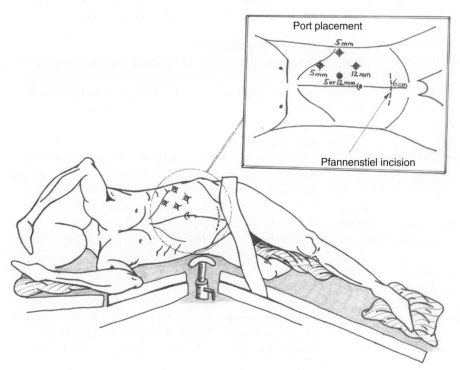

Figure 8.1 Patient position and port site placement for a left transperitoneal nephrectomy. The camera port can be 5 or 12 mm. A Pfannenstiel incision is used for donor kidney removal.

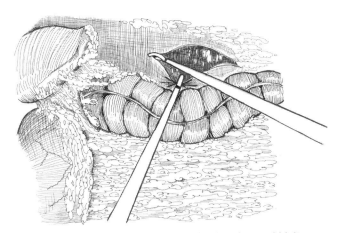

Figure 8.2 Medial mobilization of the left colon along Toldt's line.

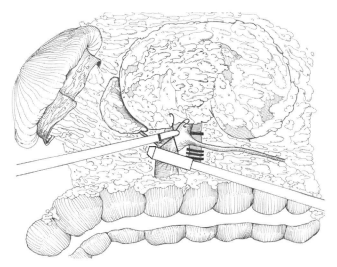

Figure 8.3 Once the renal artery is clipped, make sure that the renal vein is collapsed. A 0/0 polyglycolic acid suture is used to narrow the renal vein and assist the Endo-GIA® placement.

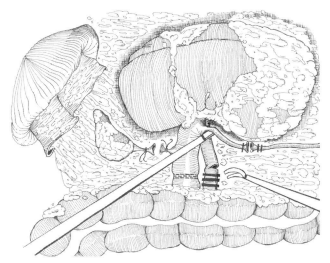

Figure 8.4 The renal vein and renal artery are ligated only on the patient side, preserving maximal vessel length.

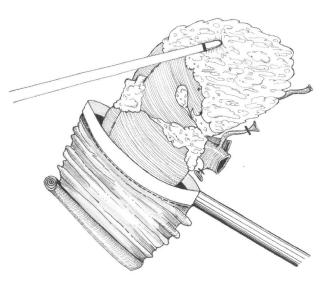

Figure 8.5 The kidney is placed into a 15 mm Endo-Catch® bag for removal from the enlarged caudal port site or the Pfannenstiel incision (donor nephrectomy).

Chapter 9
Transperitoneal Laparoscopic Adrenalectomy

M. Zacharias, P. Fornara, and J.-U. Stolzenburg

Introduction

Minimally invasive techniques have changed the surgical approach to the adrenal gland. Adrenal surgery is already a success story of laparoscopy in the realm of urology and surgery. Since the introduction of laparoscopic adrenalectomy, we cannot find another approach for an ablative surgical operation that provides, so completely, such a clear discrepancy between the extended incision in traditional adrenalectomy and the smaller size of the targeted organ [1–3,5].

Since Gagner's initial report on the laparoscopic approach for adrenalectomy in 1992, several authors have reported on the feasibility and effectiveness of the laparoscopic technique for the treatment of different adrenal diseases. More than 10 years after the first report of laparoscopic adrenalectomy, this operation is presently considered to be the standard technique for most adrenal diseases requiring surgery [3,5,6].

The advantages of laparoscopic adrenalectomy over open adrenalectomy are well documented and include a shorter hospital stay, a decrease in postoperative pain, a shorter interval between surgery and return to preoperative activity level, and improved cosmesis. A variety of laparoscopic approaches to the adrenal gland exist.

The lateral transperitoneal, anterior transperitoneal, lateral retroperitoneal, and posterior retroperitoneal techniques have been described. The lateral transperitoneal approach is the technique most often used for laparoscopic adrenalectomy [1–3,5,6].

Indications

• Functional adrenal tumors, including aldosteronomas, glucocorticoid- and androgen- or estrogen-producing adenomas, and small to moderate-sized solitary pheochromocytomas.
• Selected cases of bilateral adrenal hyperplasia (bilateral LA).
• Incidentalomas >4 cm.
• Nonfunctional tumors >3 cm that demonstrate growth on serial imaging studies.

Contraindications

• Although size is not a definite contraindication, laparoscopy may not be generally advisable for adrenal tumors larger than 10 cm, unless an experienced laparoscopist is available.
• Invasive adrenal cortical carcinomas requiring en bloc resection of the kidney and perinephric fat, spleen, tail of pancreas, diaphragm, and lymph nodes should be managed via an open approach.
• Pheochromocytomas, which demonstrate malignant behavior with multiple sites or metastatic nodes, should not be removed laparoscopically (^{123}I-MIBG scintigraphy should be performed in all pheochromocytomas preoperatively!).
• Serious cardiac conditions (intracardiac shunts, and severe aortic or mitral valve insufficiency).
• Severe cardiac insufficiency (NYHA V).
• Uncorrected coagulopathy.

Preoperative management

• Intravenous single dose antibiotics (cephalosporin) at induction.
• Bowel preparation is not necessary.
• Thrombosis prophylaxis (low molecular weight heparin).

Pharmacological management

Pheochromocytoma

Give preoperatively (5–14 days):
• Phenoxybenzamine hydrochloride (α-adrenergic blocker): an initial divided dose of 20–30 mg is given orally and is increased by 10–20 mg/day (up to 160–320 mg/day).
• Propanolol (β-adrenergic blocker) 20–40 mg three or four times daily (tachycardia >100/min).

Cushing's disease (unilateral adrenalectomy, bilateral subtotal adrenalectomy)

Hydrocortisone given 100 mg/day intraoperatively, and 20–

30 mg/day (plus 0.05–0.2 fludrocortisone) postoperatively with continual dose reduction.

Conn's disease (aldosteronoma)

· Spironolactone 200–300 mg/day for 2–3 weeks preoperatively (improvement of blood pressure).
· Potassium substitution.

Anesthesia

General anesthesia given; intraoperative invasive monitoring involves an intra-arterial line, and central venous pressure monitoring in pheochromocytomas.

Special instruments/suture material

· Laparoscopic standard tower (Olympus) (Fig. 9.1).
· 0° optical system (30° optional).
· 1 × dissection forceps (monopolar current), 1 × bipolar forceps, 1 × endoscissors, 1 × 5 or 10 mm clip applicator.
· 1 × retractor, 1 × Lap-sac, 1 × suction device.
· LigaSure (Tyco Healthcare) is optional.
· *Technique A* (Zacharias, Fornara, Halle): 4 × 12 mm trocars with a Visiport system (Tyco Healthcare) (advantage: all instruments including the optic can be introduced through all the trocars, with maximum flexibility).
· *Technique B* (Stolzenburg, Leipzig): 2 × 5 mm and 2 × 12 mm trocars (advantages: only two 12 mm trocars are needed; for 5 mm trocars there is no need to close the fascia at the end of the procedure; reduced costs).

Operative technique

Position the patient on the operative table, with the arms secured using an arm support or placed beside the trunk. The patient is secured with cloth tapes across the hips and legs.

Technique A (semilateral decubitus position)

· A back support is placed under the side of operation to bring the body to 30°.
· The table is rolled to a horizontal position for entry into the abdomen.
· A Veress needle is introduced above the umbilicus to insufflate the abdomen for closed trocar placement.
· The abdominal cavity is insufflated to 12 mmHg using CO_2.
· Insert the optical trocar.
· The peritoneal space is explored with a 0° laparoscope.
· The patient is rolled to the semilateral position (total 60°) for additional trocar placement.
· Two trocars are placed along the medioclavicular line (pararectal line), one trocar 2 cm below the costal margin and one trocar at the level of the umbilicus.
· The third trocar is placed below the xiphoid (for the retractor).

Technique B (classic flank position)

· Peritoneal access is gained initially with a Veress cannula into the anterior axillary line 2 cm below the costal margin (position of the later 5 mm trocar).
· Insufflation of the peritoneal cavity with CO_2 at 12 mmHg pressure and insert a 12 mm safety trocar (Versaport) into the pararectal line at the umbilical level. If any problem occurs during CO_2 insufflation or with an inexperienced laparoscopist, the patient is repositioned horizontally and a mini-laparotomy is performed at this site for safe trocar placement.
· Insert the optics (assistant) and place the other three trocars under direct vision: one 5 mm trocar into the position of the Veress needle (assistant), one 5 mm trocar into the mid or posterior axillary line (operator) at the level of the umbilicus, and one 12 mm trocar into the anterior axillary line (operator) at the level of the iliac crest.

Left (lateral) transperitoneal adrenalectomy

· Toldt's line is incised from the splenic flexure to the sigmoid junction.
· The left colon is reflected medially.
· The phrenicocolic and the lienorenal ligaments are incised.
· The splenic attachments to the abdominal side wall and the diaphragma are released.
· Mobilize and visualize the upper pole of the left kidney.
· Identify, clip, and divide the main adrenal vein (left side = inferior vein!) where it drains into the renal vein.
· The venous stump is used to gently lift the adrenal gland.
· Clip and divide the small medial and superior adrenal vessels.
· The adrenal gland is freed from its lateral and medial attachments.
· The specimen is extracted intact in an endobag.

Right (lateral) transperitoneal adrenalectomy

· Mobilize and make a trans-section of the triangular ligament.
· Cephalad retraction of the liver.
· The posterior peritoneum is transversely incised high along the under surface of the liver, extending from Toldt's line laterally up to the inferior vena cava medially.
· The duodenum is mobilized medially to expose the renal pedicle.
· Identify, clip ligate, and divide the main adrenal vein (right side = medial vein!).
· Clip and divide the small inferior and superior adrenal vessels.
· The adrenal gland is entrapped in the sack and removed after the complete mobilization.

Tips

· The periadrenal tissue containing tiny arterial and venous branches can be safely controlled with the harmonic scalpel (SonoSurge, Olympus; UltraCision, Ethicon) or the LigaSure device (Tyco), instead of clipping.

• A 30° lens can be helpful to improve visualization in difficult patients.

Postoperative care

• Hormone substitution (hydrocortisone, see above).
• Intensive care monitoring is mandatory for patients with pheochromocytoma.

Troubleshooting

• Injury of the vena cava:
  • small lesion: press with an endopeanut for few minutes, then place a hemostyptika over the defect;
  • suturing: close the injury with forceps, insert another 5 mm port, and suture the defect;
  • large defect: conversion with an incision between the two pararectal trocars (no median laparotomy).
• Bleeding from small vessels: increase the pressure to 18 mmHg and use bipolar coagulation.

• Pleural injuries: suture (beware of pneumothorax and check with X-ray after the procedure).
• Visceral injuries (spleen, liver): argon-beam coagulator, bipolar coagulation, and hemostyptika.

References

1 Del Pizzo JJ. Transabdominal laparoscopic adrenalectomy. Curr Urol Rep 2003;4:81–6.
2 Gill IS. The case for laparoscopic adrenalectomy. J Urol 2001;166:429–36.
3 Guazzoni G, Cestari A, Montorsi F, Lanzi R, Rigatti P, Gill IS. Current role of laparoscopic adrenalectomy. Eur Urol 2001;40: 8–16.
4 Heniford BT, Arca MJ, Walsh RM, Gill IS. Laparoscopic adrenalectomy for cancer. Semin Surg Oncol 1999;16:293–306.
5 McKinlay R, Mastrangelo MJ Jr, Park AE. Laparoscopic adrenalectomy: indications and technique. Curr Surg 2003;60(2):145–9.
6 Suzuki K, Kageyama S, Hirano Y, Ushiyama T, Rajamahanty S, Fujita K. Comparison of three surgical approaches to laparoscopic adrenalectomy: a nonrandomized, backround matched analysis. J Urol 2001;166:437–43.

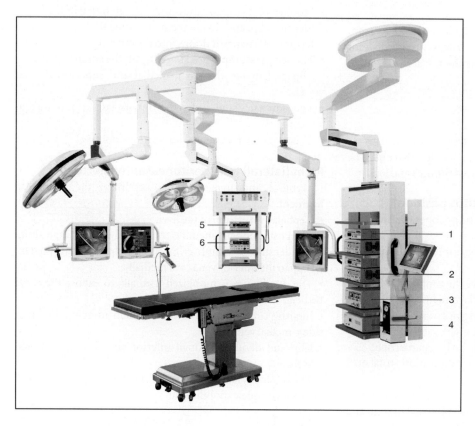

Figure 9.1 Operating room equipment: 1, video camera system supporting digital recording (DV output) and connection of videoendoscopes; 2, light source, 300 W xenon lamp; 3, high flow insufflation unit (35 L/min); 4, integrated endosurgery control system; 5, ultrasonic cutting and coagulation system; 6, HF unit.

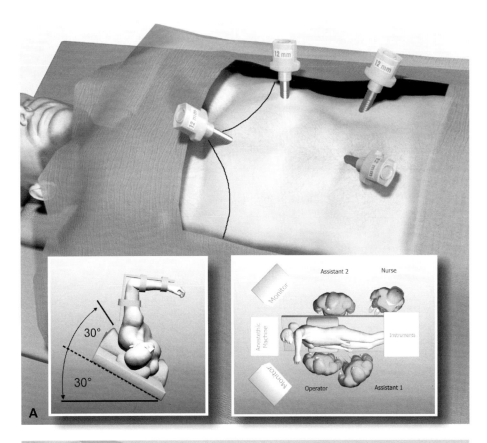

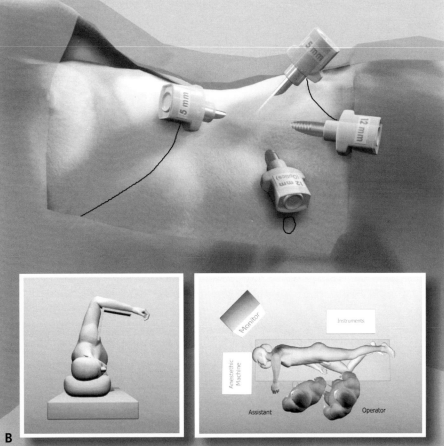

Figure 9.2 Room set-up and trocar positions for laparoscopic adrenalectomy. (A) The semilateral decubitus position with the side of the lesion elevated at 60° and trocar placement of: 2 × 12 mm trocars into the mid-line, and 2 × 12 mm trocars into the pararectal line (PRL, mediclavicular line). (B) Classic flank position (90°) trocar placement: 1 × 12 mm trocar (optical trocar) into the PRL, 1 × 12 mm and 1 × 5 mm trocar into the anterior axillary line, and 1 × 5 mm trocar into the mid or posterior axillary line depending on the size of the patient.

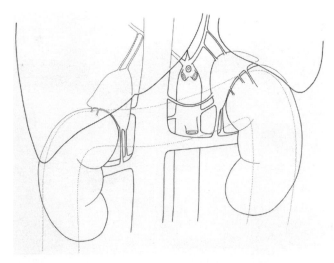

Figure 9.3 Anatomy of the adrenal glands.

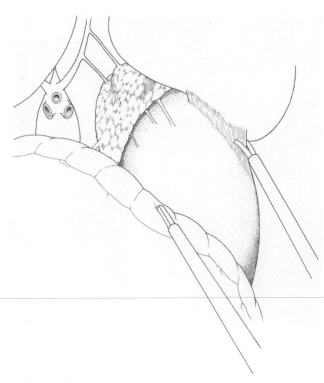

Figure 9.5 Division of the lienorenal ligament after mobilization of the splenic flexure of the colon.

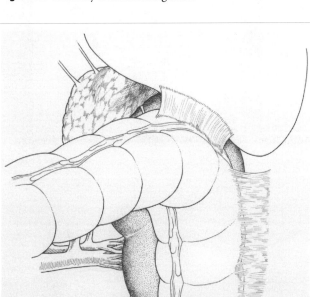

Figure 9.4 The relationship of the left adrenal with the left colic (splenic) flexure.

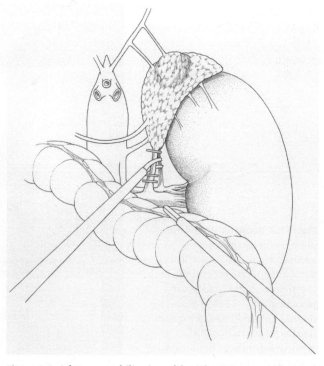

Figure 9.6 Adequate mobilization of the colon is necessary for good visualization of the renal vein and the left main (inferior) adrenal vein, which is then clipped and divided from the renal vein.

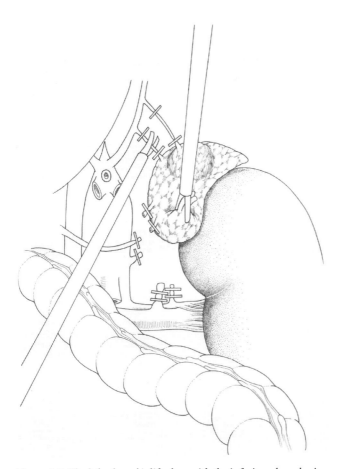

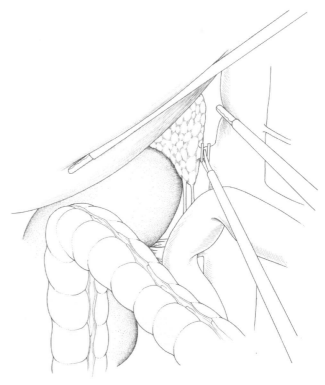

Figure 9.8 Identification, clipping, and division of the clipped right main (medial) adrenal vein after mobilization of the right colic flexure and duodenum.

Figure 9.7 The left adrenal is lifted up with the inferior adrenal vein, followed by clipping and division of the smaller medial and superior periadrenal vessels. Bipolar coagulation is useful to control minor bleeding.

Chapter 10
Partial Nephrectomy in Cold Ischemia

J. Steffens and U. Humke

Introduction

Nephron-sparing surgery for renal malignancy in patients with tumors in a solitary kidney, synchronous bilateral tumors, or renal failure in the opposite kidney (imperative indications) is the only alternative to radical nephrectomy followed by hemodialysis or transplantation [1].

Nephron-sparing surgery is usually performed under ischemia. Warm ischemia is used for short resection times (<30 min) while cold ischemia is preferable for larger, less accessible, central or intraparenchymal tumors. If long operation times on the renal parenchyma are expected, perfusion cooling can be used as an alternative to the frequently practiced cold ischemia with surface cooling only [1,2,7–10]. The technique of perfusion cooling is the fastest and most physiological form of cooling, immediately cools the renal medulla, removes any blood left in the kidney and prevents intravascular coagulation, and improves intraoperative visibility for resection, as clear fluid instead of blood comes out of the injured vessels.

The technique has been established in clinical practice for many years, is a reserve procedure for select cases, and makes the previously used *ex vivo* workbench surgery followed by autotransplantation unnecessary [5].

Patient counseling and consent

- There is a risk of temporary postischemic renal failure, and a transient need for hemodialysis is possible.
- Unexpected need for nephrectomy is always possible.
- Endstage renal failure is rare.
- Postoperative formation of hematoma and urinary fistula.

Anesthesia

General anesthesia.

Indications

Indications are larger, less accessible central or intraparenchymal tumors in a solitary kidney. Also optionally in benign diseases: heminephrectomy or complicated open surgery for calculous disease.

Limitations and risks

Large tumors of more than two-thirds of the whole kidney.

Contraindications

- Tumor extension into the renal vein and vena cava.
- Bad renal function (creatinine more than 4 mg%).
- Resectable tumors in the presence of lung metastases are only relative contraindications.
- Disseminated metastatic disease of renal cell carcinoma.

Preoperative management

- CT scan is usually sufficient (Figs 10.1, 10.2); 3D reconstruction may be helpful in selected cases.
- Arteriography in selected cases only, because tumor location and extension, not vascular anatomy, are leading parenchymal and vascular dissection.
- Occasionally selective renal venography or MRI in patients with large tumors is needed to evaluate for intrarenal and intracaval venous thrombosis.

Preischemic conditioning

Generally, the following nephroprotective measures are employed before every operation with planned warm or cold renal ischemia. The aim is to reduce intra- and postischemic renal vasoconstriction in order to ameliorate reperfusion and postischemic recovery [6].

- Preoperative hydration of the patient for 12 h with isotonic electrolyte solution (1.5 L). No diuretics are given during this period.

- After induction of anesthesia, positioning of the patient, and establishment of stable hemodynamics, administration of 1.25 mg IV of the angiotensin-converting enzyme inhibitor enalaprilate (at least 30 min before the start of ischemia). This dose is halved in patients with previous hypotension.
- Additional administration of 20% mannitol (1 mL/kg body weight).
- Good intraoperative hydration.
- Give heparin (2000 IU) as a bolus IV 2–5 min before the beginning of ischemia.

Special instruments/suture material

- Right-angle curved vascular clamps or Satinsky clamps.
- Venous cannula (16 G, 1.7 mm) or PDA (peridural anesthesia cannula for arterial perfusion.
- Brain dissector.

Surgical approach

Retroperitoneal (lateral recumbent position) access with optional extension into the intrathoracic and/or intra-abdominal space.

Operative technique

- Perform cystostomy (in men) or the placement of a transurethral bladder catheter for postoperative monitoring of the fluid balance.
- The kidney is mobilized on all sides (leaving the perirenal fat intact) to interrupt retrograde renal perfusion from the adrenals and the perirenal fat.
- The renal vein and renal artery are identified and dissected free avoiding traction on the vessels (danger of vasospasm). The vessels are exposed up to their junctions with the aorta and vena cava.
- If possible, the tumor is identified on the surface of the kidney and the perirenal fat around the tumor is removed to determine the incision line.
- A vascular clamp is placed on the ureter and gonadal vessels to interrupt retrograde perfusion.
- The renal artery and renal vein are separately occluded proximally, close to the large vessels (Fig. 10.3).
- A small arteriotomy (stab incision) is performed close to the kidney with a spring lancet. A venous cannula (16 G, 1.7 mm) or PDA cannula is introduced into the renal artery in a central direction, i.e. away from the operator and towards the vascular clamp (Fig. 10.3). An infusion set is connected to the cannula and the kidney perfused with 500 mL cooled (4°C) Ringer's lactate. On no account should preservation solutions with a high potassium content (e.g. Euro Collins, University of Wisconsin solution) be used *in situ* (danger of cardiac arrest!). Maintenance of a perfusion pressure of 120 mmHg is monitored via a pressure cuff. The direction of flow is reversed in the

artery and reaches all segmental vessels in an antegrade direction.
- A venotomy (renal vein) is performed on the right side with a lancet to drain the perfusate (Fig. 10.3). On the left side, the gonadal vein is divided and left open. The color of the perfusate is checked, the perfusate is suctioned off, and hypothermia of the kidney is verified.
- After 500 mL of cold perfusion, the perfusate is clear and the kidney cold. The cannula is removed from the renal artery. The arteriotomy is closed with a superficial (vascular adventitia, a little media) suture of 5/0 to 6/0 Prolene. The venotomy on the right is closed with the same vascular suture. The left gonadal vein is ligated.
- Crushed sterile ice is wrapped in flat compresses around the kidney to maintain the cooling.
- The renal capsule is incised with a scalpel or electrocautery (Fig. 10.4) and the tumor is dissected out of the parenchyma with scissors and/or a brain dissector (Fig. 10.5).
- Tissue specimens from the resection surface of the remaining kidney are sent for frozen section analysis to prove completeness of resection. The surgical safety margin of the resected tumor should be at least some millimeters of macroscopically healthy, peritumoral tissue [11].
- Small vessels are suture ligated with 4/0 or 5/0 absorbable sutures. The renal collecting system is closed with continuous absorbable sutures. The resection site is closed with 2/0–0 Vicryl rapid U sutures (Fig. 10.6). Tabotamp or remnants of perirenal fat are placed in the parenchymal defect and the resection margins are approximated and fixed by tying the parenchymal sutures crosswise (Fig. 10.7).
- If the collecting system has been opened wide, a 7 or 8.5 Fr double-J ureteral stent is inserted through the opened collecting system or an additional pyelotomy. Alternatively, a pyelostomy can be used (Figs 10.6, 10.7).
- All vascular clamps (venous clamp first) are removed to restore renal perfusion (Fig. 10.8). The resection site is checked for bleeding, and the parenchyma is checked for homogenous perfusion.

Postoperative care

- The maintenance of stable hemodynamic parameters intra- and postoperatively is important for optimal reperfusion of the kidney (mean arterial pressure ≥ 100 mmHg). If necessary, low dose dopamine (<3 μg/kg/min) may be given postoperatively.
- Drainage is removed on day 3 to 4 or later, depending on the amount of secretion.
- If a ureteral stent has been placed, the bladder catheter is left in place for 10 days; otherwise it can be removed earlier after mobilization if the patient is voiding without residual urine.
- An excretory urogram is performed on day 10 to document

renal function and an intact morphology of the collecting system.

Complications

The complication rate of nephron-sparing renal tumor surgery reaches 7–16% and is comparable to that of radical tumor nephrectomy [3–5]. The following should be mentioned:
- *Postoperative hemorrhage*: if the patient is hemodynamically stable, the interventional radiologist should attempt superselective embolization. If this is not possible, operative reintervention is necessary, which often results in nephrectomy.
- *Urinary fistula*: diagnosed by the measurement of the creatinine level in the drainage fluid. Insert a double-J ureteral stent and leave the cystostomy or create a new one.
- *Urinoma*: diagnosed by ultrasound and CT. Use antibiotic therapy and the insertion of a double-J stent. If there is an increase in size or abscess formation, operative reintervention is necessary.
- *Temporary postischemic acute renal failure in a solitary kidney*: use hemodialysis.
- *Arterial thrombosis after renal artery puncture*: this differential diagnosis must be considered if there is no diuresis, acute flank pain, or fever. However, the risk of this complication is very low because of the stab incision, the direction of the cannula insertion from peripheral to central, and the use of a thin cannula.

Results

- *n* = 65.
- Time of cold ischemia: 49 ± 37 min.
- pT1 = 16.4%   G1 = 24.6%.
- pT2 = 67.2%   G2 = 60.7%.
- pT3 = 16.4%   G3 = 14.8%.
- Postoperative transient hemodialysis: 6.2%.

To do

- Operate with sufficient arterial pressure only (more than 100 mmHg mean arterial pressure); instruct anesthetist.
- Always perform a stab incision of the arterial wall before cannula insertion as this prohibits intimal dissection.
- Use a thin perfusion cannula.
- The direction of the arterial cannula insertion should be from peripheral to central.

- Close the arteriotomy immediately after completion of the cold perfusion.

Not to do

- Do not use repetitive vascular clamping, to avoid arterial thrombosis and to minimize postischemic reperfusion injury.
- Tumor excision within the pseudocapsule.

References

1 Adkins KL, Chang SS, Cookson MS, Smith JA Jr. Partial nephrectomy safely preserves renal function in patients with a solitary kidney. J Urol 2003;169:79–81.
2 Black P, Filipas D, Fichtner J, Hohenfellner R, Thüroff JW. Nephron-sparing surgery for central renal tumor: experience with 33 cases. J Urol 2000;163:737–41.
3 Corman JM, Penson DF, Hur K, et al. Comparison of complications after radical and partial nephrectomy: results from the National Veterans Administration Surgical Quality Improvement Program. Br J Urol Int 2000;86:782–9.
4 Fergancy AF, Hafez KS, Novick AC. Long-term results of nephron-sparing surgery for localized renal cell carcinoma: 10 years followup. J Urol 2000;163:442–5.
5 Ghavamian R, Cheville JC, Lohse CM, Weaver AL, Zincke H, Blute ML. Renal cell carcinoma in the solitary kidney—an analysis of complications and outcome after nephron-sparing surgery. J Urol 2002;168:454–9.
6 Humke U. Die pharmakologische Blockade des Renin-Angiotensin-Systems in der Prävention des postischämischen akuten Nierenversagens. Akt Urol 1999;30:476–504.
7 Moll V, Becht E, Ziegler M. Kidney preserving surgery in renal cell tumors: indications, techniques and results in 152 patients. J Urol 1993;150:319–21.
8 Steinbach F, Stöckle M, Müller SC *et al.* Conservative surgery of renal cell tumors in 140 patients: 21 years of experience. J Urol 1992;148:24–7.
9 Stephenson AJ, Hakimi AA, Snyder ME, Russo P. Complications of radical and partial nephrectomy in a large contemporary cohort. J Urol 2004;171:130–4.
10 Uzzo RG, Novick AC. Nephron-sparing surgery for renal tumors: indications, techniques and outcomes. J Urol 2001;166:6–18.
11 Zucchi A, Mearini L, Mearini E, Costantini E, Vivacqua C, Porena M. Renal cell carcinoma: histological findings on surgical margins after nephron-sparing surgery. J Urol 2003;169:905–8.

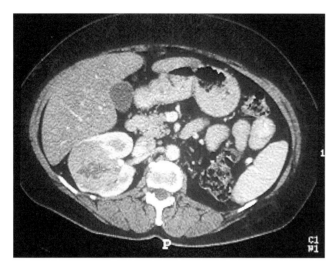

Figure 10.1 CT scan of a large central tumor in a solitary right kidney.

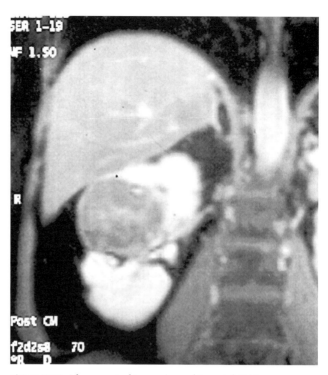

Figure 10.2 A large central tumor in a solitary right kidney.

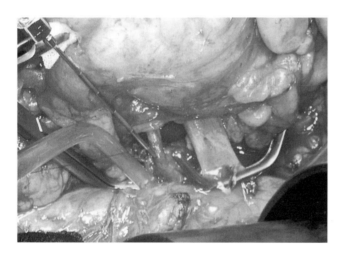

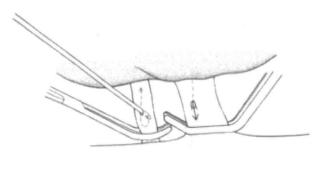

Figure 10.3 *In situ* perfusion of the kidney: after clamping the hilar vessels and arteriotomy, perfuse with cooled Ringer's lactate via an intra-arterial inserted cannula. Drainage of the perfusate is via a venotomy.

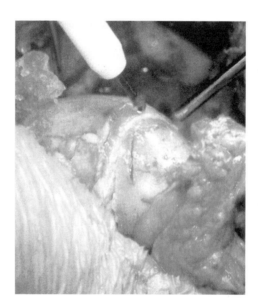

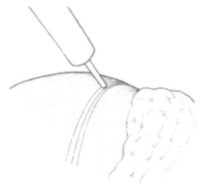

Figure 10.4 Transparenchymal tumor resection by incision of the renal capsule, with a safety margin of about 10 mm.

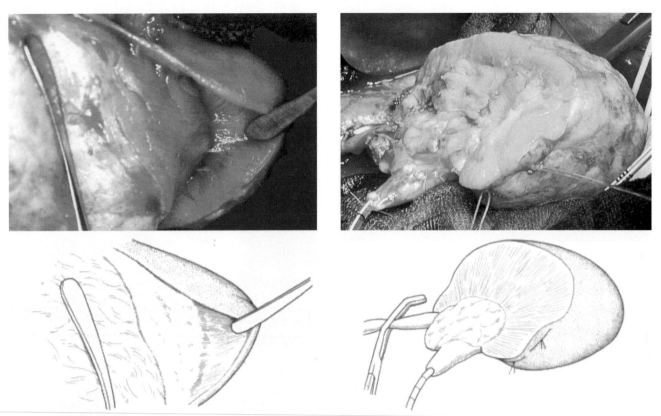

Figure 10.5 Complete tumor resection: retractor into the hilum and exploration for tumor location, intraparenchymal vessels, and collecting system.

Figure 10.6 Caudal third of the kidney after complete tumor resection: reconstruction of the hilar structures, renal pelvis, and parenchyma. The pyelostomy is in place.

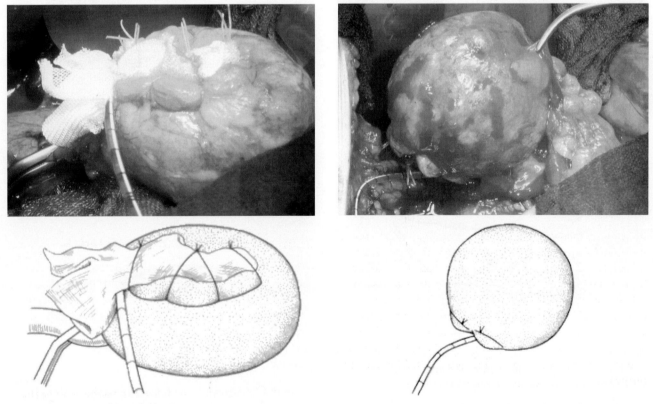

Figure 10.7 Closure of the parenchymal defect by tying sutures over a bolster, with a clamp at the renal vein still *in situ*.

Figure 10.8 Release of renal perfusion: complete perfusion of the remnant kidney without relevant bleeding.

Chapter 11
Minimal Access Approach for Cardiopulmonary Bypass and Circulatory Arrest for Renal Cell Carcinoma with IVC Involvement

J. Libertino, A. Sorcini, and L. Svensson

Introduction

Renal cell carcinoma has the propensity to infiltrate the venous system and propagate into the inferior vena cava (IVC). The incidence of IVC extension has been reported in 4–13%. In 2–4% of cases, the tumor thrombus may reach the suprahepatic IVC. The use of cardiopulmonary bypass and deep hypothermic circulatory arrest for suprahepatic tumor thrombi provides controlled conditions and a bloodless field, facilitating the complete resection of the thrombus and, in some cases, of the infiltrated venous wall. The main cause of operative mortality associated with this procedure is due to pulmonary embolism. In order to prevent distal embolization related to the procedure we changed the traditional surgical strategy, whereby the dissection of the kidney and the radical nephrectomy is performed only after cardiopulmonary bypass, circulatory arrest, caval thrombectomy, and caval reconstruction.

For the last 4 years we have utilized a minimal access approach for cardiopulmonary bypass and deep circulatory arrest. Adopting this strategy and techniques, we verified a marked decrease in total operative time, postoperative length of stay on a ventilator and in the intensive care unit, and use of postoperative narcotics. There were no embolic events, and when compared to the procedures performed with the traditional strategy, the blood loss was equal.

Indications

Indications include renal cell carcinoma with IVC tumor thrombus above the hepatic veins, and absence of diffuse metastatic disease demonstrated by preoperative radiologic testing and intraoperative assessment. In cases of resectable solitary metastasis, the procedure is still indicated. In a few cases of patients with acceptable performance status and severe symptoms, such as recurrent pulmonary embolisms, severe pain, severe edema secondary to the renal cell tumor, and caval extension, the procedure is indicated for palliative purposes.

Contraindications

- Diffuse metastatic disease demonstrated on preoperative radiologic evaluation or at intraoperative exploration.
- Aortic regurgitation.
- Coronary artery disease requiring simultaneous coronary artery bypass graft through a median sternotomy (in this case the traditional approach is indicated).

Preoperative management

- Metastatic work-up: abdominal CT scan, chest X-ray/CT, and bone scan.
- Evaluation of cranial level of tumor thrombus: MRI of abdomen and chest with gadolinium, and inferior cavogram to improve accuracy of the MRI in selected cases.
- Cardiac evaluation: echocardiogram, and cardiac catheterization with coronarogram.
- Neurologic evaluation: EEG and placement of electrodes for continuous intraoperative EEG monitoring.
- Renal artery embolization.
- Preoperative hydration (dextrose + KCl + mannitol).

Anesthesia

Volatile gas and pentothal 10 mg/kg just before circulatory arrest.

Special instruments/suture material

- Bookwalter retractor for the abdominal incision.
- Widlander retractor for the subclavicular incision.
- Finocchietto retractor for the right parasternal incision.
- Suture material: 4/0 and 5/0 Prolene for caval reconstruction and atrial closure; 6/0 Prolene for subclavian artery closure; and 8 mm Dacron vascular graft in obese patients.

Surgical approach

- Transabdominal transverse 'chevron' incision.
- 5 cm right subclavicular incision for arterial cannula.
- 6 cm right parasternal incision at the level of fourth and fifth ribs.

Operative technique

- The patient is placed in the supine position. The lower extremities are in the 'frog position' to allow for a potential need for great saphenous vein retrieval.
- Place the intravesical and intraesophageal thermometers.
- Prepare with Betadine from the neck to the ankles.
- Make a chevron incision: two finger breaths below the costal arcade, from the tip of the 11th rib on the side of the tumor to the lateral margin of the rectus muscle on the contralateral side. The incision can be extended to the tip of the contralateral 11th rib once the absence of metastases is established.
- Explore the abdomen with examination and palpation of the liver, palpation of the periaortic lymphadenopathy, and evaluation of tumor resectability.
- Dissect the hepatic colonic flexure.
- Perform medial mobilization of the duodenum and head of the pancreas by the Kocher maneuver.
- Re-evaluate tumor resectability and the presence of lymph node metastases.
- Dissect the hepatic caudate lobe from the anterior aspect of the IVC with ligation of the minor hepatic veins.
- The inferior margin of the liver is retracted upward to expose the IVC.
- In case of a need for wider exposure because of extensive invasion of the caval wall, the right triangular ligament can be incised and the right hepatic lobe mobilized medially either at this time or during circulatory arrest.
- At this point, if the absence of metastatic disease is confirmed, the cardiac portion of the operation can be started:
  - a 5 cm incision is made one finger-breadth below and parallel to the right clavicle;
  - incise the attachment of the pectoralis magnum to access the right subclavian;
  - dissect the right subclavian artery;
  - make a right parasternal incision (two finger-breadths lateral from the sternal margin) at the level of the heads of the third and fourth ribs;
  - disarticulate and resect the heads of the third and fourth ribs;
  - place the Finocchietto retractor;
  - make a longitudinal incision of the pericardium and exposure of the heart;
  - the pericardium is sutured to the skin;
  - place a pursestring suture at the level of the auricle of the right atrium;

- perform a transverse arteriotomy and place a 14 Fr arterial cannula;
- incise the right atrium and place a venous cannula;
- use systemic heparinization;
- institute cardiopulmonary bypass;
- the patient temperature is lowered down to 16–18°C (the heart is in fibrillatory arrest at 24–26°C).

When continuous EEG monitoring shows an isoelectric trace, deep hypothermic circulatory arrest has been obtained. The patient is exsanguinated and the blood kept in the heart–lung machine. From this point the urology and cardiac surgery team work simultaneously.

Urology team

- The inferior cavotomy starts 6–7 cm above the origin of the renal vein and 1 cm from the lateral margin of the vena cava and is directed to the junction of the cava and the renal vein with the tumor thrombus in it. An elliptic incision is made around the renal ostium of the affected side. Prolong the cavotomy for about 4–5 cm below the origin of the renal vein.
- Dissect the tumor thrombus from the caval wall using scissors and blunt dissection.
- Incise the posterior aspect of the caval wall around the renal ostium; on a few occasions a larger resection of the caval wall may be necessary. In those cases, retrieval of a patch of pericardium may be used to reconstruct the vena cava.
- Use endoscopic control of the vena cava with a flexible cystoscope to rule out the presence of residual thrombus infiltrating the wall and/or extending into the hepatic veins.
- Close the vena cava with a 4/0 Prolene running suture.

Cardiac surgery team

- Perform a longitudinal atriotomy.
- Dissect the tumor thrombus from the atrial wall.
- Amputate the tumor thrombus if the distal tip is larger than the caval lumen.
- Dissect the tumor thrombus from the intrapericardial caval wall.
- Close the atrial wall using a 4/0 Prolene running suture in two layers.
- Cardiopulmonary is re-established and the patient is warmed.
- Isolate, ligate with 0 silk, and divide the renal artery, which was embolized preoperatively.
- Isolate, ligate, and divide the ureter.
- Incise the posterior peritoneum superior, lateral, and inferior to the kidney.
- Perform careful renal and adrenal dissection and radical nephrectomy.
- Close the pericardium with the placement of a 24 Fr chest tube in the pleural space.
- Place a laminar dram in the renal fossa.
- Reapproximate the pectoralis muscles to the sternal edge.
- Close the abdominal wall in layers.

Complications

Intraoperative complications

• *Pulmonary embolism* is the most frequent cause of intraoperative death. It is usually due to excessive manipulation of the kidney and/or vena cava prior to deep hypothermic circulatory arrest. Minimizing the caval dissection and performing the nephrectomy after the caval thrombectomy appears to prevent embolic events.

• *Intraoperative hemorrhage* is usually the result of a wide tumor resection and the coagulopathy associated with the cardiopulmonary bypass and deep hypothermic circulatory arrest. Performing the nephrectomy after the tumor thrombectomy does not increase the requirement of blood transfusions.

• *Intraoperative cardiac complications* are rare. Every patient is worked up preoperatively with cardiac catheterization and an echocardiogram. In cases of surgically correctable coronary artery disease, the aortic–coronary bypass is performed during the cooling phase of the cardiopulmonary bypass.

Postoperative complications

• *Respiratory insufficiency:* usually, after a cardiopulmonary procedure, the patient remains intubated for 12–24 h. When the requirement for blood products is elevated, a longer time may be needed on the ventilator.

• *Sepsis:* in cases of prolonged intensive care unit stay, sepsis is a potential complication.

• *Neurologic injury:* the incidence of neurologic injuries is related to the length of deep hypothermic circulatory arrest. A safe limit for hypothermic arrest is 40 min.

• *Renal failure:* if the preoperative creatinine is normal, postoperative renal failure is a rare event. The kidney is usually well protected by hypothermia. In cases of prolonged circulatory arrest, acute tubular necrosis is the most frequent cause of reversible renal failure.

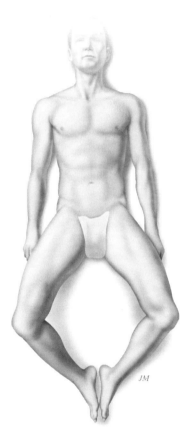

Figure 11.1 Position of the patient on the operating room table.

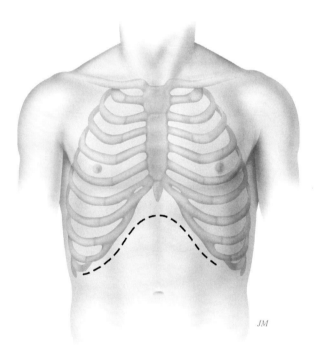

Figure 11.2 Chevron incision for the abdominal portion of the procedure.

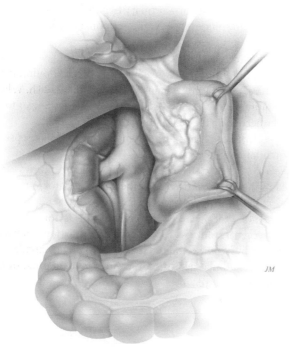

Figure 11.3 Duodenal mobilization allowing exposure of the inferior vena cava.

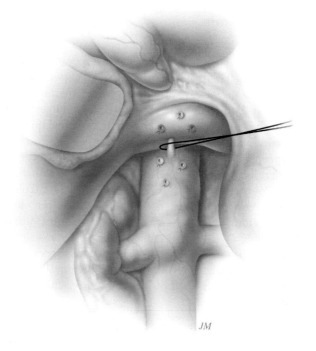

Figure 11.5 Ligation of the minor hepatic veins.

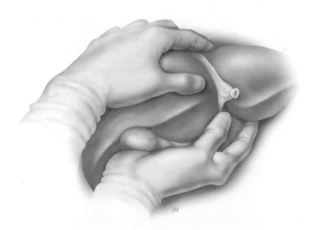

Figure 11.4 Palpation and mobilization of the liver.

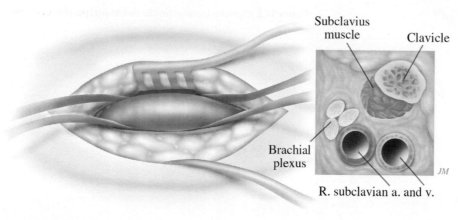

Subclavius muscle

Clavicle

Brachial plexus

R. subclavian a. and v.

Figure 11.6 Exposure of the right subclavian artery.

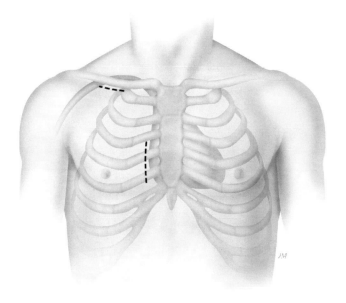

Figure 11.7 Right parasternal incision over the fourth and fifth ribs.

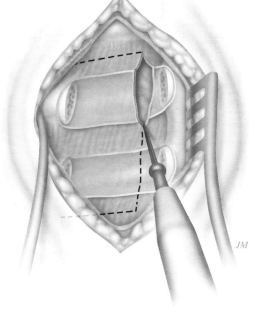

Figure 11.9 Parasternal rib resection.

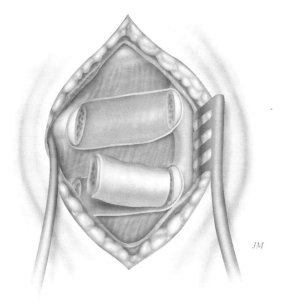

Figure 11.8 Resection of the heads of the fourth and fifth ribs.

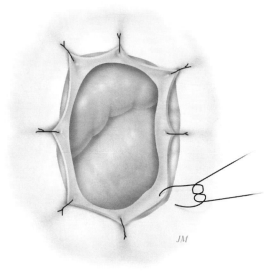

Figure 11.10 Preparation of the pericardial window.

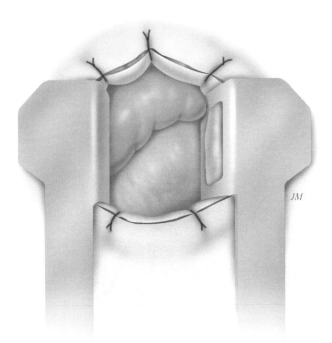

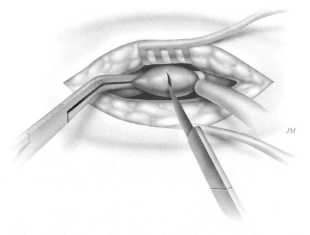

Figure 11.13 Incision of the right subclavian artery for the arterial inflow cannula.

Figure 11.11 Placement of the retractor for atrial exposure.

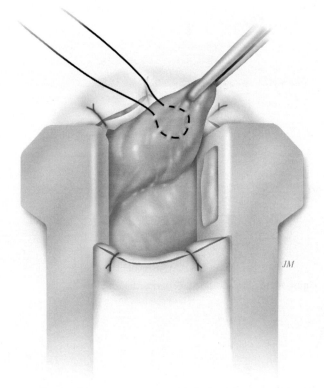

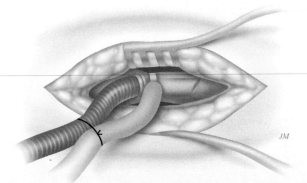

Figure 11.14 Placement of the right subclavian arterial cannula.

Figure 11.12 Placement of the atrial pursestring suture.

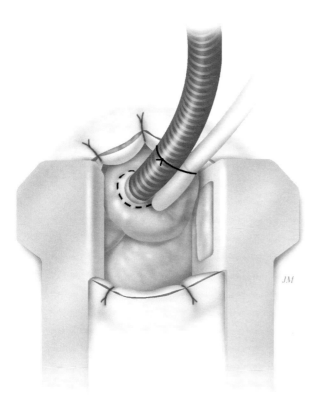

Figure 11.15 Placement of the atrial cannula for the venous out-flow.

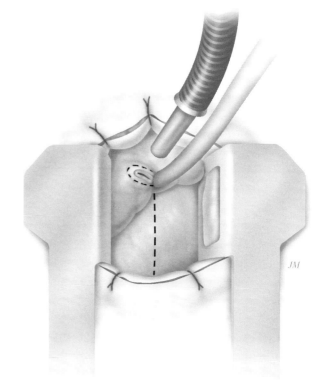

Figure 11.17 Insertion of the atrial cannula for the venous outflow.

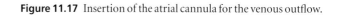
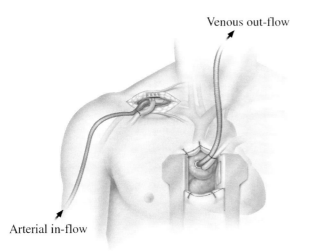

Venous out-flow

Arterial in-flow

Figure 11.16 Venous outflow from the atrium to pump with arterial inflow into the right subclavian artery.

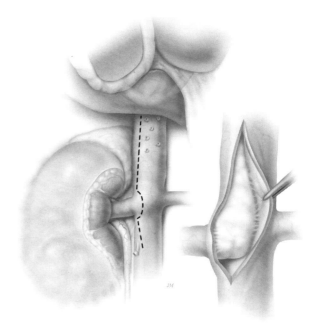

Figure 11.18 Venacavotomy for tumor thrombectomy.

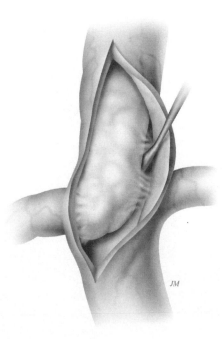

Figure 11.19 Use of the endarterectomy spatula to mobilize the tumor thrombus.

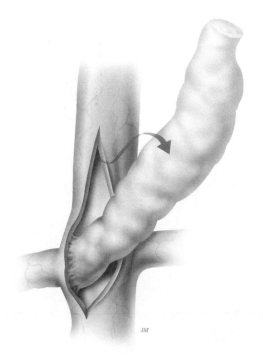

Figure 11.21 Extraction of the tumor thrombus from the inferior vena cava.

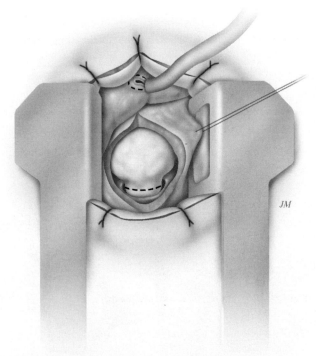

Figure 11.20 Division of the head of the tumor thrombus extending into the right atrium.

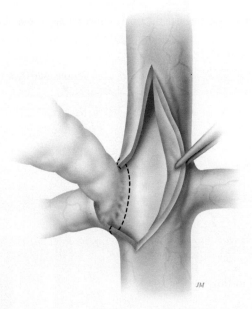

Figure 11.22 Resection of the ostium of the right renal vein with a cuff of inferior vena cava.

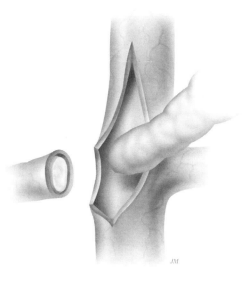

Figure 11.23 Resection of the posterior wall of the right renal vein and tumor thrombectomy.

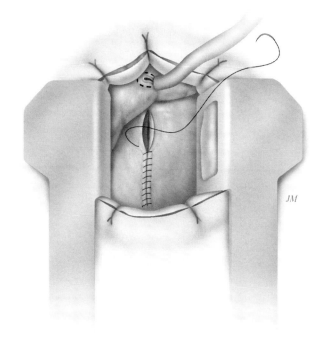

Figure 11.25 Closure of the right atrium.

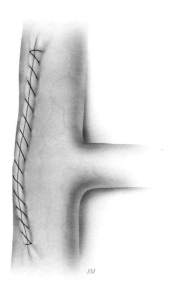

Figure 11.24 Closure of the inferior vena cava with 4/0 Prolene.

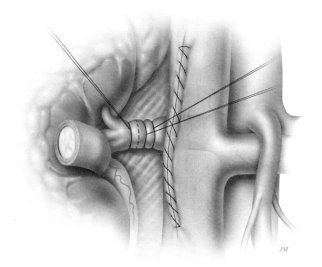

Figure 11.26 Division of the right renal artery.

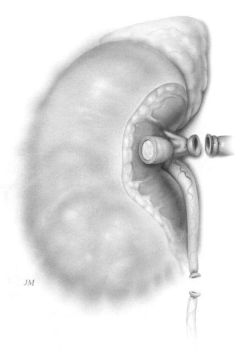

Figure 11.27 Ligation of the right ureter.

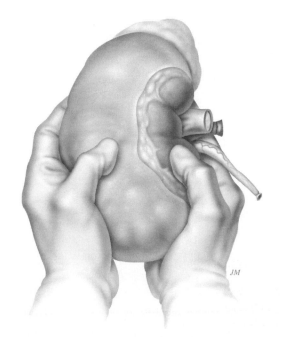

Figure 11.29 Removal of the right kidney.

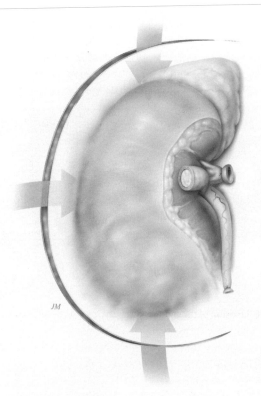

Figure 11.28 Mobilization of the right kidney after division of the artery, vein, and ureter.

Chapter 12
Reconstructive Renovascular Surgery

U. Humke and M. Ziegler

Introduction

Renal artery diseases such as stenoses, occlusions, or anomalies may lead to arterial hypertension and, later, to progressive deterioration of renal function. Pathophysiologically, a close connection exists between these two symptoms. Firstly, the decrease in renal bloodflow leads to activation of the renin–angiotensin system and other intrarenal vasoactive components that try to maintain glomerular filtration. Secondly, a further decrease of renal bloodflow caused by progressive renal artery disease exceeds the humoral compensatory mechanisms and glomerular filtration drops significantly. Hypertension and deterioration of kidney function are closely associated with the incidence of myocardial infarction, apoplectic insults, and peripheral arterial vascular disease—all of which are of increasing importance for overall national health, especially if the increasing age of the population worldwide is taken into account. The prevalence of renovascular hypertension is estimated at 1–20%, with with a greater incidence in the age groups under 10 and over 40 years old. The incidence of the disease is about 5% [5,8].

Pathology of the renal artery

• *Stenosis* from atherosclerosis (most frequent), fibromuscular dysplasia (intimal, medial, perimedial fibroplasia), arteriitis, or neurofibromatosis.
• *Renal artery aneurysm* (rare, tends to rupture with increasing size (>2 cm), causes hypertension and peripheral intrarenal microembolism).
• *Acute renal artery occlusion* through arterial embolism (emboli of cardial origin) or arterial thrombosis (following blunt kidney traumas with rupture of the intimal and medial layers of the renal artery wall).

Indications

Today surgical treatment for renal artery disease is indicated much less frequently than it was 10–15 years ago. The causes are improvements in medical antihypertensive therapy options and—most of all—an enormous progress in, and widespread use and availability of, interventional radiologic techniques [4].
• *Pharmacological therapy*: this is obligatory for the symptomatic treatment of renal hypertension. Long-term monotherapy poses a significant risk for progression of atherosclerosis and stenosis, including deterioration of renal function.
   • *Percutaneous transluminal angioplasty* (PTA) [4]: therapy of choice for fibromuscular stenoses and atherosclerotic stenoses located in the middle part of the renal artery.
• *PTA with insertion of an endovascular stent* [4] for near-aortic, so-called ostial atherosclerotic stenoses (long-term results and prospective randomized comparisons with surgical procedures are still being waited for).
• Further techniques of *interventional radiology*: intravascular lysis therapy for arterial thrombi and selective embolization for small aneurysms.
• *Surgial revascularization of the renal artery*:
   • as a primary treatment alternative for severe atherosclerotic ostial renal artery stenosis (probably in younger patients because of its superior long-term results);
   • as primary treatment in simple or multiple stenoses of segmental renal arteries or their origins from the mainstem renal artery;
   • as primary treatment in renal artery aneurysms with a diameter >2 cm;
   • as secondary or tertiary treatment after an unsuccessful PTA (recurrent stenoses >60%);
   • as secondary and emergency treatment for complications during PTA (approximately 3%, indicated for the rescue of renal function, with the indication dependent on individual patient morbidity and the benefit : risk ratio).

Preoperative management

• Diagnosis and quantification of renal artery stenosis with color-coded Doppler sonography; renal scintigraphy (with or without captopril); bilateral determination of plasma renin activity in the renal venous blood; aortic and renal arteriography; and arteriography of the iliac vessels in cases of renal autotransplantation. CT or MRI for renal artery aneurysm. Excretory urography only in cases of sufficient renal function.

• Detection and, if possible, repair of coexisting coronary and/or carotid artery stenoses because of the danger for myocardial infarction and/or apoplectic insult during the decrease of blood pressure after successful restoration of renal bloodflow.

• Pharmacological conditioning of the kidney for intraoperative ischemia:

  • Preoperative hydration of the patient overnight: Ringer's lactate 1–1.5 mL/kg/h;

  • after induction of anesthesia: application of mannitol 20% 1 mL/kg IV and enalaprilate (Xanef®) 1.25 mg IV [3];

  • before clamping the renal artery: 30 U/kg heparin IV as a bolus.

Special instruments/suture material

• Standard set for kidney surgery.
• Vascular forceps.
• Blunt cannulas.
• Different vascular clamps: Satinsky clamps, bent and straight vascular clamps, bulldog clamps.
• Vascular sutures: 7/0 polyglycolic acid, 5/0 and 6/0 monofilament nonabsorbable.

Surgical approach

• *Retroperitoneal approach*: this causes only minor morbidity, especially in older patients. It is the standard approach to the left renal artery for all reconstructive procedures with good, superficial exposure of the vessel. In selected cases it is also an adequate approach to the right renal artery (e.g. iliacorenal bypass and autotransplantation).

• *Transperitoneal approach*: this is more invasive and has higher postoperative complication rates (ileus, pneumonia). It is the standard approach for bilateral renal artery reconstruction and *in situ* reconstruction of the right renal artery (e.g. aortorenal bypass).

Methods for ischemia protection of the kidney

• *Warm ischemia* for ischemia time of less than 30 min: pharmacological conditioning (see above) without further protection (e.g. for renal artery endarterectomy).

• *Cold ischemia in situ* for ischemia time of 30–90 min: pharmacological conditioning (see above) as well as cannulation (blunt cannula) of the renal artery after transection and perfusion of the kidney with Ringer's lactate (500 mL, 4–7°C). The perfusate is drained either via a small incision of the right renal

vein or via the dissected gonadal vein on the left side. Additional surface cooling of the kidney with crushed ice slows down rewarming (e.g. during bypass procedures).

• *Cold ischemia ex situ* for autotransplantation and presumed ischemia times longer than 90 min: pharmacological conditioning (see above) and harvesting of the kidney after central transection of the vessels. Extracorporeal perfusion on the workbench with either Euro-Collins (EC), University of Wisconsin (UW), or HTK Bretschneider solution (1000 mL, 4–7°C). Storage and surgical preparation of the kidney in an ice water bath on the workbench as long as necessary (e.g. for microsurgical reconstruction of hilar segmental vessels with a hypogastric artery graft).

Surgical technique

General surgical steps

• Surgical mobilization of the kidney inside Gerota's fascia is necessary only during a retroperitoneal approach (better exposure and mobility of the kidney).

• Separation of the renal artery and vein, and placement of vessel loops: during retroperitoneal access starting from the renal hilum, and during transperitoneal access starting from the aorta.

• For exposure of the renal artery, slight caudal or cranial retraction of the renal vein with a vessel loop or an eyelid retractor without compromising the venous bloodflow.

• Careful dissection of the periarterial lymphatic structures.

• Always expose the aortorenal junction for determination of the complete renal artery length.

In situ techniques

Endarterectomy

• For the correction of atherosclerotic ostial renal artery stenosis [2].

• Place the Satinsky clamp on the aorta around the renal artery orifice.

• Make a longitudinal incision of the proximal renal artery into the aorta.

• In case of significant backflow of blood from the kidney, place a distal renal artery clamp.

• Blunt circumferential freeing of the intima including the plaque with an endarterectomy probe.

• In case of loose intima margins at the distal resection site, fix the intima and media with sutures (double-armed 6/0 or 7/0 sutures, moved from inside through the vessel wall to the outside and tied outside) to prohibit later dissection of the vascular wall caused by the bloodstream.

• Close the vessel: (i) with a longitudinal 5/0 or 6/0 continuous vascular suture without narrowing the artery significantly; or (ii) with a Dacron patch using two continuous 5/0 or 6/0 vascular sutures.

Bypass techniques

- For the correction of proximal renal artery stenosis [9].
- Transection of the artery behind the stenosis and ligation of the stump (2/0 nonabsorbable sutures).
- Direct reimplantation of the renal artery into the aorta is usually impossible because of the short vessel. Therefore, a bypass-procedure is necessary.
- *Aortorenal bypass*: this uses a saphenous vein graft or synthetic graft (hypogastric artery graft in children):
  - placement of a Satinsky clamp on the anterolateral surface of the aorta distally to the renal artery. Incision of the aortic wall and end-to-side anastomosis of the aorta and graft with two continuous 5/0 vascular sutures, first establishing the posterior wall;
  - end-to-end-anastomosis between the renal artery and graft with interrupted sutures or two continuous 6/0 vascular sutures. For small vessels (<8 mm) spatulation and anastomosis is in an oval shape.
- *Splenorenal bypass*: this uses the splenic artery for the revascularization of the left kidney [1]:
  - the procedure is only feasible if there has been no previous surgery to the stomach;
  - retroperitoneal identification and dissection of the splenic artery is done craniomedial of the left kidney at the upper margin of the pancreatic tail;
  - dissect the splenic artery approaching the splenic hilum and transect after the placement of a proximal vascular clamp;
  - the spleen remains intact *in situ* and is supplied by the short gastric arteries;
  - carefully ligate the small pancreatic branches leaving the splenic artery;
  - after sufficient mobilization of the splenic artery and kidney, spatulate both the splenic and renal arteries;
  - perform an oval-shaped end-to-end-anastomosis with 6/0 vascular sutures (continuous or interrupted).
- *Iliacorenal bypass*: used for retroperitoneal revascularization of the right kidney with a venous graft via a caudally prolonged subcostal incision [6]:
  - harvest the saphenous vein from the left (contralateral) groin;
  - make an incision in the groin parallel to the inguinal ligament and vertical distal extension along the vein;
  - ligate all side branches of the saphenous vein along a length of 20 cm;
  - transect distally and proximally, marking carefully one end to later identify reliably the bloodflow direction due to the venous valves;
  - ligate the venous stumps *in situ*;
  - flush the graft with saline through a tied cannula; control any leakage;
  - spatulate the *distal* end, and perform an end-to-side anastomosis after clamping and incision of the right common iliac artery (5/0);

- perform an end-to-end-anastomosis of the graft and renal artery with interrupted or continous 6/0 vascular sutures. For small vessels (<8 mm), use spatulation and oval-shaped anastomosis.

Ex situ technique

- *Graft interposition and autotransplantation*: used for reconstruction of hilar segmental renal artery stenoses or for aneurysms of the renal artery [7]:
  - harvest an internal iliac artery graft via a contralateral suprainguinal incision after dissection of the external and internal iliac vessels;
  - carefully dissect the internal iliac artery, including its first three branches;
  - make a distal transection of the branches and proximal transection of the main stem close to the bifurcation;
  - on the workbench, in an ice water bath, adjust the graft to the renal hilum. The branches of the internal iliac artery correspond to the segmental renal arteries;
  - perform a microsurgical end-to-end anastomosis between the segmental renal arteries and the internal iliac artery branches (7/0);
  - resect and close unnecessary branches of the internal iliac artery;
  - replant the kidney into the iliac fossa, performing end-to-side anastomosis of the renal vein with the external iliac vein and end-to-side-anastomosis of the renal artery (proximal end of the internal iliac artery graft) with the external iliac artery (5/0 or 6/0);
  - implant the ureter with an extravesical, antirefluxive technique into the bladder dome. Insert an external stent and percutaneous cystostomy.

Tips

- Strict avoidance of mechanical traction on the vascular structures during vessel dissection because of the danger of severe vasospasm.
- For resolution of vasospasm, use intraoperative topical application of lidocain 1% or papaverine on the vessel.
- Microsurgical anastomosis of the internal iliac artery branches with the segmental renal arteries in an ice water bath *ex situ*, using transient insertion of a small ureteric stent into the vascular lumen (helps in the safe construction of a nonstenotic anastomosis).

Postoperative care

- After reperfusion of the kidney and during the postoperative intensive care phase, make sure there is sufficient fluid volume in the circulation and sufficient arterial blood pressure. If necessary, apply catecholamines (dopamine) in a renal dose.
- Treat metabolic acidosis with sodium bicarbonate 8.4%.

- Intravenous low dose heparine (100–500 IU/h IV, without prolongation of the prothrombin time).
- Ultrasound controls for hematoma formation.

Not to do

Never use extracorporeal perfusion solutions (e.g. EC, UW, or HTK solutions) for perfusion *in situ*. The high potassium content of these solutions can lead to an influx of potassium in the circulation and consequent cardiac arrest.

References

1 Geroulakos G, Wright JG, Tober JC, Anderson L, Smead WL. Use of the splenic and hepatic artery for renal revascularization in patients with atherosclerotic renal artery disease. Ann Vasc Surg 1997;11:85–9.
2 Hallett-JW J, Textor SC, Kos PB *et al.* Advanced renovascular hypertension and renal insufficiency: trends in medical comorbidity and surgical approach from 1970 to 1993. J Vasc Surg 1995;21:750–9.
3 Humke U. Die pharmakologische Blockade des Renin-Angiotensin-Systems in der Prävention des postischämischen akuten Nierenversagens. Akt Urol 1999;30:476–91.
4 Humke U, Uder M. Renovascular hypertension: the diagnosis and management of renal ischaemia. Br J Urol Int 1999;84: 555–69.
5 Kaplan NM. Epidemiology and clinical importance of renovascular and renal parenchymatous hypertension. In: Renovascular and Renoparenchymatous Hypertension (Lüscher TF, Kaplan NM, eds). Springer Verlag, Berlin, 1992:63–70.
6 Mulherin JL, Edwards WH. Alternative methods of renal revascularization. Ann Surg 1987;205:740–6.
7 Novick AC. Surgical management of branch renal arterial disease. In: Renovascular and Renoparenchymatous Hypertension (Lüscher TF, Kaplan NM, eds). Springer Verlag, Berlin, 1992: 259–66.
8 Vaughan ED, Jr, Sosa RE. Renovascular hypertension. In: Campbell's Urology (Walsh PC, Retik AB, Vaughan ED, Jr, Wein AJ, eds). W.B. Saunders, Philadelphia, 1998:423–59.
9 Wise KL, McCann RL, Dunnick NR, Paulson DF. Renovascular hypertension. J Urol 1988;140:911–24.

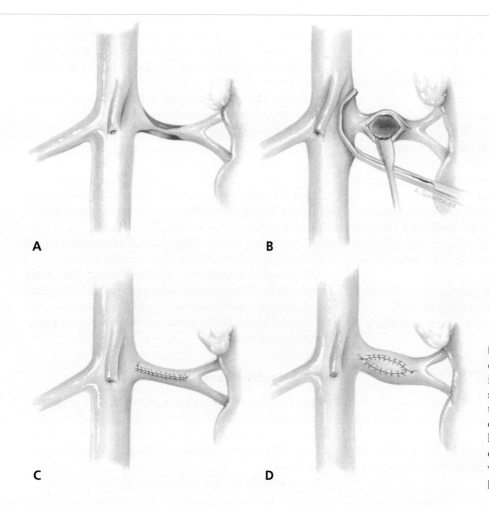

A **B** **C** **D**

Figure 12.1 Endarterectomy. (A) In cases of ostial renal artery stenosis, incise the renal artery across the stenosis after clamping and removal of the atherosclerotic plaque using an endarterectomy probe (B). Closure in large vessels should be with a continuous suture (C), or in small vessels with application of a Dacron patch (D).

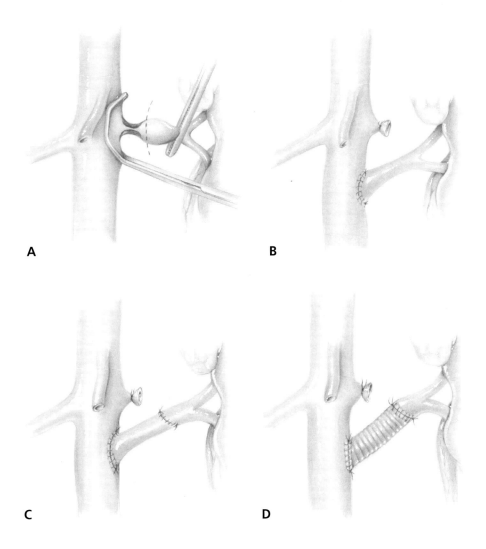

A

B

C

D

Figure 12.2 Aortorenal bypass. (A) In cases of near-aortic renal artery stenosis, clamp and transect the artery close behind the stenosis. (B) After clamping with a Satinsky clamp and incision of the aorta, perform end-to-end anastomosis with the renal artery stump if there is enough artery length left and if the kidney can be mobilized. If the remaining renal artery is too short, aortorenal anastomosis is performed with the use of a saphenous vein graft (hypogastric artery graft in children) (C) or a synthetic graft (D). Note the oval shape of the end-to-end anastomosis.

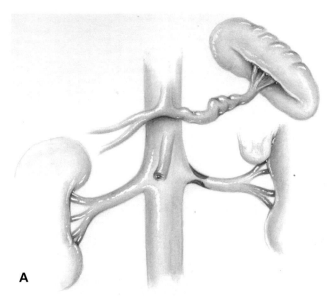

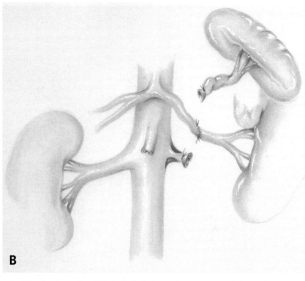

Figure 12.3 Splenorenal bypass. (A) The indication for this procedure is exclusively for left-sided, near-aortic renal artery stenosis. Use a retroperitoneal approach via a flank incision. The dissected splenic artery is transected close to the splenic hilum and the renal artery is transected close to the stenosis. (B) End-to-end anastomosis is performed in an oval shape between the splenic and renal arteries. The spleen remains *in situ*.

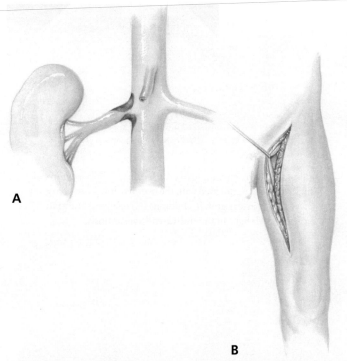

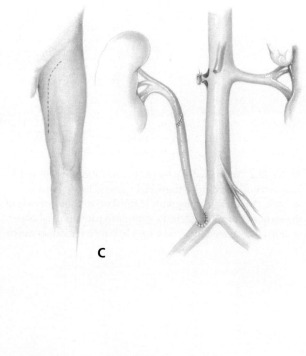

Figure 12.4 Iliacorenal bypass. (A) The indication for this procedure is for a right-sided, near-aortic renal artery stenosis, using a purely retroperitoneal approach. (B) Harvesting of the saphenous vein graft is done via a distally extended inguinal incision. (C) Implantation of the graft under consideration of the venous valves (flow direction from caudal to cranial!) with end-to-side anastomosis between the graft and common iliac artery and an oval-shaped end-to-end anastomosis between the graft and renal artery stump.

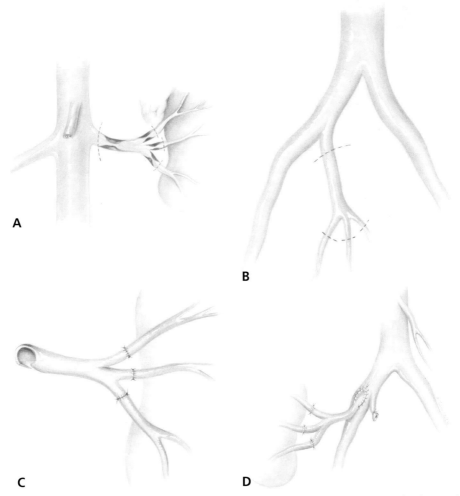

Figure 12.5 Graft interposition *ex situ* and autotransplantation. (A) This procedure is indicated for multiple segmental renal artery stenoses. (B) There is contralateral removal of the hypogastric artery with its first three branches, followed by nephrectomy, perfusion of the kidney, and excision of the diseased vessel parts in the renal hilum in an ice water bath. (C) The segmental arteries are reconstructed with a microsurgical end-to-end anastomosis with the hypogastric artery graft. (D) Autotransplantation of the reconstructed kidney into the contralateral iliac fossa with end-to-side anastomosis between the renal artery and common iliac artery, renal vein anastomosis, and antirefluxive implantation of the ureter into the bladder dome.

Part 1.2
Mid and Lower Ureter

Chapter 13
Psoas Hitch

M. Fisch

Introduction

The psoas hitch is the method of choice for ureter reconstruction. The ureter is fixed to the psoas muscle at the 'point of entrance' in order to avoid obstruction and kinking when the bladder capacity changes through filling and emptying or as children grow older. The ureter is reimplanted through a submucosal tunnel and anchored into the detrusor so it remains antirefluxive in the lower third of the ureter. This procedure is preferred in contrast to end-to-end anastomosis or ureteroureterostomy.

Patient counseling and consent

There is a possibility of urinary leakage or intermediate nephrostomy. In recurrent stenosis large bowel interposition may be necessary.

Preoperative management

Ultrasound, intravenous pyelogram, or MRI and voiding cystogram (VCU) should be performed to obtain the best information possible about the kidney function, the length of the defect, and the contralateral kidney. Estimation of bladder capacity, large bowel contrast X-ray and preparation should be performed in long strictures with risk for a change of operative procedure.

Anesthesia

General and epidural anesthesia.

Indications

- Ureter defects bridged up to 5–6 cm. In longer defects use a modified technique.
- Broad spectrum of indications: reflux in adults.
- Trauma, fistulas, or obstructions resulting from gynecological or large bowel surgery, kidney transplantation, ureteroscopy, specific inflammations, megaureter, double systems, and repeated operations.

Limitations and risks

- Kidney function >20% in adults and >10% in children (with a normal contralateral kidney).
- Previous irradiation.
- Bladder capacity is related to body height and the distance to be bridged (small patient, large bladder capacity).
- In borderline bladder capacity, combine with bladder augmentation.
- Lesion of the genitofemoralis nerve.

Contraindications

The procedure is contraindicated in low bladder capacity.

Special instruments/suture material

- Fine instruments for ureter implantation.
- Bipolar coagulation instruments.
- Suture material: 4/0 and 5/0 Monocryl.
- Cystostomy set.
- 6–10 Fr soft splints (Websinger).

Operative technique

- Make a standard parainguinal incision, extended cranially. In large defects use transperitoneal pararectal or xyphoid to symphysis incisions, kidney mobilization, bladder augmentation.
- Identify the ureter under the lateral umbilical cord crossing the iliac vessels.
- Distal preparation: preserve the longitudinal subadventitial and the branches of the gonad vessels.
- Ligate and cut the ureter above the level of obstruction or fistula area. Observe the blood supply; resect the stump until capillary arterial bleeding occurs.

- Bladder mobilization is facilitated by insertion of the digital finger after opening between stay sultures.
- Measure the distance to the ureter and direct the bladder to the psoas.
- The genitofemoralis nerve is identified and a 4/0 Maxon or PDS suture is placed. (The psoas minor is a tendinous structure located on the nerve's medial margin optimal. Although it is not always present.) Avoid deep sutures due to variations of the femoralis nerve inside the psoas muscle.
- Place the suture through the lateral corner of the detrusor, and stretch it to check the distance. Switch over to Übelhör technique (see below) for tension-free implantation.
- If needed, extend the incision to open the bladder dome.
- The submucous tunnel preparation is facilitated by four stay sutures, which mark the tunnel length of 3–4 cm.
- Perform a pull-through maneuver—nice and smoothly—if the point of entrance is wide enough.
- Tie the psoas fixation suture.
- Spatulate the ureter and cut it if needed.
- Place anchor sutures of 4/0 Monocryl at 5 and 7 o'clock deep in the detrusor, mucosa–mucosa adaptation 5/0 Monocryl at 6, 3, 9, and 12 o'clock, and insert a 6–8 Fr soft splint fixed by a 5/0 Vicryl rapid suture. Use two stab incisions for the cystostomy and the splint through the bladder, and fix this also.
- Close the bladder with running 5/0 mucous and interrupted detrusor 4/0 Monocryl sutures. The bladder mucosa is fixed at the adventitia of the ureter with two stitches.
- Check the port of entrance by a curved Overholdt clamp.

Übelhör technique
- Extend the longitudinal bladder incision down in the opposite direction to the mobilized bladder by crossing the midline. Ligate the urachus and the chorda lateralis opposite. Insert a splint into the contralateral orifice and fix it with a Vicryl rapid suture.
- Incise the anterior and posterior basis of the now triangular bladder flap with the scissors in order to elongate it.
- Follow the standard hitch procedure with the top of the triangular flap fixed to the psoas muscle.
- The antireflux implantation is performed on the medial side of the flap that is closed to a tube later on.

Results
- $n = 373$.
- Complications: 1.6%.
- Obstruction: 1.6%.
- Reflux: 1%.
- Success rate: 97.4%.

Psoas hitch repeat procedure
- $n = 29$.
- Obstruction, $n = 12$.
- Reflux, $n = 17$.
- Success rate: 96%.

Reference

1 Hohenfellner R, Leissner J, El-McKresh. Megaureter. Akt Urol 1999;30:143–54.

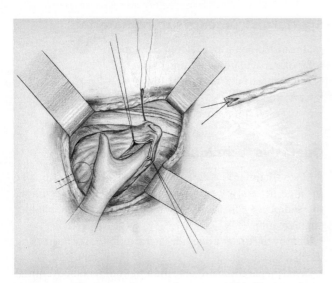

Figure 13.1 The distance between the ureter and bladder is too long for standard implantation.

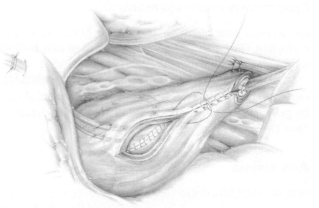

Figure 13.2 Bladder closure using two layers: running mucosa and interrupted detrusor.

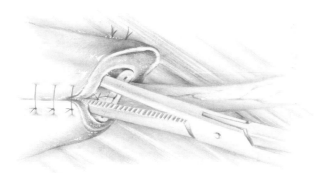

Figure 13.3 Check the port of entrance between the mucosa fixed to the adventitia of the ureter and the detrusor adaptation suture.

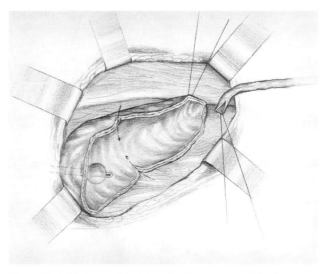

Figure 13.4 Bladder wall incisions for flap extension (Übelhör technique.)

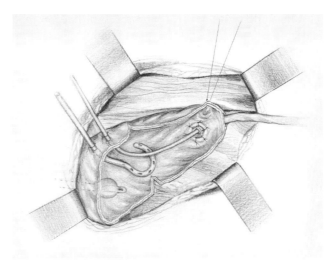

Figure 13.5 The psoas fixation suture is tied, following ureter implantation (Übelhör technique).

Chapter 14
Megaureter Surgery

M. Fisch

Introduction

The congenital primary obstructed megaureter is classified according to the location of the dilatation:
- Grade I: Ia, distal ureter; Ib, up to the iliac vessels.
- Grade II: including the ureteropelvic junction.
- Grade III: if the calyces are also dilated, often combined with malrotation, or there is so-called 'long kidney' with a polycalical system or megacaliosis and stone formation in the lower calyx.

Megaureter is often found by chance in babies with grade III, and later on in symptomatic adults with grade Ia as the ureter length increases from 15 cm up to 30 cm, with the so-called terminal dilatation left behind.

Preoperative management

Ultrasound, MRI, and voiding cystogram (VCU): reflux?

Indications

Surgery with reimplantation is indicated in recurrent high febrile urinary tract infections, flank pain, and reflux. Rare in adults.

Contraindications

Kidney function >20% in adults, and >10% in children contraindicates the use of this technique.

Operative technique

- Identify the dilated ureter with thickened walls, adjusted to the peritoneum with dense fibrous tissue.
- Careful preparation should be carried out, preserving the longitudinal vessels under the adventitia. Additional branches from the gonad vessels are found medially and parallel to the left ureter down to the crossing point with the iliac vessels. On the right side the branches cross the vena cava, making a net-work around the mid and upper ureter. Branches of the iliac vessels reach the lower third of the ureter and have to be ligated.
- The connective tissue bands that fix the loops are dissected and the ureter is ligated and cut 3 or 4 cm above the ureterovesical junction, preserving the ganglion pelvicum.
- Open the ureter longitudinally, preserving the longitudinal vessels up to the 'critical point' just above the iliac vessels where the caliber becomes significantly smaller.
- Insert a 16 Fr splint fixed with several 5/0 Vicryl rapid sutures to the mucosa.
- Ureter tapering is performed up to the critical point in cases of excessive dilatation. In borderline dilatation, where tapering is questionable, the lumen is narrowed by interrupted all-layer gather sutures only.
- Follow the standard psoas hitch procedure step by step (see Chapter 13).
- The ureter is shortened to an adequate length before tension-free antirefluxive submucous tunnel implantation. Observe capillary arterial bleeding from the ureter stump and spontaneous peristalsis.
- The port of entrance has to be wide enough to perform a nice and smooth pull-through maneuver.

Tips

- Preserve as many arterial branches as possible from the aorta and the gonadal vessels.
- Narrow the lumen to a minimal diameter of 1 cm before it shrinks. Postoperatively it shrinks by 30%.
- Cover the reconstructed ureter and the psoas hitch with the greater omentum in adults.

Postoperative care

Remove the wound drain on day 2, the bladder catheter on day 8, and the ureter splint on day 10. Close the cystostomy; remove if residual free voiding is demonstrated by ultrasound. Antibiotic treatment and prophylaxis is given later on.

Complications

- Splint not functioning: (i) asymptomatic: do not irrigate; if no dilatation is found on ultrasound, wait and see; and (ii) symptomatic: perform a percutaneous nephrostomy.
- Paralytic ileus: check for paravesical extravasation, hematoma, or epigastric vessels. Extravasation: try a puncture first, otherwise perform an open revision.
- Prolonged urine drainage: wait and see; on day 8 remove the drain step by step. Expect spontaneous closure of the fistula in the majority of cases.
- Lesion of the ramus genitalis (nervi genitofemoralis or femoralis): see Chapter 75.
- Ureter obstruction or reflux: perform nephrostomy first, and repeat the procedure 3 months later. In cases of small capacity and a short ureter, use large bowel interposition.

Remarks

- The indication for this procedure is restricted to symptomatic and refluxive patients only. Due to the risk of lesions of the pelvic ganglion with persistent neurogenic bladder dysfunction, a staged procedure is recommended with reconstruction of the bilateral side performed 8 months later.
- In extended ureter reconstruction, ureter bladder anastomosis is superior to end-to-end anastomosis or ureteroureterostomy (cross-over technique, see Chapter 15).
- Mobilize the kidney to bridge any large defects.
- In contrast to the Boari flap, the blood supply of the flap is superior because of its broad basis.
- Capillary arterial bleeding from the ureter stump and the flap is mandatory in order to prevent an ischemic obstruction.
- In addition, bladder augmentation may become necessary, using a detubularized isolated sigma segment (cup patch technique, Goodwinn technique), if the remaining bladder is too small.
- Perform a sigma interposition between the ureter stump and the psoas hitch if a tension-free anastomosis is questionable.

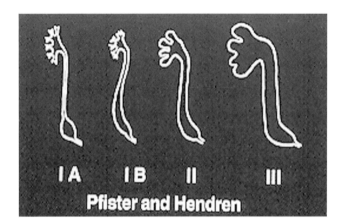

Figure 14.1 Classification of the megaureter.

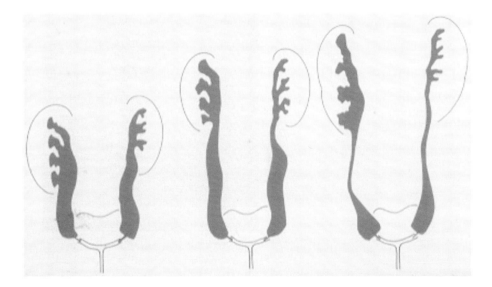

Figure 14.2 Ureter dilatation in the same patient at the ages of (left to right): 4 months, 14 years, and 25 years.

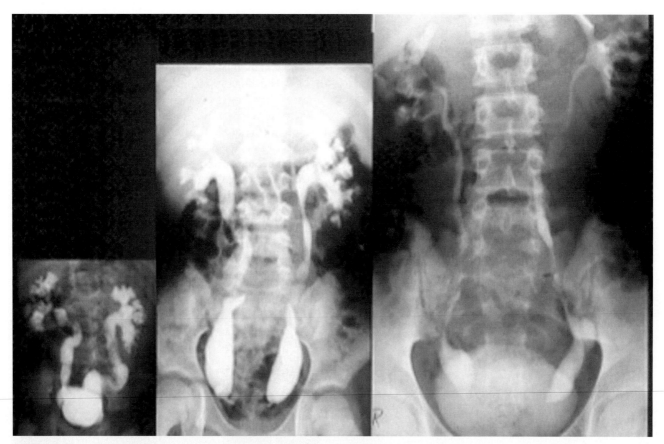

Figure 14.3 Showing ureter dilatation in the same patient shown in Fig. 14.2, at 4 months, 14 years, and 25 years (left to right).

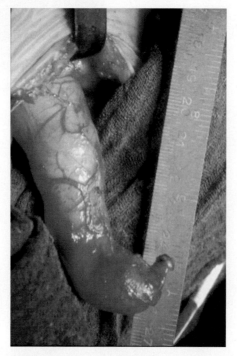

Figure 14.4 Intraoperative finding: note the narrow prevesical segment.

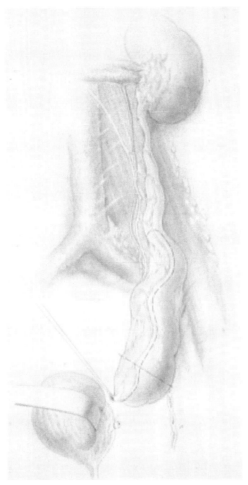

Figure 14.5 The dashed line shows the line of longitudinal incision and resection. The blood supply is from the main longitudinal subadventitious vessel, with additional supply from the gonad vessels running medially.

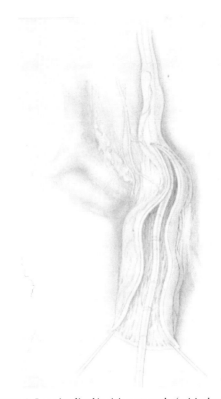

Figure 14.6 Longitudinal incision up to the 'critical point'. Note the change of caliber!

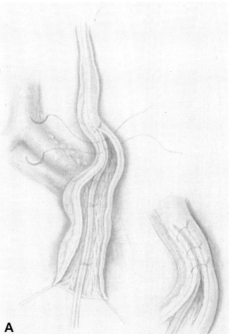

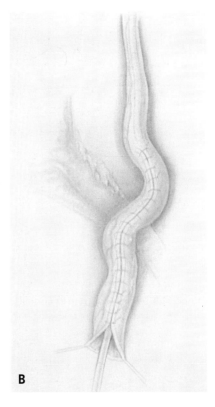

Figure 14.7 All-layer, interrupted gather sutures using 4/0 Monocryl are needed for caliber reduction.

A

B

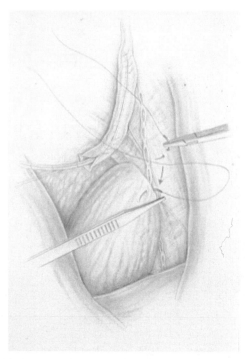

Figure 14.8 The lateral corner of the bladder is fixed to the psoas.

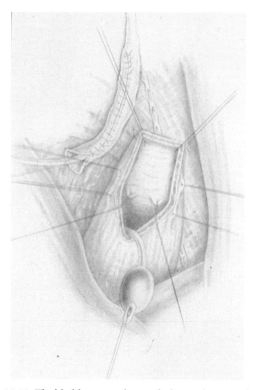

Figure 14.10 The bladder opened up to the 'port of entrance'.

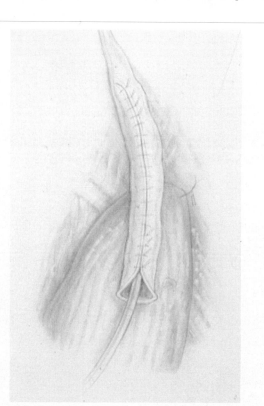

Figure 14.9 With the ureter in its normal topographic position, check that there is an adequate length for antireflux implantation.

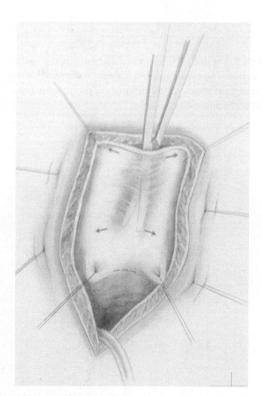

Figure 14.11 Tunnel preparation.

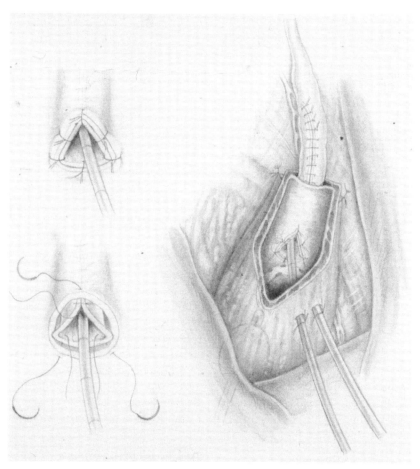

Figure 14.12 Ureter implantation.

Chapter 15
Cross-Over Technique

M. Fisch

Introduction

In selected cases a one-stage psoas hitch reimplant of both ureters can be performed.

Indications

This procedure can only be performed in children. Indications include primary bilateral obstructive refluxive megaureters, and recurrent urinary tract infections. The child should have normal bladder capacity and be slim.

Advantages

The correction can be made in one session, thus avoiding the 'yo-yo' phenomenon of uretero-ureteral reflux in transuretero-ureterostomy in dilated systems.

Limitations and risks

The cross-over should be made from right to left only (better blood supply from the right ureter), and is only suitable for a primary correction.

Contraindications

The procedure is contraindicated if the right ureter is too short for a nice, smooth cross-over, and if there is borderline bladder capacity.

Operative technique

• Make a transperitoneal midline incision.
• Achieve bladder mobilization by separation of the urachus and chorda umbilica dextra and sinistra.
• The bladder is adjusted to the left psoas.
• The right ureter is dissected close to the bladder and is mobilized carefully up to the ureteropelvic junction.
• It is important to preserve the arteria testicularis dextra, which crosses over the ureter from the lateral to medial aspect.
• Cross over intraperitoneally, from right to left through a window of the mesosigma just below the arteria mesenterica inferior.
• If the ureter is long enough to be implanted, dissect the left ureter 5 cm above the ureterovesical junction (take care not to injure the pelvic ganglion).
• Perform a side-to-side butterfly anastomosis (see also double systems, Chapter 4).
• Implant both ureters in the submucosal tunnel.

Postoperative care

Remove the wound drain on day 2, the bladder catheter on day 8, and the ureter splint starting on day 10 (one after the other). Then close the cystostomy. This can be removed if residual free voiding is demonstrated by ultrasound. Antibiotic prophylactic treatment should be given later on.

Complications

• *Splint not functioning.* If the splint is not functioning but the patient is asymptomatic, do not irrigate! If there is no dilatation on ultrasound, wait and see. If the patient is symptomatic, perform percutaneous nephrostomy. In paralytic ileus consider: paravesical extravasation, hematoma, or bleeding from epigastric vessels. Try a puncture first, otherwise consider open revision. In prolonged urine drainage, wait and see and on day 8 remove the drain step by step. Expect a spontaneous closure of fistula in the majority of cases. For lesions of the ramus genitalis nervi genitofemoralis or femoralis, see Chapter 75.
• *Ureter obstruction or reflux.* Perform a nephrostomy first, and then repeat the procedure 3 months later. In cases of small capacity and a short ureter, use large bowel interposition.

Remarks

• In extended ureter reconstruction, ureter bladder anastomosis is superior to end-to-end anastomosis or uretero-ureterostomy (cross-over technique).
• Mobilize the kidney to bridge any large defects.
• In contrast to the Boari flap, the blood supply of the triangular flap is superior because of its broad basis.
• Capillary arterial bleeding from the ureter stump and the flap is mandatory in order to prevent an ischemic obstruction.
• In addition, bladder augmentation may become necessary, using a detubularized isolated sigma segment (cup patch technique, Goodwinn procedure), if the remaining bladder is too small.
• Perform a sigma interposition between the ureter stump and the psoas hitch if a tension-free anastomosis is questionable.

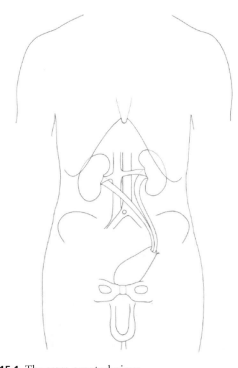

Figure 15.1 The cross-over technique.

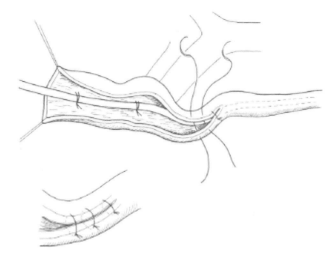

Figure 15.2 Caliber reduction of the left megaureter.

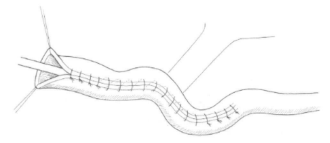

Figure 15.3 View after tapering.

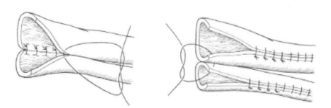

Figure 15.4 Side-to-side butterfly anastomosis of the left and right ureters.

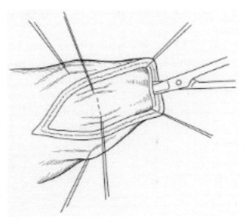

Figure 15.5 Preparation of a wide submucous tunnel.

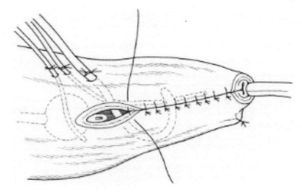

Figure 15.6 The final situation.

Chapter 16
Lich–Gregoir Procedure

M. Fisch

Introduction

This is the method of choice for primary vesicorenal reflux (VRR) in children only. It is easy to teach and is reproducible.

Patient counseling and consent

The success rate is high, but complications requiring surgery occur in 1% of cases. Nonfebrile urinary tract infections may still occur.

Indications

- Noncomplicated VRR grade II–V.
- Before puberty in nondilated single as well as double systems.

Limitations and risks

- Kidney function: MAG 3 clearance >20%.
- It is a two-stage procedure, performed over 6–8 months in bilateral VRR.
- Spontaneous resolution of contralateral reflux in >20%.
- Risk of postoperative voiding dysfunction with residual urine due to lesions of branches of the inferior pelvic ganglion.

Contraindications

The procedure is contraindicated post puberty, in terminal ureter obstruction, and in severely dilated ureters.

Preoperative management

Ultrasound MAG 3, and voiding cystogram (VCU) should be performed. MRI (intravenous pyelogram) is needed for special indications. Exclude terminal ureter obstruction.

Special instruments/suture material

Fine instruments, bipolar coagulation, and a magnification lens system are needed; 4/0 and 6/0 Monocryl is needed in bladder mucosa lesions.

Operative technique

- The ureter is dissected upward 6–7 cm from the peritoneum and down to the bladder hiatus.
- Place two stay sutures on the bladder dome at a right angle to the ureterovesical junction, and fill the bladder with 100 cm^3 saline.
- Incise the detrusor muscle with scissors, also dissecting small crossing muscle fibers, until the mucosa bulges and the ventral circumference of the hiatus is open.
- The ureter becomes embedded by emptying the bladder and closing the detrusor with 4/0 Monocryl interrupted sutures over the ureter.

Tips

- Preserve branches of the gonad vessels crossing the ureter.
- Change over to the psoas hitch procedure in cases of an unexpected dilated ureter.
- 6/0 Monocryl closes mucosa lesions watertight.
- Leave the posterior fixation of the ureter intact.
- The course of the tunnel (right angle as described in the original publication by Gregoir) is mandatory to avoid kinking later on.
- The new port of entrance has to be wide enough to avoid obstruction.

Postoperative care

Perform a kidney ultrasound and discharge the child on the same day. Remove the catheter on day 3 or 4. Repeat the kidney ultrasound. Antibiotic prophylactic treatment is continued.

Complications

In cases of mucosal lesions, remove the catheter on day 6 or 7. Place a percutaneous nephrostomy in cases of dilatation; if persistent, perform a psoas hitch 3 months later.

Results

The success rate was 98.5% in more than 1000 cases over a period of 40 years with redo operations in 1.5% and persistent reflux in 1%. In a follow-up of more than 20 years, arterial hypertension occurred in 2.1% and asymptomatic bacteriuria (ABU) in 52%. All pregnancies were undisturbed.

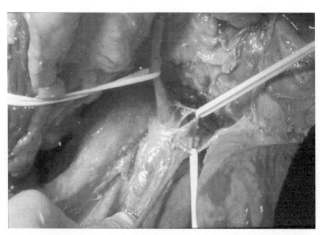

Figure 16.1 Branches of the inferior pelvic plexus are armed with vessel loops.

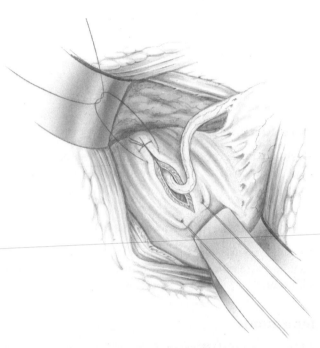

Figure 16.3 The ureter is embedded.

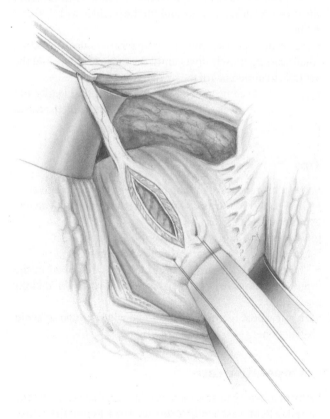

Figure 16.2 Perpendicular incision of the detrusor muscle. The mucosa remains intact.

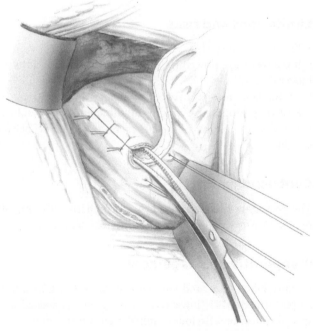

Figure 16.4 Check the width of the entrance into the tunnel.

Part 1.3
Special Techniques

Chapter 17
Surgical Therapy of Ormond's Disease

M. Fisch and R. Wammack

Introduction

Ormond's disease is a form retroperitoneal fibrosis causing ureteral obstruction. This obstruction starts at the level of the promontory and proceeds in a cranial direction. There is a progressive course of the disease, which respects the adventitia of the ureter and major vessels, thus giving a layer for dissection. Primary surgery and secondary medical treatment (cortisone and azathioprine) should be used in cases of dilatation.

Symptoms occur late, with bilateral ureteral dilatation proximal to the iliac vessels with subsequent looping of the ureters. In symptomatic dilatation and impaired renal function, there should be preoperative nephrostomy.

Patient counseling and consent

• There is increased mortality in patients previously treated with cortisone or a pigtail catheter.
• Lesions of the ureteral adventitia or longitudinal ureteral vessels, or accidental opening of the ureter, present major complications requiring peritoneal patching (with the serosa inside).
• If both ureters are injured, ureteral replacement may be required using the large bowel from left to right with antireflux-ive implantation and hitching the bladder to the psoas muscle.
• Dissection in the wrong layer can injure the aorta and vena cava and may require vascular surgery (vascular prosthesis).
• There is a risk of intrahilary recurrence when the proximal dissection is incomplete.

Indications and risks

Unilateral or bilateral asymmetric dilatation of the upper tract with classic medialization of the ureters at the level of the promontory.

Differential diagnosis

Differential diagnoses include peritoneal carcinosis (e.g. breast cancer) or lymphatic neoplasms.

Preoperative management

Ultrasonography, intravenous urography, and computer tomography should be performed. MRI with contrast medium is needed in impaired renal function. Laboratory diagnostics, including coagulation parameters, are needed.

Anesthesia

General anesthesia.

Special instruments/suture material

As for vascular surgery.

Operative technique

See Figs 17.1–17.6.

Tips

• Magnification loops (×2.5) facilitate dissection of the ureter in the right plane.
• Depending on the intraoperative and individual situation, use either a free peritoneal patch (free tissue transfer) or wrap with the omentum.
• With a split omentum both ureters can be wrapped.
• Respect the vascular situation. Badly vascularized parts of the omentum may lead to fibrosis and infection.
• If ureteral peristalsis is good and there is no leakage, the abdomen can be closed without drainage.

Postoperative care

There is intraoperative clamping of the nephrostomy tube. Intravenous urography is performed after 7 days, with removal of the nephrostomy tube, and the start of immunosuppression with cortisone and azathioprine.

To do

• Dissect in the layer between the adventitia of the vena cava/aorta/ureter and the fibrotic tissue.

• Continue the dissection cranially until reaching the renal hilus, this avoids recurrence (intrahilary Ormond's disease).
• Cover the ureters (peritoneal patch, wrapping with omentum) down to the iliac crossing.

Not to do

• Do not use badly vascularized parts of the omentum as this leads to fibrosis and infection.

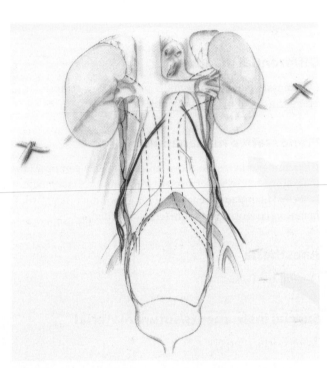

Figure 17.1 Classic medialization of the ureters at the level of, and cranial to, the promontory due to retroperitoneal fibrosis (Ormond's disease).

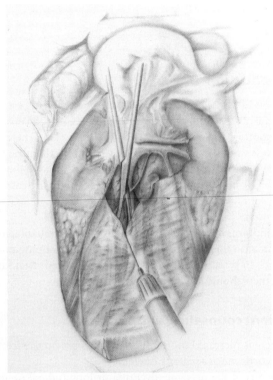

Figure 17.2 Median laparotomy, right paracolic incision, and incision along the mesenteric root up to the Treitz ligament. The bowel is moved out of the abdominal cavity and the ureter is identified. The dissection starts in the layer between the adventitia of the vena cava/right ureter and the fibrotic tissue, with the tissue elevated by a fine overhold and cut using electrocautery ('split and roll' technique). The dissection ends distal to the crossing with the iliac vessels.

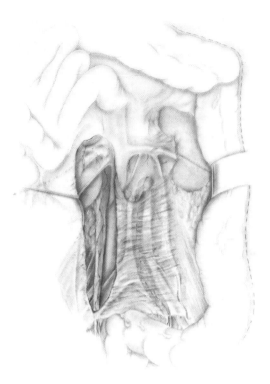

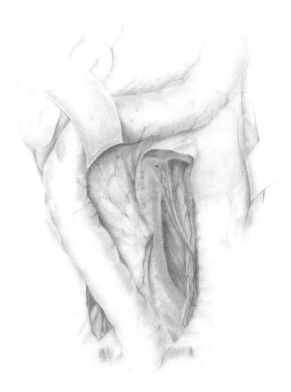

Figure 17.3 The right-sided dissection is finished. The longitudinal ureteral vessels as well as the gonadal vessels (running from left to right, marked with a vessel loop) are saved. The left ureter is dissected with a left paracolic incision.

Figure 17.4 Cranial dissection into the renal hilus avoids recurrence (intrahilary Ormond's disease).

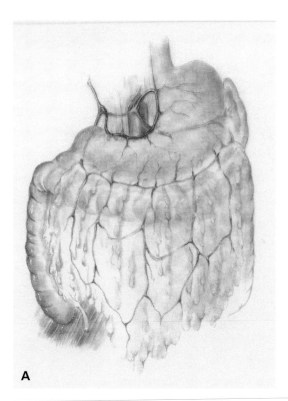

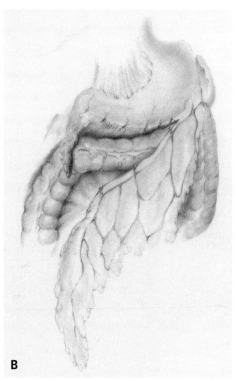

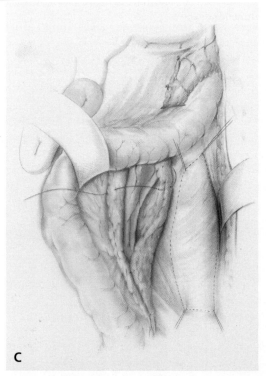

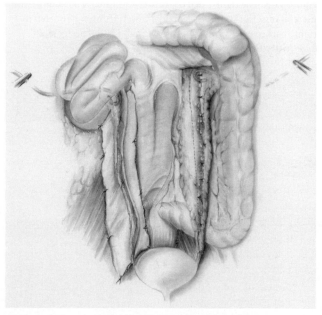

Figure 17.6 The situation after the peritoneal patch is fixed on the right; the left ureter is wrapped by omentum, and the wrapping goes down to the iliac crossing to avoid recurrence.

Figure 17.5 Wrapping the left ureter with omentum is advantageous. (A) Ligate the omentum close to the pylorus and dissect by cutting and ligating the branches of the right gastroepiploic vessels. (B) The omentum receives its blood supply from the left gastroepiploic artery through a pedicle; it is brought retroperitoneally through a mesenteric slit. On the right side, the omentum can be brought down behind the mobilized right colonic flexure. (C) Dissection of a peritoneal patch for wrapping the left ureter.

Chapter 18

Surgical Correction of Ureteral Complications after Kidney Transplantation

A. Pycha, D. Latal, and L. Managadze

Introduction

Necrosis of the ureter with the formation of a urinoma, increasing creatinine as well as urosepsis after kidney transplantation, can be seen in 1–30% of all cases [1–5]. Firstly, the renal hydronephrotic pelvis has to be drained. There are, however, no strict rules for surgical revisions. A presentation of our approach follows.

Indications

- Urinoma at the ureterovesical implantation.
- Complete or partial necrosis of the ureter.
- Stenosis of the ureterovesical junction.
- Prolapse of the transplanted kidney in a scar hernia with subsequent mechanical obstruction.
- Urinoma deriving from an unknown double ureter.

Preoperative management

- Ultrasound examination of the lower abdomen to show the relationship of the surrounding structures.
- Drainage of the hydronephrotic renal pelvis by percutaneous nephrostomy.
- Antegrade pyelography to examine the ureter and demonstrate extravasation.
- Drainage of the urinary bladder: transurethral catheter or suprapubic cystostomy.
- Cystography to give evidence of or exclude extravasation.

Anesthesia

General anesthesia.

Special instruments/suture materials

- Standard instruments for renal surgery, and a ring retractor.
- Suture materials: 2/0, 3/0, and 4/0 Vicryl, and 3/0, 4/0, and 5/0 Monocryl.

Operative technique

- Lithotomy position and cystoscopy, with retrograde examination of both the original ureters, and the introduction of two 5 Fr ureteric stents.
- After identification of the implantation orifice, attempt stenting of the transplant ureter (normally fails).
- Then change to a Lloyd-Davis position.
- The old incision, normally a parainguinal access, is opened. Layer by layer division of the original two-layered, reconstructed, lateral abdominal wall. (Take care when dividing the deeper layer as the transplanted kidney lies below in very close proximity.)
- Expose and ligate the epigastric vessels.
- Identify the ductus deferens and place a loop around it.
- Expose the lower pole of the kidney, from lateral to medial, reflecting the peritoneum in the same direction.
- Inferior to the lower pole of the kidney, the ureter is explored to the bladder—thereby opening the urinoma.
- Stay sutures are placed at the intact distal end of the ureter at 12 o'clock with 4/0 Monocryl. Distal positioning of an Overholt clamp is followed by sectioning of the ureter. The distal ureteric stump is closed with a single 2/0 Vicryl stitch.

Ureterocystoneostomy (psoas hitch)

- Mobilize the bladder until the apex can be brought tension-free to the level of the lower kidney pole.
- Expose the psoas muscle fascia (note that the anastomosis of the renal vessels is in close proximity).
- Make a longitudinal opening of the bladder over a length of 4 cm between two stay sutures of 2/0 Vicryl.
- After identifying the genitofemoral nerve, the apex of the bladder is mobilized superiorly to a point where the new ureteric implantation is feasible. The bladder is fixed with two deep stitches of 2/0 Vicryl to the psoas muscle.
- The bladder is incised at the proposed implantation site.
- Stay sutures with 4/0 Monocryl in the bladder mucosa mark the new ureteric orifice.

- A submucosal tunnel is created by incising a small window in the bladder mucosa and separating it in a longitudinal direction with scissors.
- The ureter is pulled through the submucosal tunnel, shortened, and spatulated.
- Establish the uretral anastomosis to the bladder mucosa using 5/0 Monocryl single sutures.
- Fix the adventitia of the ureter to the bladder muscle with a single 4/0 Vicryl suture.
- Stent the ureter with a 8 Fr ureteric catheter and fix with a 4/0 Vicryl rapid. A separate exit through the bladder wall is made.
- Place a suprapubic cystostomy (12 Fr balloon catheter with a central orifice).
- Close the bladder mucosa with a running 4/0 Monocryl suture.
- Close the detrusor with 2/0 Vicryl single sutures.
- Remove the preoperatively placed nephrostomy.

Pyeloplasty using the transplant ureter

- Pyeloplasty is recommended for delayed upper ureteric obstruction, which is usually caused by scar tissue.
- The pelvis is exposed, adhesions are divided, and the ureter is dissected out in the direction of the bladder.
- The stenosed area is exposed.
- After placement of 4/0 Monocryl stay sutures, the pelvis is opened.
- The stenosed part of the ureter is resected and a segment of ureter is excised to a point where arterial capillary bleeding is evident.
- The distal 2 cm of the ureter is spatulated.
- An anchor 5/0 Monocryl suture is placed at the deepest point of the opened renal pelvis and the spatulated ureter.
- The posterior wall of the renal pelvis and the ureter are anastomosed with interrupted sutures (the knots are outside).
- A 6 Fr ureter splint is placed in the ureter and passed out through the pelvis.
- The anterior wall of the renal pelvis and the ureter are anastomosed with interrupted sutures.
- The nephrostomy remains in place.

Optional

- An incision of 15 cm is made in the peritoneum between two stay sutures.
- A segment of the omentum is pulled through the peritoneal opening.
- The omentum is draped over the anastomosis and secured with interrupted 3/0 Vicryl sutures.

Pyeloplasty with the native ureter

- If the stenotic part of the ureter is too long as a result of ischemic necrosis or after excision of the affected segment, an alternative is a pyeloplasty using the ipsilateral genuine ureter. In the case of an atrophic kidney, nephrectomy could also be performed.

- Expose the stented ureter at the level of crossing the iliac vessels; prepare as proximally as possible.
- A 4/0 Monocryl stay suture is placed at the medial insertion of the ureter.
- Ligate and transect the proximal ureteric stump.
- Resect the transplant ureter with the lateral part of the renal pelvis.
- Change the nephrostomy.
- Spatulate the native ureter distally.
- The posterior wall of the renal pelvis and the ureter is anastomosed with interrupted sutures using 5/0 Monocryl (knots outside the urothelium).
- A 6 Fr ureteric stent is inserted into the ureter and passed out through the renal pelvis.
- The anastomosis on the anterior aspect is completed with 5/0 Monocryl interrupted sutures.
- Open the peritoneum, and pull-through the omentum tip.
- Surround the renal pelvis and the anastomosis with omentum.

Special case: hernia

- In rare cases, a scar hernia might result if a large kidney is transplanted into a small patient. During exploration of the hernial sac particular attention should be paid to the fact that the kidney is situated in the subcuticular area. On the medial side of the kidney, the renal vein is found early in the dissection due to the kinking of the hilus caudally.
- Completely expose the kidney.
- Completely prepare the ureter.
  Two solutions are possible:
- Reposition the kidney and repair the abdominal wall by a Mayo-plasty.
- Transposition of the kidney into the peritoneal space is the method of choice:
  - a 25 cm incision is made in the peritoneum and secured between two stay sutures of 3/0 Monocryl;
  - after opening the peritoneum, the kidney is turned slightly in a medial and cranial direction and submerged intraperitoneally;
  - the mobilized omentum is brought around the lower kidney pole and fixed on the lateral abdominal wall by 3/0 Monocryl interrupted sutures in such a way as to resemble a hammock;
  - the abdominal wall is repaired by herniaplasty.

Postoperative care

- Fluid balance and creatinine controls daily.
- Antibiotic treatment until removal of the stents, followed by long-term prophylaxis.
- Removal of the perirenal drainage between the third and fifth postoperative day.
- *In psoas hitch*: remove the suprapubic cystostomy on the

seventh postoperative day. The indwelling catheter remains in place.
- Remove the ureteral stent on day 9.
- Perform a cystogram on day 10. In the absence of extravasation, remove the indwelling catheter.
- *In pyeloplasty*: remove the ureteral stent on day 9. On the next day perform an antegrade pyelogram via the nephrostomy. In cases of good drainage and in the absence of leakage, the nephrostomy is closed. If this is well tolerated remove the nephrostomy 24 h later.
- Perform ultrasonography of the kidney the next day.

Results

From March 1, 1994 to April 1, 2000, 53 patients were treated in our institution by the above-described techniques. In 19 cases the revision was done for the first time. In 17 cases a previous revision had been performed: in 10 cases twice before, and in seven cases three times before, with an inadequate surgical result. In our cohort of patients the rate of restricture was 5.6% (3/53). In one patient the hydronephrosis did not disappear completely. The Whitaker test showed a result of 17 cm H_2O in the presence of a normal creatinine and it was therefore considered unnecessary to perform a revision. In one patient we performed a pyelocystostomy at the fourth revision. In another patient a transuretropyelostomy was performed because after the third revision the ipsilateral native ureter became necrotic.

References

1 Butterworth PC, Horsburgh T, Veitch PS, Bell PRF, Nicholson ML. Urological complications in renal transplantation: impact of change of technique. Br J Urol 1997;79:499–502.
2 Dreikorn K. Problems of the distal ureter in renal transplantation. Urol Int 1992;49:76–89.
3 Maier U, Madersbacher S, Banyai-Falger S, Susani M, Grünberger T. Late ureteral obstruction after kidney transplantation. Transpl Int 1997;10:65–8.
4 Pycha A, Latal D, Managadze C. Operative Korrektur ureteraler komplikationen nach Nierentransplantation. Akt Urol 2001;32:47–54.
5 Shoskes DA, Hanbury D, Cranston D, Morris PJ. Urological complications in 1000 consecutive renal transplant recipients. J Urol 1995;153:18–21.

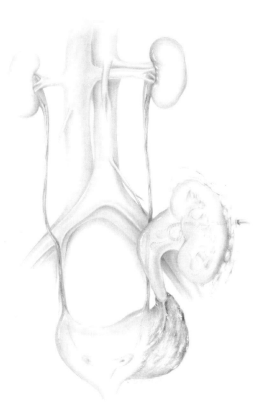

Figure 18.1 Paravesical urinoma after necrosis of the transplant ureter. The hydronephrotic transplant kidney is drained by a percutaneous nephrostomy.

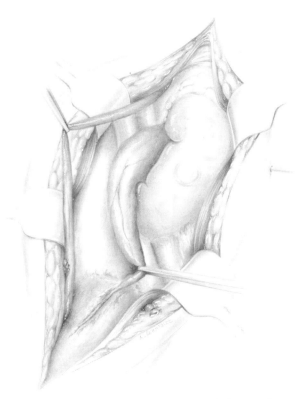

Figure 18.2 After preparation of the ureter, both the transplant ureter and the genuine ureter are wrapped, the epigastric vessels are ligated, and the urinoma is opened.

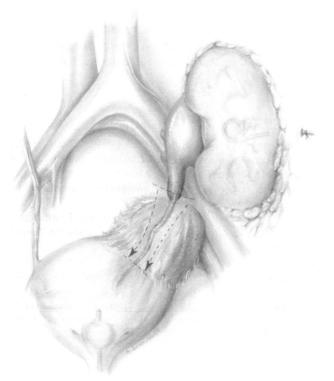

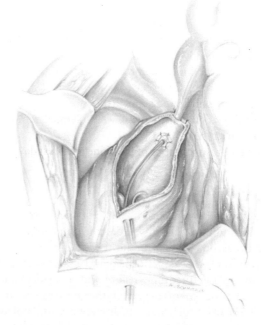

Figure 18.5 After preparation of the submucosal tunnel, the ureter is pulled through and the ureteromucosal anastomosis is performed. A cystostomy is placed and the ureter stent is led out.

Figure 18.3 Dilatation of the ureter up to the obstruction; the dashed lines mark the length of the ureter that has to be resected—a short proximal ureteric segment.

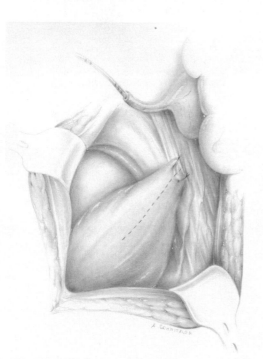

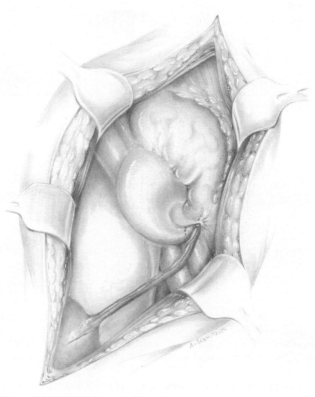

Figure 18.4 The ureter has just been shortened and drained by a ureter stent. After mobilization of the bladder, it is fixed on the psoas muscle fascia.

Figure 18.6 Scar tension on the proximal ureter causing obstruction with marked hydronephrosis.

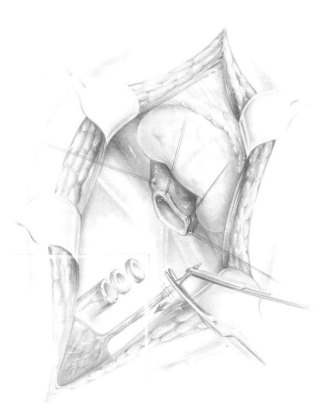

Figure 18.7 Between stay sutures, the renal pelvis is opened. The stenotic ureter segment is resected. The insert shows the ureter being shortened until adequate arterial bleeding is evident.

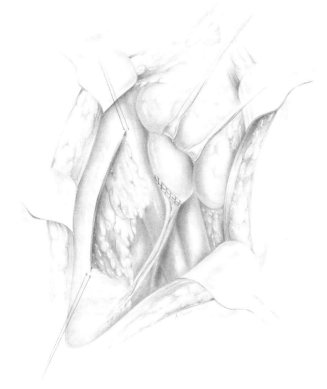

Figure 18.8 The anastomosis between the ureter and renal pelvis is finished, using interrupted sutures of 5/0 Monocryl. The peritoneum is opened between stay sutures and a tip of the omentum is pulled through.

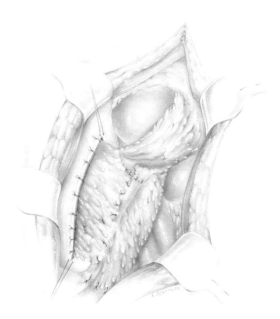

Figure 18.9 The pyeloplasty and ureter are surrounded by omentum. Single 3/0 Vicryl sutures are used for fixation on the peritoneum and the bladder.

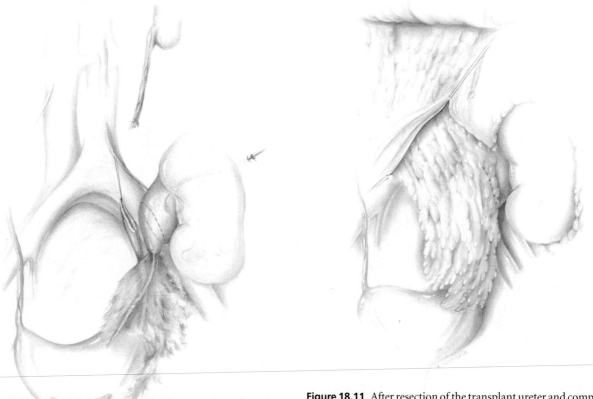

Figure 18.10 Obstructed transplant ureter with hydronephrosis and urinoma. The hydronephrosis is drained by a nephrostomy. The genuine ureter with a stay suture at 9 o'clock is shortened to the right length. In the case of an atrophic kidney, the proximal ureter is only ligated and the kidney left in place.

Figure 18.11 After resection of the transplant ureter and completed pyeloplasty, the peritoneum is opened between two stay sutures, an omentum tip is pulled through, and the pyeloplasty is coated by omentum.

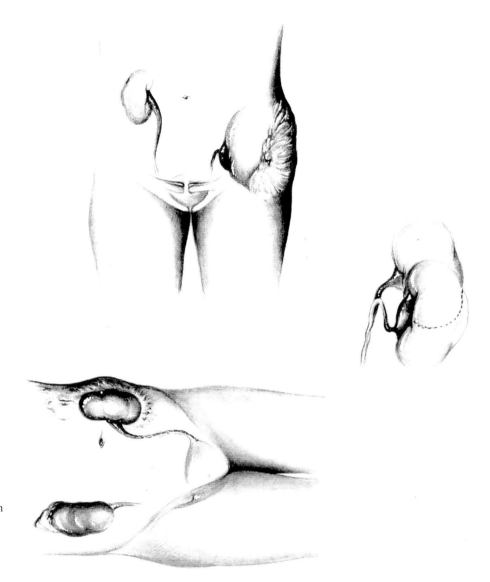

Figure 18.12 The transplant kidney lays in an abdominal wall hernia. Therefore, in the upright position, the kidney tips over the horizontal axis provoking an intermittent obstruction of the ureter. In the lying position, the kidney returns back to its original position and the obstruction is reduced.

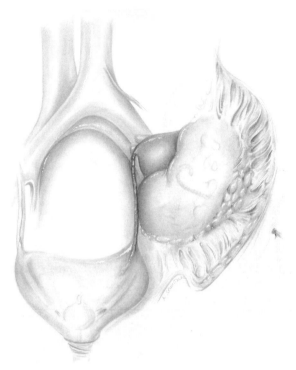

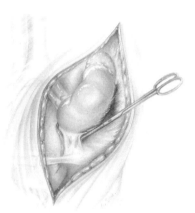

Figure 18.14 Complete exposure and preparation of the kidney. During the preparation of the hernial sac, careful attention should be paid as the abdominal muscles are rarefied and extremely thin. The kidney is situated just below the subcutis. The kidney vein can be found immediately on the medial side due to the caudal kinking of the hilus.

Figure 18.13 A kinked kidney with a sharply bent ureter. The hydronephrosis is drained by nephrostomy.

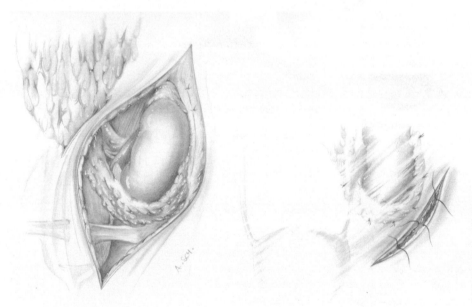

Figure 18.15 After opening the peritoneum and intraperitoneal shifting of the kidney, a hammock is constructed with omentum and fixed at the abdominal wall. This is followed by reduction of the hernia and performing a duplication of the fascia.

Chapter 19
Surgical Treatment for Traumatic Ureteral Injury

N. F. Alsikafi, S. P. Elliott, and J. W. McAninch

Introduction

Ureteral injury caused by external violent trauma is uncommon, accounting for less than 1% of all genitourinary injuries from violent trauma [4]. These injuries are most commonly caused by penetrating trauma, such as gunshot wounds and stab injuries, though blunt injuries to the ureter do occur.

In the acute setting ureteral injuries are difficult to diagnose radiographically, and are diagnosed most often at the time of emergent exploratory laparotomy for associated injuries. Patients with traumatic ureteral injuries are often acutely ill, and have other associated injuries in more than 90% of cases. Concomitant injuries commonly include the small and large bowel, although thoracic and major vascular injuries are common as well [1–8]. While hypotension is common (56% of cases in one study), it is not uniformly present, and is indicative of associated injuries rather than the ureteral injury itself [4].

The surgical treatment for ureteral injuries follows established operative principles, which include resecting devitalized injured ureteral tissue, establishing tensionless mucosal apposition over a stented ureter, isolating the anastomotic repair with omentum or fat, and placing of a drain in close proximity to the repair.

Indications

In a stable patient, any evidence of ureteral extravasation on the CT scan should be investigated with either a retrograde pyelogram with possible stent placement or open exploration depending on the severity and urgency of the associated injuries. In an unstable patient who is in the operating room for the repair of associated injuries, a high level of suspicion is essential to diagnose ureteral injuries.

Contraindications

Life-threatening hemodynamic instability intraoperatively is a contraindication for formal ureteral repair. In those cases when damage control is the overlying objective and time is critical, the proximal end of the injured ureter is clipped or tied with subsequent placement of a percutaneous nephrostomy tube several days postoperatively. Future definitive ureteral repair can then be performed under a more stable situation.

Preoperative management

The patient should be given broad-spectrum antibiotics. In a stable patient who has time to be imaged, a CT scan with intravenous contrast with delayed films should be obtained to assess for significant ureteral injury. In an unstable patient, radiographic studies are often impossible to do preoperatively. In some circumstances imaging may be performed in the operating room, although a single shot 'trauma' intravenous pyelogram unreliably diagnoses ureteral injuries. A retrograde pyelogram of the injured side is the single best test, but is often impractical to do in a polytrauma victim.

Anesthesia

General endotracheal intubation.

Special instruments/suture materials

- Standard laparotomy tray.
- Tinotomy scissors.
- Vascular forceps.
- 5/0 absorbable suture material.
- Double-J stent.
- Guidewire.

Operative technique

The operative technique is dependent upon the location of the ureteral injury.

Short proximal or mid-ureteral injury: uretero-ureterostomy

• With the patient in the supine position, mobilize the large bowel medially to visualize the injured ureter.
• Identify both ends of the ureter and mobilize the surrounding attachments of the proximal and distal ureter sharply (taking care not to injure the ureteral adventia) so that enough laxity will be present in the ureter to allow for a tension-free anastomosis (Fig. 19.1).
• Debride any nonviable tissue with tinotomy scissors and spatulate the proximal and distal ureters on opposite sides (Fig. 19.2).
• Place one stitch of 5/0 absorbable suture between the apex of the spatulation on the proximal ureter to a point exactly across from the spatulation on the distal ureter. Do the same on the opposite side of the ureter (Fig. 19.3).
• Pass one tie beneath the ureter so as to spin the ureter, facilitating exposure of the posterior aspect of the anastomosis.
• Place three equally spaced 5/0 absorbable sutures along the posterior aspect of the ureter.
• Spin the ureter back so that the anterior surface of the anastomosis is easily visualized.
• Place the guidewire into the distal ureter so as to curl it into the bladder. Pass a double-J stent over the wire into the distal ureter and bladder. Remove the wire from the stent and pass the wire into the proximal ureter so as to curl it in the renal pelvis. Pass the wire into the proximal tip of the stent, having the end of the wire exit the stent from one of its side holes along the stent shaft. Pass the proximal stent into the renal pelvis and remove the wire.
• Place three equally placed 5/0 absorbable sutures along the anterior aspect of the ureter, so as to complete the anastomosis (Fig. 19.4).
• Isolate the repair with perirenal fat or a small piece of omentum.
• Place a drain close to, but not on top of, the repair.

Long mid-ureteral injury or short mid-ureteral injury with large pelvic hematoma: transuretero-ureterostomy

• With the patient in the supine position, the large bowel is mobilized medially to visualize the ureter.
• Identify the proximal end of the ureter and debride any nonviable tissue with tinotomy scissors. Tie the distal ureter if easily accessible (Fig. 19.5).
• Mobilize the proximal ureter enough so that it can reach the contralateral ureter without tension.
• Dissect and mobilize the contralateral ureter as little as possible in the area of the anastomosis.
• Pass a long clamp from the contralateral ureter to the ipsilateral ureter under the small bowel mesentery posterior to the inferior mesenteric artery and anterior to the aorta and spine.

Pull the ipsilateral ureter to the side of the contralateral ureter (Fig. 19.6).
• Spatulate the ipsilateral ureter and make a ureterotomy on the medial aspect of the contralateral ureter.
• Place a 5/0 absorbable suture from the apex of the spatulation to the apex of the ureterotomy. Place a second 5/0 absorbable suture on the opposite side of the ureter to the opposite apex of the ureterotomy (Fig. 19.7).
• Suture the posterior aspect of the uretero-ureterostomy with equally spaced 5/0 absorbable sutures. Then tie the sutures on the outside of the ureter.
• Place a stent in the ipsilateral ureter as previously described.
• Suture the anterior aspect of the ureter with equally spaced 5/0 absorbable sutures (Fig. 19.8).
• Isolate the ureteral anastomosis with adjacent fat or omentum.
• Place a drain.

Distal ureteral injuries: ureteroneocystostomy with psoas hitch or Boari flap
Psoas hitch

• The patient is supine with a low midline incision.
• Mobilize the proximal ureter ipsilateral to the side at the level of the iliac vessels.
• Debride any devitalized tissue if present.
• Ligate the distal ureter at the level of the ureterovesical junction if it is easily found.
• Open the bladder with a curvilinear incision along the anterior, superior border of the bladder (Fig. 19.9).
• Place an index and middle finger within the bladder and stretch the bladder to the level of the psoas muscle tendon. If mobilization is restricted, ligate the contralateral bladder pedicles one by one to create enough laxity (Fig. 19.10).
• With the surgeon's fingers still within the bladder, place three 2/0 nonabsorbable sutures from the outer bladder muscle (with care taken not to enter the mucosa) and into the psoas tendon. Tie the sutures. Care is taken not to entrap the genitofemoral nerve (Fig. 19.11).
• Make a small incision in the bladder mucosa in the area of the planned ureteroneocystostomy.
• Tunnel a small clamp under the bladder mucosa and push through the bladder muscle.
• Pull the ureter through the bladder muscle and into the bladder (Fig. 19.12).
• Place six equally spaced 5/0 absorbable sutures from the ureteral mucosa to the bladder mucosa (intravesical reimplant).
• Place a single 5/0 suture extravesically from the ureteral wall to the detrusor to take any tension off the intravesical suture line.
• Place a stent by passing a guidewire up the ureter and gingerly passing the stent over the wire (Fig. 19.13).
• Close the anterior wall of the bladder in two layers using 3/0 absorbable suture (Fig. 19.14).
• Place a drain.

Boari flap

- The patient is supine with a low midline incision.
- Mobilize the proximal ureter at the level of the iliac vessels.
- Debride any devitalized tissue if present.
- Ligate the distal ureter at the level of the ureterovesical junction if it is easily found.
- Incise the anterior and superior aspects of the bladder to create a U-shaped bladder flap. Care should be taken to make the base of the bladder flap wide so as to ensure viability (Fig. 19.15).
- Make a small incision in the bladder mucosa in the area of the planned ureteroneocystostomy.
- Tunnel a small clamp under the bladder mucosa.
- Pull the ureter through the tunnel and into the bladder.
- Place six equally spaced 5/0 absorbable sutures from the ureteral mucosa to the bladder mucosa (intravesical reimplant) (Fig. 19.16),
- Place a single 5/0 suture extravesically from the ureteral wall to the detrusor to take any tension off the intravesical suture line.
- Place a stent by passing a guidewire up the ureter and gingerly passing the stent over the wire.
- Pull the edges of the bladder flap together and suture the edges together (Fig. 19.17).
- Close the anterior wall of the bladder in two layers using 3/0 absorbable sutures (Fig. 19.18).
- Place a drain.

Tips

- Debride the ends of the injured ureter until the edges bleed. This will ensure viability of the ureter.
- In a transuretero-ureterostomy care should be taken when tunneling the injured proximal ureter between the inferior mesenteric artery (IMA) and aorta. If the ureter is situated close to the junction of the IMA and aorta, a nutcracker phenomenon may result, producing obstruction of the ipsilateral kidney. This can be avoided by allowing a spacious tunnel and by placing the ureter inferior to the take off of the IMA.
- Small closed suction drains (e.g. the Jackson–Pratt drain) can perpetuate urine fistulas if placed directly onto the ureteral anastomosis. In all patients the anastomotic repair is isolated by fat or omentum to prevent the drain from lying on the anastomosis and hence to reduce urinary fistula formation. Alternatively a nonsuction drain (e.g. the penrose drain) may be used. The rate of ureteral fistula formation is presumed to be less because of the absence of suction.

Postoperative care

A plain abdominal X-ray is taken in the recovery room to assess for proper stent position. The catheter is removed on day 5–7, and the drain is removed between 24 and 72 h after the procedure.

Complications

Our sources of complications from the uretero-ureterostomy (Table 19.1) include: (i) one patient with a concomitant ureteral and pancreatic injury who developed a periureteral abscess (the abscess was drained percutaneously); (ii) one patient who developed a bilateral urinoma after bilateral ureteropelvic junction avulsions, which were initially treated with stents but ultimately were treated definitively with open repair; (iii) one patient who had a urinoma form after a stent was pulled too early for unknown reasons (the urinoma resolved after re-stenting); (iv) one patient who developed a leak from the anastomosis after the Jackson–Pratt drain was placed over it (the uretero-ureterostomy healed after the drain was taken off suction); (v) and one patient who did not return to us until 3 years after his injury and presented with a completely encrusted stent necessitating open removal. The single complication associated with the ureteral reimplant was a pulmonary embolus postoperatively.

Table 19.1 The results of 38 ureteral injuries at the San Francisco General Hospital.

Type of repair	Number of cases	Complications
Uretero-ureterostomy	16	6
Reimplant	5	1
Primary closure	12	0
Stenting only	2	0
Boari	1	0
Transuretero-ureterostomy	1	0
Nephrectomy	1	0
Other	0	0
Observation	0	0
Total cases	38	7 (18%)

Troubleshooting

If the output from the drain is high postoperatively, a fluid creatinine level can be sent to determine the presence of urine.

Results

The results from a 25-year experience at the San Francisco General Hospital reveals that out of 38 patients with traumatic ureteral injury, all were repaired successfully, though there was an 18% complication rate (listed in Table 19.1), attesting to the critical nature of injuries associated with ureteral trauma.

References

1 Azimuddin K, Milanesa D, Ivatury R *et al.* Penetrating ureteric injuries. Injury 1998;29:364–7.
2 Carlton CE, Scott R, Guthrie AG. The initial management of ureteral injuries: a report of 78 cases. J Urol 1971;105:335–40.
3 Eikenberg H, Amin M. Gunshot wounds to the ureter. J Trauma 1976;16:562–5.
4 Elliott SP, McAninch, JW. Ureteral injuries from external violence: the 25-year experience at San Francisco General Hospital. J Urol 2003;170:1213–16.
5 Liroff SA, Pontes JES, Pierce JM. Gunshot wounds of the ureter: 5 years of experience. J Urol 1977;118:551–3.
6 Peterson NE, Pitts JC. Penetrating injuries of the ureter. J Urol 1981;126:587–90.
7 Steers WD, Corriere JN, Benson GS *et al.* The use of indwelling ureteral stents in managing ureteral injuries due to external violence. J Trauma 1985;25:1001–3.
8 Velmahos GC, Degiannis E, Wells M *et al.* Penetrating ureteral injuries: the impact of associated injuries on management. Am Surg 1996;62:461–8.

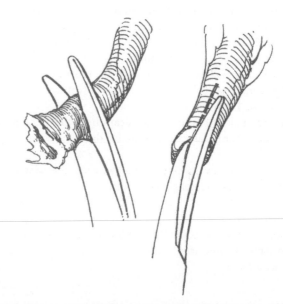

Figure 19.2 Any nonviable tissue is debrided with tinotomy scissors and the proximal and distal ureters are spatulated on opposite sides. (Reproduced with permission from Presti JC Jr, Carroll PR. Intraoperative management of the injured ureter. In: Perspectives in Colon and Rectal Surgery (Schrock TR, ed.). Quality Medical, St Louis, 1988:98–106.)

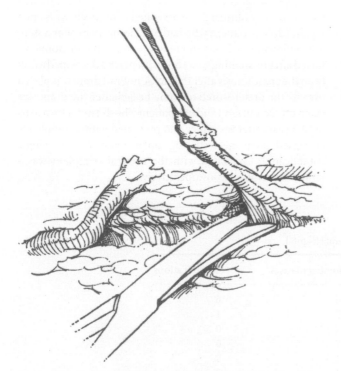

Figure 19.1 Both ends of the ureter are identified. The surrounding attachments of the proximal and distal ureter are mobilized sharply. (Reproduced with permission from Presti JC Jr, Carroll PR. Intraoperative management of the injured ureter. In: Perspectives in Colon and Rectal Surgery (Schrock TR, ed.). Quality Medical, St Louis, 1988:98–106.)

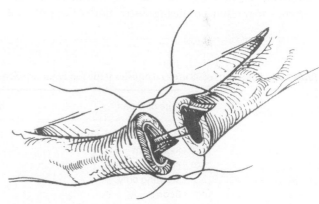

Figure 19.3 A 5/0 absorbable suture is placed between the apex of the spatulation on the proximal ureter to a point exactly across from the spatulation on the distal ureter. The same is done on the opposite side of the ureter. (From Guerriero WG. Urologic Injuries. Appleton-Century Crofts, Norwalk, CT, 1984.)

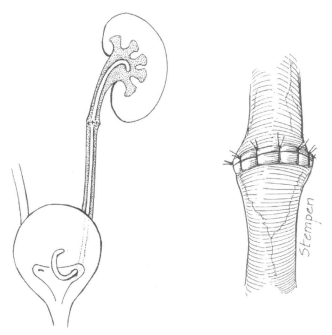

Figure 19.4 Three equally placed 5/0 absorbable sutures are placed along the anterior aspect of the ureter, so as to complete the anastomosis. (Reproduced with permission from Presti JC Jr, Carroll PR. Intraoperative management of the injured ureter. In: Perspectives in Colon and Rectal Surgery (Schrock TR, ed.). Quality Medical, St Louis, 1988:98–106.)

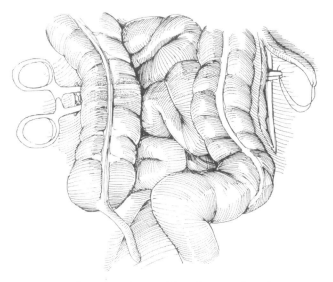

Figure 19.6 A long clamp is passed from the contralateral ureter to the ipsilateral ureter under the small bowel mesentery posterior to the inferior mesenteric artery and anterior to the aorta and spine. The ipsilateral ureter is pulled to the side of the contralateral ureter. (Reprinted from Hinman F Jr. Ureteroureterostomy. In: Atlas of Urologic Surgery, Vol. I, 1989:681, with permission from Elsevier.)

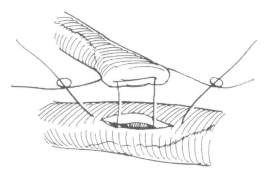

Figure 19.7 A 5/0 absorbable suture is placed from the apex of the spatulation to the apex of the ureterotomy. A second 5/0 absorbable suture is placed on the opposite side of the ureter to the opposite apex of the ureterotomy. (Reprinted from Hinman F Jr. Ureteroureterostomy. In: Atlas of Urologic Surgery, Vol. I, 1989:681, with permission from Elsevier.)

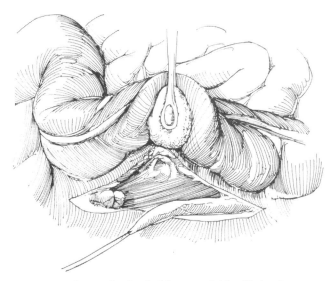

Figure 19.5 The proximal end of the ureter is identified and any nonviable tissue is debrided with tinotomy scissors. The distal ureter is tied if easily accessible. (Reprinted from Hinman F Jr. Ureteroureterostomy. In: Atlas of Urologic Surgery, Vol. I, 1989:681, with permission from Elsevier.)

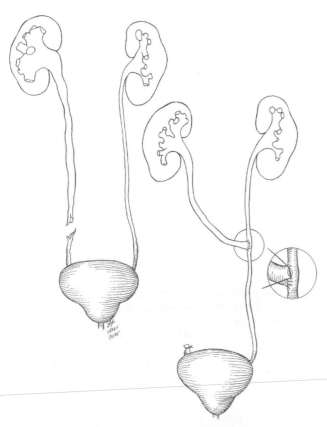

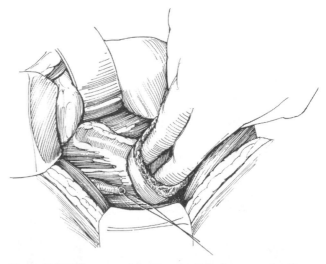

Figure 19.10 The surgeon's index and middle finger are placed within the bladder and the bladder is stretched to the level of the psoas muscle tendon. (Reprinted from Hinman F Jr. Psoas hitch procedure. In: Atlas of Urologic Surgery, Vol. I: 1989:666, with permission from Elsevier.)

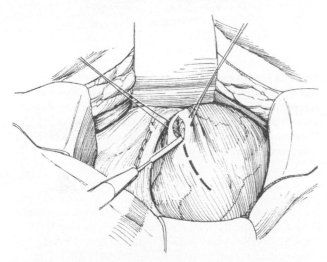

Figure 19.8 The anterior aspect of the ureter is sutured with equally spaced 5/0 absorbable sutures. (Reprinted from McAninch JW. Traumatic and Reconstructive Urology, Vol. I, 1996, fig. 13.6, with permission from Elsevier.)

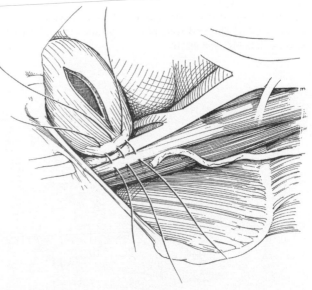

Figure 19.11 Three 2/0 nonabsorbable sutures are placed, with the surgeon's fingers still within the bladder, into the bladder muscle (with care taken not to enter the mucosa) and psoas tendon. The sutures are tied. (Reproduced with permission from Presti JC Jr, Carroll PR. Intraoperative management of the injured ureter. In: Perspectives in Colon and Rectal Surgery (Schrock TR, ed.). Quality Medical, St Louis, 1988:98–106.)

Figure 19.9 The bladder is opened with a curvilinear incision along the anterior–superior border of the bladder. (Reprinted from Hinman F Jr. Psoas hitch procedure. In: Atlas of Urologic Surgery, Vol. I: 1989:666, with permission from Elsevier.)

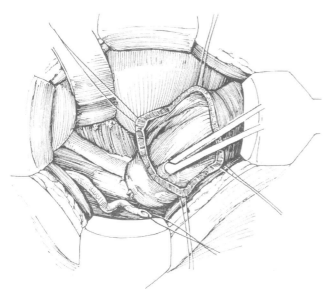

Figure 19.12 The ureter is pulled through the bladder muscle and into the bladder. (Reprinted from Hinman F Jr. Psoas hitch procedure. In: Atlas of Urologic Surgery, Vol. I: 1989:666, with permission from Elsevier.)

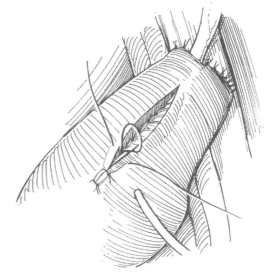

Figure 19.14 The anterior wall of the bladder is closed in two layers using 3/0 absorbable sutures. (Reproduced with permission from Presti JC Jr, Carroll PR. Intraoperative management of the injured ureter. In: Perspectives in Colon and Rectal Surgery (Schrock TR, ed.). Quality Medical, St Louis, 1988:98–106.)

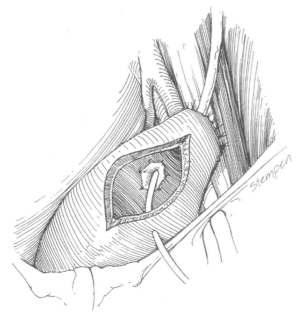

Figure 19.13 A stent is placed by passing a guidewire up the ureter and carefully passing the stent over the wire. (Reproduced with permission from Presti JC Jr, Carroll PR. Intraoperative management of the injured ureter. In: Perspectives in Colon and Rectal Surgery (Schrock TR, ed.). Quality Medical, St Louis, 1988:98–106.)

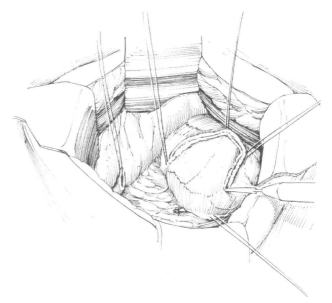

Figure 19.15 The anterior and superior aspects of the bladder are incised to create a bladder flap. Care should be taken to make the base of the bladder flap wide so as to ensure viability. (Reprinted from Hinman F Jr. Psoas hitch procedure. In: Atlas of Urologic Surgery, Vol. I: 1989:670, with permission from Elsevier.)

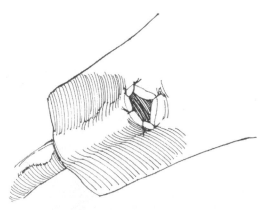

Figure 19.16 Six equally spaced 5/0 absorbable sutures are placed from the ureteral mucosa to the bladder mucosa (intravesical reimplant). (Reprinted from Hinman F Jr. Psoas hitch procedure. In: Atlas of Urologic Surgery, Vol. I: 1989:671, with permission from Elsevier.)

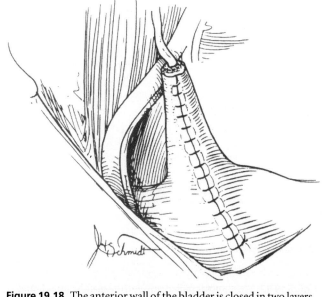

Figure 19.18 The anterior wall of the bladder is closed in two layers using 3/0 absorbable suture. (From Guerriero WG. Urologic Injuries. Appleton-Century Crofts, Norwalk, CT, 1984.)

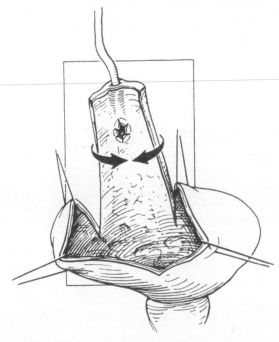

Figure 19.17 The edges of the bladder flap are pulled together and the edges are sutured together. (From Guerriero WG. Urologic Injuries. Appleton-Century Crofts, Norwalk, CT, 1984.)

Chapter 20
Surgical Repair of Ureteral Hernia

R. Homberg and A. Kollias

Introduction

Ureteral hernias are very rare. Most common are the cases of inguinal, scrotal, femoral, and obturatorial herniations. In these areas there are two anatomical types. Most of them are acquired and paraperitoneal, that is, a loop of herniated ureter extends alongside, always medial, to the peritoneal hernia sac. Only a minority are extraperitoneal and congenital, without a peritoneal sac. Internal hernias of the ureter are even more exceptional. They could be both acquired or congenital. Reports have been published of sciatic hernia (suprapiriformis, infrapiriformis) into the sciatic foramen and of herniation between the psoas muscle and the iliac vessels. In general, ureteral hernias can mimic colic, diverticulosis, or irritable bowel syndrome, or they may be asymptomatic. In cases of sciatic herniation, back pain or neurologic deficiency is possible.

The surgical method has to be chosen depending on the location of the hernia. If the ureter shows sign of inflammation or trophic disturbances, then ureterolysis, probably partial cut, reimplantation, and hernioplasty should be carried out. Furthermore, laparoscopic methods are established.

Indications

Absolute indication in cases of hydronephrosis, incarceration, or neurologic deficiency. Otherwise, necessity of surgical intervention depends on the severity of the symptoms.

Limitations and risks

Age; there are also risks with obesity and after irradiation.

Contraindications

Small bladder capacity is a relative contraindication.

Preoperative management

Regular ultrasonography of the upper urinary tract. Retrograde cystography is necessary to estimate bladder volume for the ureterocystoneostomy procedure. Intravenous and retrograde ureterography show the course of the ureter and are able to prove, for example, a kinking. CT and MRT may be helpful in diagnosis but are not obligatory. Give one bottle of x-prep the day before the procedure. Provide antibiotic coverage and preoperative ureter stenting.

Anesthesia

General and peridural anesthesia.

Special instruments/suture material

- Bipolar coagulation.
- Powerstar scissors.
- 7 Fr Mono-J and 12 Fr suprapubic catheter.
- 5/0 Vicryl (ureter implantation), 4/0 Monocryl (mucosa running suture), 3/0 Vicryl (detrusor muscle), 3/0 PDS (traction suture at the psoas muscle).
- For hernia repair: Prolene mesh (e.g. VIPRO II).

Operative technique

- Make a suprainguinal incision with extraperitoneal access to the ureter.
- After double ligature and cut of the inferior epigastric vessels, the chorda umbilicalis has to be cut to find the ureter below.
- In women, ligature and cut of the rotundum ligament is necessary.
- Follow the ureter, often imbedded in scar tissue, by blunt and sharp dissection as far as possible.
- In the hernia, complete ureterolysis is necessary before resecting the elongated ureter.
- Resection should be carried out until capillary bleeding

from the proximal ureter stump and spontaneous peristaltic and urine ejaculation can be demonstrated.

• Estimate the distance between the ureter stump and the bladder to be fixed at the psoas muscle.

• A standard psoas hitch procedure is then performed (see Chapter 13).

• If required, the ureter undergoes partial tailoring or tapering.

• In cases of inguinal, scrotal, femoral, or obturatorial hernia, a general surgical technique with complete removal of the hernia sac and preperitoneal interposition of a Prolene mesh is suggested.

Postoperative care

Remove the urethral catheter on day 5–7, and the Mono-J on day 8–10. After inconspicuous intravenous urography, allow urination. Remove the suprapubic catheter when bladder voiding is satisfactory. Perform regular ultrasonography of the upper urinary tract.

Complications

• Postoperative urinary leakage or obstruction after ureterocystoneostomy with or without urinary infection.

• Late ureter stenosis due to scars.

• Unnoticed destruction of the ureter during hernioplasty.

• Urinary infection may occur after removal of the Mono-J: give antibiotics. If it is prolonged, coinciding with hydronephrosis, combine the antibiotics with percutaneous nephrostomy and antegrade ureteral stenting to bypass the obstruction.

• In cases of urinary leakage, leave the suprapubic catheter until it stops.

Results

One 61-year-old woman was suffering from back pain and weakness of the right leg due to ureterosciatic hernia with compression of the sciatic nerve. At the time of discharge there was full recovery.

To do

See Chapter 13.

Not to do

• 'Stripping' of the vessels belonging to the ureter.

• Exaggerated hook pressure on the psoas muscle, for example because of little skin incision, with indirect irritation of the femoral nerve.

• Avoid fixation of the mesh by suture otherwise the risk of injury increases due to the stitches.

References

1 Colville JAC, Power RE, Hickey DP, Lane BE, O'Malley KJ. Intermittent anuria secondary to a stone in an ureterofemoral hernia. J Urol 2000;164(2):440–1.

2 Gee J, Munson JL, Smith JJ. Laparoscopic repair of ureterosciatic hernia. Urology 1999;54(4):730–3.

3 Giuly J, Francois GF, Giuly D, Leroux C, Nguyen-Cat RR. Intrascrotal hernia of the ureter and fatty hernia. Hernia 2003;7(1): 47–9.

4 Luke P, Singal RK, Morton T, Sales JL. Presentation of ureteral colic in a patient with an ureteroinguinal hernia. Can J Urol 1997;4(3): 429–30.

5 Noller MW, Noller DW. Ureteral sciatic hernia demonstrated on retrograde urography and surgically repaired with boari flap technique. J Urol 2000;164(3):776–7.

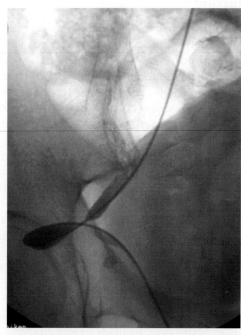

Figure 20.1 Fixed kinking of the ureter with a guidewire in retrograde ureterography.

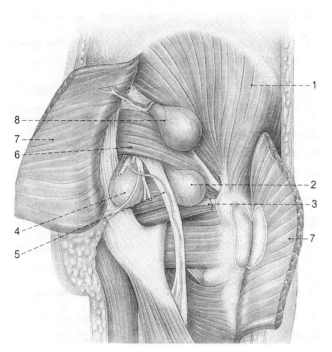

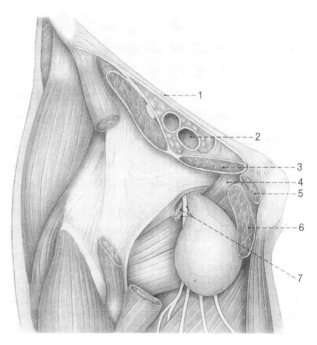

Figure 20.2 Hernia ischiadica: topography. 1, M. gluteus medius; 2, hernia infrapiriformis; 3, M. obturator internus, Mm. gemelli; 4, hernia spinotuberosa; 5, N. ischiadicus; 6, M. piriformis; 7, M. gluteus maximus; 8, hernia suprapiriformis. (Reprinted from Kremer K. et al. (eds) Chirurgische Operationslehre, Vol. 7. Thieme, Stuttgart, 1994:134–6.)

Figure 20.3 Hernia obturatoria: topography. 1, Lig. inguinale; 2, V. femoralis; 3, M. pectineus; 4, M. obturator externus; 5, M. adductor longus; 6, M. adductor brevis; 7, N. obturatorius, A., V. obturatoria. (Reprinted from Kremer K. et al. (eds) Chirurgische Operationslehre, Vol. 7. Thieme, Stuttgart, 1994:134–6.)

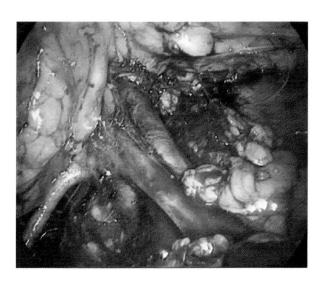

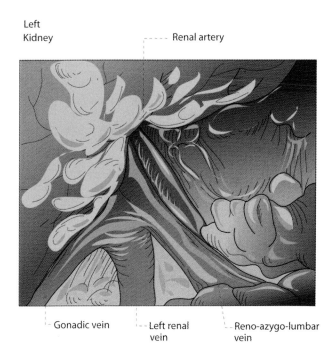

Left
Kidney ----- Renal artery

---- Gonadic vein ---- Left renal
vein ---- Reno-azygo-lumbar
vein

Plate 7.3 View of the left renal pedicle.

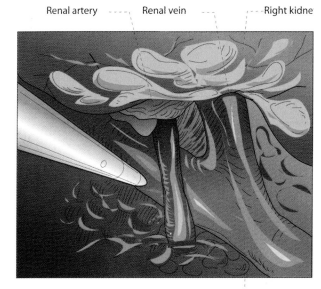

Renal artery ----- Renal vein ----- ----Right kidney

Inferior vena cava ----

Plate 7.4 View of the right renal pedicle.

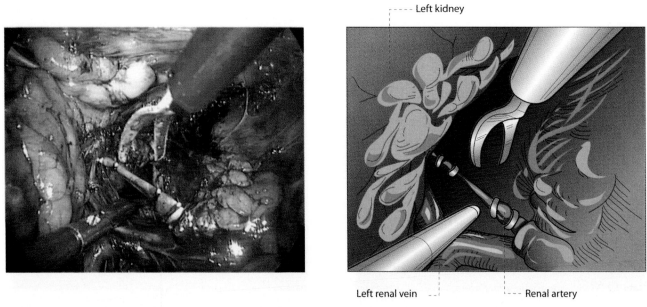

Plate 7.5 Clipping (9 mm metallic clips, three clips proximally and two clips distally) and sectioning of the renal artery.

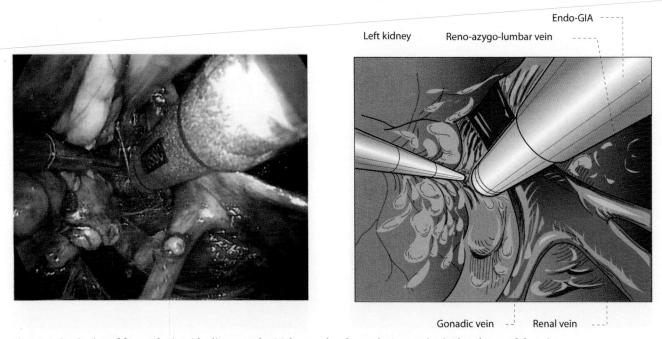

Plate 7.6 Sectioning of the renal vein with a linear stapler. Make sure that the stapler is completely closed around the vein.

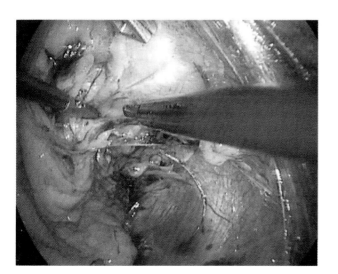
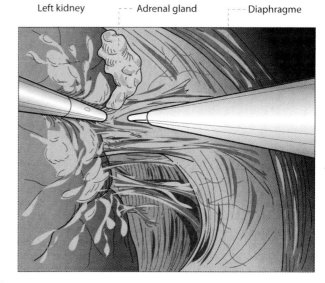

Left kidney --- Adrenal gland --- Diaphragme

Plate 7.7 Mobilization of the kidney from the posterior to the cephalad direction.

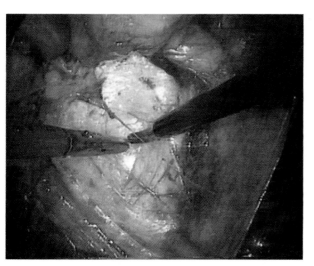
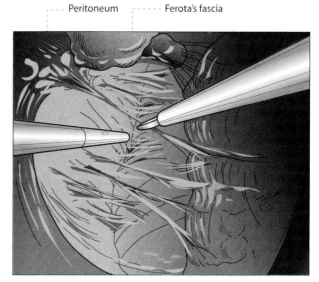

Peritoneum --- Ferota's fascia

Plate 7.8 Mobilization of the kidney is continued anteriorly between the peritoneum and Gerota's fascia.

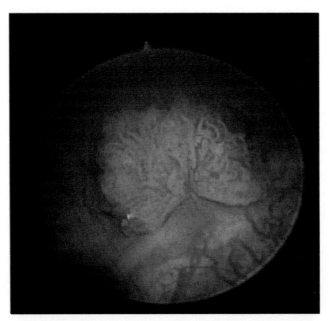

Plate 21.1 Papillary tumor on the left bladder wall.

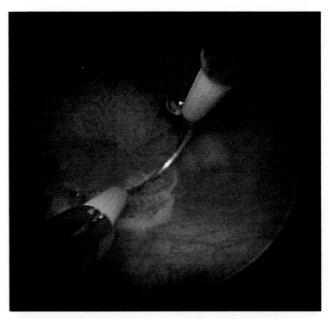

Plate 21.3 Starting with the flat loop to cut the mucosa and penetrate into the detrusor.

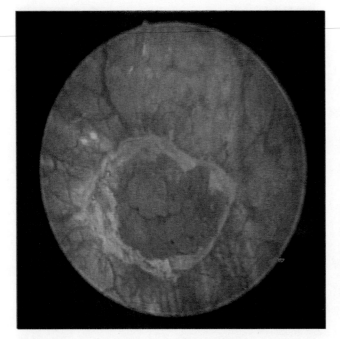

Plate 21.2 Circular coagulation mark around the tumor.

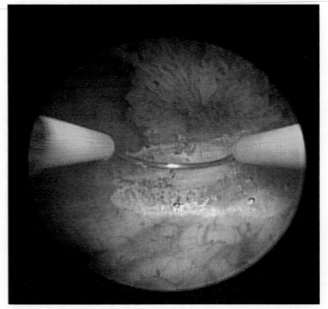

Plate 21.4 Deep resection in the horizontal plane in the muscle layer.

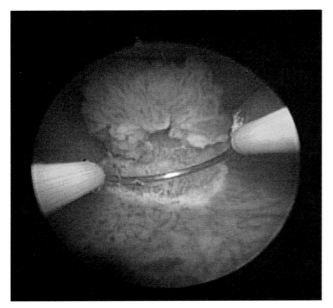

Plate 21.5 Resection enlarged and nearly completed.

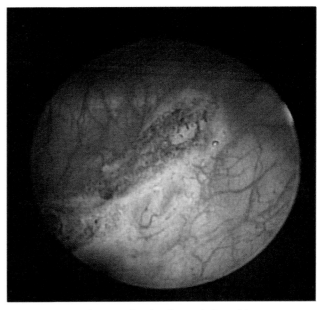

Plate 21.7 Resection completed and coagulation of the tumor ground.

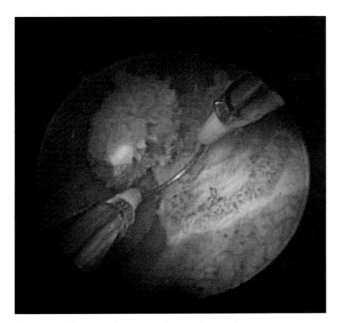

Plate 21.6 The posterior mucosal layer about to be cut.

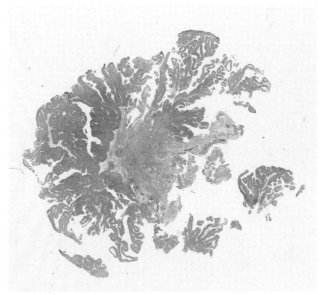

Plate 21.8 Histological section of a resected specimen of transitional cell carcinoma, stage pTa, grade 2.

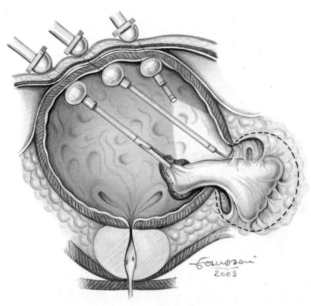

Plate 22.4 Three Entec trocars inserted in the bladder in order to perform the diverticulectomy.

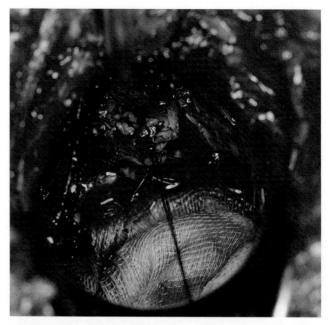

Plate 28.2 The resected left neurovascular bundle.

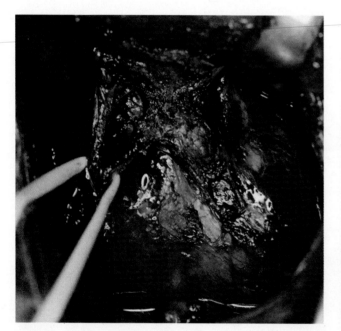

Plate 28.1 A deep blue stained right neurovascular bundle armed by a vessel loop.

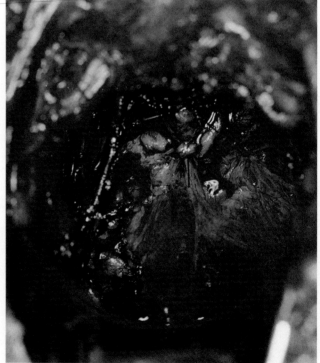

Plate 28.3 The final situation.

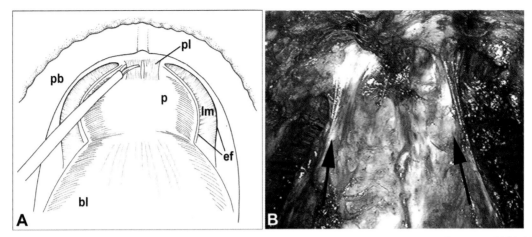

Plate 29.6 Exposure of the bladder neck, incision of the endopelvic fascia, and dissection of the puboprostatic ligaments. bl, bladder; ef, endopelvic fascia (dissected); lm, levator ani muscle; p, prostate; pb, pubic bone; pl, puboprostatic ligaments (arrows).

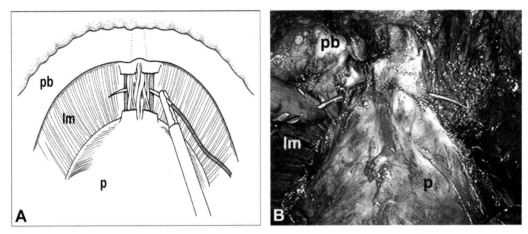

Plate 29.7 Ligation of the Santorini plexus (0/0 Vicryl, MH+ needle). Alternatively, the dorsal vein complex can be dissected with Ultracision® or the SonoSurg ultrasound device without prior ligation during the apical dissection. For abbreviations, see Plate 29.6.

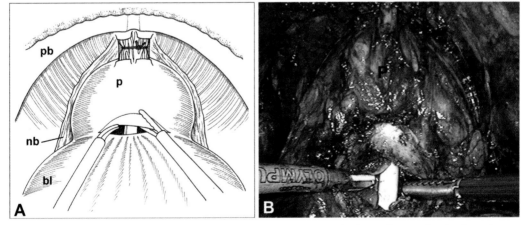

Plate 29.8 Anterior bladder neck dissection. The bladder neck overlaps the prostate in the shape of a triangle. The dissection starts at a 12 o'clock position at the tip of this triangle. For abbreviations, see Plate 29.6; nb, neurovascular bundles.

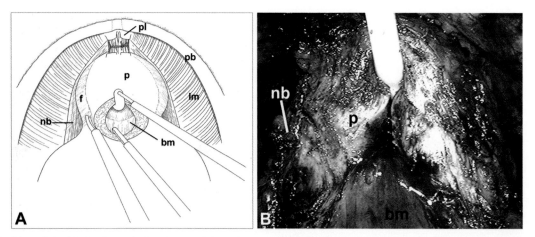

Plate 29.9 Incision of the thin fascia overlaying the anteriolateral aspect of the prostate to mobilize the neurovascular bundles before sectioning of the dorsal bladder neck. bm, bladder mucosa; f, fascia; lm, levator ani muscle; nb, neurovascular bundles; p, prostate; pb, pubic bone; pl, puboprostatic ligaments (dissected).

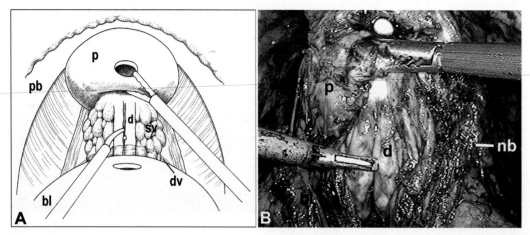

Plate 29.10 Sectioning of the ampullary portions of the vasa deferentia. The prostate is elevated anteriorly in the direction of the symphysis by the assistant. bl, bladder; d, ampulla of vas deferens; dv, anterior Denonvilliers' fascia (dissected); nb, neurovascular bundles; p, prostate; pb, pubic bone; sv, seminal vesicle.

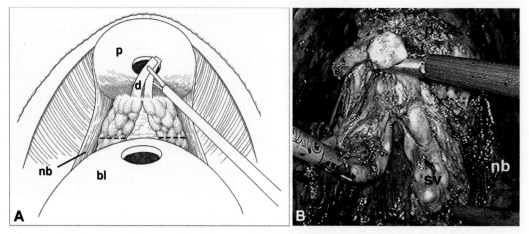

Plate 29.11 Dissection of the seminal vesicles. Traction on the vasa deferentia (by the assistant) is helpful to identify the seminal vesicles in a slightly lateral and caudal direction. The seminal vesicle are completely dissected or cut along the interrupted line to preserve the bundles lying very close to the tip of the seminal vesicles. For abbreviations, see Plate 29.10.

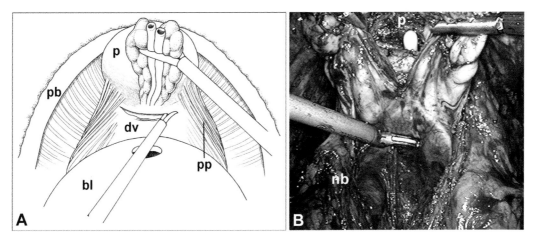

Plate 29.12 Incision of the posterior Denonvilliers' fascia. For abbreviations, see Plate 29.10; dv, posterior Denonvilliers' fascia; pp, prostate pedicle.

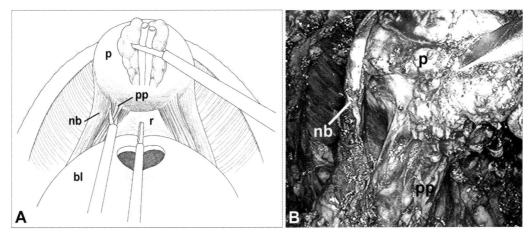

Plate 29.13 Dissection of the cranial prostatic pedicles with preservation of the neurovascular bundles. During preparation of the left side the assistant retracts the prostate to the right side; during preparation and dissection on the right side the surgeon retracts the prostate to the left. For abbreviations, see Plate 29.10; pp, prostate pedicle; r, rectum (prerectal fatty tissue).

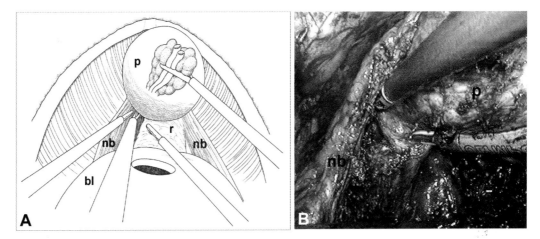

Plate 29.14 Dissection of the caudal prostatic pedicles and separation of the neurovascular bundles on the left side. For abbreviations, see Plate 29.10; r, rectum (prerectal fatty tissue).

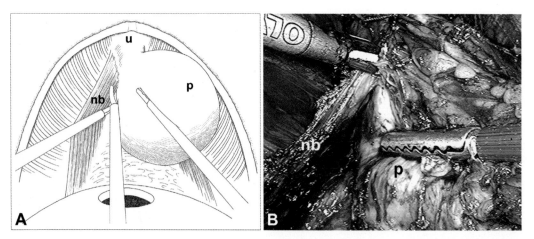

Plate 29.15 Preparation of the neurovascular bundles close to the apex of the prostate and the urethra is done anterolaterally, in contrast to the dorsal preparation at the base of the prostate. The assistant pulls the prostate to the right side for preparation of the left neurovascular bundle and vice versa. nb, neurovascular bundles; p, prostate; u, urethra.

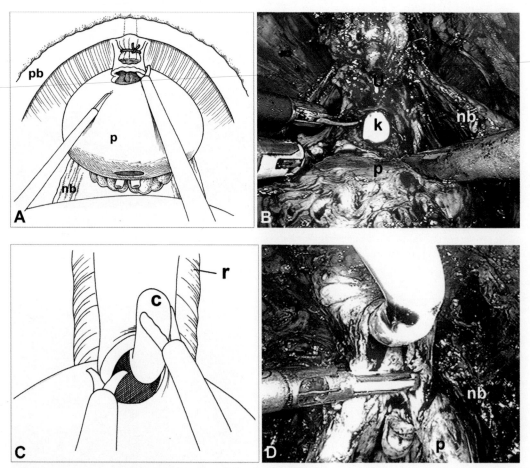

Plate 29.16 Apical dissection: sectioning the Santorini plexus, the external sphincter, and the urethra ventrally (A and B) and dorsally (C and D). c, catheter; nb, neurovascular bundles; p, prostate; pb, pubic bone; r, rectum.

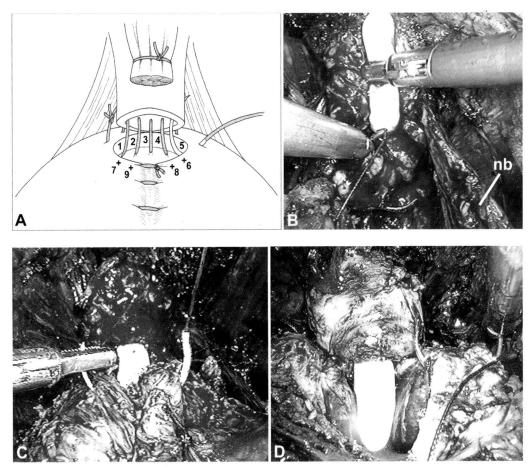

Plate 29.17 Urethrovesical anastomosis (interrupted sutures, 2/0 Vicryl, UR-6 needle). (A) The stitches are always performed 'outside–in' at the bladder neck and 'inside–out' at the urethra, and always tied extraluminally in the given order (1–9). (B) Technique of the dorsal anastomosis. (C) In the case of a nonbladder-neck-preserving procedure, the bladder neck is reconstructed at a 12 o'clock position. (D) Anterolateral and ventral anastomosis is performed with an inserted catheter. nb, neurovascular bundles.

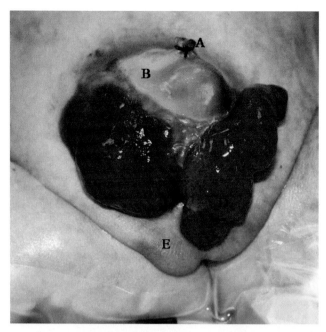

Plate 69.1 Preoperative appearance of a newborn male with cloacal exstrophy.

Key for Plates 69.1–69.12 A, umbilical cord; B, omphalocele; C, bladder plate; D, intussuscepted terminal ileum; E, scrotum; F, penis (right and left); G, urethral plate; H, glans penis; I, appendix (right and left); J, small bowel; K, hindgut; L, ileocecal valve; M, colostomy; N, ureteral orifices; O, corpus cavernosum (right and left); P, ureteral stent; Q, penile skin (internal aspect); R, sutures through the urethral plate and corpus spongiosum; S, deep paravesical dissection (right and left); T, reapproximation of the dorsal urethra and corpus spongiosum; U, suprapubic catheter.

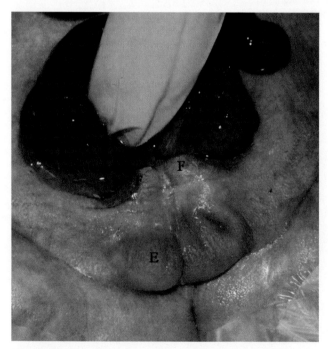

Plate 69.2 Preoperative appearance of the external genitalia in a male newborn with cloacal exstrophy when the intussuscepted bowel (D) is retracted.

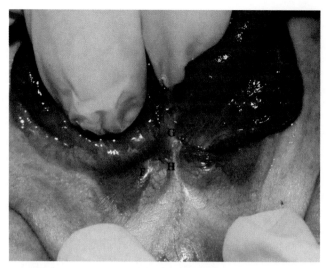

Plate 69.3 Close up of genitalia including a hemi-penis (F), glans penis (H), and urethral plate (G).

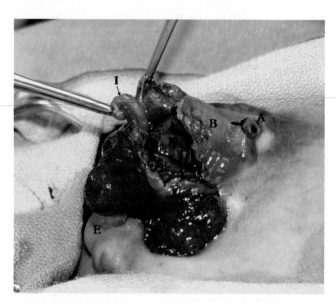

Plate 69.4 The dissection is started below the omphalocele.

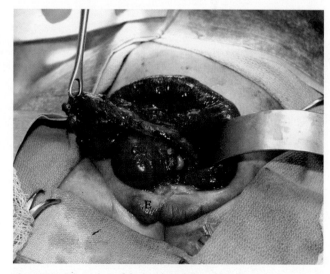

Plate 69.5 Dissection of the hindgut (K) and small gut (J).

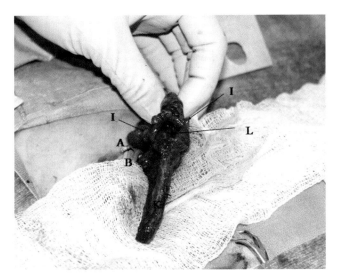

Plate 69.6 Complete release of the hindgut (K), showing the ileocecal valve (L) and split appendix (I).

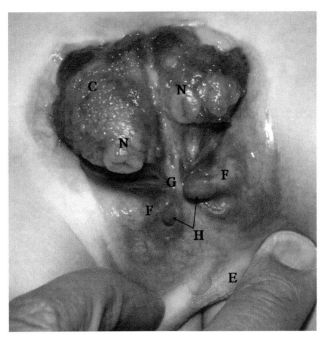

Plate 69.9 Appearance before the second-stage surgery.

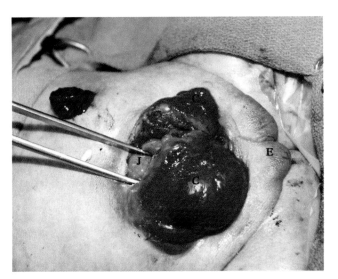

Plate 69.7 The surgical field after construction of the colostomy (M).

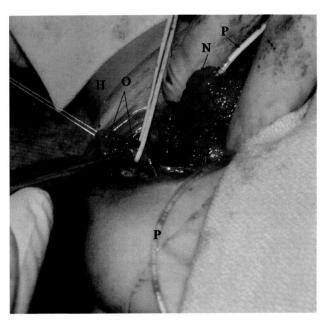

Plate 69.10 Dissection of the corpora cavernosa.

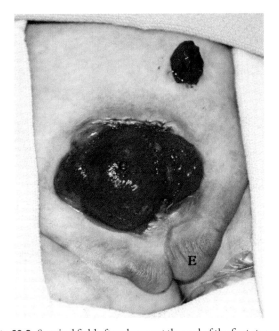

Plate 69.8 Surgical field after closure at the end of the first stage.

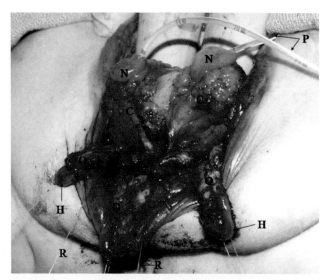

Plate 69.11 Complete penile disassembly.

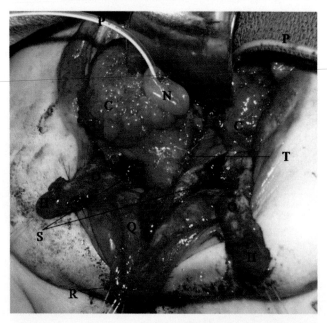

Plate 69.12 Deep dissection lateral to the urethra and bladder neck.

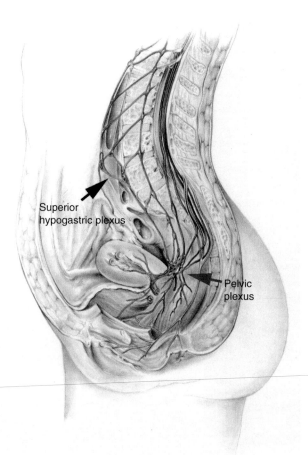

Plate 76.1 Pelvic plexus and innervation of the bladder: green, sympathetic nerves; blue, parasympathetic nerves; yellow, pudendal nerve; red arrow, pelvic plexus; black arrow, superior hypogastric plexus.

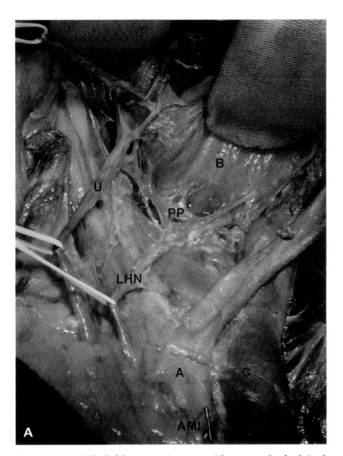

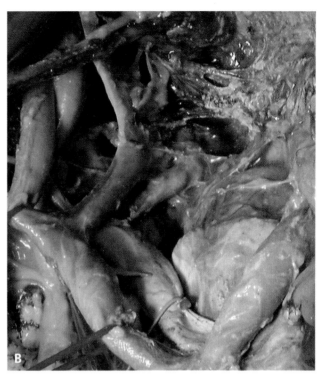

Plate 76.3 (A) The left hypogastric nerve with a network of pelvic plexus nerve bundles. Branches run to the distal ureter (U) and bladder (B) trigones. A, aorta; AMI, inferior mesenteric artery; C, inverior vena cava; LHN, left hypogastric nerve; PP, pelvic plexus. (B) Nerve bundles of the left hypogastric nerve and pelvic plexus are visualized with methylene blue staining.

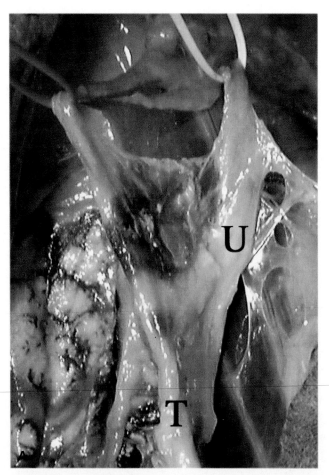

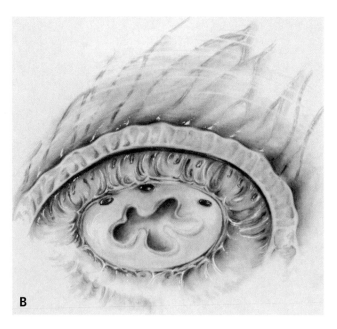

Plate 76.4 (A) The layer of the mesoureter between the ureter (U) and the testicular vessels (T). In this layer the ureter can be dissected without compromising the blood supply and without damaging the nerve structures. (B) Layers of the ureter beginning from the center: lumen, lamina muscularis, adventitia with blood vessels, mesoureter, and nerve structures.

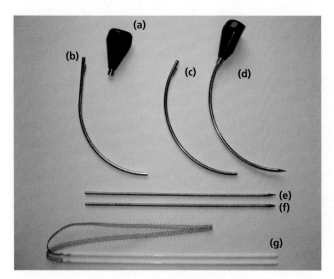

Plate A1 Instruments for retropubic (Chapter 42) and infracoccygeal (Chapter 45) approaches. (a) Handle. (b) 'Straight' introducer with perforations. (c) 'Curved' introducer. (d) Handle, introducer, and tip assembled. (e) Pointed tip. (f) Blunt (security) tip. (g) Tip with guide.

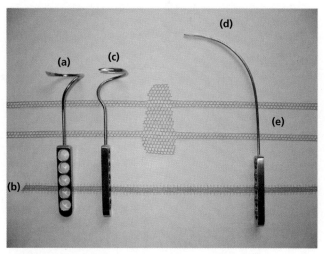

Plate A2 (a) Helix-shaped instrument and (b) tape for transobturator tape procedures (Chapter 43). (c) XXL-Helix and (d) Serasis V instruments, and (e) SerATOM-Implant for prolapse surgery (Chapter 45).

Section 2
Bladder

Chapter 21
En Bloc Transurethral Resection of Bladder Tumors

M. Lodde and A. Pycha

Introduction

Transurethral resection (TUR) of the bladder is carried out for the grading and staging of bladder tumors. Conventionally it is performed 'piece by piece' so the pathologist is confronted with a certain number of tumor fragments, more or less damaged by the procedure. Histological examination is difficult and the microanatomy of the papillary tumor is destroyed. Histopathologic evaluation becomes hard, especially when determining the exact penetration depth of the tumor. To overcome this problem *en bloc* resection with a flat loop electrode is an alternative method.

Patient counseling and consent

The patient should be warned of the possibility of perforation (intra- and extraperitoneal) and of the development of TUR syndrome.

Indications

The procedure is indicated in all superficial, papillary lesions of transitional cell carcinoma with a diameter up to 2.5 cm situated on the trigone, bladder bottom, and lateral bladder wall.

Limitations and risks

- Lesions bigger than 2.5 cm.
- Lesions in the bladder dome, anterior wall, and upper posterior wall.
- Bladder perforation.

Contraindications

The procedure is contraindicated in cases of low bladder capacity and irradiated bladder.

Preoperative management

- Take a full history.
- Clinical investigation.
- Urine cytology and/or additive urine bound tests.
- Intravenous pyelogram.
- Preoperative endoscopy and documentation of the lesions in an appropriate schema.
- Single-shot antibiosis.

Anesthesia

General and spinal anesthesia.

Special instruments/suture material

- Visual obturator with a 0° optical system.
- 24 Fr resectoscope.
- 0°, 30°, and 70° optical systems.
- Flat and angulated loop electrodes.
- 100 mL syringe.
- Diathermia of last generation.
- High power light source.
- Photographic documentation system.
- 18 Fr irrigation Nelaton catheter.
- Glycine irrigation system.

Operative technique

- The patient should be placed in the lithotomic position and entry made into the bladder with a visual obturator.
- Make a primary check of the bladder; the number and position of the lesions are recorded and compared to the initial findings.
- Check if *en bloc* resection is feasible.
- Reduce the cutting power to one-third of the normal value.
- A circular coagulation mark at a distance of 5 mm from the tumor pedicle is put around the lesion.

- At this mark, an incision in the bladder wall is made, down to the deep muscular layer.
- Using the coagulation mark as a lateral landmark and pushing the specimen backwards with the shaft, the resection proceeds in little steps using the cutting power.
- Bleeding from the bladder wall is immediately coagulated.
- Resection is completed with the specimen free floating in the bladder.
- The tumor is retrieved using the 100 mL syringe.
- Coagulation of the tumor ground is done with a ball-end coagulation electrode.
- Make a last check of the bladder with a 70° lens system.
- Place an 18 Fr irrigation Nelaton catheter.
- Normally, no use of continuous irrigation is needed.
- The data are entered in the database.

Tips

- Evaluate half and maximal bladder capacity with one hand on the lower abdomen before starting the resection.
- The irrigation jet pushes the lesion upwards and the view is much better.
- Using a duck-beak resectoscope sheath, the lesion can be pushed in any position (note that this can only be used with a 30° optical lens).

Postoperative care

- Check fluid balance for 24 h.
- Blood count and creatinine control 6 h after intervention and during the next day.
- Catheter removal after 24–48 h.
- Ultrasonography of the kidneys the day after the procedure.
- After removal of the catheter, check the post voiding residual volume twice.
- Antibiotic treatment for 1 week.
- In cases of perforation, a cystogram should be performed after 3 days and in any case before catheter removal.

Complications

- Uncontrolled perforation.
- Obstruction of the catheter with consecutive overextension of the bladder.
- Make sure postoperative fluid is monitored.

Troubleshooting

- In cases of bleeding: this is avoidable with an accurate circular coagulation around the tumor before starting with TUR of the bladder. During resection coagulation is easily performable using the flat loop. After resection, irrigation should not be necessary.
- Bleeding that requires irrigation for more than 24 h needs an operative revision under anesthesia.
- Extraperitoneal perforation: use meticulous coagulation and prolonged placement of the transurethral catheter. Take care to avoid postoperative irrigation.
- Intraperitoneal perforation: use a middle inferior laparotomy and placement of an intraperitoneal and an extraperitoneal drain in cases of small lacerations. In cases of large perforation, a primary bladder suture is mandatory.

Results

In a period from April 2001 to June 2002, a total of 37 patients (32 males and five females) with a mean age of 64.7 years (range 47–87 years) underwent *en bloc* resection of bladder tumors using a flat loop electrode.

In 37 patients, 62 lesions were removed by one surgeon. All lesions were superficial, papillary, and equal or less than 2.5 cm in diameter. In three cases the thin pedicle tore away from the papillary portion of the tumor during excavation with the syringe. Nevertheless in all cases, tissue slides permitted correct determination of the depth of cancer invasion (pTa).

As a complication we have to report an extraperitoneal bladder perforation. After careful coagulation and specimen evacuation a catheter was placed and could be removed on the third day after a negative cystogram. No uncontrollable bleeding or perforation occurred in the other cases.

References

1 Barnes RW, Bergman RT, Hadley HL, Love D. Control of bladder tumors by endoscopic surgery. J Urol 1967;97:864–8.
2 Herr HW, Reuter VE. Evaluation of new resectoscope loop for transurethral resection of bladder tumors. J Urol 1998;159: 2067–8.
3 Kawada T, Ebihara K, Suzuki T, Imai K, Yamanaka H. A new technique for transurethral resection of bladder tumors: rotational tumor resection using a new arched electrode. J Urol 1997;157: 2225–6.
4 Lodde M, Lusuardi L, Palermo S, Signorello D, Maier K, Hohenfellner R. En bloc transurethral resection of bladder tumors: use and limits. Urology 2003;63(3):472–5.
5 Saito S. Transurethral en bloc resection of bladder tumors. J Urol 2001;166:2148–50.
6 Ukai R, Kawashita E, Ikeda H. A new technique for transurethral resection of superficial bladder tumor in one piece. J Urol 2000;163:878–9.

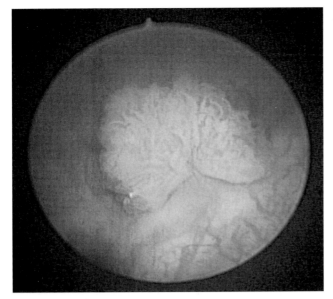

Figure 21.1 Papillary tumor on the left bladder wall. (For color, see Plate 21.1, between pp. 112 and 113.)

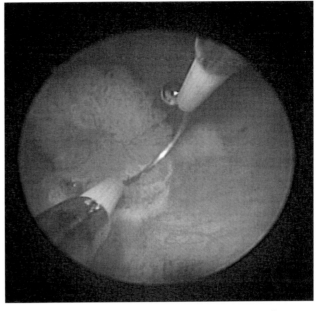

Figure 21.3 Starting with the flat loop to cut the mucosa and penetrate into the detrusor. (For color, see Plate 21.3.)

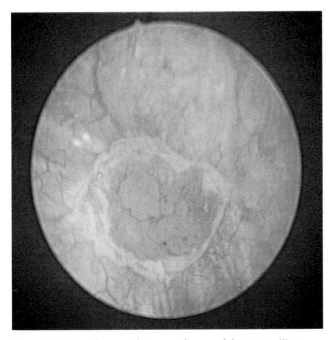

Figure 21.2 Circular coagulation mark around the tumor. (For color, see Plate 21.2.)

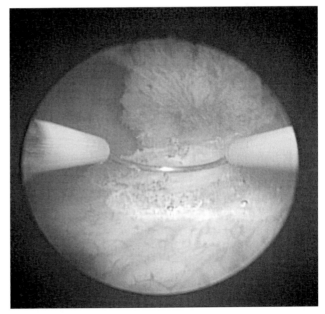

Figure 21.4 Deep resection in the horizontal plane in the muscle layer. (For color, see Plate 21.4.)

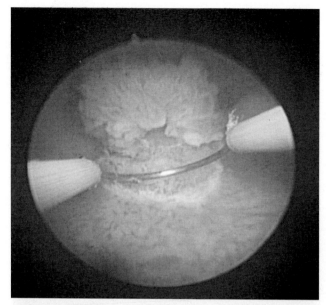

Figure 21.5 Resection enlarged and nearly completed. (For color, see Plate 21.5, between pp. 112 and 113.)

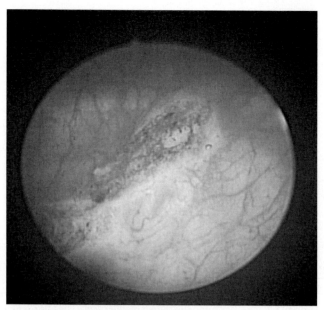

Figure 21.7 Resection completed and coagulation of the tumor ground. (For color, see Plate 21.7.)

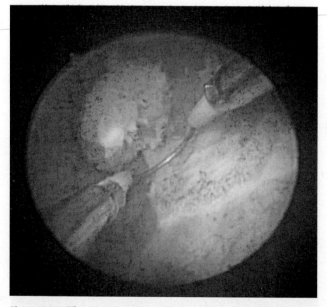

Figure 21.6 The posterior mucosal layer about to be cut. (For color, see Plate 21.6.)

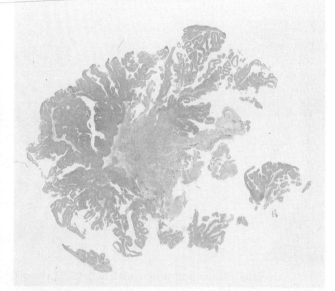

Figure 21.8 Histological section of a resected specimen of transitional cell carcinoma, stage pTa, grade 2. (For color, see Plate 21.8.)

Chapter 22
Laparoscopic Bladder Diverticulectomy

V. Pansadoro

Introduction

Bladder diverticulum is the hernia of the bladder mucosa, through a weak point of a hypertrophied muscular wall, due to a bladder outlet obstruction. Bladder diverticula can be congenital but, more frequently, are acquired.

The diverticulum wall includes an inner mucosal layer and an outer fibrous reactive layer. In 1922 Geraghty demonstrated that removing the mucosal layer was sufficient to obliterate the cavity delimited by the fibrous layer.

The author's method of choice is the transvesical laparoscopic removal of the inner mucosal layer, reproducing the open procedure, with very limited trauma to the patient.

Patient counseling and consent

Informed consent is needed for a laparoscopic procedure.

Indications

The procedure is indicated in diverticula over 4–5 cm in diameter.

Limitations and risks

A small bladder capacity can be a limiting factor.

Contraindications

- Diverticula positioned on the dome.
- Multiple diverticula.
- Hutch diverticula.

Preoperative management

Suprapubic and transrectal ultrasounds are needed, as well as sterile urine and routine exams.

Anesthesia

Blended, general, and peridural anesthesia.

Special instruments/suture material

Three 5 mm Entec trocars with a self-retaining balloon are needed, and a 5 mm 0° optic.

Operative technique

- With the patient in general anesthesia, a cystoscopy is performed to localize the diverticulum's ostium and its relationships with the ureters. Under ultrasound and endoscopic control three 5 mm Entec trocars are introduced (Fig. 22.1). The trocar that will be used for the 5 mm 0° optic is introduced on the midline and the remaining two on the opposite side of the diverticulum.
- Water is substituted with air and the diverticulum orifice is circumscribed. The cleavage plan between the mucosa and fibrous layer is easily developed using a monopolar hook (Fig. 22.2). Once completely released from the fibrotic capsule, the intact diverticulum is recovered from the bladder cavity through a transurethral resectoscope.
- A small Redon drainage is introduced in the bladder through one of the trocars. At the same time, through an extravesical separate stab wound, a Kelly clamp is introduced in the residual cavity and the drainage is positioned in an extravesical location.
- The defect in the bladder wall is sutured with two running sutures, 3/0 Vicryl for the muscle and 5/0 Vicryl for the mucosa. Trocars are substituted with 14 Fr Foley catheters.
- In cases of a small prostate, a transurethral resection of the prostate (TURP) is performed in the same setting. If the prostate is large, the TURP is postponed for 1 week.

Tips

- The combination of ultrasound and endoscopic control ensures the appropriate placement of the three trocars avoiding the peritoneal cavity.

• In the case of a large prostate, postponement of the TURP seems reasonable.

• The use of the Entec trocars, with a self-retaining balloon, allows the surgeon to fix the bladder wall to the abdominal wall, thus avoiding the possibility of loosing the bladder in case a deflation occurs (Fig. 22.2).

Postoperative care

The transabdominal Foley catheters and the drainage are removed after 48 h, and the urethral catheter 24 h later. Patients are dismissed the day after that.

Complications

Ultrasound control of free ureteral drainage is advisable.

Troubleshooting

Indico carmine is injected intravenously during the procedure to ensure proper function. Laparoscopic suturing is required.

Results

Patient satisfaction is very high.

To do

Make sure there is a proper indication with a bladder of reasonable capacity.

References

1 Das S. Laparoscopic removal of bladder diverticulum. J Urol 1992;148:1837–9.
2 Nadler RB, Pearle MS, McDougall EM, Clayman RV. Laparoscopic extraperitoneal bladder diverticulectomy: initial experience. Urology 1995;45:524–7.
3 Orandi A. Transurethral fulguration of bladder diverticulum: new procedure. Urology 1977;10:30.
4 Parra RO, Jones JP, Andrus CH, Hagoor PG. Laparoscopic diverticulectomy: preliminary report of a new approach for the treatment of bladder diverticulum. J Urol 1992;148:869–71.
5 Porpiglia F, Tarabuzzi R, Cossu M et al. Sequential TurP and laparoscopic bladder diverticulectomy: comparison with open surgery. Urology 2002;60(6):1045–9.
6 Vitale PJ, Woodside JR. Management of bladder diverticula by transurethral resection: re-evaluation of an old technique. J Urol 1979;122:744.

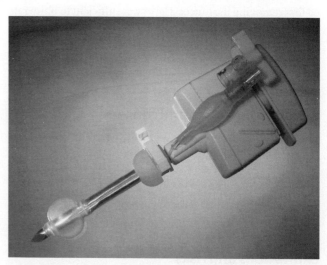

Figure 22.2 The Entec trocar with the stopcock slid down.

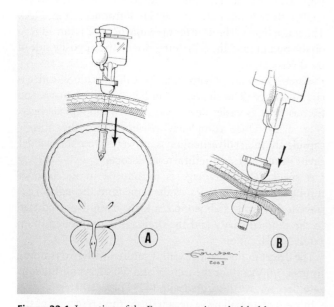

Figure 22.1 Insertion of the Entec trocar into the bladder.

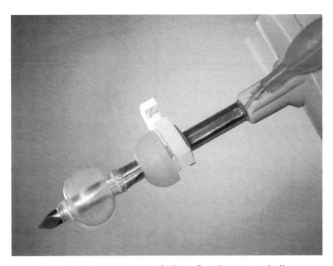

Figure 22.3 The Entec trocar with the inflated retention balloon.

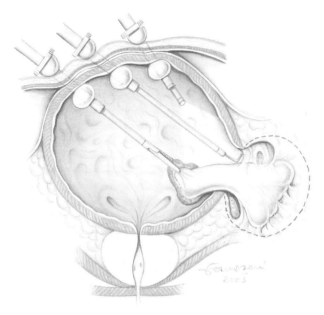

Figure 22.4 Three Entec trocars inserted in the bladder in order to perform the diverticulectomy. (For color, see Plate 22.4, between pp. 112 and 113.)

Chapter 23
Treatment of Abnormalities of the Urachus

P. J. Bastian and P. Albers

Introduction

The urachus is an embryonic remnant of the primitive bladder dome. It consists of a fibrous cord stretching from the umbilicus to the bladder dome. Abnormalities of the urachus are uncommon but usually represent its incomplete regression. Most anomalies present during early childhood [2,12]. The etiology of urachal anomalies is undefined at present [7].

Four clinical abnormalities of the urachus have been described: urachal sinus, urachal cyst, patent urachus, and vesicourachal diverticulum. Urachal abnormalities can be associated with other genitourinary conditions, such as vesicoureteral reflux, hypospadia, or crossed renal ectopia [7,20,26]. Malignant urachal lesions occur, but they are even more rare than the benign lesions.

Treatment of urachal abnormalities is surgical excision of the abnormality with a bladder cuff to avoid recurrence or development of a carcinoma in the unresected tissue [7].

Main abnormalities of the arachus

Urachal sinus

Persistence of the urachal apex results in a blind external sinus that opens at the umbilicus. The lesion presents with intermittent discharge from the umbilicus, which can be purulent. Generalized pain, fever, periumbilical pain, or redness may be associated. Differential diagnosis includes other urachal abnormalities, umbilical granuloma, omphalomesenteric remnants, and omphalitis.

Voiding cystourethrogram, ultrasound, and excretory urograms can be of diagnostic value. A sinogram is diagnostic in all cases [7].

Urachal sinus occurs in 49% of patients with urachal abnormalities [7].

Urachal cyst

Urachal cysts may form within the urachal canal if the lumen is enlarged from epithelial desquamation or degeneration [12]. They present as painless midline swellings below the umbilicus with vague abdominal symptoms, voiding symptoms, or fever. Most commonly the cyst manifests because of infection and drainage through the umbilicus or bladder. Other manifestations are calcification of the cyst wall [22], caliculus formation of the cyst [10], acute abdominal pain secondary to hemorrhage into the cyst [9], and intraabdominal rupture with or without peritonitis [1,24,29,33]. *Staphylococcus aureus* (82%) is the most common organism isolated [7,12,14,23].

Infected cysts usually occur in adults [5,32], but they have also been described in infants [13,17].

Differential diagnosis includes other urachal abnormalities [14], appendiceal abscesses, or suture granuloma [30].

Voiding cystourethrograms and computed tomography can be of diagnostic value. Ultrasound is diagnostic in all cases [7]. Computed tomography may determine the extent and the possible involvement of surrounding organs [4], but should be limited to patients in whom a malignant anomaly is suspected [28].

In a recent study, urachal cysts were diagnosed in 31% of patients with urachal abnormalities [2].

Patent urachus

Persistence of the urachus is usually recognized in the neonate. The patent urachus results when there is a failure of obliteration of the urachal remnant. A patent urachus may present with discharge of urine and diagnosis may be prompted by catheterization. Umbilical cord enlargement with delayed slough is suspicious for a patent urachus. Persistence of the urachus acting as a safety valve has been attributed to intrauterine bladder outlet obstruction, but only 14% of the patients with urachal abnormalities present with bladder outlet obstruction [12].

Differential diagnosis includes omphalomesenteric duct [7] and umbilical hernia.

Voiding cystourethrograms, excretory urograms, and ultrasound can be of diagnostic value, although clinical examination alone may be sufficient. A sinogram may help to distinguish patent urachal from omphalomesenteric duct [7].

Analysis for urea and creatinine of the drainage confirms the diagnosis.

Patent urachus occurs in 15% of patients with urachal abnormalities [7].

Vesicourachal diverticulum

Urachal diverticulum is an incidental radiographic finding, which does not require further treatment [12]. Massive lesions in adults requiring percutaneous drainage or surgery have been described [4,21]. Urachal diverticulum may be associated with prune belly syndrome [21] or diverticula calculi [3,25].

Urachal carcinoma

Urachal carcinomas are exceedingly rare malignant lesions. Most carcinomas are adenocarcinomas, but transitional cell carcinomas and sarcomas have also been described. The most common finding is hematuria [15]. Additional signs are a palpable suprapubic mass, abdominal pain, initiation of voiding symptoms, or mucous passage in the urine [31]. Umbilical discharge is not necessarily found in urachal carcinoma.

A cystogram is the leading diagnostic tool, showing a filling defect in the bladder dome with stipple calcifications. Computerized tomography might help to locate the origin and extent of the lesion. Histology can be established with cystoscopy.

The treatment of choice is radical cystectomy with pelvic lymphadenectomy and *en bloc* excision of the urachus and the umbilicus [12]. In small, well-differentiated tumors partial cystectomy with *en bloc* excision of the urachus and the umbilicus is adequate treatment. Radiation [31] and chemotherapy [12] are not effective in these tumors.

Urachal carcinoma progresses by local invasion but also metastasizes to the iliac and inguinal lymph nodes, omentum, liver, lung, and bone [8,31]. Local recurrence is found in 50% of the cases, and metastatic lymph node involvement in 30% [18,35].

A follow-up every 6 months with clinical examination, urine cytology, ultrasound, cystoscopy, and abdominal computerized tomography is recommended [16].

Long-term prognosis is poor due to the late diagnosis and treatment [31]. Five-year survival rates between 10 and 43% are reported [15,31]. The stage at diagnosis is the limiting factor for survival time after surgery [16,27].

Special instruments/suture material

- Retracting device, e.g. Bookwalter retracting system.
- 2/0 and 3/0 Vicryl, 5/0 Monocryl, and 4/0 and 5/0 Vicryl rapid.

Surgical technique

Benign urachal abnormalities

- Under general anesthesia, place the patient in a supine position.
- To ease identification of the urachal lesion, place a catheter or a feeding tube into the umbilical portion. If they do not pass, an injection of dilute methylene blue may be of help.
- Fill the bladder to full extension with saline.
- Perform a transverse skin crease incision halfway between the umbilicus and the symphysis pubis. This incision gives access to the umbilicus and the bladder dome to resect the dome of the bladder and the urachal abnormality.
- Divide the rectus sheath vertically in the midline. Identify the dome of the distended bladder and isolate the urachus with a surgical clamp or vessel loop. Place two stay sutures in the adjacent bladder wall at the urachal insertion. While resecting the urachus towards the umbilicus the umbilical arteries become visible on either side. Delineate the proximal urachus and, if necessary, remove a bladder cuff with the urachal insertion.
- Close the bladder in a watertight, two-layered fashion (5/0 Monocryl, 2/0 Vicryl).
- Dissect the urachus distally in an extraperitoneal fashion and ligate it at the obliterated portion. All urachal tissue, with the umbilical arteries, should be removed and, if possible, the navel should remain intact. Close the umbilical defect in two layers from inside (3/0 Vicryl).
- Following dissection from the surrounding tissues and the peritoneum, a large urachal sinus or cyst may require a circumferential cut around the stoma of the sinus. Place two Allis clamps on the stoma and dissect the tract.
- Ligation of the hypogastric vessels may be necessary if they are encountered.
- A vertical midline incision gives exposure for massive inflammatory lesions as well. Elliptical excision of the umbilicus may be necessary if it is involved in the inflammatory lesion.
- Perform skin closure with 4/0 and 5/0 Vicryl rapid absorbable sutures and skin clips.

Postoperative care

Postoperative transurethral or suprapubic bladder drainage is dependent on the extent of the bladder resection. Postoperative drainage of the prevesical space is recommended. The postoperative recovery depends on the patient's preoperative condition. Wound infections in the umbilical area are most commonly superficial.

Laparoscopic approach

The laparoscopic approach to urachal abnormalities may be preferred to open surgery due to cosmetic reasons. The laparoscopic approach, however, is transperitoneal and the surgical trauma of open surgery is minimal.

- General anesthesia, a Foley catheter, and a nasogastric tube are needed.
- Place the patient in a supine position.
- Trocar placement:
  - camera device at the level of the umbilicus or midway between the umbilicus and the right anterior iliac crest;
  - the Veress needle (11 mm) lateral to the border of the rectus muscle to insufflate the abdomen;
  - 10–12 mm trocar at the superior margin of the umbilicus or a little above after visualizing the urachal abnormality, the medial urachal ligament, and the bladder;
  - a 5 mm trocar, as necessary, along the right lateral rectus border superior or inferior to the Veress needle.
- Establish a pneumoperitoneum to a pressure of 15 mmHg after inserting the Veress needle.
- Blunt and sharp resection of the urachal abnormality and medial umbilical ligaments towards the umbilicus and bladder.
- Distend the bladder and the umbilical ligaments.
- Incise the peritoneum along the plane between the urachal abnormality and the bladder dome.
- Divide the medial umbilical ligaments with clips.
- Separate the urachal abnormality.
- Divide the attachment of the urachus to the umbilicus or/and bladder with an Endo-GIA stapler (introduced through the 10–12 mm trocar site).
- Resect a bladder cuff if necessary, using a two-layer closure with 2/0 Vicryl.
- Place the specimen in a laparoscopic sack and remove it through the 10–12 mm trocar site. Remove the laparoscopic sack through a Pfannenstiel incision (about 4 cm) if necessary.
- Close the port sites in a standard fashion (2/0 absorbable polyglycolic acid). Skin closure with 4/0 subcuticular absorbable sutures and Steri-Strips.

Special laparoscopic technique in children

The technique in school-age children is the same as in adults. In children less than 8 years of age, the working distance between the abdominal wall and the organs of the abdominal cavity is shorter, requiring smaller trocar sheath units (5 mm diameter units) [11].

Empty the bladder before laparoscopic procedures in children. The bladder is in a more intra-abdominal position and thus may be injured more easily in children younger than 3 years of age [11].

- Insert the Veress needle and the initial trocar sheath unit at a midpoint halfway between the umbilicus and anterior superior iliac spine [34].
- Establish pneumoperitoneum slowly with a pressure of only 10–12 mmHg (reduced abdominal space).

- Lower the intra-abdominal pressure to 5 mmHg to detect bleeding sites.
- Suture all cannula sites under optical control to prevent bowel herniation (3/0 Vicryl).

References

1 Agatstein EH, Stabile BE. Peritonitis due to intraperitoneal perforation of infected urachal cysts. Arch Surg 1984;199:1269–73.

2 Atala A, Retik AB. Patent urachus and urachal cysts. In: Gellis and Kagan's Current Pediatric Therapy (Burg FD, Ingelfinger JR, Wald ER, eds). W.B. Saunders, Philadelphia, 1993:386–7.

3 Bandler CG, Mitbed AH, Alley JL. Urachal caicutus. NY State J Med 1942;42:2203.

4 Berman SM, Totia BM, Laor E, Reid RE, Schweizerhof SP, Freez SZ. Urachal remnants in adults. Urology 1988;31:17–21.

5 Blichert-Toft M, Nielson OV. Disease of the urachus simulating intraabdominal disorders. Am J Surg 1971;122:123–8.

6 Cadeddu JA, Boyle KE, Fabrizio MD, Schulam PG, Kavoussi LR. Laparoscopic management of urachal cysts in adulthood. J Urol 2000;164:1526–8.

7 Cilento BG, Jr, Bauer SB, Retik AB, Peters CA, Atala A. Urachal anomaly: defining the best diagnostic modality. Urology 1998;52:120–2.

8 Cothren CC, Ferucci P, Harken AH, Veve RF, Finlayson CA, Johnson JL. Urachal carcinoma: key points for the general surgeon. Am Surg 2002;68:201–3.

9 Davidson BR, Brown NJ, Neoptolemos JP. Haemorrhage into a urachal cyst presenting as a 'acute abdomen'. Postgrad Med J 1987;63:493–4.

10 Diehl K. A rare case of urachal calculus. Br J Urol 1991;67:327–8.

11 Fahlemkamp D, Winfield HN, Schönberger B, Mueller W, Loeninng SA. Role of laparoscopic surgery in pediatric urology. Eur Urol 1997;32:75–84.

12 Gearhart JP, Jeffs RD. Urachal abnormalities. In: Campbell's Urology, 7th edn (Walch PC, Retik AB, Vaughan ED, Wein AJ, eds). W.B. Saunders, Philadelphia, 1998:1984–7.

13 Geist D. Patrent urachus. Am J Surg 1952;84:118.

14 Guarnaccia SP, Mullins TL, Sant GR. Infected urachal cysts. Urology 1990;36:61–5.

15 Henly DR, Farrow GM, Zincke H. Urachal cancer: rote of conservative surgery. Urology 1993;42:635–9.

16 Herr HW. Urachal carcinoma: the case for extended partial cystectomy. J Urol 1991;151:365–6.

17 Hinman F, Jr. Surgical disorders of the bladder and umbilicus of urachal origin. Surg Gynecol Obstet 1961;113:605.

18 Kakizoe T, Matsumoto K, Andoh M et al. Adenocarcinoma of the urachus. Urology 1983;21:360–6.

19 Katz PG, Crawford JP, Hackler RH. Infected suture granuloma simulating mass of urachal origin: case report. Urology 1986;135:782–3.

20 Lane V. Congenital patent urachus associated with complete (hypospadiac) duplication of the urethra and solitary crossed renal ectopia. J Urol 1982;127:990–1.

21 Lattimer JK. Congenital deficiency of the abdominal musculature and associated genitourinary anomalies. Report of 22 cases. J Urol 1958;79:343.

22 Leyson JFJ. Calcified urachal cyst. Br J Urol 1984;56:438.

23 MacNeilly AE, Koleilat N, Kiruluta HG *et al*. Urachal abscesses: protean manifestations, their recognition and management. Urology 1992;40:530–5.

24 Neir KPN. Mucous metaplasia and rupture of urachal cyst as a rare cause of acute abdomen. Br J Urol 1987;59:281–2.

25 Ney C, Friedenberg RM. Radiographic findings in the anomalies of the urachus. J Urol 1968;99:288–91.

26 Rich RH, Hardy BE, Filter RM. Surgery for anomalies of the urachus. J Pediatr Surg 1983;18:370–3.

27 Santucci RA, True LD, Lange PH. Is partial cystectomy the treatment of choice for mucinous adenocarcinoma of the urachus? Urology 1997;49:536–40.

28 Sarno RC, Klauber G, Carter BL. Computer assisted tomography of urachal abnormalities. J Comput Assist Tomogr 1983;7:674–6.

29 Savanelli A, Cigliano B, Esposito G. Infected and ruptured urachal cyst causing peritonitis. Z Kinderchir 1984;39:267–8.

30 Sawczuk IS, Brown W. Appendiceal abscess presenting as an infected urachal cyst. NY State J Med 1992;92:365.

31 Sheldon CA, Clayman RV, Gonzales R, Williams RD, Fraley EE. Malignant urachal lesions. J Urol 1984;131:1–8.

32 Sterling JA, Goldsmith R. Lesions of urachus which appear in the adult. Ann Surg 1953;137:120.

33 Valda V, Conn MJ. Spontaneous rupture of non infected urachal cyst. J Pediatr Surg 1991;26:747–8.

34 Waldschmidt J. Besonderheiten der Laparoskopie im Neugeborenen- und Säuglingsalter. In: Laparoskopische Urologie (Fahlenkamp D, Lonning SA, eds). Blackwell Scientific, Berlin, 1993:53–62.

35 Whitehead ED, Tester AN. Carcinoma of the urachus. Br J Urol 1971;43:468–76.

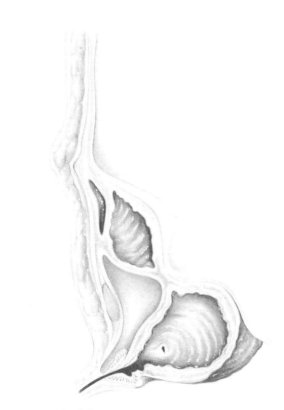

Figure 23.2 Urachal cyst.

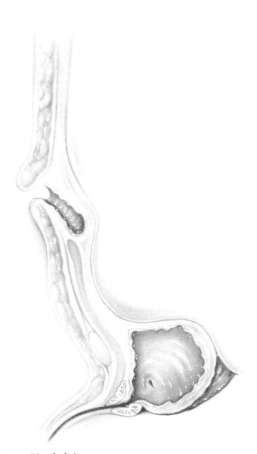

Figure 23.1 Urachal sinus.

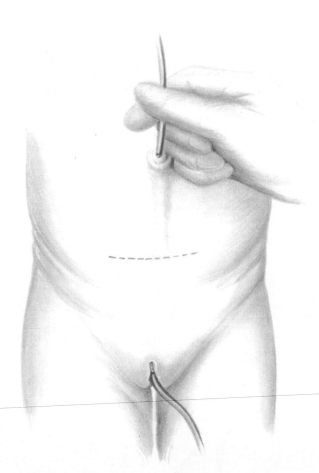

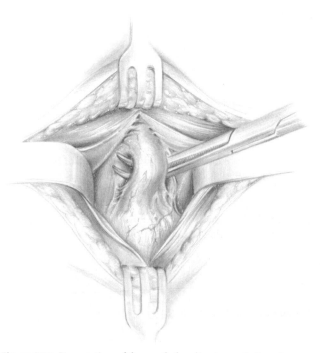

Figure 23.5 Preparation of the urachal ending towards the urinary bladder.

Figure 23.3 Catheter to locate the urachus. The catheter is placed in the urinary bladder. A transversal skin incision is then performed.

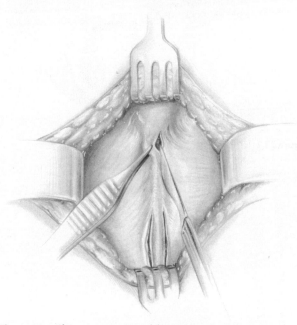

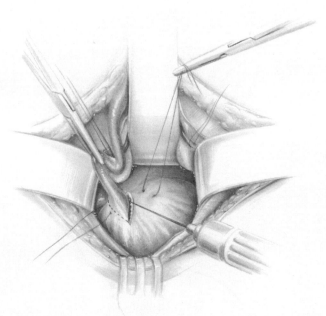

Figure 23.6 Excision of the urachal remnant and bladder cuff.

Figure 23.4 Sharp preparation of the urachus from the rectus sheath.

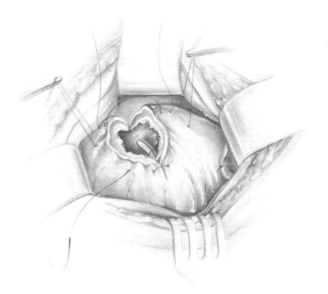

Figure 23.7 Two-layer closure of the urinary bladder.

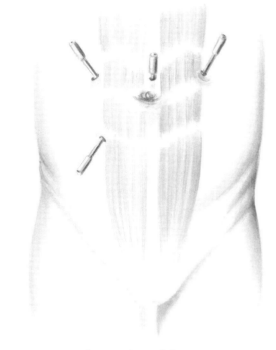

Figure 23.9 Trocar placement in an adult.

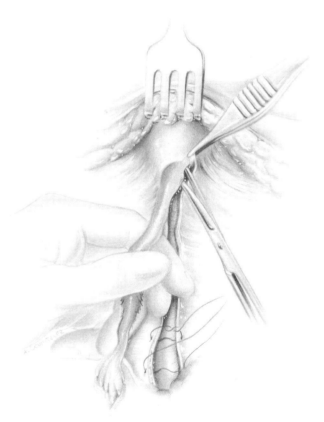

Figure 23.8 Preparation and removal of the urachal remnant, followed by closure of the defect and fixation of the umbilicus.

Chapter 24
Ureterocystoplasty

R. Stein and R. Hohenfellner

Introduction

Various kinds of intestinal segments have been used for bladder augmentation, each with its advantages and disadvantages [12]. All segments, however, share the risk of developing metabolic complications and late malignancies [8,11]. The ureter, lined with native urothelium, should be the ideal material to augment the bladder and should incur no long-term risk of metabolic complications or secondary malignancies. Patients with a megaureter, a poorly functioning kidney, and a small bladder capacity are the ideal candidates for such an operation. Unfortunately, this is a relatively rare constellation. In 1973 Eckstein and coworkers described the technique of ureterocystoplasty in a patient with urethral valves, who received a renal transplantation 6 years later [5]; 22 years after the ureterocystoplasty, the patient was completely continent with a normally functioning graft [6]. At the beginning of the 1990s, several authors discovered the ureter again and today the ureterocystoplasty is gaining in popularity [1–3,7,9,14]. The megaureter is also used after transuretero-ureterostomy for patients with two functioning kidneys [4,13]. Even if there is no megaureter, a tissue expander can be used to dilate the ureter [10]. At the current time we see no indication for the use of ureter at any price, given the known long-term complications of transuretero-ureterostomies.

Indications

The procedure is indicated in noncompliant bladders with a megaureter and a poorly functioning kidney.

Anesthesia

General anesthesia.

Special instruments/suture materials

- Standard instruments for bladder augmentation.
- 4/0 and 5/0 Monocryl.
- 4/0 polyglycolic acid (e.g. PDS).

Operative technique

- Expose the poorly functioning kidney through an extraperitoneal flank incision or dorsal lumbotomy.
- Dissect the megaureter, avoiding injury to the longitudinal vessels running inside Waldeyer's sheath.
- Ligate the renal artery and vein, dissect the proximal ureter, and perform a nephrectomy of the poorly functioning or nonfunctioning kidney.
- Pass the ureter distally, and close the incision.
- Make a parainguinal or Pfannenstiel incision.
- Perform extraperitoneal mobilization of the distal ureter.
- Carefully dissect the longitudinal fibers along the ureter with preservation of the blood supply.
- Spatulate the ureter parallel to the longitudinally running ureteral vessels in an area of decreased vascularity.
- Open the bladder dome.
- Coapt the lateral edges of the ureter to construct a large ureteral plate.
- Resect the cranial segment of the megaureter if there is any doubt about its blood supply.
- Augment the spatulated bladder with the ureteral plate using, for example, 4/0 polyglycolic acid.
- Insert a cystostomy tube.
- Close the incision.

Tips

- The main blood supply to the ureter comes from the vessels running longitudinally in Waldeyer's sheath.
- Additional blood supply on the *left side*: artery direct from the aorta running medial to the ureter with variable branches to the ureter.
- Additional blood supply on the *right side*: artery crossing the vena cava at the level of the promotorium with branches to the proximal and distal segments of the ureter.

References

1 Bellinger MF. Ureterocystoplasty: a unique method for vesical augmentation in children. J Urol 1993;149(4):811–13.

2 Ben CJ, Partin AW, Jeffs RD. Ureteral bladder augmentation using the lower pole ureter of duplicated system. Urology 1996;47:135–7.

3 Churchill BM, Jayanthi VR, Landau EH, McLorie GA, Khoury AE. Ureterocystoplasty: importance of the proximal blood supply. J Urol 1995;154(1):197–8.

4 Dewan PA, Condron SK. Extraperitoneal ureterocystoplasty with transureteroureterostomy. Urology 1999;53(3):634–6.

5 Eckstein HB, Chir M, Martin R. Uretero-Cystoplastik. Akt Urol 1973;4:255–7.

6 Etker S. Eckstein's ureterocystoplasty: Notes. In: Contemporary Issues in Pediatric Urology in Memoriam Herbert B. Eckstein (Williams DI, Etker S, eds). Pediatric Cerrahi Dergisi, Istanbul, 1996:213–15.

7 Hitchcock RJ, Duffy PG, Malone PS. Ureterocystoplasty: the 'bladder' augmentation of choice. Br J Urol 1994;73(5):575–9.

8 Kälble TWS, Berger MR, Waldherr R et al. Karzinomrisiko in verschiedenen Formen der Harnableitung unter Verwendung von Darm. Akt Urol 1993;24:1–7.

9 Landau EH, Jayanthi VR, Khoury AE et al. Bladder augmentation: ureterocystoplasty versus ileocystoplasty. J Urol 1994:716–19.

10 Liatsikos EN, Dinlenc CZ, Kapoor R, Bernardo NO, Smith AD. Tissue expansion: a promising trend for reconstruction in urology. J Endourol 2000;14(1):93–6.

11 McDougal WS. Metabolic complications of urinary intestinal diversion. J Urol 1992;147:1199–208.

12 McDougal WS. Use of intestinal segments and urinary diversion. In: Campbell's Urology, 7th edn (Walsh PC, Retik AB, Vaughan ED, Wein AJ, eds). W.B. Saunders, Philadelphia, 1998:3121–61.

13 Talic RF. Augmentation ureterocystoplasty with ipsilateral renal preservation in the management of patients with compromised renal function secondary to dysfunctional voiding. Int Urol Nephrol 1999;31(4):463–70.

14 Wolf JJ, Turzan CW. Augmentation ureterocystoplasty. J Urol 1993;149(5):1095–8.

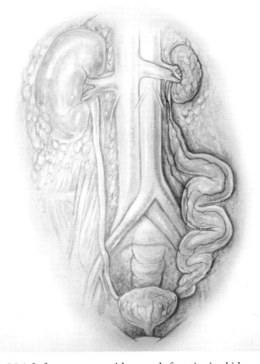

Figure 24.1 Left megaureter with a poorly functioning kidney and a small capacity bladder.

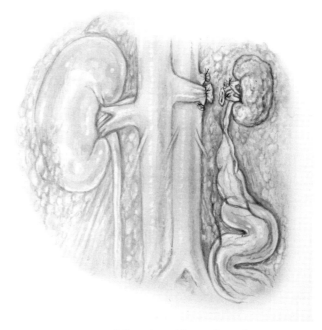

Figure 24.2 Ligation and dissection of the renal vessels.

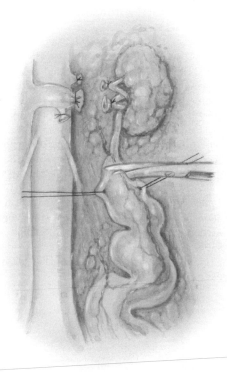

Figure 24.3 Placement of two stay sutures at the cranial end of the ureter and dissection of the ureter above the stay sutures, with removal of the kidney.

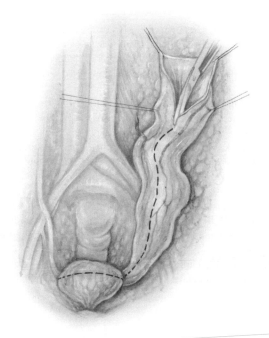

Figure 24.5 Spatulation of the ureter in an avascular area and vertical opening of the bladder.

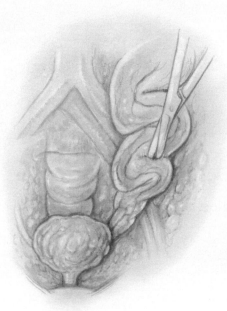

Figure 24.4 Careful dissection of östling's folds.

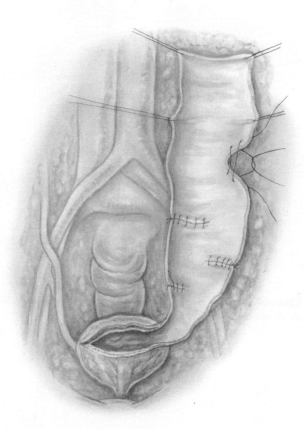

Figure 24.6 Coaptation of the edges of the ureter with 5/0 PDS in the area of previous folding to create a large ureteral plate.

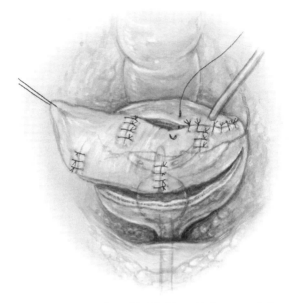

Figure 24.7 Augmentation of the bladder with the ureteral plate, and insertion of a cystostomy tube in addition to the Foley catheter.

Chapter 25
Sigma Diverticulitis with Bladder Fistula: Sigma Resection and Resection of the Fistula

M. Fisch

Introduction

Inflammation of an acquired sigma diverticula is one of the most common diseases of the large bowel. It can result in sigma bladder fistula formation.

Patient counseling and consent

Temporary colostomy may be necessary. In cases of unexpected malignancy, radical surgery has to be performed.

Indications

This procedure is indicated in fistula formation and large bowel obstruction.

Limitations and risks

Intra-abdominal sigma perforation and peritonitis in cases of 'wait and see'.

Contraindications

In cases of intra-abdominal perforation a three-stage procedure is needed: (i) colostomy; (ii) sigma resection and fistula resection; and (iii) closure of the colostomy.

Preoperative management

- Tap water enema with water-soluable contrast medium.
- Colonoscopy.
- Computed tomography.
- Cystoscopy.
- Bowel preparation.

Anesthesia

General and epidural anesthesia.

Special instruments/suture materials

See Chapter 54.

Operative technique

- Perform a laparotomy: xiphoid to symphysis.
- Sigma mobilization: ligate the vas deferens and preserve the seminal vessels. The left ureter is identified; the ureter and vas deferens are armed with vessel loops.
- Mobilization of the conglomerate tumor: start laterally and proceed cranially until healthy colon, still carrying non-inflamed diverticula, is reached.
- The proximal line of resection is marked by stay sutures and the bowel is dissected.
- Continue preparation distally and medially close to the bowel; ligate branches from the mesenteric and cranial rectal arteries step by step.
- The bladder now becomes separated from the sigma and the fistula is marked by stay sutures.
- Continue distally until healthy rectum is reached; dissect between stay sutures.
- The conglomerate tumor is removed and sent for histology: look for malignancy.
- Open the bladder, and check for spontaneous urine ejaculation.
- Excise the fistula.
- Close the bladder using running mucosa 5/0 Monocryl and interrupted detrusor 4/0 PDS.
- Perform end-to-end anastomosis of the sigma and rectum. Tension-free anastomosis is achieved by mobilization of the left flexure.
- Interpose the mobilized greater omentum in between the bladder and colon.

Tips

- Observe capillary arterial bleeding from the stumps of the rectum and sigma and cut the diverticula at the level of the mucosa before anastomosis starts.

• In cases of a short greater omentum, complete mobilization from the right to the left (left gastroepiploic artery) becomes necessary, brought retroperitoneally through a mesenteric window.

• Large mesenteric windows are covered with a free parietal peritoneal flap taken from the left lateral side.

• In cases of even partial ureter lesions, reimplantation by the psoas hitch is the method of choice.

Postoperative care

Postoperative care is as standard. The catheter is removed on day 7 after a cystogram.

Complications

No complications were observed in a series of 21 patients.

Results

The operation was successful in 21 patients. The follow-up mean was 70 (8–215) months. There were no cases of recurrence, and a temporary colostomy was necessary in only one patient. (See Chapter 54 for more details.)

References

1 Alapont Perez FM, Gil Salom M, Esclapez Valero JP *et al.* Acquired enterovesical fistulas. Arch Esp Urol 1994;47(10):973–7.

2 Benchimol D, Lagautriere F, Richelme H. Vesico-sigmoidal fistulas of diverticular origin. Ann Urol 1995;29(1):26–30.

3 Hsieh JH, Chen WS, Jiang JK, Lin TC, Lin JK, Hsu H. Enterovesical fistula: 10 years experience. Chung Hua I Hsueh Tsa Chih (Taipei) 1997;59(5):283–8.

4 King RM, Beart RW, McIlrath DC. Colovesical and rectovesical fistulas. Arch Surg 1982;117(5):680–3.

5 Kirsh GM, Hampel N, Shuck JM, Resnick MI. Diagnosis and management of vesicoenteric fistulas. Surg Gynecol Obstet 1991;173(2):91–7.

6 Kremer K, Lierse W, Platzer W, Schreiber HW, Weller S. Chirurgische Operationslehre. Kapitel 6. Thieme, Stuttgart, 1992:204–17.

7 Krompier A, Howard R, Macewen A, Natoli C, Wear JB. Vesicocolonic fistulas in diverticulitis. J Urol 1976;115(6):664–6.

8 Larsen A, Bjerklund Johansen TE, Solheim BM, Urnes T. Diagnosis and treatment of enterovesical fistula. Eur Urol 1996;29(3):318–21.

9 Mileski WJ, Joehl RJ, Rege RV, Nahrwold DL. One-stage resection and anastomosis in the management of colovesical fistula. Am J Surg 1987;153(1):75–9.

10 Moss RL, Ryan JA. Management of enterovesical fistulas. Am J Surg 1990;159(5):514–17.

11 Pontari MA, McMillen MA, Garvey RH, Ballantyne GH. Diagnosis and treatment of enterovesical fistulae. Am Surg 1992;58(4):258–63.

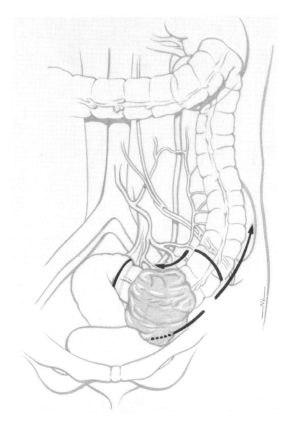

Figure 25.1 Anatomical overview.

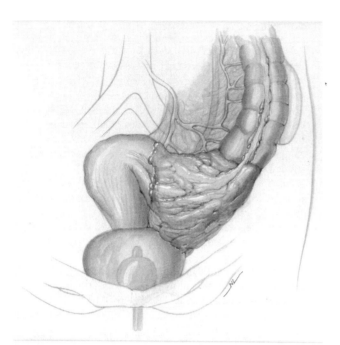

Figure 25.2 Conglomerate tumor of the sigma and bladder.

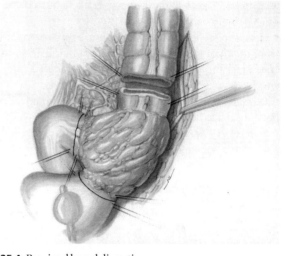

Figure 25.4 Proximal bowel dissection.

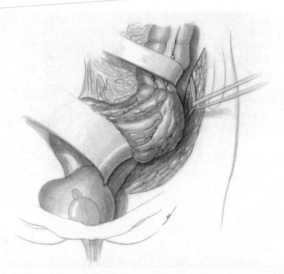

Figure 25.3 Conglomerate lateral mobilization with the ureter armed.

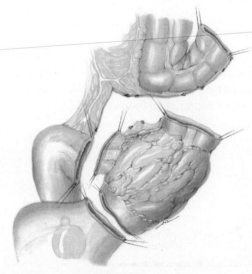

Figure 25.5 The completed resection.

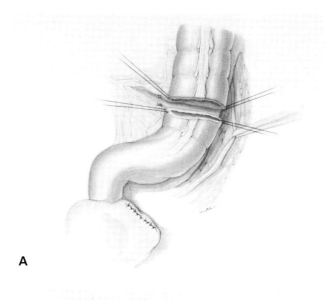

A

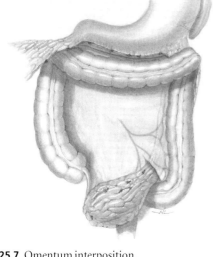

Figure 25.7 Omentum interposition.

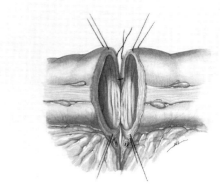

B

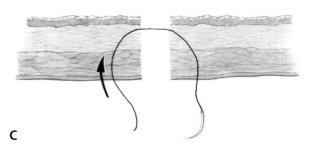

C

Figure 25.6 Bowel anastomosis: stay sutures facilitate end-to-end anastomosis (A), beginning at the back wall (B) using interrupted seromuscular single stitches (C).

Section 3
Prostate

Postoperative care

The care has been described for bladder surgery...

References

Figure 26.1 Exposure of the bladder outlet with Kocher retractors. The distal capsule suture in the region of the puboprostatic ligaments and the proximal suture of the bladder outlet are tied. The vesicoprostatic bundles are ligated and transected on both sides.

Figure 26.3 Tissue partial excision of the ventral prostatic capsule and overcircumcision of the bladder outlet with electrocautery between the preliminary sutures.

Figure 26.4 Sharp dissection of the adenoma from the dorsal median inside, visible to posterior and extension of the dorsal prostatic capsule.

Chapter 26
Millin Retropubic Prostatectomy

J. M. Fitzpatrick

Introduction

Terence Millin, a leading surgeon of his time, described the retropubic approach to enucleate the benign adenoma from the prostate in an article in the *Lancet* in 1945. His description is absolutely clear in the original paper, and is well worth reading even at the present time. His retropubic approach, not only to the prostate but also to other pelvic operations, was revolutionary in its time. Most of the points that he wrote under the heading 'Features of the operation' are still relevant, although the postoperative stay in hospital is now in the region of 5 days or less. The catheter need only be left *in situ* for 3–4 days, and the patient can be discharged from hospital on the day the catheter is removed.

Indications

The procedure is indicated in benign prostatic hyperplasia with a prostatic weight of >80 g, and in coexistent intravesical pathology such as a large stone.

Special instruments/suture material

- Standard instruments for pelvic operations.
- Millin retractor and other instruments devised by Millin.
- Suture material: 3/0, 2/0, and 1/0 polyglycolic acid.

Surgical approach

The patient is placed in the standard supine position. A moderate amount of breaking of the operating table may be helpful. A Pfannenstiel incision gives excellent access to the pelvis between the two bellies of the rectus abdominus muscle, which are spread apart. A self-retaining retractor is then inserted and the prostate is exposed.

Operative technique

- If there is fat lying anterior to the prostate, it can be removed by dissecting with a gauze wipe in an up and down direction rather than in a side-to-side direction. This prevents tearing the superficial dorsal vein of the penis, which should then be clearly visible and can be diathermized and cut.
- The bladder neck can be seen clearly and 1 cm distal to this a transverse incision should be made with a size 15 blade on a long scalpel. The capsule will bleed easily, and the bleeding vessels should be diathermized carefully with a thick Kidd–Riches diathermy forceps.
- A Metzenbaum scissors is inserted into the plane between the capsule and the adenoma. This is easily found. The blades of the scissors can then be opened fully to define carefully the plane anteriorly.
- The index finger of the right hand is then inserted into this plane and spread around the adenoma. Sometimes, particularly posteriorly, the prostatic adenoma can be adherent to the capsule. The enucleation need not be done too fast, and if necessary any adhesions between the adenoma and the capsule can be cut with the scissors under direct vision.
- At the apex of the adenoma, the urethra can be cut with the dissecting scissors. The adenoma can then be lifted out from the prostatic cavity using a Millins forceps, and the posterior surface of the adenoma is separated from the capsule.
- It is important to ensure that a large middle lobe component is carefully removed. The entire adenoma is then removed after the bladder neck fibers are separated from it, anteriorly and posteriorly.
- Any excess trigone can be removed with the dissecting scissors, and the residual trigone should then be sutured, using a 3/0 polyglycolic acid suture, to the posterior capsule.
- Starting on the side of the bladder neck, a 1/0 polyglycolic acid suture is used to close the incision in the prostatic capsule. This is run continuously and the incision is closed. A size 22 Fr hematuria catheter is inserted into the bladder, and 30 mL of fluid is left in the balloon.
- A Robinson drain is used to drain the retropubic space.

Postoperative care

The catheter can be removed on the third or fourth day postoperatively.

Reference

1 Millin T. Retropubic prostatectomy: a new extravesical technique. Report on 20 cases. Lancet 1945;Dec. 1:693–6.

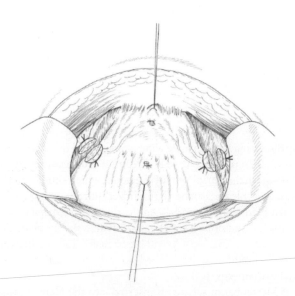

Figure 26.1 Exposure of the bladder outlet with Kader retractors. The distal capsule suture in the region of the puboprostatic ligaments and the proximal suture of the bladder outlet are tied. The vesicoprostatic bundles are ligated and transected on both sides.

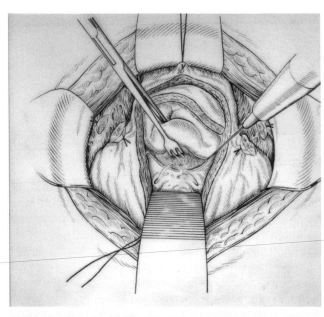

Figure 26.3 Broad partial excision of the ventral prostate capsule and overcircumcision of the bladder outlet with electrocautery between the preliminary sutures.

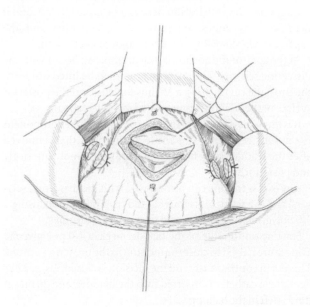

Figure 26.2 Circumcision of the adenoma distal to the ureteral orifices, showing the situation immediately before digital enucleation of the adenoma. The position and function of the ureteral orifices are marked with intravenous indigo carmine.

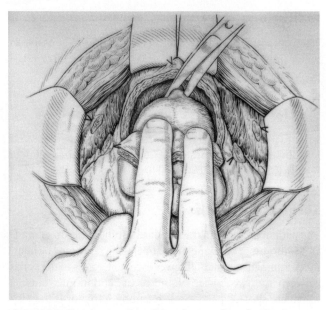

Figure 26.4 Sharp separation of the adenoma from the distal urethra, made possible by prior broad excision of the ventral prostate capsule.

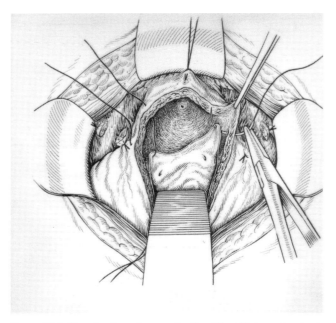

Figure 26.5 The situation after enucleation. The 1/0 chromic catgut gathering sutures are brought into position on both sides to reduce the volume of the fossa and transpose the trigone.

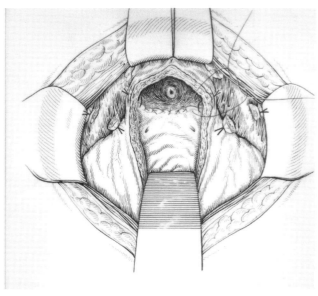

Figure 26.6 Deep retrigonization to create a wide nonobstructive junction from the fossa to the bladder.

Chapter 27
Radical Perineal Prostatectomy

J. Fichtner and W. Stackl

Introduction

This procedure is our method of choice for locally confined cancer of the prostate. When prostate-specific antigen (PSA) is >10 ng/mL or the biopsy Gleason score is above 6, a laparoscopic lymph dissection is performed prior to the procedure. If the PSA is >7 and >10 ng/mL, there is a lymph node negative predictive value of 98%.

This is a quick procedure (average 62 min), with a low rate of blood transfusion (3%).

Patient counseling and consent

There is a risk of incontinence equal to that in retropubic surgery, however early continence is better (73%). Bilateral perineal nerve sparing results in approximately 52% intercourse rate without additional measures.

Indications

The procedure is indicated in locally confined cancer of the prostate.

Limitations and risks

Prostate size more than 80–100 g.

Contraindications

• See above.
• Prior rectal surgery (e.g. rectal amputation) is *not* a contraindication.
• The perineal approach is easier following abdominal bowel surgery or endoscopic hernia repair.

Preoperative management

• Retrograde urethrogram or urethrocystoscopy to exclude urethral strictures.

• An enema on the evening prior to surgery.
• Type and screen.

Anesthesia

General or epidural anesthesia only (L4/5).

Special instruments/suture material

Straight and curved Lowsley tractors, a Young retractor, and a self-retaining retractor (e.g. Omintract or Bookwalter) are needed.

Operative technique

See Figs 27.1–27.39.

Tips

• Place the finger in the rectum for the approach to the apex whilst learning the technique.
• Dorsal pressure to the curved Lowsley tractor brings the apex of the prostate to the surface of the perineum.
• In large glands more space is gained when the prostate is placed back into the wound and is then displaced laterally.
• Mobilize the seminal vesicles initially from the dorsal aspect when possible; this facilitates later dissection of the bladder neck.
• Use curved 5/8 needles and double-armed sutures for the anastomosis.

Postoperative care

Remove the drainage tube on day 2 and start oral feeding on day 1. Check the anastomosis with a cystogram on day 7 (it is watertight in 91%) and remove the catheter when no extravasation is noted.

Complications

• If the urethral catheter falls out it can usually be replaced easily; use fluoroscopy when necessary.
• In rare cases a perineal hematoma develops postoperatively; when this is large it should be removed surgically.

Troubleshooting

• After removal of the catheter approximately 3–5% of patients develop urinary retention. Transient placement of a suprapubic catheter solves the problem within 3–4 days.
• Replace the Foley catheter when urinary extravasation through the perineal wound is noted after catheter removal (0.5–1%).

Results

• $n = 532$.
• pT2 = 73%.
• pT3 = 27%.
• Margin positive in pT2 = 8%.
• Margin positive in pT3 = 33%.
• Early continence = 73%.
• No pads after 1 year = 93%.

• Potency with bilateral nerve sparing sufficient for intercourse without Sildenafil = 52%.

To do

• Elevate the perineum until the horizontal position is reached.
• Operate with two assistants or with one if a self-retaining retractor is used.
• Use magnifying loops and an xenon headlight for better visualization, particularly in nerve sparing.
• Place a cystostomy tube prior to the procedure to avoid urinary drainage to the operative field.
• Carefully inspect the rectum to exclude rectal injury.

Not to do

• Do not insert the curved Lowsley tractor with pressure or force; when resistance is noted use rectal digital guidance or perform endoscopy.
• Do not use electrocautery in the area of the bundles when nerve sparing is performed.
• Do not choose epidural anesthesia in obese patients (respiratory problems).

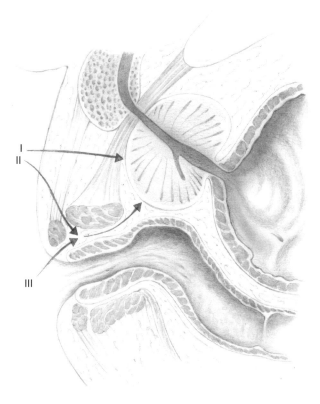

Figure 27.1 Perineal approaches: I, Young (extrasphincteric); II, Belt (subsphincteric); III, Hudson (trans-sphincteric).

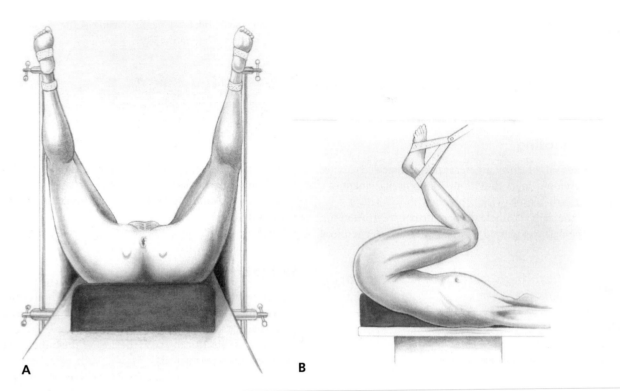

A   **B**

Figure 27.2 Positioning in extreme lithotomy with a horizontally elevated perineum.

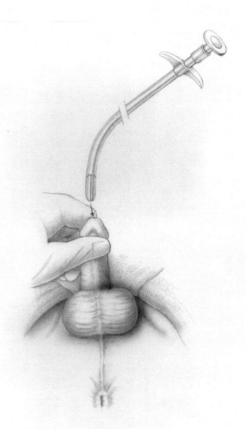

Figure 27.3 Insertion of the curved Lowsley tractor.

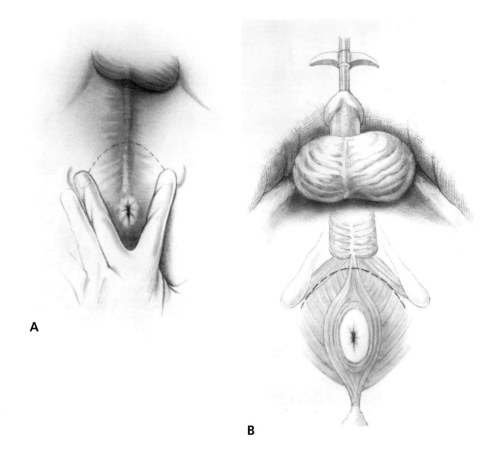

A

B

Figure 27.4 The curved skin incision with the ischial bones as lateral margins.

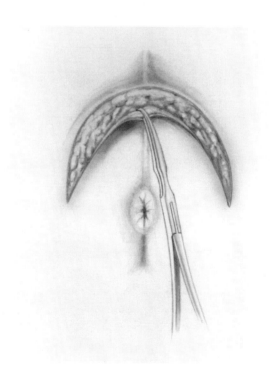

Figure 27.5 Tracting to the lower edge of the incision.

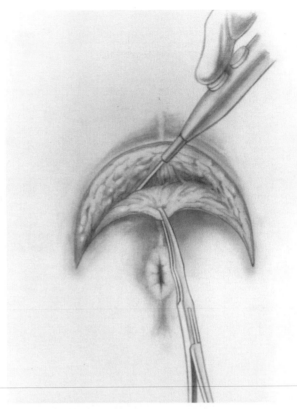

Figure 27.6 The subcutaneous tissue and the central tendon are divided with electrocautery.

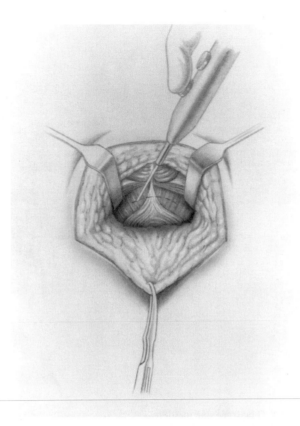

Figure 27.8 Transverse incision below the bulb and above the external anal sphincter.

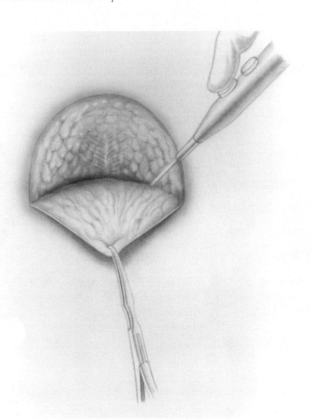

Figure 27.7 Further incision and dissection of the bulb.

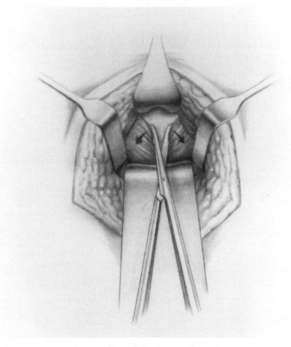

Figure 27.9 Lateral spreading of the levator branches.

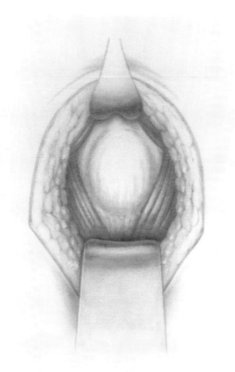

Figure 27.10 Separation of the dorsal part of the prostate with blunt dissection and traction to the vaginal speculum.

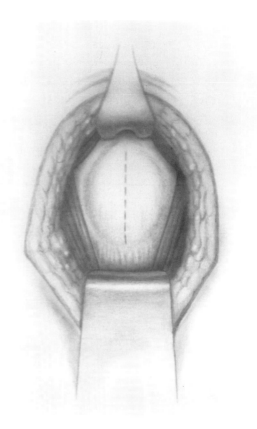

A

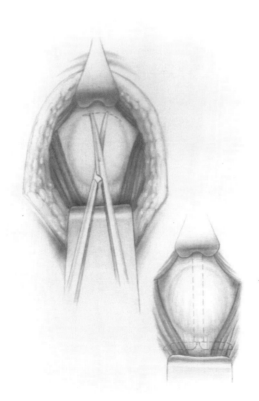

Figure 27.11 Transverse incision of Denonvilliers' fascia at the apical area.

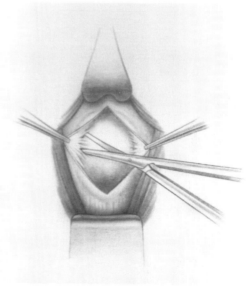

B

Figure 27.12 When nerve sparing is planned, Denonvilliers' fascia should be incised longitudinally and both neurovascular bundles should be laterally dissected.

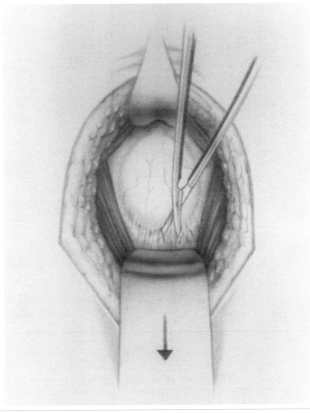

Figure 27.13 Alternatively, the entire Denonvilliers' fascia is left on the prostate and is only transversally incised at the basal part of the prostate to dissect the seminal vesicles.

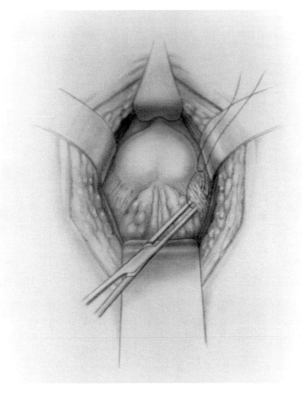

Figure 27.15 Stepwise dissection and ligation of both lateral pedicles.

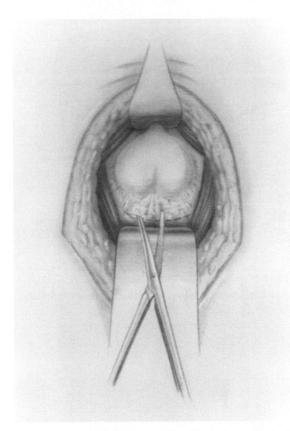

Figure 27.14 Incision of Denonvilliers' fascia is at the level of the seminal vesicles.

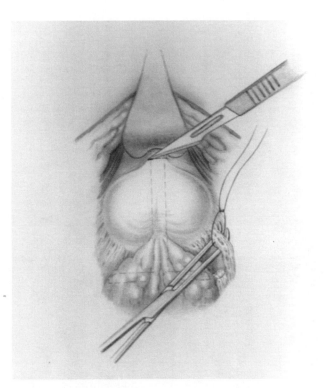

Figure 27.16 Incision of the membranous urethra 3 mm distal to the apex.

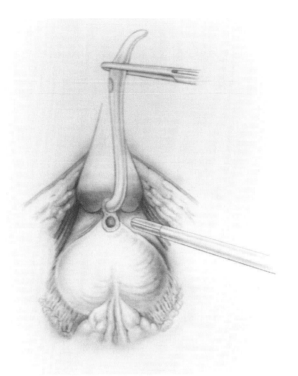

Figure 27.17 Insertion of a Foley catheter and the straight Lowsley tractor to visualize the ventral half of the urethra.

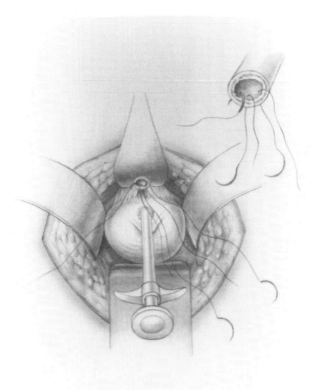

Figure 27.19 Three anastomotic sutures are placed to the ventral part at 10, 12, and 2 o'clock.

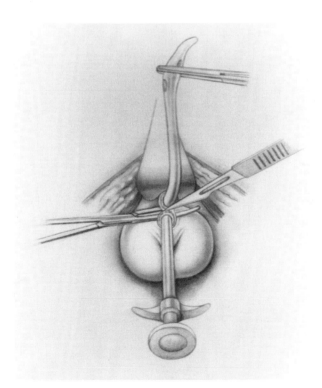

Figure 27.18 The urethra is completely separated.

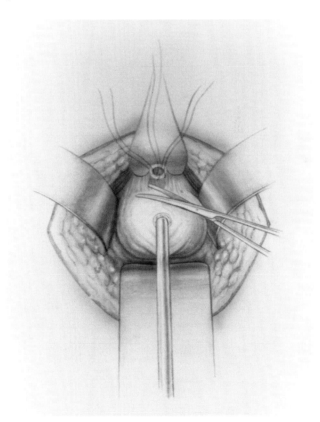

Figure 27.20 Separation of the puboprostatic ligaments.

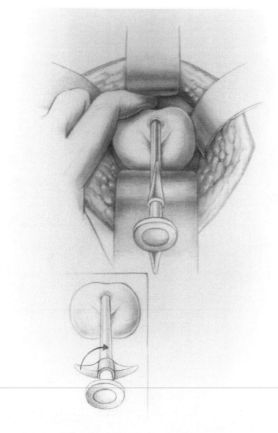

A

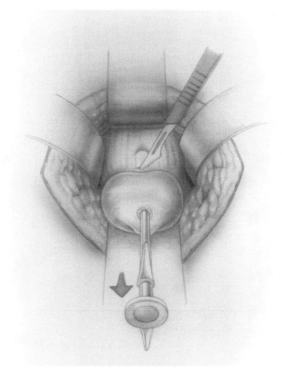

Figure 27.22 Incision of the bladder neck.

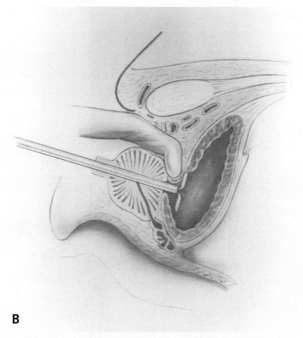

B

Figure 27.21 Rotation of the Lowsley tractor by 90° and digital dissection of the ventral part.

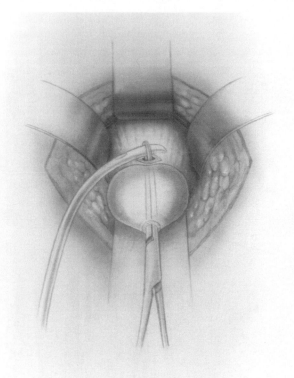

Figure 27.23 Insertion of a 14 Fr catheter for traction to the prostate.

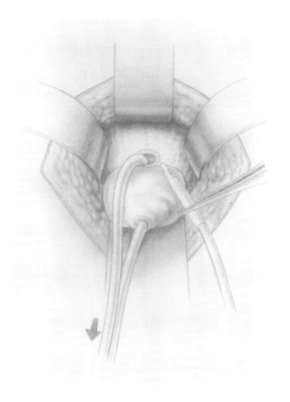

Figure 27.24 An 18 Fr Foley catheter is placed into the bladder.

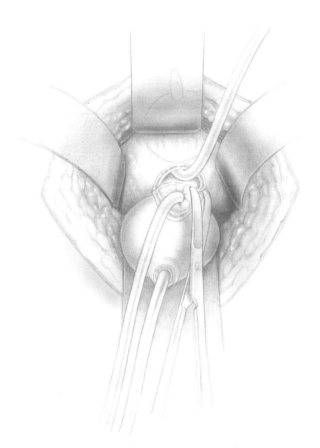

Figure 27.26 Separation of the dorsal part of the bladder neck with Satinsky scissors (only incise dorsally, to avoid damage to the trigone).

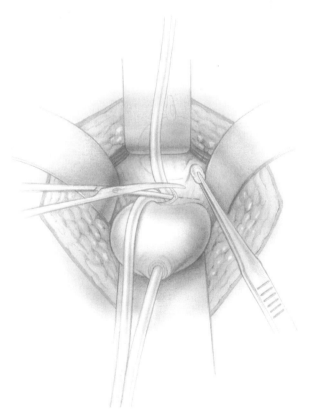

Figure 27.25 The ventral aspect of the bladder neck is opened.

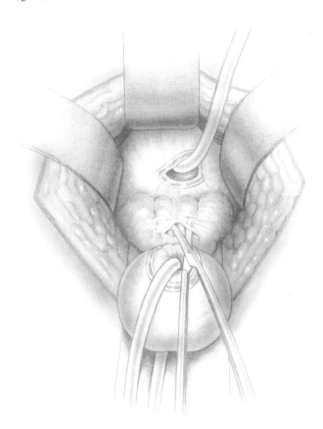

Figure 27.27 Visualization of the seminal vesicles.

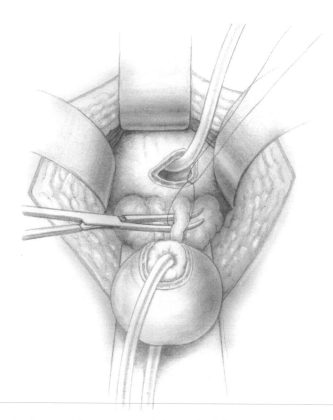

Figure 27.28 Separation and division of both ducts.

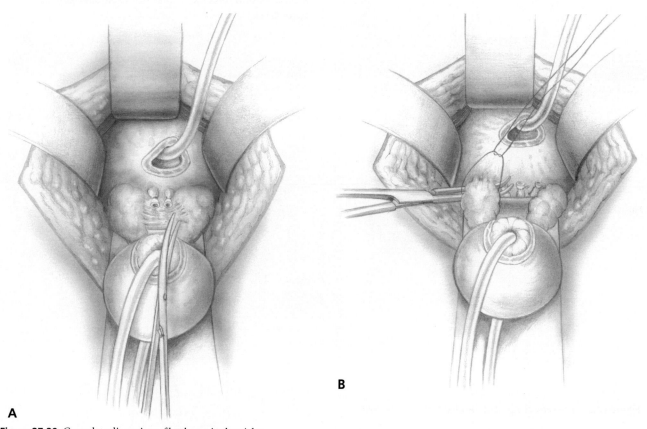

A

B

Figure 27.29 Complete dissection of both seminal vesicles.

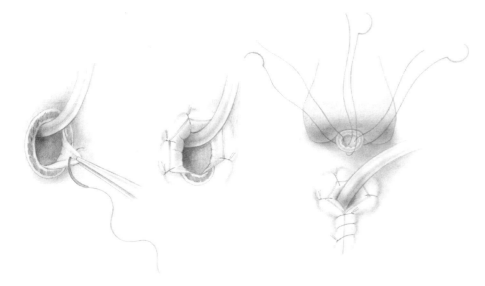

Figure 27.30 Eversion of the bladder mucosa and reconstruction of the bladder neck.

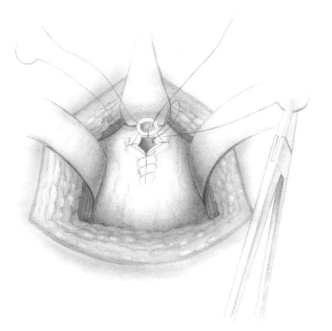

Figure 27.31 Anastomosis of the three ventrally placed sutures.

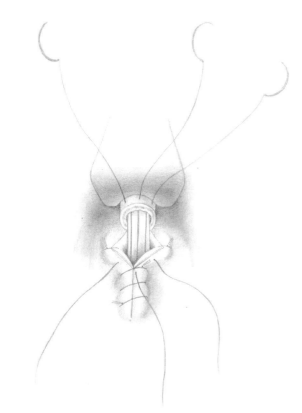

Figure 27.32 Anastomosis of the dorsal circumference of the urethra with three or four sutures.

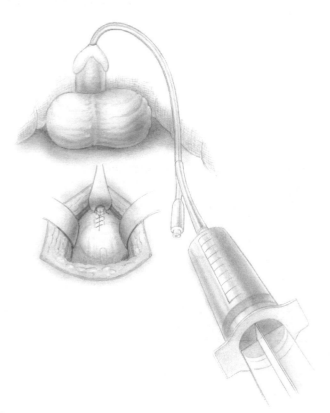

Figure 27.33 The anastomosis is checked to see if it is watertight after instillation of 300–400 cm³ of saline.

Figure 27.35 Wound closure after placement of a drainage tube.

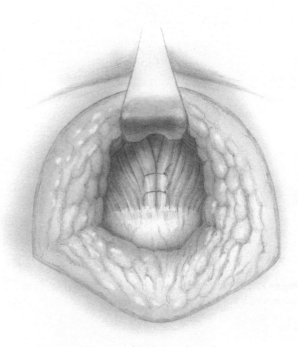

Figure 27.34 Approximation of the levator branches.

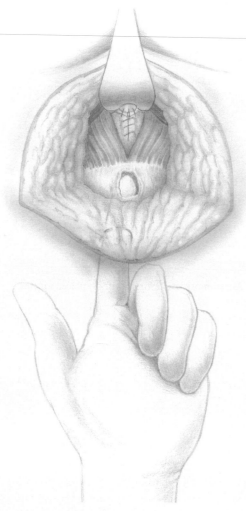

Figure 27.36 Rectal digital control to exclude rectal injury (when rectal injury is noted see Fig. 27.37).

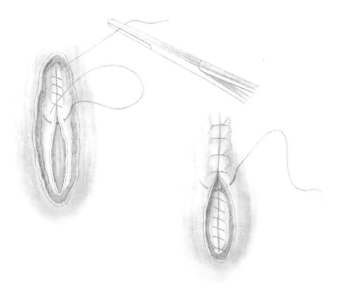

Figure 27.37 Primary two-layer closure (6/0 mucosa running, 5/0 seromuscular interrupted sutures).

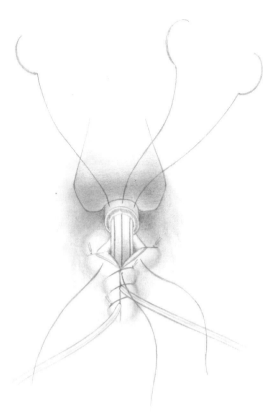

Figure 27.39 The stent is brought out through the reconstructed bladder neck.

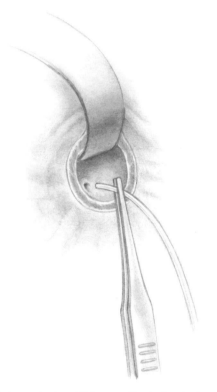

Figure 27.38 A stent is placed if the resection is close to the ureteral orifice.

Chapter 28
Use of Intraoperative Methylene Blue Staining (IMBS) in Nerve-Sparing Perineal Radical Prostatectomy

M. Lodde and A. Pycha

Introduction

Developed by Ehrlich (1885) as the so-called 'supravital staining method' used to identify peripheral nerves in cadaver preparation, intraoperative methylene blue staining (IMBS) is now used in maxillofacial and otorhinopharyngeal surgery. Identification of the pelvic ganglion by IMBS and preservation of bladder function was demonstrated later on in pelvic surgery. IMBS also facilitates the identification of the neurovascular bundle (NVB) for experienced surgeons and to teach residents in nerve-sparing radical perineal prostatectomy.

Methylene blue (a guanylate cyclase inhibitor) is well known in emergency medicine and is cheap and has no adverse side effects. The technique is easy to perform and is reproducible.

Operative technique

The first steps follow the standard technique of Young [2].
• After incision of the posterior layer of Denonvilliers' fascia at the level of the bulbi ductus deferentis, the seminal vesicles are prepared.
• The part of Denonvilliers' fascia that covers the prostate is incised in the middle line. Caution should be taken to avoid causing a lesion to the NVB located laterally and between the anterior and posterior layer of the fascia.
• Methylene blue is then put on the tissue of interest using a little swab. After 2 min the color is washed out by saline solution. Nerves and vessels remain deep blue in color, in contrast to the surrounding tissue, which returns to its normal color or to a light blue.
• The identified NVB is then isolated using the harmonic scalpel, as far as the urethra.
• This is followed by division of the prostatic pedicles.
• The urethra is divided preserving the laterally attached NVBs.

• Standard preparation is continued and a urethrovesical anastomosis is performed.

Tips

• Use the original concentration of methylene blue.
• Use a swab fully soaked with methylene blue.
• Color the tissue with the swab.
• Wait 2 min and then clean the tissue with saline solution.
• If the blue is bleached after 30–60 min repeat the same procedure if needed.

Results

Deep blue staining of the NVB occurred in all 33 patients. In comparison with the initial identification, a broad spectrum of discrepancies were registered. Connective tissue and topographic anatomical variations were the major causes of misinterpretation in this training program.
The initial identification, as performed by the resident, could only be confirmed by IMBS in 12 patients (36%).

References

1 Lang J. Neuroanatomy of the optic, trigeminal, facial, gonopharyngeal, vagus, accessory and hypogonadal nerves. Arch Otorhinolaryngol 1981;231:1–69.
2 Young HH. The early diagnosis and radical cure of carcinoma of the prostate—a study of 40 cases and presentation of a radical operation that was carried out in 4 cases. Johns Hopkins Hosp Bull 1905;16:315.

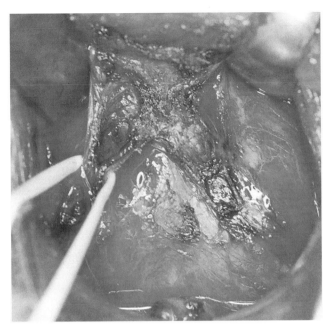

Figure 28.1 A deep blue stained right neurovascular bundle armed by a vessel loop. (For color, see Plate 28.1, between pp. 112 and 113.)

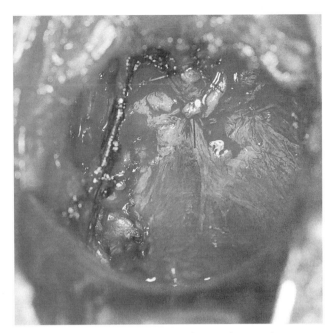

Figure 28.3 The final situation. (For color, see Plate 28.3.)

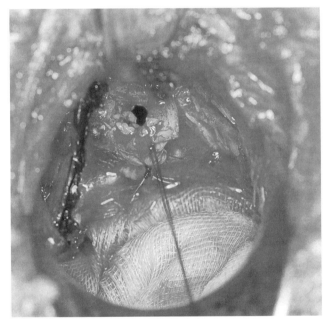

Figure 28.2 The resected left neurovascular bundle. (For color, see Plate 28.2.)

Chapter 29

Nerve-Sparing Endoscopic Extraperitoneal Radical Prostatectomy

J.-U. Stolzenburg

Introduction

Laparoscopic radical prostatectomy (LRPE) has become the operative procedure of choice for patients with clinically localized prostate cancers in selected and specialized urological centers around the globe [1,2]. The technique was developed in an attempt to duplicate the high success rates achieved with retropubic and perineal prostatectomy while offering the advantages of minimally invasive laparoscopy. However, a major drawback of LRPE is the transperitoneal route of access to the extraperitoneal organ of the prostate. The principal disadvantages of LRPE are potential intraperitoneal complications, such as ileus, bowel injury, intraperitoneal bleeding, intraperitoneal urinary leakage, or postoperative adhesion formation, and concomitant small bowel obstruction. Endoscopic extraperitoneal radical prostatectomy (EERPE) is a further advancement of minimal invasive surgery as it overcomes the limitations of LRPE by using the strictly extraperitoneal route of access, combining the advantages of minimal invasive surgery with the advantages of an extraperitoneal procedure [3–6].

Indications

The procedure is indicated in localized prostate cancer, although there are no specific selection criteria. Experienced surgeons only should deal with patients with a prior hernia repair with mesh placement.

Contraindications

• Absolute contraindications for laparoscopy in general are those associated with increased intra-abdominal and intra-thoracic pressure: serious cardiac conditions (intracardiac shunts, severe aortic or mitral valve insufficiency), severe cardiac insufficiency (NYHA III–IV), or high intracranial and intraocular pressure (risk of intracranial or retinal hemorrhage).
• Uncorrected coagulopathy.

• Moderate cardiac insufficiency or obstructive lung diseases are relative contraindications depending on the individual condition of the patient.

Preoperative management

• Both oral bowel preparation and an enema are used the day before the operation.
• Cross-matching of blood is optional.
• Intravenous single dose antibiotic at induction.

Anesthesia

General anesthesia. Invasive intraoperative monitoring (central line, invasive arterial blood pressure monitoring) is unnecessary.

Special instruments/suture material

• Standard laparoscopic tower: high flow (carbon dioxide) insufflator, monitor, camera (Olympus VISERA camera OTV-S7), light source CLV-S40, video laparoscope (EndoEye) with 0° optic 10 mm for a VISERA control unit OTV-S7V-B set, and SonoSurg G2 generator (ultrasonic surgical system).
• Trocars: 1 × Ballontrokar PDB 1000 (Tyco), 1 × Hassan-type optical trocar, 1 × 12 mm trocar with converter (downsizer), and 3 × 5.5 mm trocars insulated with thread.
• Instruments (Olympus): 2 × dissection forceps (HiQ+, 5 × 330 mm straight), 1 × grasping forceps (HiQ+, 5 × 330 mm), 1 × grasping forceps (HiQ+, 5 × 330 mm, wave type), 1 × laparoscopic Metzenbaum scissors, 1 × SonoSurg scissors (5 mm), 1 × bipolar forceps (Ethicon), 1 × needle holder, and 1 × Endo-Bag.

Operative technique

• The patient is placed in a dorsal supine position with a 10–15° head-down tilt and a Foley catheter inserted.
• A 15 mm right infraumbilical incision—a stab incision of

the anterior rectus fascia — is followed by horizontal extension of this incision with scissors and retractors, parting the right rectus muscle with the retractors and blunt finger dissection of the preperitoneal space along the posterior rectus sheath.

• Balloon trocar dilatation is performed under direct visual control (landmark: epigastric vessels).

• Stay sutures are placed on either end of the anterior rectus sheath incision.

• The balloon trocar is exchanged for an optical trocar (Hassan type), with CO_2 insufflation (pressure 12 mmHg) of the preperitoneal space.

• The second trocar (5 mm) is placed two finger-breadths left lateral to the midline, one-third of the distance from the umbilicus to the pubic symphysis (roughly 3–4 cm below the umbilicus).

• All subsequent trocars placed in a line between the umbilicus and the anterior superior iliac spine.

• Two 5 mm trocars are placed in the right side of the abdomen: trocar number 3 is two finger-breadths medial to the right superior iliac spine and trocar number 4 is on the right pararectal line (beware of the epigastric vessels).

• Operating bimanually through trocars number 3 and 4, the dissection is continued into the left preperitoneal space. Follow the pubic arch from right to left and then identify the iliac vessels and spermatic cord. Dissect underneath the epigastric vessels.

• Trocar number 5 (12 mm) is placed three finger-breadths medial to the left superior iliac spine.

• If indicated, pelvic lymph node dissection is performed as a staging procedure within the following anatomical landmarks: the external iliac vessels (lateral border), bifurcation of the common iliac artery (cranial border), the pubic bone (caudal border), and the obturator nerve (posterior border).

• Incise the endopelvic fascia at both sides.

• Section the puboprostatic ligaments, exposing the dorsal vein complex and the urethra.

• Ligate the dorsal vein plexus.

• Anterior bladder neck dissection: start at 12 o'clock at the tip of the triangle formed by folding the bladder tissue over the prostate; enlarge and deepen the incision from 10 to 2 o'clock; identify the longitudinal musculature of the bladder neck; open the bladder neck mucosa anteriorly; and retrieve and fix the catheter into the retropubic space.

• Lateral bladder neck dissection: dissection is continued laterally in the plane between the bladder neck and prostate (visualizing the bladder mucosa for orientation).

• In nerve-sparing procedures incise the thin fascia overlying the anterolateral aspect of the prostate.

• Dorsal bladder neck dissection: complete dissection of the dorsal bladder neck in a straight dorsal direction to avoid intraprostatic extension.

• Identify both ampullary portions of the vasa deferentia as anatomical landmarks.

• Incise the thin anterior layer of Denonvilliers' fascia and section the vasa deferentia.

• Free the seminal vesicles.

• Make a horizontal incision of the posterior layer of Denonvilliers' fascia, freeing the prerectal fatty tissue from medial to lateral at the dorsal surface of the prostate.

• Separate the neurovascular bundles and dissect the prostatic pedicles.

• Apical dissection in stages: (i) divide the dorsal vein plexus; (ii) divide the anterior urethral wall (external striated sphincter); and (iii) identify, preserve, and open the longitudinal smooth muscle layer of the urethra anteriorly. Cut the lateral wall of urethra, identify the urethral crest, and finally cut the dorsal wall.

• The specimen is placed into an Endo-Bag, positioned at the left iliac fossa.

• Urethrovesical anastomosis: the first stitch is placed at the 8 o'clock position (backhand: bladder neck; backhand: urethra) followed by stitches at the 7, 6, and 5 o'clock positions (forehand, backhand), and the 4 o'clock position (forehand, forehand).

• Place the catheter into the bladder.

• Two further sutures are placed at the 3 and 9 o'clock positions.

• Bladder neck reconstruction at a 12 o'clock position if necessary.

• The final two anastomotic sutures are placed at 11 and 1 o'clock (left side: backhand, backhand; right side: forehand, forehand).

• Check the water tightness of the anastomosis and placement of the drainage.

• Remove the prostate via trocar number 5 in the left iliac fossa. The skin and fascia are enlarged depending on the size of the prostate.

• Closure of the fascia is necessary for the sites of trocar number 1 (optic trocar) and 5 (left iliac fossa specimen extraction site). All the other port sites require skin closure only.

Tips

• In cases of a large middle lobe or prior extensive transurethral resection of the prostate, the insertion of double-J catheters is helpful to avoid injury of the ureteral orifices intraoperatively.

• The use of ultrasound devices (e.g. SonoSurg, Olympus, Winter & IBE, Hamburg, Germany) makes procedures such as bladder neck dissection, sectioning the vasa deferentia, freeing the seminal vesicles, and prostatic pedicles dissection easier and quicker. If hemostasis is incomplete use bipolar forceps.

• The neurovascular bundles are completely separated from the prostate during the prostatic pedicle dissection with the help of the ultrasound devices. Alternatively, small vessels can be divided between endoclips.

• Do not use monopolar current in neurovascular bundle

separation and apical dissection. (We do not use monopolar diathermy at all in our department.)

Postoperative care

The drain is removed 24–48 h after the procedure and the catheter is removed on day 5 or 6.

Complications

Anastomotic leakage is rare if the correct technique of anastomosis is used and can be managed by prolonging the period of catheterization.

Troubleshooting

- *Injury of epigastric vessels* (mostly caused by incorrect trocar placement into the right pararectal line): use coagulation, clips, or suturing (long and straight needles, stitch from the outside into the preperitoneal space and return, with extracorporal knot tying; cut the suture 2 days later).
- *Trocar placement in patients with extensive adhesions of the preperitoneal space* (prior multiple surgeries in the lower abdomen including hernia repair with mesh placement): a partial intraperitonealization of the procedure is helpful. The adherent peritoneum is incised along a length of 2–3 cm to make the placement of the lateral trocars possible under visual control.
- *Reduced preperitoneal space*: check that there is sufficient muscle relaxation of the patient with anesthesiologist (a peritoneal injury with resulting capnoperitoneum alone does not minimize the preperitoneal space).
- *Bleeding Santorini plexus*: short-term increase of CO_2 pressure to 18 mmHg and (extensive) bipolar coagulation.
- *Rectal injury*: double layer suturing laparoscopically.
- *Postoperative lymphocele after drainage removal*: if asymptomatic, use antibiotic prophylaxis (for 2–3 weeks); and if symptomatic, use ultrasound-guided puncture or drainage for 3–5 days. Laparoscopic fenestration if the problem persists.

Results

- $n = 500$.
- Mean operative time = 140 min, including lymphadenectomy, in 232 patients.
- No conversion.
- Transfusion rate = 0.8%.
- Mean time of catheterization = 6.6 days.
- Positive surgical margin rate: 9% (pT2), 30% (pT3).
- Continence rate (no pad): 37% (on day 10), 74% (after 3 months), and 86% (after 6 months).
- Major complications: three early reinterventions (two for bleeding, and one for preperitoneal hematoma), five late reinterventions (four for fenestrations of lymphocele, one for colostomy caused by rectal fistula, and one for bladder neck incision caused by anastomotic stricture).

References

1 Guillonneau B, el-Fettouh H, Baumert H *et al*. Laparoscopic radical prostatectomy: oncological evaluation after 1,000 cases in a Montsouris Institute. J Urol 2003;169:1261–6.
2 Guillonneau B, Vallancien G. Laparoscopic radical prostatectomy: the Montsouris technique. J Urol 2000;163:1643–9.
3 Stolzenburg JU, Do M, Pfeiffer H, König F, Aedtner B, Dorschner W. The endoscopic extraperitoneal radical prostatectomy (EERPE): technique and initial experience. World J Urol 2002;20: 48–50.
4 Stolzenburg JU, Do M, Rabenalt R *et al*. Endoscopic extraperitoneal radical prostatectomy (EERPE) — initial experience after 70 procedures. J Urol 2003;169:2066–71.
5 Stolzenburg JU, Truss MC, Bekos A *et al*. Does the extraperitoneal laparoscopic approach improve the outcome of radical prostatectomy? Curr Urol Rep 2004;5:115–22.
6 Stolzenburg JU, Truss MC, Do M *et al*. Evolution of endoscopic extraperitoneal radical prostatectomy (EERPE)–technical improvements and development of a nerve-sparing, potency-preserving approach. World J Urol 2003;21:147–52.

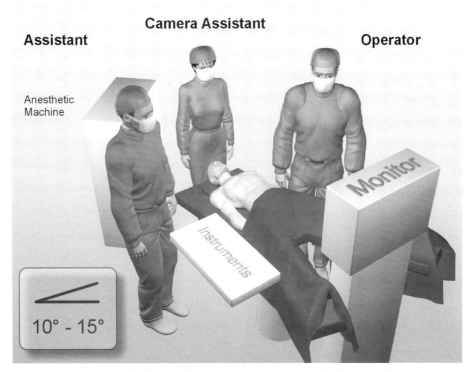

Figure 29.1 Room set-up for EERPE. The straddled legs of the patient make placement of the laparoscopic tower closer to the surgeon's eye level possible.

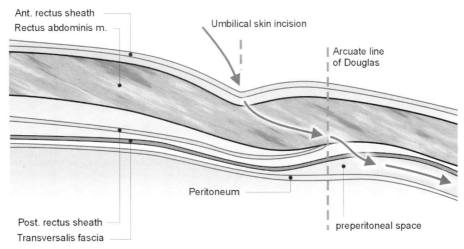

Figure 29.2 Dissection of the preperitoneal space.

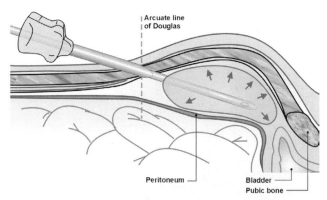

Figure 29.3 Preparation of the preperitoneal space by balloon trocar insufflation.

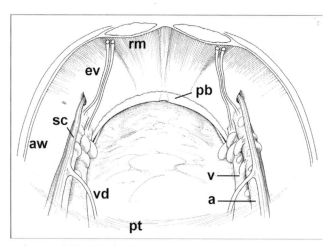

Figure 29.5 Anatomical landmarks of the preperitoneal space: a, external iliac artery; aw, abdominal wall; ev, epigastric vessels; pb, pubic bone; pt, peritoneum; rm, rectus muscle; sc, spermatic cord; v, external iliac vein; vd, vas deferens.

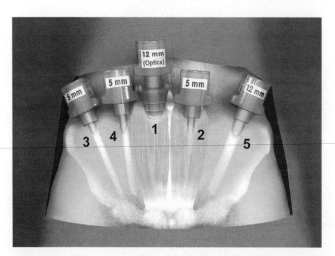

Figure 29.4 The sequence of placement of trocars for EERPE. In extremely obese or very tall patients, all trocars should be placed 1–3 cm caudally for optimal access to the retropubic space.

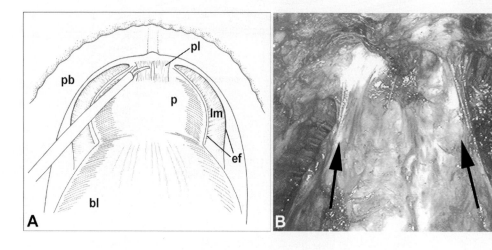

Figure 29.6 Exposure of the bladder neck, incision of the endopelvic fascia, and dissection of the puboprostatic ligaments. bl, bladder; ef, endopelvic fascia (dissected); lm, levator ani muscle; p, prostate; pb, pubic bone; pl, puboprostatic ligaments (arrows). (For color, see Plate 29.6, between pp. 112 and 113.)

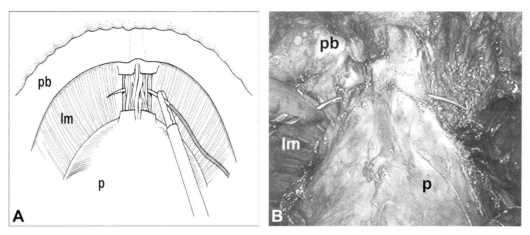

Figure 29.7 Ligation of the Santorini plexus (0/0 Vicryl, MH+ needle). Alternatively, the dorsal vein complex can be dissected with Ultracision® or the SonoSurg ultrasound device without prior ligation during the apical dissection. For abbreviations, see Fig. 29.6. (For color, see Plate 29.7, between pp. 112 and 113.)

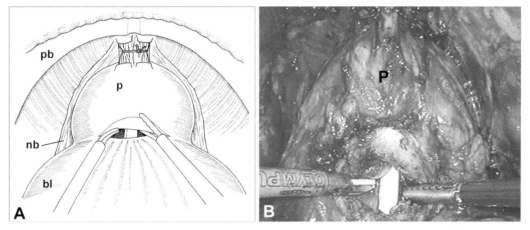

Figure 29.8 Anterior bladder neck dissection. The bladder neck overlaps the prostate in the shape of a triangle. The dissection starts at a 12 o'clock position at the tip of this triangle. For abbreviations, see Fig. 29.6; nb, neurovascular bundles. (For color, see Plate 29.8.)

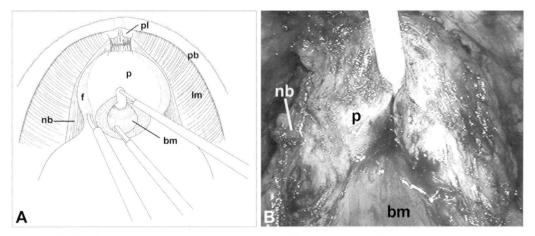

Figure 29.9 Incision of the thin fascia overlaying the anteriolateral aspect of the prostate to mobilize the neurovascular bundles before sectioning of the dorsal bladder neck. bm, bladder mucosa; f, fascia; lm, levator ani muscle; nb, neurovascular bundles; p, prostate; pb, pubic bone; pl, puboprostatic ligaments (dissected). (For color, see Plate 29.9.)

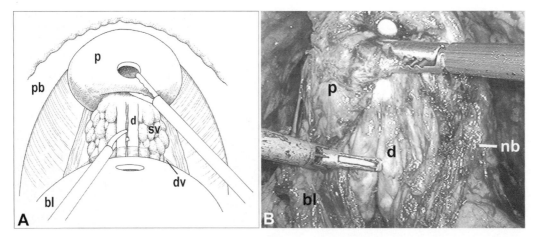

Figure 29.10 Sectioning of the ampullary portions of the vasa deferentia. The prostate is elevated anteriorly in the direction of the symphysis by the assistant. bl, bladder; d, ampulla of vas deferens; dv, anterior Denonvilliers' fascia (dissected); nb, neurovascular bundles; p, prostate; pb, pubic bone; sv, seminal vesicle. (For color, see Plate 29.10, between pp. 112 and 113.)

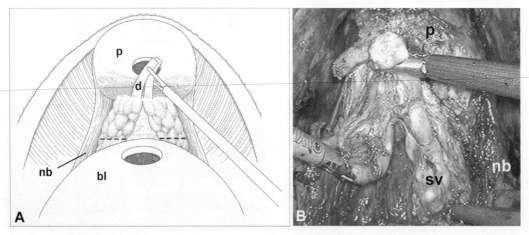

Figure 29.11 Dissection of the seminal vesicles. Traction on the vasa deferentia (by the assistant) is helpful to identify the seminal vesicles in a slightly lateral and caudal direction. The seminal vesicle are completely dissected or cut along the interrupted line to preserve the bundles lying very close to the tip of the seminal vesicles. For abbreviations, see Fig. 29.10. (For color, see Plate 29.11.)

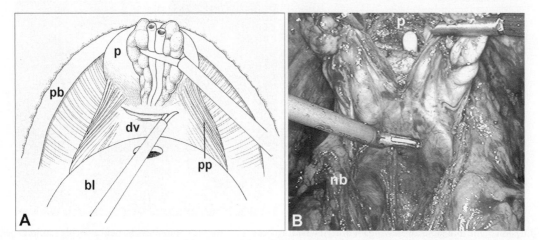

Figure 29.12 Incision of the posterior Denonvilliers' fascia. For abbreviations, see Fig. 29.10; dv, posterior Denonvilliers' fascia; pp, prostate pedicle. (For color, see Plate 29.12.)

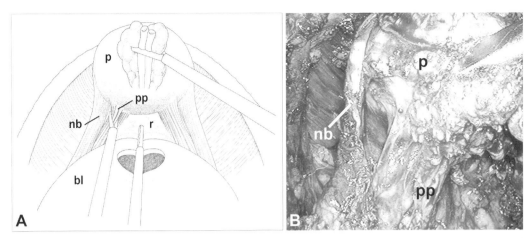

Figure 29.13 Dissection of the cranial prostatic pedicles with preservation of the neurovascular bundles. During preparation of the left side the assistant retracts the prostate to the right side; during preparation and dissection on the right side the surgeon retracts the prostate to the left. For abbreviations, see Fig. 29.10; pp, prostate pedicle; r, rectum (prerectal fatty tissue). (For color, see Plate 29.13, between pp. 112 and 113.)

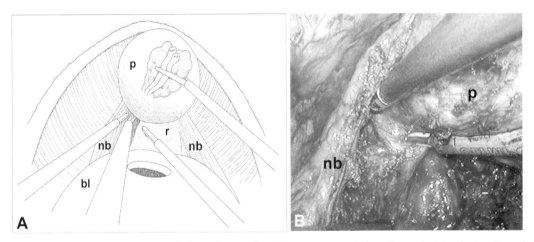

Figure 29.14 Dissection of the caudal prostatic pedicles and separation of the neurovascular bundles on the left side. For abbreviations, see Fig. 29.10; r, rectum (prerectal fatty tissue). (For color, see Plate 29.14.)

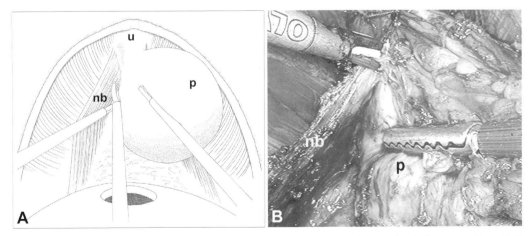

Figure 29.15 Preparation of the neurovascular bundles close to the apex of the prostate and the urethra is done anterolaterally, in contrast to the dorsal preparation at the base of the prostate. The assistant pulls the prostate to the right side for preparation of the left neurovascular bundle and vice versa. nb, neurovascular bundles; p, prostate; u, urethra. (For color, see Plate 29.15.)

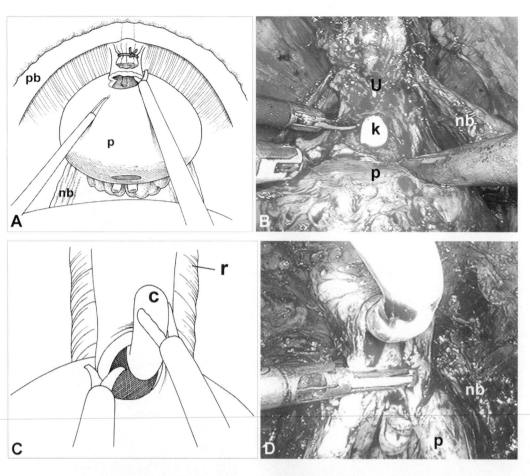

Figure 29.16 Apical dissection: sectioning the Santorini plexus, the external sphincter, and the urethra ventrally (A and B) and dorsally (C and D). c, catheter; nb, neurovascular bundles; p, prostate; pb, pubic bone; r, rectum. (For color, see Plate 29.16, between pp. 112 and 113.)

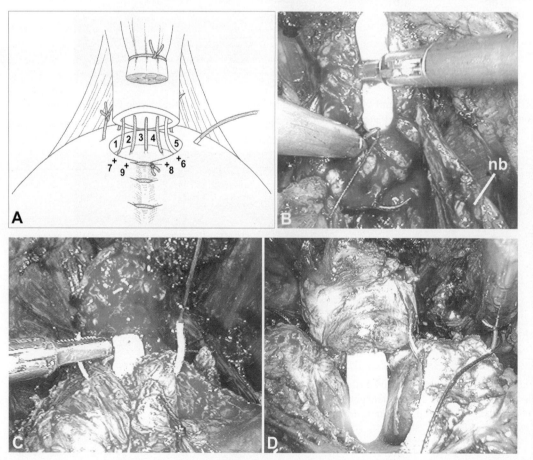

Figure 29.17 Urethrovesical anastomosis (interrupted sutures, 2/0 Vicryl, UR-6 needle). (A) The stitches are always performed 'outside–in' at the bladder neck and 'inside–out' at the urethra, and always tied extraluminally in the given order (1–9). (B) Technique of the dorsal anastomosis. (C) In the case of a nonbladder-neck-preserving procedure, the bladder neck is reconstructed at a 12 o'clock position. (D) Anterolateral and ventral anastomosis is performed with an inserted catheter. nb, neurovascular bundles. (For color, see Plate 29.17.)

Chapter 30
Laparoscopic Radical Prostatectomy Technique

A. P. Steinberg and I. S. Gill

Introduction

In 1997, Schuessler *et al.* described the first series of nine patients who underwent laparoscopic radical prostatectomy (LRP) but the authors were discouraged by lengthy operative times [7]. The French team of Guillonneau and Vallencien ultimately pioneered the technique, reducing it to an efficient, day-to-day practice [6]. Other European teams have since added to the overall experience of LRP [1] and have confirmed the feasibility and efficacy of LRP in terms of both early oncologic outcome and postoperative functional status. At the Cleveland Clinic, we have developed the technique to bring it in line with the principles of open radical retropubic prostatectomy as performed in the United States today.

Indications

Patients need to fulfill criteria for undergoing laparoscopy and criteria for undergoing prostatectomy (clinically localized prostate cancer).

Contraindications

The surgical treatment of advanced stages of cancer (T3, T4) remains controversial. Prior hormonal treatment (androgen blockade) or localized radiation therapy will raise the level of difficulty of the procedure and increase the potential for operative morbidity. Other relative contraindications include multiple abdominal surgeries, morbid obesity, and uncorrected coagulopathy.

Preoperative management

- On the day prior to surgery, the patient is started on a diet of clear fluids and instructed to drink two bottles of magnesium citrate.
- Parenteral antibiotic prophylaxis (first generation cephalosporin).
- Bilateral sequential compression devices.

Operative technique

Anterior transperitoneal technique

- The patient is placed in a modified lithotomy (thighs abducted) position with the arms adducted by the side.
- A Foley catheter (22 Fr) is inserted.
- Primary port placement (12 mm) is infraumbilical. In total, five laparoscopic ports are used in an inverted V shape.
- Pelvic lymph node dissection (only when indicated; prostate-specific antigen (PSA) $\geq$ 10, Gleason score $\geq$ 8, large volume tumors or stage $\geq$ T3).
- The bladder is distended with 200 mL of saline.
- An inverted U-shaped peritoneotomy is made to enter the space of Retzius.
- The endopelvic fascia is incised bilaterally, leaving the puboprostatic ligaments intact.
- The Foley catheter is replaced by a metallic urethral dilator (22 Fr).
- Ligate the dorsal venous complex with two passes of 2/0 Vicryl on a CT-1 needle.
- A similar stitch is placed over the base of the prostate (back bleeding stitch).
- The anterior and posterior bladder necks are sequentially incised with J-hook electrocautery.
- The posterior plane is dissected with electrocautery until the vasa are visualized.
- Vas deferens and seminal vesicles dissection: the vasa are clipped and transected. With continuous traction on the vasa, the seminal vesicles are freed. A harmonic scalpel is used to dissect the lateral border of the seminal vesicles. The vesicular artery is secured with a hemolock (Weck) clip.
- The Denonvilliers' fascia is incised beyond the seminal vesicles.
- Transect the lateral pedicles with an Endo-GIA (non-nerve sparing) or clips and harmonic scalpel (nerve sparing).
- Transect the dorsal vein complex, urethra, and apical dissection. The dorsal vein complex is transected with J-hook electrocautery or a harmonic scalpel. If bleeding begins, a figure-of-eight stitch is placed. Urethral transection and

prostatic apical dissection is performed using sharp dissection.
- The specimen is placed in an Endo-Catch bag.
- The bladder neck is reconstructed in a 'tennis racket' fashion, if necessary.
- Urethrovesical anastomosis: two-stitch running method using 2/0 Vicryl stitches on UR-6 needles. The first stitch starts at 5 o'clock and runs in a clockwise direction until the 11 o'clock position. The urethral dilator has a hollowed tip and is used to guide the needle into the urethral stump. At this point the dilator is replaced by a 22 Fr Foley catheter. The second stitch is placed at 5 o'clock and runs in a counterclockwise direction.
- Alternatively, two 25 cm lengths of 2/0 Monocryl (UR-6 needle) are tied together at the tips. Both needles are passed outside–in at the bladder neck (6 o'clock). The ends are then run in opposite directions and tied to each other at 12 o'clock.
- The specimen is extracted through a circumumbilical extension of the primary port site.
- A Jackson–Pratt drain is placed through a port site, and the remaining port sites are closed.

Nerve-sparing modifications

- In order to minimize trauma to the neurovascular bundle (NVB), we use no thermal energy near the tip of the seminal vesicles. Instead, a hemostatic locking clip (Weck clip) is used to secure the vesicular artery.
- The lateral prostate fascia is incised superficially with 'cold' endoshears to release the tethering of the NVB.
- The lateral pedicles are controlled by clipping (Weck clip) and cold cutting or with a harmonic scalpel.
- The tissue lateral to the urethra, which contains the NVB, is dissected off the urethra and apex prior to urethral transection. Additionally, dissection distal to the prostate apex is minimized, so as to better preserve this nerve-rich, sphincter-active zone.

Tips

- Bladder neck dissection: by tenting the dorsal vein stitch towards the symphysis pubis, the prostate is displaced anteriorly and the bladder is seen tethered posteriorly. This aids in identifying where the perivesical fat ends, signifying the prostatovesical junction. Repeated in-and-out movements of the urethral dilator can aid in visualization of the bladder neck.
- Ligation of the dorsal venous complex: contact of the needle and dilator alerts the surgeon that the stitch is placed through the urethra.
- To improve postoperative continence, retropubic urethropexy is performed by suspending the sutures to the puboprostatic ligaments above.

Postoperative care

The hospital stay is, on average, between 1 and 2 days. A cystogram is performed on the third postoperative day. If there is no anastomotic leak, the Foley catheter can be removed. If contrast extravasation is noted, the Foley catheter is left for drainage and the cystogram is repeated in 1 week.

Results

- *Intraoperative data*:
  - At the Cleveland Clinic, our first 50 cases averaged 5.4 h, while the next 100 cases averaged 3.7 h [8]. Our current operative times range from 2 to 3.5 h.
  - In a pooled analysis of 1228 patients undergoing LRP at six European centers, the average blood loss was 488 mL with a transfusion rate of 3.5% [9].
- *Postoperative recovery*: hospital stay after LRP at the Cleveland Clinic has decreased to an average of 1.5 days [8], and following discharge from the hospital only two patients (4%) required narcotics [10]. By 2 weeks postoperatively, 68% of patients reported they could return to work.
- *Perioperative complications*:
  - At the Cleveland Clinic, a major complication rate of 6% was reported in the first 50 cases: pulmonary embolism with death (one patient), rectal injury (one patient), and ureteral injury (one patient). Minor complications were seen in 14% of cases: shoulder abrasion (two patients), prolonged (1 week) urinary drainage (two patients), paralytic ileus (two patients), and port-site hematoma (one patient) [10].
  - Similarly, Guillonneau *et al.* reported 3.7% major and 14.6% minor complication rates in a review of 567 patients undergoing LRP [5].
- *Oncologic control*:
  - Surgical pathology: Guillonneau *et al.* examined 1000 consecutive patients who underwent LRP and reported positive surgical margins in 6.9, 18.6, 30, and 34% for pathologic stages pT2a, pT2b, pT3a, and pT3b, respectively [4].
  - Biochemical (PSA) recurrence: the overall actuarial biochemical progression-free survival rate, in the group above, was 90.5% at 3 years [4].
- *Urinary continence*: Guillonneau *et al.*, using self-administered questionnaires reported on their first 133 patients with a 1 year or greater follow-up [2]. Total continence (no protection needed during day or night) was reported in 85.5% of patients with another 10.7% wearing only one pad per 24 h. Five patients (3.8%) were classified as severely incontinent.
- *Potency*: Guillonneau *et al.* reviewed 73 patients who had either bilateral (46 patients) or unilateral (27 patients) nerve-sparing LRP with a follow-up ranging from 2 to 12 months [3]. An impressive 74% spontaneous erection rate was reported in

the bilateral nerve-sparing group and 51% in the unilateral group.

References

1 Abbou CC, Salomon L, Hoznek A *et al.* Laparoscopic radical prostatectomy: preliminary results. Urology 2000;55:630.

2 Guillonneau B, Cathelineau X, Doublet JD *et al.* Laparoscopic radical prostatectomy: the lessons learned. J Endourol 2001;15:441.

3 Guillonneau B, Cathelineau X, Doublet JD *et al.* Prospective assessment of functional results after laparoscopic radical prostatectomy. J Urol 2001;165(Suppl):614A.

4 Guillonneau B, El-Fettouh H, Baumert H *et al.* Laparoscopic radical prostatectomy: oncological evaluation after 1,000 cases in a Montsouris Institute. J Urology 2003;169:1261–6.

5 Guillonneau B, Rozet F, Cathelineau X *et al.* Perioperative complications of laparoscopic radical prostatectomy: the Montsouris 3-year experience. J Urol 2002;167(1):51.

6 Guillonneau B, Vallancien G. Laparoscopic radical prostatectomy: the Montsouris experience. J Urol 2000;163:418.

7 Schuessler W. Laparoscopic radical prostatectomy: initial short-term experience. Urology 1997;50:854.

8 Steinberg A, Gill I, Farouk A *et al.* 150 laparoscopic radical prostatectomies (LRP): learning curve in the United States. Can J Urol 2002;9:Abstract.

9 Sulser T, Guillonneau B, Gaston R *et al.* Complications and initial experience with 1228 laparoscopic radical prostatectomies at 6 European centers. J Urol 2001;165(Suppl):615A.

10 Zippe CD, Meraney AM, Sung GT *et al.* Laparoscopic radical prostatectomy in the USA: Cleveland Clinic series of 50 patients. J Urol 2001;165(Suppl):1341A.

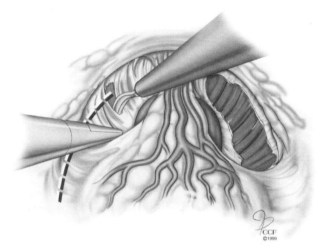

Figure 30.2 Incision of the endopelvic fascia is performed bilaterally until the puboprostatic ligaments are visualized.

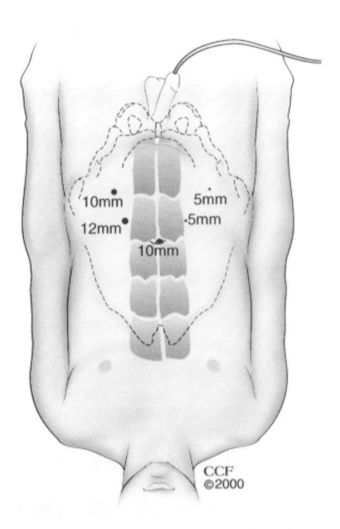

Figure 30.1 Port placement, showing the five-port 'fan array' transperitoneal approach.

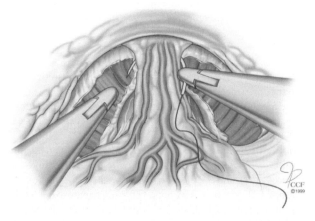

Figure 30.3 Two dorsal vein stitches are placed. Retropubic urethropexy is then performed by suspending these sutures from the puboprostatic ligaments above.

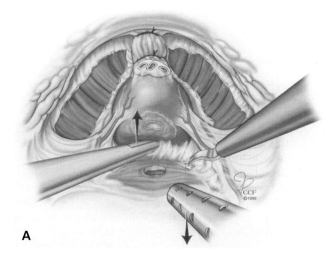

A

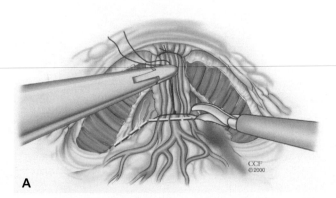

A

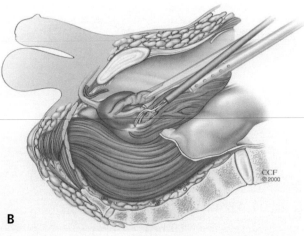

B

Figure 30.5 Dissection of the seminal vesicles. (A) The plane between the posterior base of the prostate and the bladder neck is dissected until the vas deferentia are seen. (B) Sagittal view.

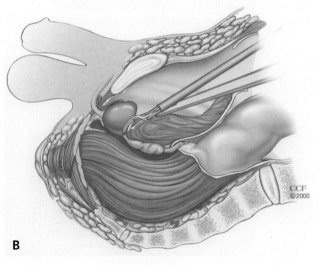

B

Figure 30.4 Transection of the bladder neck. (A) The back bleeding stitch is placed (CT-1 needle, 2/0 Vicryl) and the bladder neck is transected. The dashed line demonstrates the plane of dissection between the base of the prostate and the anterior bladder neck. (B) Sagittal view.

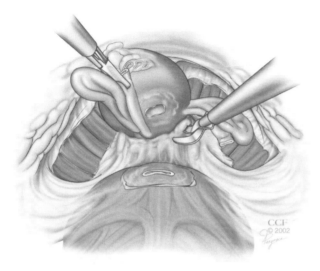

Figure 30.6 Incision of Denonvilliers' fascia. The incision is performed with 'cold' endoshears and extreme care is taken to avoid injury to the rectum.

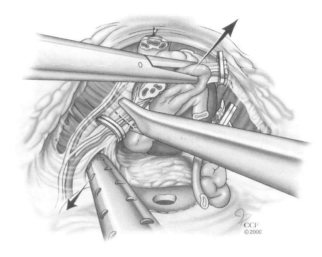

Figure 30.8 Transection of the lateral pedicles (nerve-sparing technique). Meticulous clip ligation and cold cutting or transection with a harmonic scalpel is employed immediately adjacent to the prostate to preserve the neurovascular bundle.

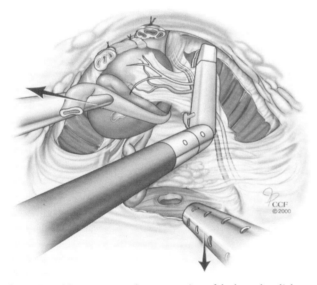

Figure 30.7 Non nerve-sparing transection of the lateral pedicles. The articulating Endo-GIA stapler is used to widely transect the lateral pedicle and neurovascular bundle from the prostate.

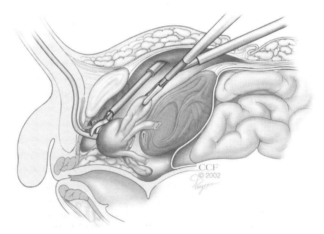

Figure 30.9 Transection of the urethra. Urethral transection and prostatic apical dissection is carefully performed using cold-cutting endoshears.

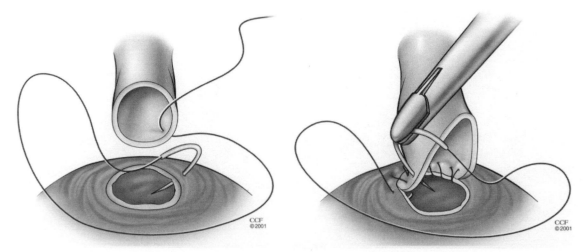

Figure 30.10 First anastomotic stitch. The first stitch starts at 5 o'clock and runs in a clockwise direction until the 11 o'clock position.

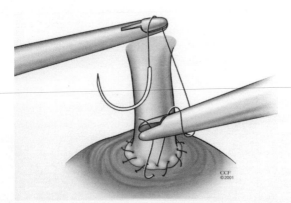

Figure 30.11 Second anastomotic stitch. The two stitch ends are tied at 12 o'clock, allowing immediate watertight approximation.

Section 4
Genitalia

Chapter 31
Anterior Urethral Stricture Repair and Reconstruction of Hypospadia

F. Schreiter and B. Schönberger

Introduction

Anterior urethral strictures may involve the fossa navicularis, the pars pendulans of the urethra, and part of the bulbar urethra. These strictures can be caused by inflammatory disease, including lichen sclerosis or balanitis xerotica obliterans of the corpus spongiosum [1], traumatic scarring after a blunt trauma or traumatic catheterization, long-term indwelling catheter treatment and forced bougination, as well as in congenital anomalies (hypospadias, epispadias, and hypospadia cripples) as a result of multiple previous reconstructions. The use of scrotal or genital skin can lead to hair growing, inflammation, stone formation, and diverticula.

Since the use of buccal mucosa [8] is included in urethral stricture repair, there is a clear tendency for one-stage free graft repairs to occur in pedicle flap procedures [4–7].

Free prepucial grafts of the inner sheet of the foreskin—a moist full-thickness skin graft lacking hair follicles—seem to represent similar good long-term results [2]. The easy harvesting and transfer of the grafts, which are free of hair, may be the greatest advantage.

Hypospadia patients who have undergone multiple previous procedures of urethral reconstruction develop severe scars and present an operative challenge (Fig. 31.1). The problems develop from the absence of healthy tissue that can be used for urethral reconstruction. In those cases a two-stage procedure is recommended, which can either be performed by using buccal mucosa in a two-stage procedure [3] or using a free split skin graft, the so-called two-stage mesh graft procedure [6].

Preoperative management

A complete bowel preparation should be performed the day before surgery. A special liquid diet is recommended. On the day of surgery the genital area and the perineum are shaved.

Special instruments/suture material

- Fine surgical instruments.
- Magnifying glasses 1 : 2.5 to 1 : 3.5.
- Dilatation set up to 30 Fr.
- Bipolar electrocoagulation.
- Submucosal injection (epinephrine 1 : 100,000).
- Scott retractor.
- Cystoscope.
- Suture material: 4/0 to 6/0 absorbable.
- Nonadhesive wound dressing.

One-stage meatoplasty: buccal mucosa or foreskin graft urethroplasty

Indications

This procedure is indicated in short meatal strictures within the glans penis or hypospadia meatal stenosis.

Operative technique (Fig. 31.2)

- The strictures are fully opened.
- A buccal mucosa graft (if available) is harvested from the lower lip or the cheek. If foreskin is available it can be harvested from the inner sheet as well.
- The graft is sutured to the left rim of the opened navicular fossa.
- The graft is rotated over the urethral plate and sutured to the right rim of the glandular urethra with the mucosal or epithelial surface facing the urethra.
- The glans is closed over the graft and a 20 Fr catheter or silicon stent is left in place for 10 days.

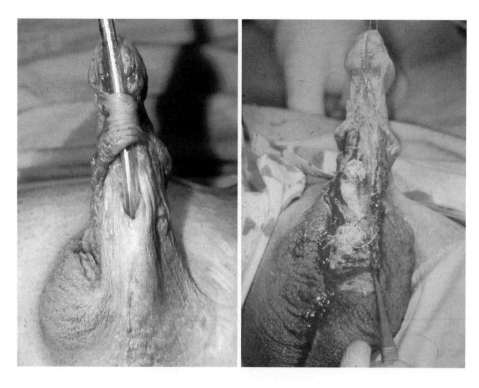

Figure 31.1 Hypospadia patients undergo multiple surgical reconstructions (lack of skin, hair, and stone formations).

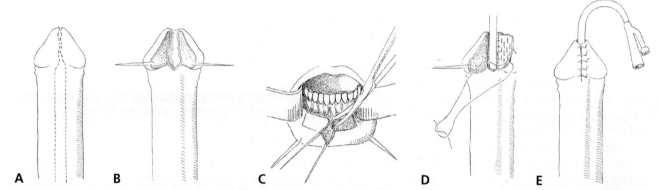

A   B   C   D   E

Figure 31.2 (A) Meatal stricture. (B) Open the meatal stricture until healthy spongious tissue is reached. (C) Harvest the buccal mucosa. (D) Suture the graft to the urethral rim on both sides. (E) The glans is closed over the graft.

One-stage meatoplasty: pedicled flap urethroplasty (Jordan flap)

Indications

The flip-flap technique (Jordan flap) gives excellent cosmetic and functional results. This technique is used for meatal strictures extending beyond the glans penis.

Operative technique (Fig. 31.3)

• The flap is prepared crosswise on the ventral side of the distal penile shaft.

• Open the stricture until healthy tissue of the corpus spongiosum is reached.

• The pedicle has to be prepared as long as the flap can be rotated 90°.

• The rotated flap is sutured to the rim of the urethral plate.

• The penile shaft skin is sutured over the Jordan flap using an asymmetric penile skin flap (Bayar's flap).

• Or, if possible, the edges of the glans are sutured over the Jordan flap.

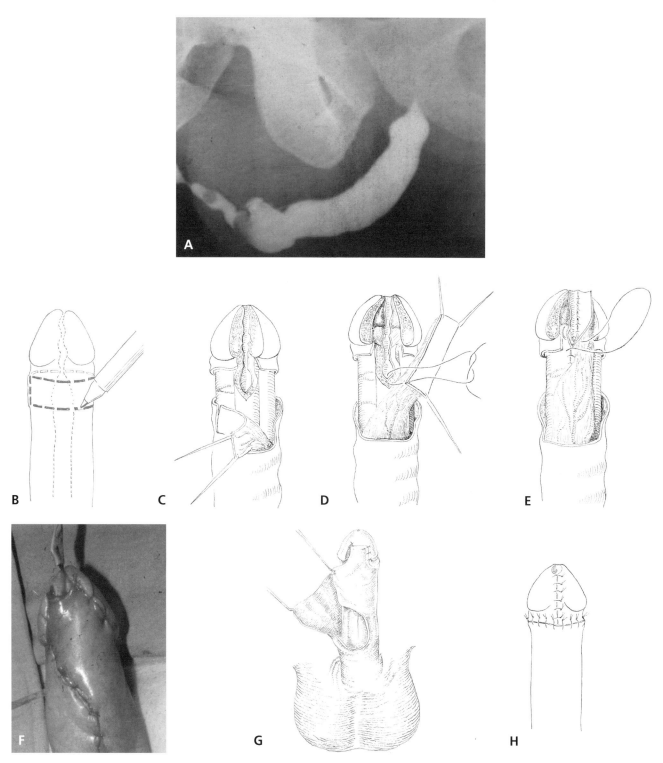

Figure 31.3 (A) Anterior stricture including the meatal part of the urethra. (B) Meatal plasty (Jordan flap): preparation of a broad-based pedicled penile skin flap. (C) The skin island flap is elevated with a long pedicle and the stricture is opened. (D) The flap is rotated and sutured to the rim of the urethra. (E–G) The penile skin and glans are closed over the urethra using a Bayars' flap. (H) If possible, the edges of the glans are covered over the flap and the skin is sutured to the rim of the prepuce.

Pedicled penile flap urethroplasty (Quartey and Orandi–Devine techniques)

Indications

This technique is recommended in patients with extended penile strictures with or without strictures of the fossa navicularis. Enough penile skin has to be available for it to be possible. This technique is used especially for patients who have to avoid harvesting of the buccal mucosa and in circumcised patients. A transverse penile skin flap can be prepared with a long vascularized pedicle that can be rotated 90° and can be pulled through the undermined scrotum to reach the bulbar urethra (Quartey technique). A longitudinal penile flap (Orandi–Devine technique) is easy to prepare with a short pedicle that allows the flap to be rotated with its epithelial surface to the marsupialized urethral plate.

Quartey operative technique (Fig. 31.4)

- Make a midline incision in the raphe of the penis and deglove the penile skin.
- Transversely dissect the penile flap.
- Carefully dissect the tunica dartos pedicle between the two layers of penile skin vessels.
- Split the strictured urethra.
- Trim the flap to the length of the stricture and suture first to the left rim of the stricture and thereafter to the right side of the stricture over a 20 Fr indwelling catheter.
- Cover all the suture lines with the tunica dartos tissue.
- The penis is then covered with the outer penile skin.
- For repair of *bulbar strictures* (Fig. 31.5), the long pedicled flap is pulled through the undermined scrotum.
- The flap is sutured to both rims of the opened urethral stricture using a running 5/0 resorbable suture material.

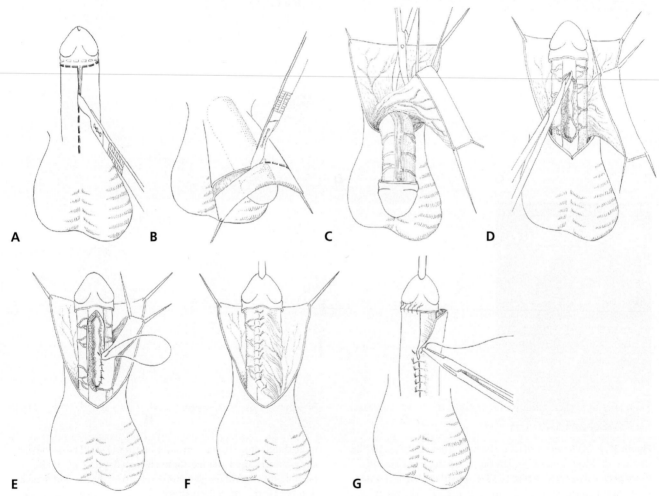

Figure 31.4 (A) Deglove the penile skin and make a midline incision of the skin in the raphe. (B) Transverse dissection of the penile skin flap. (C) Dissection of the tunica dartos pedicle between the two layers of skin vessels. (D) Open the stricture. (E) Rotate the flap over the split urethra and suture to the rims. (F) Cover the suture lines with the tunica dartos pedicle tissue. (G) The penile skin is sutured covering the penile shaft.

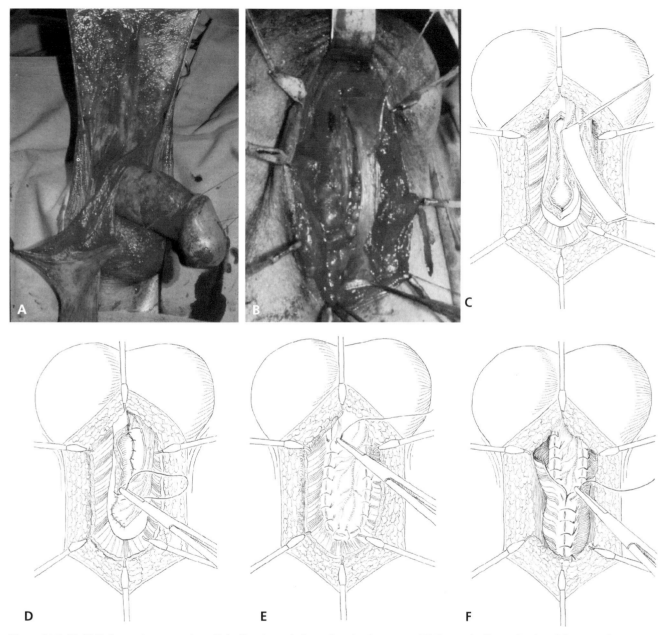

Figure 31.5 (A, B) Bulbar stricture repair: pull the flap through the undermined scrotum. (C) Suture the flap to the rim of the opened stricture. (D, E) Cover the suture lines with the tunica dartos of the pedicle. (F) The urethra is covered using the bulbocavernous muscle.

• The tissue of the pedicle (tunica dartos) is used to cover the sutures of the flap to prevent fistulas.
• Cover the bulbocavernosus muscle and close the wound.

Orandi–Devine operative technique
(Fig. 31.6)

• Peritomy of the flap in the middle of the penile shaft. For long strictures the flap can be lengthened by cutting the flap further on subcoronally.

• A short pedicle is prepared so that the rotation of the flap is without tension.
• The flap is rotated and sutured to the rim of the strictured urethra on both sides.
• The tunica dartos is sutured over the flap to cover all the suture lines and to prevent fistulas.
• The skin is placed over the flap. Sometimes a rotated Byars' flap is necessary to reconstruct the skin.

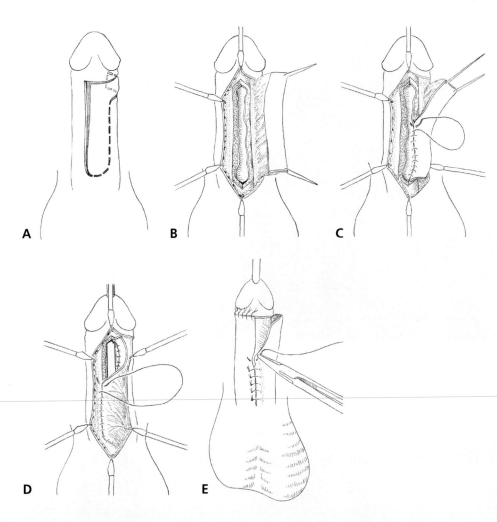

Figure 31.6 (A) Prepare a long penile skin flap, occasionally extended subcoronally. (B) Dissection of a short pedicle. (C) Rotate and suture the flap to the rim of the urethra. (D) Cover the suture lines with the tunica dartos. (E) Cover the penile skin over the flap.

Dorsal buccal mucosa graft (Barbagli technique)

Indications

This technique is suggested for the repair of penile urethral strictures only in patients with a normal corpus spongiosum of the urethra. It is rarely performed in anterior strictures.

Operative technique (Fig. 31.7)

- Totally strip the penile skin, including the tunica dartos.
- Ventral opening of the corpus spongiosum to healthy tissue.
- Incise the urethral plate in the midline dorsally and mobilize the lateral wings of the urethral plate.
- The gap of the urethral plate is covered using a buccal mucosa or free prepucial graft using 6/0 interrupted resorbable sutures.

- The corpus spongiosus is sutured over a 20 Fr catheter.
- The glans and penile skin are closed covering the urethra with the dartos tissue underlying the penile skin.

Two-stage buccal mucosa graft (Bracka technique)

Indications

This technique is recommended in patients with hypospadia features and strictures resulting from lichen sclerosis or balanitis xerotica obliterans, where the urethral plate is absent or has to be removed completely. With this technique a complete replacement of the urethra is possible. In very long defects, the harvesting of buccal mucosa may be limited to the length of the stricture.

The two-stage mesh graft procedure may become reasonable.

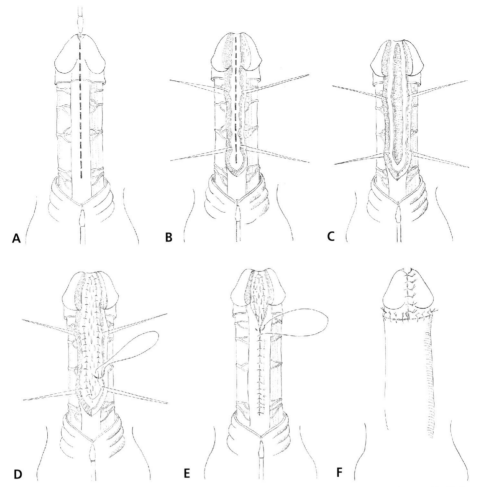

Figure 31.7 (A) Deglove the penile skin. The dashed line shows the midline incision of the corpus spongiosum. (B, C) Open the urethra and incise the urethral plate. (D) Suture the graft into the split dorsal wall of the urethral plate. (E) Close the urethra. (F) Cover the urethra with the penile skin.

Operative technique (Fig. 31.8)

• In the first stage the urethral plate is removed until healthy tissue is reached.
• A buccal mucosa graft is sutured into the defect covering Buck's fascia of the corpora cavernosa. The graft is fixed to the rim of healthy penile skin.
• The graft is healed and stable 3–6 months after the first stage.
• A pertomy of the graft has to be done, with the skin laterally and slightly mobilized and the neourethra sutured using 5/0 resorbable monophilic suture material.
• The mobilized penile skin is sutured over the neourethra.
• No catheter is necessary, and suprapubic urinary diversion is recommended.

Dorsal onlay graft urethroplasty (Barbagli technique)

Indications

This procedure is indicated in rather short and bulbar or near-bulbar strictures of all origins. The advantage of this technique is a stable widening of the strictured urethra and the lack of diverticula formation.

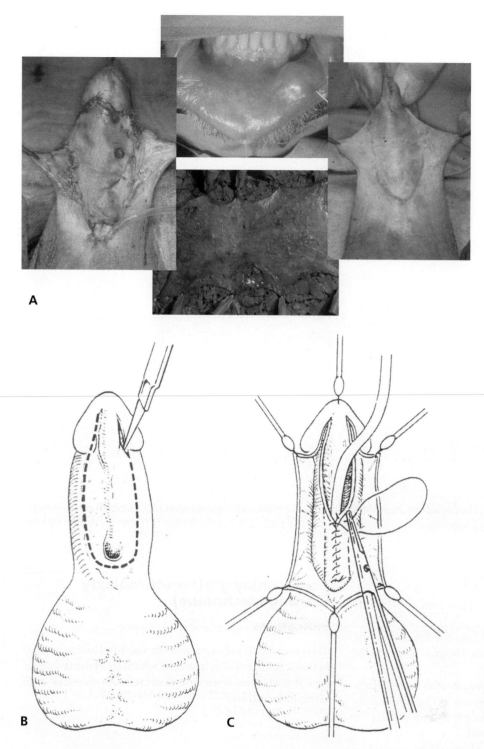

A

B

C

Figure 31.8 (A) Removal of the urethral plate and grafting the defect with buccal mucosa. (B, C) Reconstruction of the neourethra from the graft.

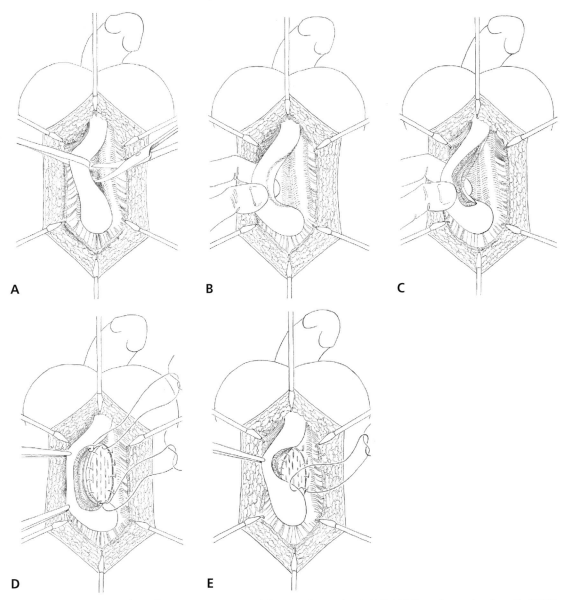

Figure 31.9 (A) Dissect the urethra from the corpora cavernosa. (B) Rotate the urethra (180°). (C) Open the urethra dorsally. (D) The trimmed graft is sutured to the corporal bodies. (E) The urethra is sutured to the graft and is rotated back to cover the graft.

Operative technique (Fig. 31.9)

· A midline perineoscrotal incision is made. The bulbocavernous muscle is split.

· The strictured part of the urethra is mobilized.

· The mobilized urethra is rotated 180°.

· The stricture is opened dorsally.

· A buccal mucosa graft or a prepuse graft is trimmed to the length of the stricture and sutured to Buck's fascia of the corpora cavernosa.

· The rim of the opened urethra is sutured, splayed, and quilted to the rim of the graft using 6/0 resorbable suture material.

Dorsal augmented anastomotic urethroplasty (Fig. 31.10)

Indications

This procedure is indicated in strictures of the bulbar or penile urethra that are too long for simple anastomotic repair.

Operative technique

· A penile or perineoscrotal incision is performed and the bulbocavernous muscle is split. The beginning of the stricture is located using a bougie.

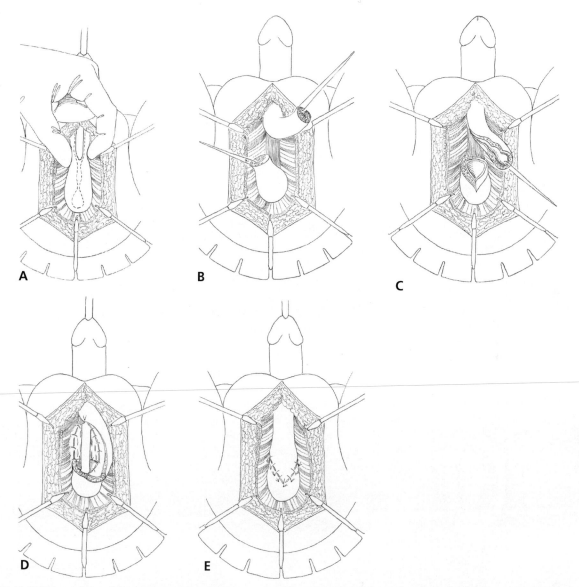

Figure 31.10 (A) Transection of the urethra and opening over an indwelling bougie. (B) Dissection of the urethra from the corporal bodies and resection of the stricture. (C) Spatulation of the edges of the urethra. (D) Suture the graft to the corporal bodies and the lower edge of the urethra and suture the urethra to the graft. (E) Rotation of the urethra to cover the graft.

- The urethra is mobilized and totally dissected. The urethra edges are freed from the corporal bodies.
- The urethral stumps are spatulated.
- A buccal mucosa graft or prepuce skin graft is sutured to the rim of the spatulated distal stump and is fixed to the corporal bodies.
- The distal spatulated stump is rotated 180° to cover the graft and spatulated distal stump and is sutured using 6/0 resorbable suture material.
- At the end of the procedure the grafted area is covered entirely by the urethra. A 20 Fr catheter is left in for 3 weeks.

Tips

- Use fine or microsurgical instruments.
- Use magnifying glasses.
- Prepare the stricture until healthy tissue of the corpora spongiosus is reached.
- Mobilize the urethra widely over the length of the stricture. This is most important in anastomotic repair.
- Do not underestimate the length of the stricture. In urethrograms they look shorter than they really are. Use additional diagnostic procedures such as combined MCU and retrograde urethrogram as well as ultrasound using a 10 MHz probe.

Ultrasound is the best method for visualizing the length of the spongiofibrosis.

- Put the patient in the right position on the operating table. Use the lithotomy position for all bulbar strictures and a flat position for distal strictures. Be aware that sometimes you have to change the position of the patient if you have to go from a distal procedure to a proximal part of the urethra.
- Take into account the shrinking of the free transplanted grafts. The shrinkage can be up to 30%.
- Take special care over the dressing. The dressing should be easily removable (use fatty gaze or other nonadhesive wound dressings).
- Do not remove the dressing before the fifth postoperative day. In cases of two-stage procedures do not remove it before the 10th day.

Postoperative care

- Keep the urine sterile during the first postoperative period.
- Avoid heavy movement of the patient.
- Remove the dressing gently and carefully.
- Do not remove the catheter or suprapubic tube before the urethra is watertight, as shown in a retrograde urethrogram or voiding micturition cystogram.

Complications

In general, penile urethroplasties are more intrinsically prone than anastomotic reconstructions to complications like hematoma, infections, or fistula—especially in enlarged flap procedures that disturb blood circulation of the outer skin. Following shrinkage of the flaps and grafts, the penis can undergo torsion or curvature. Alteration of sexual function may also occur. This is seen less when using buccal mucosa grafts. It is not recommended to use buccal mucosa as a circular tube as this would lead to more failure. As the use of genital or extra-genital skin mainly fails in cases of lichen sclerosis, the use of buccal mucosa is mandatory as skin grafts become affected by the underlying inflammatory disease.

Remarks

The use of free flaps in urethral reconstructive surgery is easier to perform than flap procedures. The complication rate is lower and the free graft procedures require no extensive training in tissue transfer procedures as flap procedures do. If the long-term results reach our expectations, the free buccal mucosa graft will come to predominate the penile flap. But the question of when to use a free graft procedure or a more difficult flap or two-stage procedure cannot yet be answered finally. A surgeon who is involved in urethral reconstruction surgery must have all the choices of surgical technique available in order to respond to the complexity, etiology, size, and location of the stricture.

References

1 Barbagli G, Palminteri E, Lazzeri M, Turini D. Lichen sclerosus of the male genitalia involving anterior urethra. Lancet 1999;354: 429.
2 Barbagli G, Selli C, Tosto A, Palminteri E. Dorsal free graft urethroplasty. J Urol 1996;155:123–6.
3 Brakka A. Hypospadia repair: the two stage alternative. Br J Urol 1995;76:31–41.
4 Jordan GH. Rconstruction of the fossa navicularis. J Urol 1987; 138:102–4.
5 Jordan GH, Devine PC. Surgery following the failed urethral reconstruction. In: Difficult Problems in Urologic Surgery (Scott McDougal W, ed.). Yearbook, Chicago, 1989:289–309.
6 Orandi A. One-stage urethroplasty: 4 years follow-up. J Urol 1972: 107:977.
7 Quartey JKM. One-stage penile/preputial island flap urethroplasty for urethral stricture. J Urol 1985;134:474.
8 Schreiter F. The two-stage meshgraft urethroplasty using split-thickness skin. Atlas Urol Clin N Am 1997;5:104–8.
9 Stein R, Fichtner J, Fillipas D, Hohenfellner R. Harnröhrenrekonstruktion mit Mundschleimhaut. Akt Urol 1999;30:287–94.

Chapter 32
Organ-Sparing Surgery of Penile Carcinoma

A. Bracka

Introduction

Partial penectomy is often performed for penile cancer, but large parts of the penile shaft have to be sacrificed to obtain a sufficient skin flap for coverage of the penile stump.

Fractionated radiotherapy provides an alternative treatment with increased morbidity and a prolonged course of the disease. It also produces bad cosmetic results, uncertain long-term prognosis, and aggravation of balanitis xerotica obliterans as the patient's immunocompetent cells are downregulated.

Organ-sparing surgery is an alternative to radical intervention in cases of cancer restricted to the penile glans and the surrounding tissue, as the tunica albuginea is a natural barrier for penile cancer.

The benefits of preserving good function, cosmesis, and self-esteem are incalulable. A 17-year experience has yielded cure rates comparable with more radical traditional operations. Furthermore, no local tumor recurrence has occurred, even when histological clearance margins have been as little as 1 mm.

Indications

This procedure is indicated in penile cancer of the glans or coronal sulcus without infiltration of corporal bodies, and in mutilation of the glans penis due to trauma, irradiation, or other destructive processes.

Preoperative management

Use MRI to determine the exact tumor extension and to exclude infiltration of corporal bodies. Intraoperative application of antibiotics such as amoxycillin is needed.

Anesthesia

Regional or general anesthesia.

Special instruments/suture material

- Dermatome.
- Bipolar diathermy.
- Absorbable 6/0 and 5/0 sutures.
- 6/0 silk suture.

Operative technique

See Figs 32.1–32.8.

Tips

- To achieve excellent cosmetic results, the skin graft should not be meshed and windows should not be created.
- The quilting stitches guarantee direct contact of the free graft with the corporal bodies, otherwise small hematoma or seroma can lead to elevation of the free graft and graft necrosis.
- The quilting stitches should be tied with light adaptation; high tension will lead to necrosis and scars.
- The blood supply of the graft is achieved by 'bridging phenomena'; the distance to the blood vessels has to be less than 5 mm.
- Silk sutures have excellent material characteristics (important for the right tension of knots) and are easy to remove.
- When the tourniquet is removed, bleeding stops spontaneously.

Postoperative care

- Insert a transurethral catheter with fixation to the abdominal wall to avoid any movement.
- A dressing is not required.
- The donor area is covered by a moist alginate compress (0.5% bupivacaine) and compressive dressing, which can be removed after 10 days.
- The silk sutures are removed on day 5 or 6 postoperatively to avoid scars.

• Smaller incrustations can be removed; small dark areas are remnants of insufficiently reabsorbed hematomas.
• Absorbable sutures should be left.
• The patient should rest in bed (for 5–6 days) until the free graft has taken (also use antithrombotic stockings and low-dose heparin).
• At discharge, mupirocin-containing cream is locally applied to the sites of sutures and smaller wound dehiscence.
• Advise no intercourse for a minimum of 6 weeks.

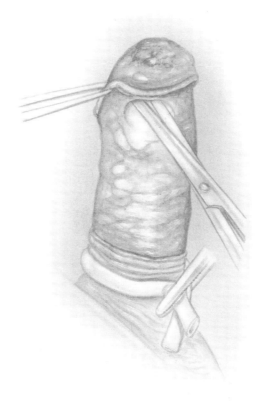

Figure 32.2 Place a tourniquet around the base of the penis. Perform a circular incision proximal to the coronal sulcus, with sharp dissection and separation of the glans from the tip of the corporal bodies.

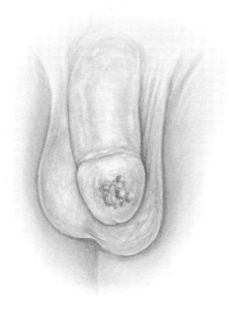

Figure 32.1 Carcinoma of the penile glans, showing the incision line.

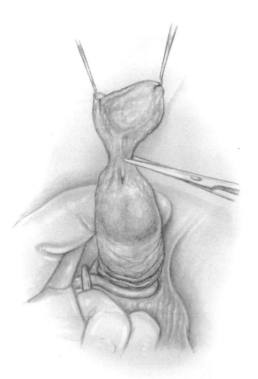

Figure 32.3 The urethra and corpus spongiosum are cut at the level of the tip of the corporal bodies. Fixation of the ureteral stump is in between the two corpora cavernosa, with absorbable suture material, to create a split-like meatus.

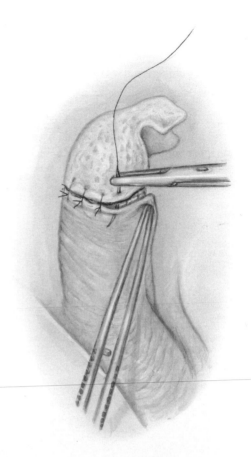

Figure 32.5 Reconstruction of a 'pseudoglans' using a split skin graft (from the thigh): the corporal tips are covered with the free graft and the graft is fixed to the penile skin. Fixation is also around the neomeatus and there is resection of excessive tissue.

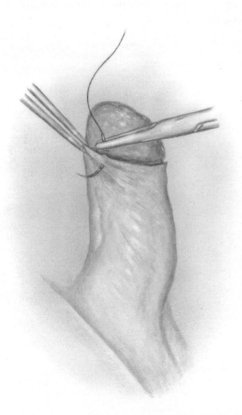

Figure 32.4 A new sulcus is created by anastomosis of the penile skin and corporal bodies; the tip of the bodies remain uncovered.

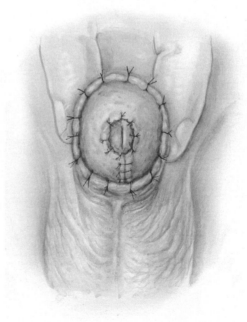

Figure 32.6 The final result after removal of the tourniquet.

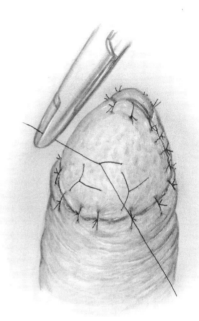

Figure 32.7 The free graft is fixed with quilting stitches of 6/0 silk, loosely tied.

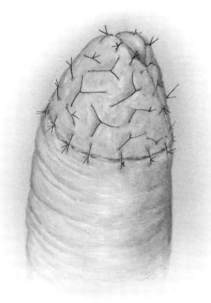

Figure 32.8 The reconstructed neoglans before the insertion of a transurethral catheter, and removal of the tourniquet.

Chapter 33

Meshed Unexpanded Split-Thickness Skin Grafting for the Reconstruction of Penile Skin Loss

P. C. Black, L. H. Engrav, and H. Wessells

Introduction

Split-thickness skin grafting (STSG) has become the standard method of covering penile skin loss. Unmeshed sheet grafts are believed to provide optimal cosmetic and functional results in potent men [5]. Sheet graft survival, however, is frequently compromised by fluid accumulation and graft bed contamination.

Meshed STSG allows fluids to drain through the graft without lifting the graft off its bed. This offers several potential advantages: better accommodation of the graft to the contours of the graft bed, easier application, and excellent take in difficult, often contaminated, wounds [4,5].

Meshing of STSG is usually avoided in penile coverage, as it is thought to be associated with contraction and unsatisfactory cosmesis [5]. McAninch describes the use of meshed grafts to the penis in impotent patients, in whom contraction will have no functional consequences [5]. Contraction, however, is more related to graft expansion than to meshing. An unexpanded mesh graft can be expected to contract no more than a nonmeshed graft [3]. This chapter describes the use of unexpanded meshed grafts on the penis regardless of erectile function [1].

Patient counseling and consent

Patients will initially experience some tightness around the corona or base of the penis during erection, but this will resolve by 6 months. The mesh pattern remains visible for several months but diminishes over time.

Indications

The procedure is indicated in penile skin loss regardless of etiology or erectile function.

Contraindications

Gross contamination needs to be treated prior to coverage, and any coagulopathy should be corrected.

Preoperative management

Fournier's gangrene or other infectious processes should be debrided, followed by specialized wound care until the wound is covered by healthy granulation tissue (3–6 weeks). In patients with elective penoscrotal reconstruction, the penile skin and soft tissue is excised down to Buck's fascia immediately prior to grafting.

Anesthesia

General or spinal anesthesia.

Special instruments/suture material

- Guillion.
- Pneumatic dermatome (10 or 12.5 cm).
- Shur Clens® (ConvaTec, Skillman, NJ).
- Sutures: 3/0 Prolene, 3/0 chromic catgut.
- 16 Fr Foley catheter.
- Dressings:
  - Telfa® (The Kendall Co., Mansfield, MA);
  - Duoderm® (ConvaTec Ltd, Princeton, NJ);
  - Tegaderm® (3M Health Care Ltd, St Paul, MN);
  - Sulfamylon® (Bertek Pharmaceuticals Inc, Sugar Land, TX);
  - nonadherent petroleum gauze (Xeroform®, Sherwood Medical, St Louis);
  - Acticoat® (Smith & Nephew, London);
  - fine mesh gauze (The Kendall Co., Mansfield, MA);
  - Kling® (Johnson & Johnson Medical, New Brunswick, NJ);
  - Kerlix® (Tyco Healthcare Group, Exeter, NH).

Operative technique

This procedure needs a joint team of a urologist and a plastic surgeon.

• Give prophylactic intravenous antibiotics (first generation cephalosporin).

• Place the patient in the low lithotomy or frog leg position.

• Shave and prepare the thigh circumferentially on the side intended for skin donation; place a sterile stocking below the knee on this side to allow intraoperative repositioning of the entire lower extremity.

• Insert a Foley catheter on the operative field and cap so as to be used for penile positioning.

• Excise the thick granulation tissue sharply prior to grafting in patients with previous debridement (Fig. 33.1).

• Determine graft length by measuring the shaft circumference and adding an additional 3–5 cm overlap of ventral skin to allow a zigzag closure.

• The preferred donor site is on the posterolateral thigh where the skin is thicker than the medial thigh and allows better re-epithelialization.

• Inject normal saline intradermally if skin laxity at the proposed donor site prevents proper graft harvesting.

• Harvest donor skin from the patient's thighs using a 10 or 12.5 cm wide pneumatic dermatome after an application of Shur Clens® with a graft thickness of 0.014–0.016 inches.

• Cover the donor site with Telfa® soaked in epinephrine.

• Mesh the graft in a 1 : 1 ratio.

• Anchor the prepubic and scrotal skin to the base of the penis with buried nonabsorbable sutures.

• Apply grafts without expansion of the mesh.

• Orientate the meshed slits transversely on the penis (Fig. 33.2).

• Make a zigzag juncture on the ventral surface (Fig. 33.2B).

• Anchor the grafts around the periphery with interrupted 4/0 chromic sutures and intervening tacking sutures as required, to obtain full graft apposition.

• Place grafts in a similar fashion to cover additional scrotal, perineal, and abdominal wounds.

• Soak the dressing in Sulfamylon®.

• Apply a multilayer compressive dressing: fine mesh gauze covered with Kling®, followed by Kerlix® and a second layer of Kling®.

• Cover the donor site with Acticoat® at the end of the procedure.

Tips

• Remove the penile skin completely to the corona in order to prevent subsequent edema and constriction.

• The graft thickness (≥0.012 inches) is important in preventing contracture.

• A ventral zigzag graft juncture prevents longitudinal con-

tracture of the penis [5,7]; it is placed ventrally for optimal cosmetic outcome.

• Tacking sutures at the penile base are critical in preventing penile retraction during the healing phase, which can lead to a buried penis or graft loss.

• Avoid expansion of the graft during application, as this leads to persistence of the meshed pattern and possible constriction.

• The application of a suitable bulky dressing is essential for graft immobilization.

• Once the graft take has occurred, postoperative erections are welcomed as a natural method of tissue expansion [5].

Postoperative care

• Bed rest for 3–5 days.

• Use a Foley catheter while the patient is in bed.

• Give intravenous pain medication if necessary.

• Keep the dressing moist with Sulfamylon® — add every 4 h.

• Remove the dressing after 3–5 days and cover with Xeroform® gauze; change this daily.

• Use vitamin E cream to soften the grafted penis starting after the first postoperative clinic visit (2–3 weeks).

• The Acticoat® covering on the donor site is allowed to dry out and the edges are trimmed as they peel up.

Complications

• Graft loss is the principal potential complication.

• Patchy areas can be managed conservatively: cover with Xeroform® and await secondary epithelialization.

• Extensive graft loss requires regrafting.

Results

• The results are based on nine consecutive patients with penile skin loss [1].

• Fournier's gangrene occurred in four cases, chronic penoscrotal lymphedema in two, severe penile skin deficiency from prior surgeries in two, and Crohn's disease with perineal fistula in one.

• All patients had a complete graft take (Fig. 33.3).

• One patient experienced partial distal graft loss secondary to self-manipulation.

• All other patients had a satisfactory cosmetic result (Fig. 33.3).

• None of the donor sites required grafting.

• The mean follow-up was 6 (1.2–19.8) months.

• There were no scar contractures at the circumferential margins or ventral graft juncture.

• One patient developed a pinpoint urethrocutaneous fistula at the coronal margin, which resolved with nonoperative management.

• Glanular edema persisted in two patients after grafting, resulting in intermittent spraying of the urinary stream.

• Four of the nine patients could achieve postoperative erections (intercourse successful in two); three patients had poor erections pre- and postoperatively (unchanged); and no information was available in the other two patients.

References

1 Black PC, Friedrich J, Engrav L, Wessells H. Meshed unexpanded split thickness skin grafting for reconstruction of penile skin loss. J Urol 2004;172:976.

2 Dandapat MC, Mohapatro SK, Patro SK. Elephantiasis of the penis and scrotum. A review of 350 cases. Am J Surg 1985;149:686.

3 Fifer TD, Pieper D, Hawtof D. Contraction rates of meshed, non-expanded split-thickness skin grafts versus split-thickness sheet grafts. Ann Plast Surg 1993;31:162.

4 Housinger TA, Keller B, Warden GD. Management of burns of the penis. J Burn Rehab 1993;14:525.

5 McAninch JW. Management of genital skin loss. Urol Clin N Am 1989;16:387.

6 Morey AF, Meng MV, McAninch JW. Skin graft reconstruction of chronic genital lymphedema. Urology 1997;50:423.

7 Troshev K. Free skin graft in the treatment of penile skin defects. Acta Chir Plast 1981;23:235.

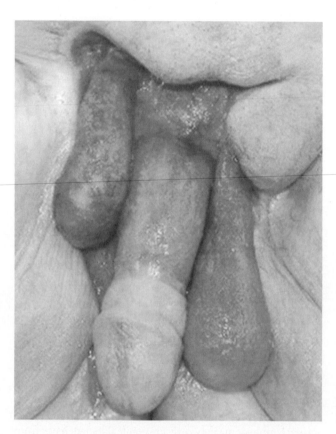

Figure 33.1 Sample preoperative photograph of a patient with Fournier's gangrene after granulation of the debrided wound.

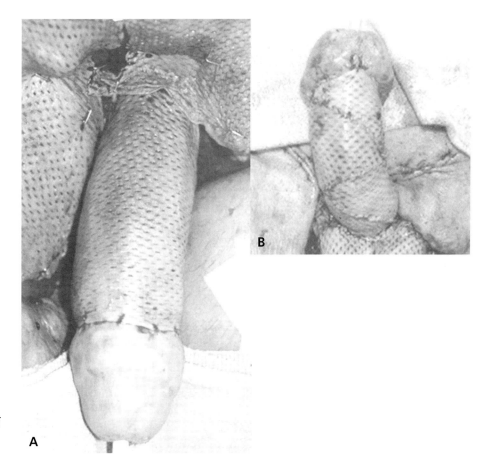

Figure 33.2 Sample intraoperative photographs of the unexpanded meshed STSG: (A) the dorsal aspect of penis; and (B) the ventral zigzag closure.

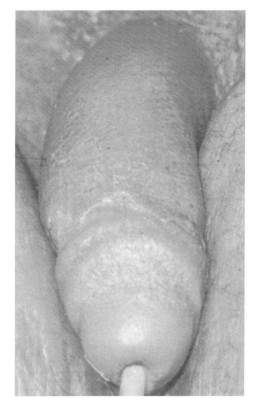

Figure 33.3 Postoperative appearance of one of the patients at 3 months.

Chapter 34
Epispadias Repair: Complete Penile Disassembly

M. E. Mitchell, P. C. Black, and R. W. Grady

Introduction

Male patients with epispadias can undergo complete separation of the corpora cavernosa and corpus spongiosum without compromising blood supply. Complete penile disassembly facilitates the anatomic reconstruction, whereby the medial rotation of the corpora cavernosa reverses the dorsal curvature without the need for corporotomies in most cases. Complete mobilization of the urethral wedge allows the urethra to be brought ventrally with resultant orthotopic positioning of the meatus. This also reduces dorsal tension on the corporal bodies thereby limiting dorsal chordee. The planes of dissection extend to the bladder neck, thereby facilitating concomitant bladder neck reconstruction if required. Furthermore, the mobilization of the bladder neck and urethra afforded by complete disassembly allows improved anatomical positioning of these structures. Complete penile disassembly yields a satisfactory cosmetic and functional outcome with reduced need for revisions. With an optimal repair, dorsal chordee are corrected, the patient is given a straight urethra, and normal erectile function is maintained [1–3].

Indications

- Primary proximal epispadias.
- Bladder exstrophy.
- Cloacal exstrophy.
- Reoperation of patients with epispadias–exstrophy complex.

Limitations and risks

- Repair within 24–72 h for proximal epispadias and distal forms associated with incontinence; distal epispadias with continence can be repaired after 6 months.
- When associated with exstrophy, the epispadias can be repaired at the time of primary bladder closure (single-stage reconstruction).

- An interval of at least 6 months should be left for reoperation.
- It can be used as a salvage procedure for older children, often requiring dorsal dermal graft for penile straightening, as long as previous exstrophy skin flaps have not been used.

Contraindications

Previous surgery in which the urethral plate was completely divided.

Preoperative management

A single preoperative dose of ampicillin and gentamicin should be given.

Anesthesia

General anesthesia with caudal injection.

Special instruments/suture material

- Small tray with fine instruments.
- Surgical loupes ($\times$ 2–4 magnification).
- Tungsten electrocautery (Colorado tip, Biomed Inc., Evergreen, CO).
- 8 Fr urethral stent.
- Sutures: 4/0 to 7/0 PDS®, Maxon®, Monocryl®, and Vicryl®; and 5/0 chromic catgut.
- Dressings: Telfa® (The Kendall Company Ltd, Mansfield, MA), Duoderm® (ConvaTec Ltd, Princeton, NJ), Tegaderm® (3M Health Care Ltd, St Paul, MN), Steri-Strips.

Operative technique

This procedure is described for male epispadias.
- Place 5/0 Monocryl® stay sutures transversely in each hemiglans (will become sagittal with rotation of the corpora).

- Mark the incision along the urethral wedge (the urethra and underlying corpora spongiosa) and around the meatus.
- Make an incision around the urethral wedge with Colorado tip electrocautery (minimizes blood loss); extend the incision ventrally around each hemiglans.
- Penile degloving: starting with a ventral penile circumcising incision, dissect between Buck's fascia and the dartos on the ventral and lateral aspects of the corpora, taking care not to injure the neurovascular bundles (located laterally) or devascularize the skin.
- Place 5/0 Monocryl® stay sutures through the ventral preputial hood (optional).
- Release the urethral wedge from the corpora cavernosa, coming from both sides on Buck's fascia.
- Extend the incision around the distal end of the urethral wedge, thereby completely releasing it from the corpora cavernosa; the urethral blood supply is proximal (this is also possible in patients with prior primary bladder closure for exstrophy).
- Separate the two hemiglans and corpora cavernosa in the midline; the blood supply to each hemiglans is through paired neurovascular bundles.
- Tubularize the urethra in two layers with 6/0 Maxon® and 5/0 Vicryl® over an 8 Fr urethral stent (or 3.5 Fr ureteral catheters if combined with an exstrophy repair); ventral transposition of the meatus.
- Medially rotate both corpora cavernosa so that the neurovascular bundles come to lie dorsally; the previously placed horizontal glanular stay sutures rotate medially so that they become vertical.
- Reapproximate the corpora cavernosa in the midline with interrupted 6/0 PDS® sutures, taking care to avoid injury to the neurovascular bundles.
- Position the urethra in the groove between both corpora and fix the neomeatus with 6/0 or 7/0 Vicryl® to the glans.
- Maturate the neomeatus using standard hypospadias techniques.
- Reconstruct the glans with 5/0 or 6/0 PDS® for shaping and 6/0 or 7/0 Vicryl® for reapproximation of the epithelial edges; the glans may need trimming to achieve conal form.
- Close the penile skin, with reverse Byars' flaps as necessary, using 6/0 chromic or 6/0 Vicryl®.
- Fix the urethral splint with 5/0 Monocryl®.
- Apply a three-layer dressing with Telfa®, Duoderm®, and Tegaderm®, and fix onto the abdominal wall.

Tips

- Marking the urothelium with methylene blue facilitates later dissection of the urethral wedge.
- When the urethral wedge has been mobilized in one area, the passage of a vessel loop between the wedge and the corporal bodies allows gentle retraction for further dissection.

- During closure of the urethral wedge, the suture line should come to lie on the corpora cavernosa.
- Avoid excessive mobilization and handling of the neurovascular bundles.
- A Scott retractor improves exposure in older patients.
- Subcutaneous fixation of the penis shaft skin with 5/0 or 6/0 PDS® at the base of the penis reduces tension and resultant thinning of the shaft skin.

Postoperative care

- Urine is drained into the diaper through the open catheter.
- Prophylactic antibiotics are given: ampicillin and gentamicin (if no renal impairment) until they can be taken orally, then trimethoprim/sulfamethoxazole until the tubes are out.
- Acute pain service consultation; continuous morphine infusion.
- The patient is allowed to bath/shower after 48 h, whereby the dressing is easily removed.
- Remove the catheter/splints after 10 days.

Complications

The high rate of reoperation reflects the level of technical complexity. Complications include: 10–20% urethrocutaneous fistula (typically dorsally at the base of the penis, where tissue coverage is most tenuous), persistent chordee, difficulty with urethral catheterization, and erectile dysfunction [2,3].

Troubleshooting

- For inadequate urethral length, the neomeatus is established on the proximal penile shaft and a hypospadias repair is performed later (redundant ventral foreskin is left in place for the urethroplasty), or a distal urethroplasty is performed primarily with preputial skin or buccal mucosa.
- The creation of a Mitrofanoff channel allows patients who require clean intermittent catheterization (CIC) of their bladders to do so easily despite tortuous neourethras following urethral reconstruction (especially with exstrophy).

References

1 Grady RW, Mitchell ME. Complete primary repair of exstrophy [Comments]. J Urol 1999;162:1415.
2 Mitchell ME, Bagli DJ. Complete penile disassembly for epispadias repair: the Mitchell technique. J Urol 1996;155:300–4.
3 Zaontz MR, Steckler RE, Shortliffe LMD, Kogan BA, Baskin L, Tekgul S. Multicenter experience with the Mitchell technique for epispadias repair. J Urol 1998;160:172–6.

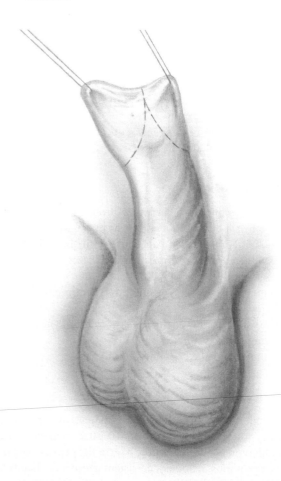

Figure 34.1 Transversely placed stay suture on each hemiglans (5/0 Monocryl®), with the ventral incision marked.

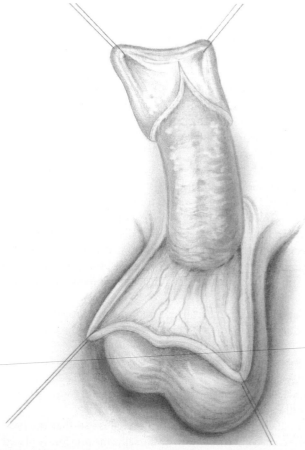

Figure 34.3 Degloving of the penis, including the ventral foreskin, with stay sutures through the ventral preputial hood (5/0 Monocryl®).

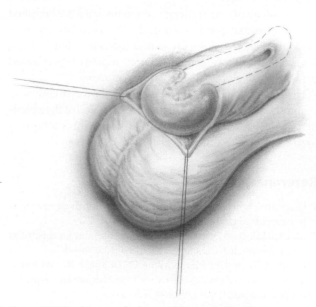

Figure 34.2 Incision marked around the urethral wedge.

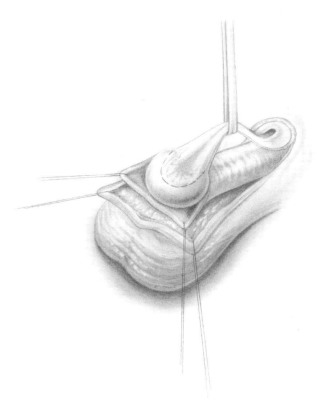

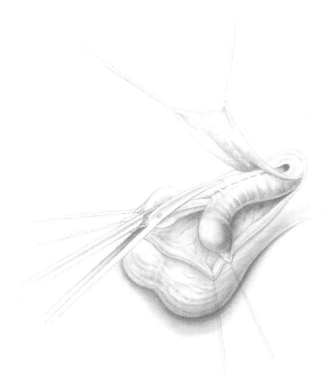

Figure 34.4 Dissection of the urethral wedge and elevation with a vessel loop. (Note that the 'urethral plate' is actually a wedge of tissue proximally that extends between the corpora cavernosa.)

Figure 34.5 After release of the urethral wedge, both glans halves are separated and so is the corpora cavernosa.

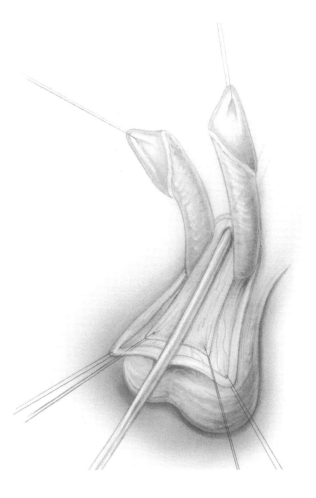

Figure 34.6 Tubularization of the urethral wedge over an 8 Fr urethral stent.

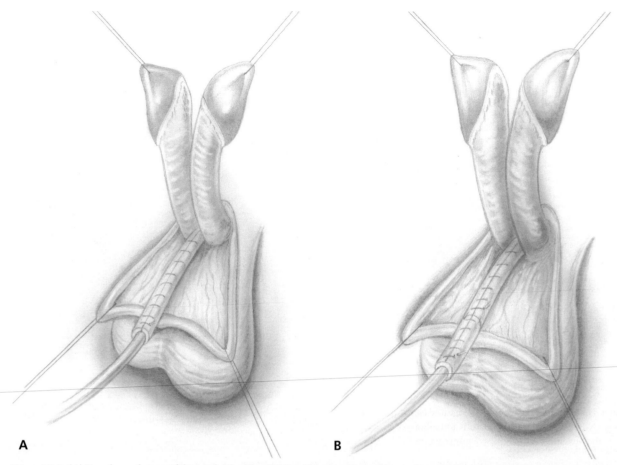

Figure 34.7 (A) Two-layer closure of the urethral wedge. (B) Possible extension of the urethra with buccal mucosa.

A

B

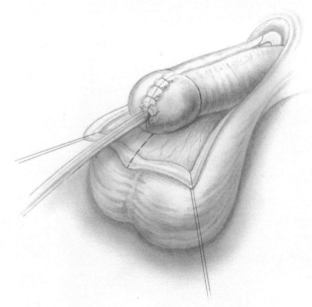

Figure 34.8 Reapproximation of the corpora cavernosa and glansplasty.

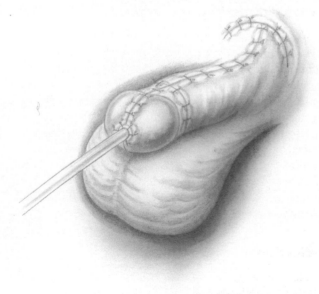

Figure 34.9 Coverage of the penis with shaft skin (Byars' flaps).

Chapter 35
Penoscrotal Transposition

S. V. Perovic

Introduction

Penoscrotal transposition is a rare anomaly of the external genitalia characterized by malposition of the penis in relation to the scrotum. There are two forms. In incomplete transposition, which is more common, the penis lies in the middle of the scrotum. In complete transposition, the scrotum covers the penis, which emerges from the perineum. Both forms are often associated with hypospadias, chordee, and cryptorchidism. Repair of isolated penoscrotal transpositions depends on their form and is usually performed as a one-stage procedure.

Penoscrotal transposition associated with hypospadias is more difficult to repair and can be performed as a one- or two-stage procedure.

Patient counseling and consent

Penoscrotal transposition may be associated with micropenis as well as with signs of intersexuality, usually due to partial or complete androgen insensitivity. Parents have to be informed that definite sex determination depends on several factors: genetic, anatomical, hormonal, psychological, sex of upbringing, and sex of perception, which cannot be determined before adolescence. There is a possibility of recessive inheritance of anomaly. The complication rate depends on the form of transposition, the associated anomalies, and surgical experience, and ranges from 15 to 50% and is mainly related to urethral reconstruction. There is no significant difference in complication rate between one- or two-stage procedures.

Indications

• Isolated incomplete penoscrotal transposition.
• Isolated complete penoscrotal transposition.
• Penoscrotal transposition with chordee without hypospadias.
• Penoscrotal transposition with chordee and hypospadias.

Limitations and risks

• Repair of anomaly before 6 months of age.
• Cases with micropenis or/and intersexuality: sex reassignment surgery should not be performed in childhood.
• Poor experience in this field of surgery.

Preoperative management

• Determine the severity of the penoscrotal transposition.
• Define the associated anomalies (hypospadias, chordee, cryptorchidism, etc.).
• Estimate the available penile and scrotal skin as well as their vascularization.
• Exclude intersexuality, especially in cases of penoscrotal transposition associated with hypospadias and cryptorchidism.
• Give local or parenteral dihydrotestosterone administration to stimulate growth of the penis and to improve vascularization of the skin.
• Release prepucial adhesions at least 3 months before surgery combined with local corticosteroids.
• Investigate partial or total androgen insensitivity either by histological examination or a clinical trial of testosterone therapy.

Anesthesia

General anesthesia combined with pain control techniques: caudal/epidural analgesia or penile block.

Special instruments/suture material

• Microsurgical instruments with magnifying glasses (×2–4 magnification).
• Ultracision harmonic knife.
• Rapid absorbable suture material.
• Scott retractor (self-holding retractor).

Operative technique

See Figs 35.1–35.36.

Tips

Penoscrotal transposition in general

• Penile transposition should be performed in the normal anatomical position without scrotal movement.
• Preserve the anterior abdominal vascular pedicle during the longitudinal skin incision on the place where the penis will be transposed.
• Reconstruction of the bifid scrotum requires excision of the thin and hairless skin in the midline, to avoid middle grove formation. Joining of both testes is recommended.
• Suture fixation of the elastic compressive dressing to the penile skin prevents it sliding off.

Penoscrotal transposition with hypospadias

• Preserve all spongiosal tissue during dissection of the urethral plate and hypospadiac urethra, even if it is fiibrotic.
• An erection provoked by prostaglandin E1 is recommended in adolescents and adults. It is useful for easier dissection of the penile entities, permanent checking during curvature repair, and the design of a proper size of the flaps/grafts for both urethroplasty and penile body reconstruction.
• Glans closure should be started at the coronal level to avoid possible strangulation of the neourethral vascular pedicle.
• The lowest parts of the corporeal bodies are fixed to the base of the penile skin, using U-shaped sutures, in order to avoid postoperative retraction of the penis.
• During the penile disassembly technique, dissection of the penile entities is made under Buck's fascia, as close as possible to the tunica albuginea, to avoid injury of the urethra and neurovascular bundle.
• Dissection of the neurovascular bundle includes sharp division of the triangular ligament located dorsally at a subcoronal level, which firmly fixes the neurovascular bundle.
• The inner layer of the prepuce is very useful for penile body skin reconstruction due to insufficient remaining penile skin.

Postoperative care

• Scrotal drainage for 2–3 days.
• Wet the dressing and change it on the first postoperative day.
• Suprapubic cystostomy (2 weeks in children, 3 weeks in adults) when urethroplasty is performed.
• Urethral splint for 10–12 days.
• Elastic compressive dressing for 2–4 weeks.
• If a dressing is applied during erection, it is necessary to change it when the penis becomes flaccid.
• In tubularized urethroplasty, calibration of the neourethra during the healing process should be performed, especially of its glanular part, in order to prevent temporary stenosis and urethral diverticulum.

Complications

• Incomplete repair of penoscrotal transposition.
• Skin flap necrosis (very rare).
• Fistula (mostly spontaneous occlusion).
• Urethral stricture (meatal/proximal anastomosis).
• Urethral diverticulum.
• Penile recurvation.
• Chronic lymphedema of the subcutaneous tissue with secondary fibrosis.
• Wound infection (especially in adolescents and adults, rarely in childhood).
• The complication rate is 15–20%.

Troubleshooting

• If the dressing causes excessive penile compression and ischemia it should be immediately removed or changed.
• Large hematomas should be evacuated and drainage re-established.
• Early fistula formation should be treated with prolonged suprapubic urinary drainage.
• Extensive penile skin edema is treated with prolonged compressive dressing.

Results

• Age: 6 months to 27 years (median 2.7 years).
• $n = 136$.
• Isolated transposition = 14.
• Associated with hypospadias = 122.
• One-stage procedure = 118.
• Two-stage procedure = 18.
• One-stage procedure complication rate = 18%.
• Two-stage procedure complication rate = 15%.
• Satisfactory esthetic and functional results = 91%.

To do

• Place the patient in the lithotomy position.
• Use endoscopic evaluation of possible intersexuality, despite negative results of genitography.
• If transurethral catheter placement is not possible (utriculus, vagina), use endoscopy for bladder filling to establish suprapubic urinary drainage.
• Use magnifying loops and a headlight for better tissue visualization.
• In spongiosal bleeding, use prolonged compression or harmonic ultrascision for hemostasis.
• Use an illumination technique to determine the distribution and development of prepucial and penile skin vascularization.

- Use a tourniquet only during glans reconstruction.
- In associated cryptorchidism, perform simultaneous orchidopexy through the scrotal or inguinal approach.
- In cases with a small penis, use ventral grafting for curvature repair in order to avoid penile shortening.
- If buccal mucosal graft is used, staged urethroplasty is recommended.
- If the neourethra is too long, perform a complete repair of the anomaly and leave the urethral fistula in the place of the proximal anastomosis for later closure.
- Perform the penile body skin reconstruction according to the remaining, well-vascularized preputial and penile skin.
- Use silastic foam dressings if available.

Not to do

- Inexperienced surgeons should not perform this procedure.
- Do not use electrocautery for spongiosal bleeding.
- Do not use a tourniquet during the operation.
- In cases of intersexuality with a very large vagina, do not perform a vaginectomy before there is definite sex determination.

- In cases of a micropenis, do not perform a feminizing operation during childhood.
- Avoid tubularized urethroplasty if onlay techniques are possible.
- Do not use a one-stage repair in complex cases of anomaly.

References

1 Ehrich RM, Scardino PT. Surgical correction of scrotal transposition and perineal hypospadias. J Urol 1982;17:175–7.
2 Glassberg KI, Hansbrough F, Horowitz M. The Koyonagi–Nonomura 1-stage bucket repair of severe hypospadias with and without penoscrotal transposition. J Urol 1998;160:1104–7.
3 Kolligian ME, Franko I, Reda EF. Correction of penoscrotal transposition: a novel approach. J Urol 2000;164:994–7.
4 Perovic S. Penoscrotal transposition. Akt Urol 1998;29:I–XVIII.
5 Perovic S, Vukadinovic V. Penoscrotal transposition with hypospadias: one-stage repair. J Urol 1992;148:1510–13.
6 Pinke LA, Rathbun SR, Husmann DA, Kramer SA. Penoscrotal transposition: review of 53 patients. J Urol 2001;166:1865–8.

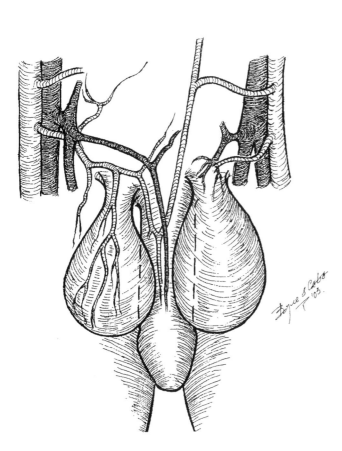

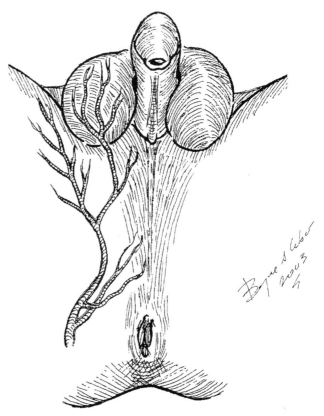

Figure 35.2 The posterior scrotal skin is supplied by scrotal branches of the perineal artery.

Figures 35.1–35.3 Penoscrotal transposition.
Figure 35.1 Deep and superficial branches of the external pudendal artery supply the penile and anterior scrotal skin.

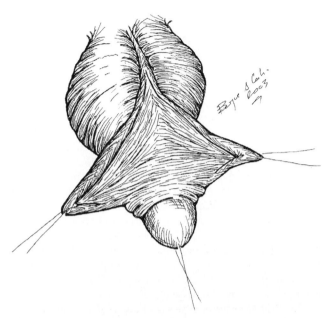

Figure 35.3 Penile skin exists only on the dorsal side of the penis, as a triangle.

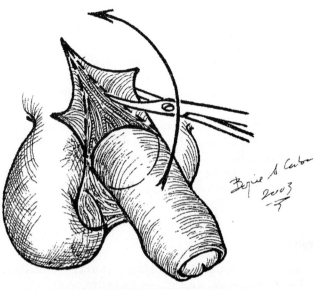

Figure 35.5 Dissection and excision of the triangular skin flaps. Care should be taken to avoid injury of the penile skin blood supply.

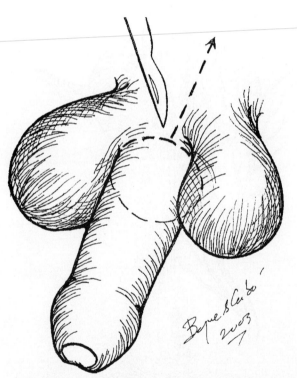

Figures 35.4–35.9 Isolated incomplete and complete penoscrotal transposition.

Figure 35.4 A circumferential incision around the penile base is extended longitudinally to the mons pubis, where the penis will be transposed.

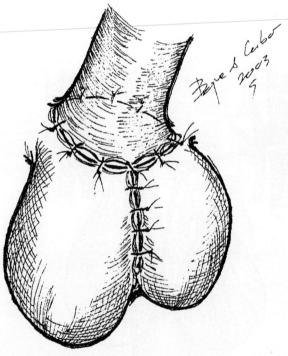

Figure 35.6 The penis is transposed to the area of incision on the mons pubis. The scrotal skin and raphe are reconstructed.

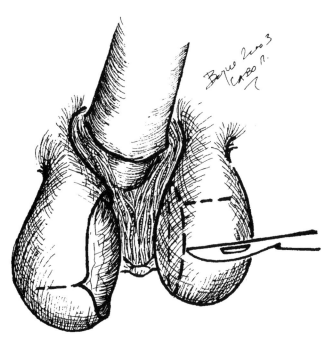

Figure 35.7 Bifid scrotum: the thin and hairless skin between both the hemiscrotums is excised. A transversal scrotal incision is done for further reconstruction.

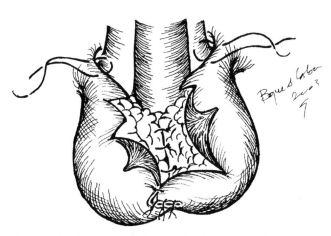

Figure 35.8 Midline testes joining with subcutaneous tissue approximation in two layers. The lowest part of the corporeal bodies are fixed to the base of the penile skin using a U-suture.

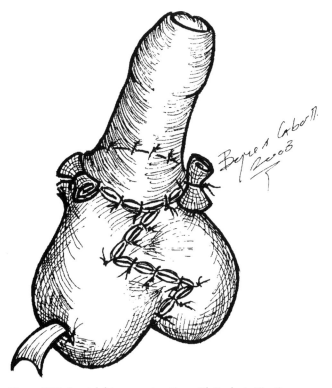

Figure 35.9 Scrotal skin reconstruction with Z-plasty. Fixation sutures of the cavernosal bodies are knotted over a bolster to prevent postoperative retraction of the penis.

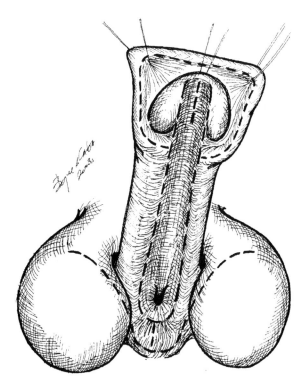

Figures 35.10–35.20 Penoscrotal transposition with severe hypospadias.
Figure 35.10 The dashed lines show the planned incisions.

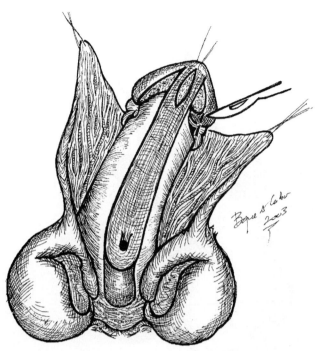

Figure 35.11 The penile and scrotal skin are mobilized. The urethral plate is preserved. The coronal parts of the glanular wings and inner prepucial layer are excised, in order to achieve a conical shape of the glans. The glanular urethral plate is incised in the midline to allow it to be folded during glanuloplasty.

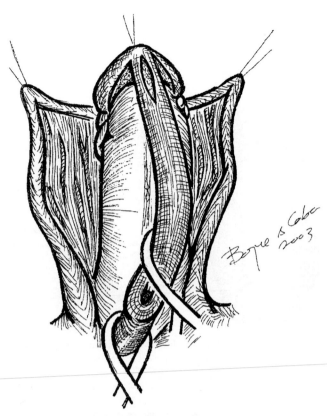

Figure 35.12 The urethral plate is completely dissected, including part of the normal urethra.

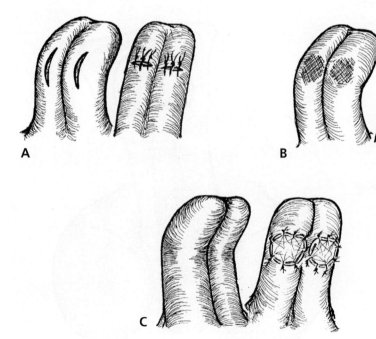

Figure 35.13 There are three types of ventral curvature repair: (A) dorsal corporoplasty by longitudinal corporotomy with transversal closure; (B) simple dorsal plication of the wounded tunica albuginea, which consists of numerous net-like incisions, without penetrating the tunica albuginea; and (C) ventral transversal corporotomy of the tunica albuginea and grafting with autologous material.

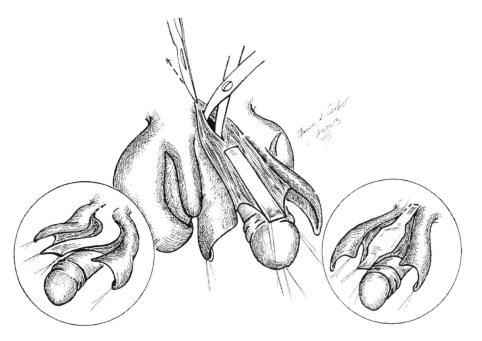

Figure 35.14 A vascularized island flap is formed on the dorsal penile skin. An additional incision is made on the skin of the mons pubis. A hole is formed by blunt dissection in the area of the mons pubis, avoiding anterior abdominal middle vascular pedicle injury. If a long urethra is necessary, a spiral skin flap is formed (left inset). In the formation of island flaps in cases of urethral plate division, the flap is wider in the middle so it can be tabularized later (right inset).

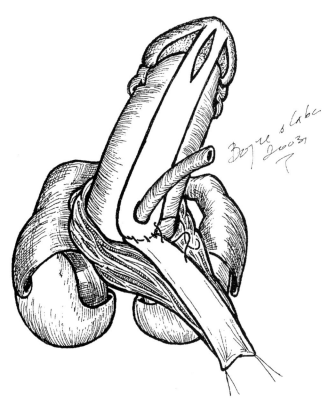

Figure 35.15 The island flap is transposed to the ventral side of the penis by a buttonhole maneuver. The island flap and urethral plate are anastomosed using 6/0 or 7/0 interrupted and/or running absorbable sutures.

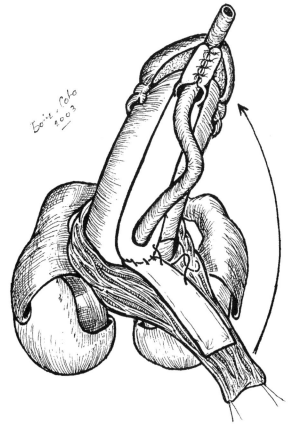

Figure 35.16 A variant of onlay urethroplasty: the deep glanular grove is tubularized and the suture line is covered with the vascularized tissue of the island flap.

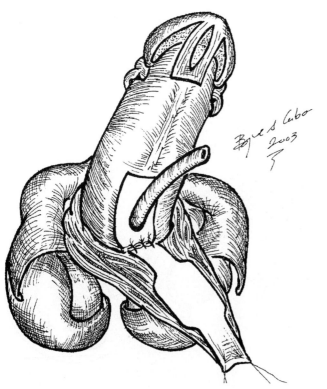

Figure 35.17 In cases with severe hypospadias, the thin and poorly developed urethral plate must be divided. Both ends of the divided urethral plate are onlayed with the island flap. The island flap is tubularized in the middle where the urethral plate is absent. The advantages of onlay urethroplasty are maintained.

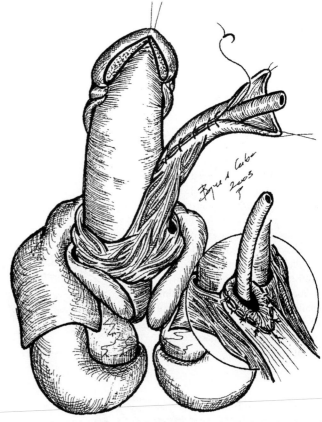

Figure 35.19 Tubularized urethroplasty: tubularization of the island flap by a subepidermal running suture. A long elliptical anastomosis is formed between the hypospadiac and new urethra (inset).

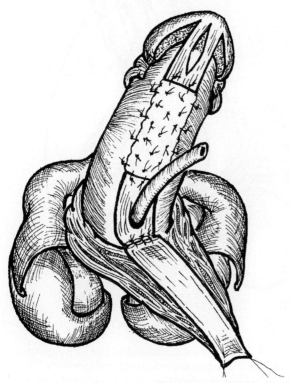

Figure 35.18 Inlay–onlay urethroplasty: the gap created after the division of the urethral plate is inlayed with a buccal mucosa graft, which is quilted to the corporeal bodies. Onlay urethroplasty follows.

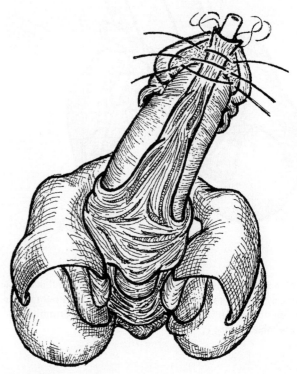

Figure 35.20 The neourethra is completely covered with well-vascularized subcutaneous tissue of the island flap. The glans wings are closed in two layers.

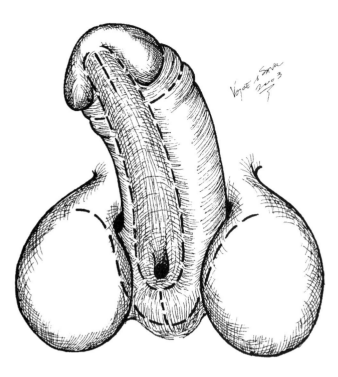

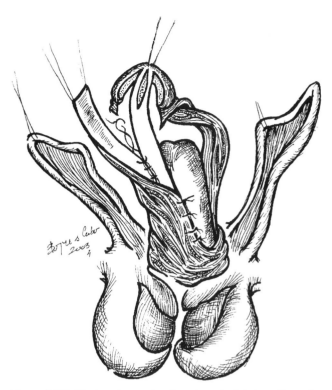

Figures 35.21–35.25 Penoscrotal transposition with severe hypospadias and chordee.

Figure 35.21 The boundaries of the incision are indicated by the dashed lines.

Figure 35.23 Urethroplasty using the onlay principle is performed.

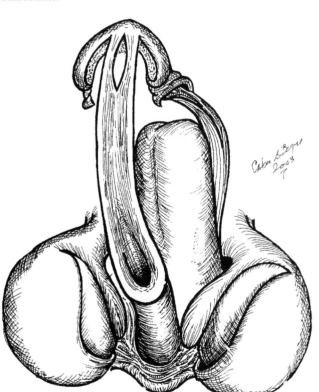

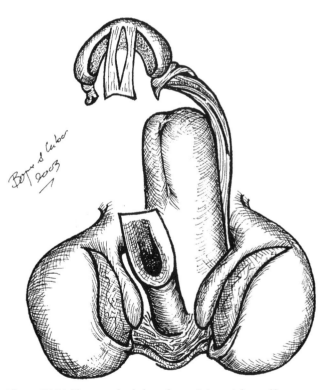

Figure 35.22 The penis is completely straightened using the penile disassembly technique. The blood supply to the glans cap derives from a completely preserved, mobilized neurovascular bundle.

Figure 35.24 Short urethral plate: the penis is straightened by disassembly and there is division of the raised short urethral plate.

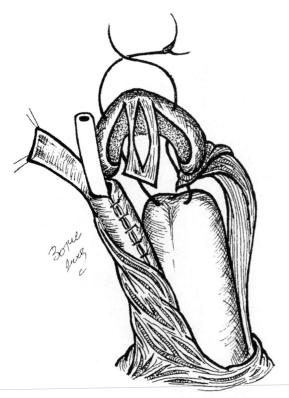

Figure 35.25 Urethroplasty using tube between two onlays is made.

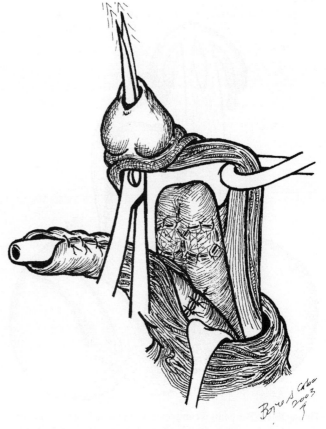

Figure 35.27 Straightening of the penis is achieved by penile disassembly combined with ventral grafting at the distal third of the cavernosal bodies. The native urethra is lengthened by tubularization of the urethral plate (inset). This way, the distance between the glans and native urethra is shortened.

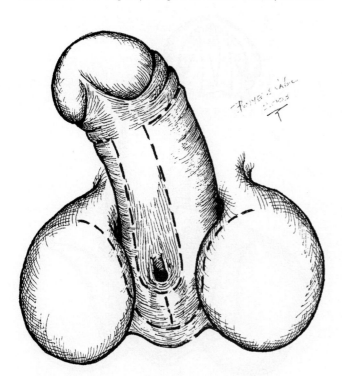

Figures 35.26–35.29 Penoscrotal transposition with severe hypospadias, chordee, and small penis.
Figure 35.26 An incision is made along the dashed lines.

Figure 35.28 Urethroplasty is completed by tubularization of the island flap. The glans channel is made.

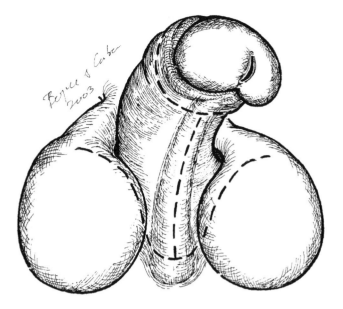

Figures 35.30–35.32 Penoscrotal transposition with chordee and short urethra but without hypospadias.

Figure 35.30 The dashed lines show the incisions.

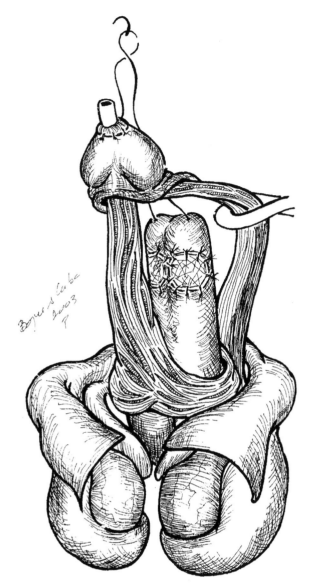

Figure 35.29 The new urethra is brought to the top of the glans. The glans cap is fixed to the tips of the corporeal bodies using U-sutures.

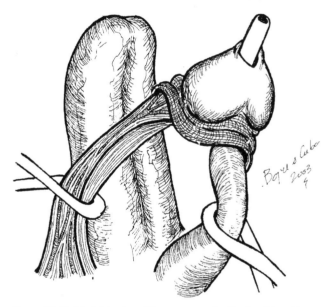

Figure 35.31 Straightening of the cavernous bodies is achieved by penile disassembly.

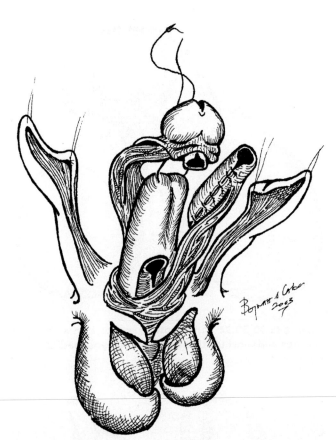

Figure 35.32 The short urethra is divided and the gap is bridged by tubularized urethroplasty.

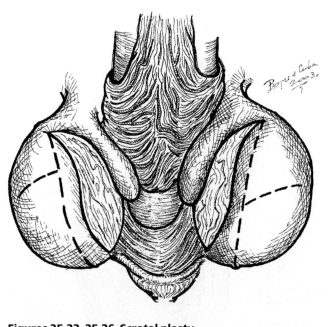

Figures 35.33–35.36 Scrotal plasty.
Figure 35.33 Excision of the medial, thin and hairless, hemiscrotal skin. The oblique scrotal dashed lines indicate the place of incision for Z-plasty.

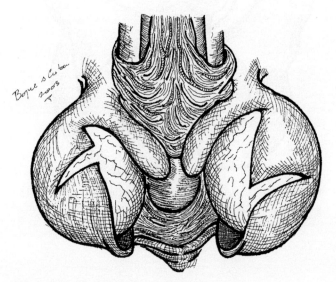

Figure 35.34 The flaps for the Z-plasty are created.

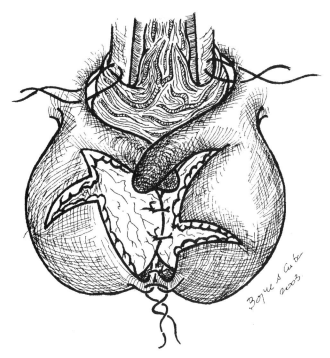

Figure 35.35 Both testes and the subcutaneous tissue are joined.

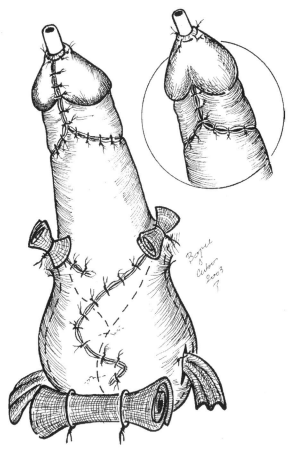

Figure 35.36 A subglanular portion of the penile body skin is reconstructed from the inner surface of the prepuce via the mucosal collar technique. The proximal penile body skin is reconstructed by two lateral sliding flaps. Z-plasty and drainage of the scrotum are then performed. Fixation sutures of the testes exiting the scrotum are knotted over a bolster to prevent retraction. If the glans is well shaped, then the glanular channel technique could be used (inset). The corporeal bodies are fixed to the base of the penile skin over bolsters.

Chapter 36
Autotransplantation of Intra-abdominal Testis by Microvascular Techniques

J. Zumbé, R. A. Bürger, M. Braun, and U. Engelmann

Introduction

Microsurgical techniques have improved dramatically over the last few years, and autotransplantation of intra-abdominal testis has become the therapy of choice. Surgical correction of the undescended testis should be performed within the first 2 years.

Patient counseling and consent

- Risk of testicular atrophy.
- Risk of secondary semicastration.
- Risk of endocrine and exocrine hormonal dysfunction with life-long substitution.
- Risk of infertility.
- Risk of bleeding.

Indications

- Surgical correction within the first 2 years.
- Bilateral intra-abdominal testes.
- Unilateral intra-abdominal testis and contralateral atrophy.
- Failed correction after conventional procedure.

Limitations and risks

Hypoplastic testicular vessels.

Contraindications

See limitations.

Preoperative management

- Ultrasonography.
- Magnetic resonance tomography.
- Retrograde phlebography of the plexus pampiniformis.
- Diagnostic laparoscopy.

- Test of hormonal stimulation in cases of bilateral impalpable testes.

Anesthesia

General anesthesia.

Special instruments/suture material

- Optical instruments: magnifying glasses and a surgical microscope.
- Surgical instruments:
  - microsurgical instruments;
  - angular bipolar coagulation (11 mm, sharp, Fa. Fischer, Freiburg, Germany);
  - Scoville microvascular clip (4 and 10 mm, Fa. Fischer, Freiburg, Germany);
  - bulldog vascular clamp/Senning (45 mm, Fa. Fischer, Freiburg, Germany);
  - Teflon G26 cannula (Fa. Critikon, Norderstedt, Germany).
- Suture materials:
  - 9/0 and 10/0 nylon suture, round needle (Fa. Ethicon, Norderstedt, Germany);
  - 10/0 and 11/0 nylon suture, double-armed (Sharpoint, Reading, PA, USA).

Operative technique

See Figs 36.1–36.6.

Tips

- Careful preparation with a bipolar pinsetter.
- Leave some fat tissue around the testicular vessels.
- Mark the vessels with different clips in order to identify them.
- Speed up the anastomosis by starting with the veins.
- Use single knots.

- The ischemia time should be less than 1 h.
- Use intratesticular measurement of the oxygen pressure.

Postoperative care

- Digital examination.
- Doppler/duplex ultrasound.
- Exocrine and endocrine functional tests.
- Perfusion study after 3 months.

Complications

Complications include thrombosis of the anastomosis and bleeding.

Troubleshooting

- Venous interposition (vena epigastrica inferior) in cases of short testicular vessels.
- Early reanastomosis in cases of thrombosis.

Results

The long-term success rates range in a small series between 25 and 78%.

To do

- Use a pararectal incision for a unilateral abdominal testis.
- To increase venous bloodflow, perform the anastomosis with both venae testicularis.

Not to do

- Avoid rarefying testicular vessels.
- Do not use running sutures, as these will minimize the diameter of the anastomosis.

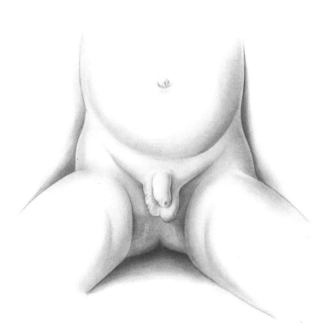

Figure 36.1 Perform a pararectal incision in a case of right lateral intra-abdominal testis.

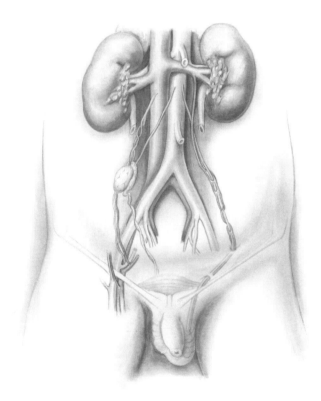

Figure 36.2 Intraperitoneal site of an undescended testis with the testicular vessels.

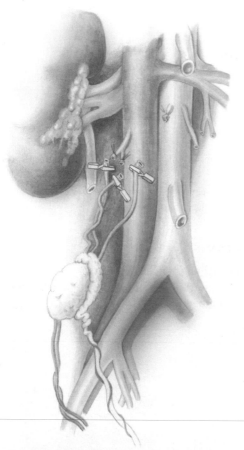

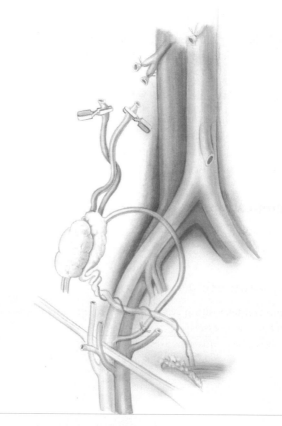

Figure 36.4 Preparation and dissection of the vasa epigastrica and the prepared anastomosis.

Figure 36.3 The most proximal ligation of the testicular vessels.

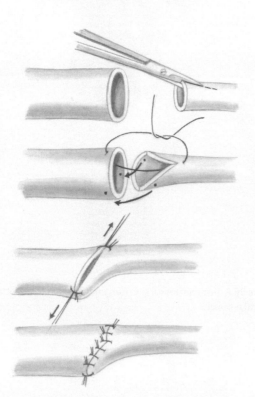

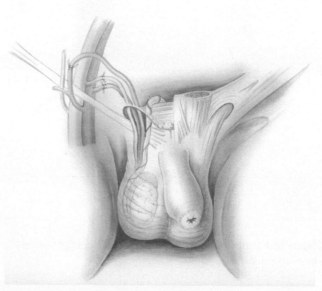

Figure 36.6 Orchiopexy of deep scrotal testicular homotransplantations.

Figure 36.5 Spatulated vessels for recompensation of different lumina, using single suture knots (10/0).

Section 5
Urethra

Chapter 37
Reconstruction of the Bulbar and Membranous Urethra

F. Schreiter, B. Schönberger, and R. Olianas

Introduction

Destruction or rupture of the posterior urethra is caused mainly by forces that occur during traumatic pelvic rupture. This trauma results in partial or complete rupture of the urethra. A complete rupture often results in destruction of the posterior urethra and may damage the sphincteric structures, while always damaging the neurovascular bundles, which results in impotence and incontinence.

For a long time, conventional urologic wisdom was that urethral rupture in men occurs at the prostatomembranous junction by a shearing force that avulses the prostatic apex from the urogenital diaphragma. Recent studies suggest that this traditional belief may be a misconception. The urethral sphincter extends from the bladder neck to the perineal membrane (diaphragma urogenitale). The muscular lining and surrounding of the membranous urethra are directly continuous with similar muscle fibers of the prostatic urethra and end abruptly at the perineal membrane.

Hence, the weakness may lie in the bulbomembranous junction rather than the prostatomembranous junction at which the posterior urethra is liable to rupture (Fig. 37.1). As the sphincteric component remains intact, incontinence occurs only when the bladder neck is impaired (post-transurethral resection of the prostate, TURP) or when the bladder neck is involved in the traumatic rupture, which occurs mainly in children.

Acute management of posterior urethral trauma

Although the urethral injury is seldom the main problem of these often multiply and severely traumatized patients, the consequences of the urethral trauma such as urethral strictures, erectile dysfunction, and (in some cases) urinary incontinence may be problems with life-long ramifications for the patients.

In this connection, primary urologic treatment should be directed at preventing early complications and minimizing the risk of the aforementioned potential problems. A satisfactory outcome is dependent on a correct diagnosis, along with thorough and well-planned urologic therapy.

Meanwhile, the controversy surrounding immediate versus delayed treatment of urethral injuries is still unresolved. The perfect treatment plan still remains to be developed; the value of the different approaches, including recent evolutions of innovative endourologic techniques to achieve urethral continuity, needs to be determined.

The following treatment strategies are available for acute management:

- Primary open suturing of the disrupted urethra.
- Endoscopic or surgical realignment by insertion of a transurethral 'railroad' catheter.
- Suprapubic cystostomy and delayed repair.

Acute surgical intervention is indicated for the following:

- Concomitant rectal tear.
- Bladder neck laceration.
- Serious, life-threatening bleeding, mainly from the inferior or superior gluteal arteries.

A large gap between the bladder neck and the disrupted urethra, also known as 'pie in the sky bladder' is a relative indication for open surgical exploration (Fig. 37.2).

Nevertheless, immediate surgical exploration does not necessarily indicate exploration of the urethral injury site. Exploration of the urethral injury also involves release of the tamponade effect of the hematoma in the small pelvis and may compromise control of the venous bleeding. Attempts to suture both ends of the urethra are challenging—dissection of the periurethral and prostatic tissues can cause additional damage to the neurovascular bundles and the intrinsic urethral sphincter structures. Due to the increased risk of iatrogenic impotency and incontinence, primary anastomotic repair is no longer recommended. Reconstructive procedures should be limited to open surgical placement of the transurethral catheter and suprapubic drainage of the bladder.

So for primary therapy of posterior urethral injury, we recommend urinary diversion using a suprapubic catheter and/or by endoscopically inserting a transurethral catheter. Several researchers have described a number of different 'railroading' techniques to manipulate the catheter across the urethral gap into the bladder. It may be useful to 'railroad' the prostate to the urethra by using a suprapubic sound or an endoscope. Sometimes it is also useful to drain the pelvic hematoma via the endoscope.

Additional traction, obtained by applying additional weight to the transurethral catheter, has been shown to produce pressure damage to the bladder neck and to subsequently increase the risk of urinary incontinence. In addition, the traction may pull the prostatic gland into an abnormal position, causing misalignment or malrotation. For these reasons, traction has been abandoned, as well as 'vest sutures', which are introduced through the prostatic apex and brought out through the perineum.

The purpose of the realignment is to reduce the number of secondary urethral strictures, and to decrease the stricture length in comparison to both suprapubic cystostomy and delayed repair. Although the ultimate value of this procedure is still under discussion, there is clear evidence that realignment can significantly decrease the incidence of strictures (Koraitim [7]: 53% vs 97%). On the other hand, this procedure may be associated with an increased risk of erectile dysfunction (Koraitim [8]: 36% vs 19%). In another study (Morey & McAnninch [9]), the incidence of erectile dysfunction was reported as up to 55% after immediate realignment.

Delayed repair

There is a widespread acceptance of a 'hands-off' policy in the acute management of posterior urethral injury, i.e. limiting initial treatment to placing a suprapubic cystostomy, which necessitates later stricture repair in most cases. Spontaneous healing after 2–3 weeks may be expected only if the urethral rupture is incomplete.

Thus end-to-end anastomosis remains the golden standard in repairing obliterated membranous urethral strictures. Experts are divided on the other treatment options. Endosurgical procedures such as 'cutting to the lights' have very limited indications and value. In most cases, they do not cure the stricture.

Indications

• Partial or incomplete rupture of the bulbar urethra following a primary straddle trauma or the secondary development of a stricture.
• Rupture (distraction) of the membranous urethra, usually as a result of pelvic fracture.
• Short strictures (e.g. iatrogenic or inflammatory) of the bulbar and membranous urethra.

Contraindications

• Stricture length greater than 3 cm (watch out for penile curvature or shortening).
• Injuries to the membranous urethra, involving the prostate and the bladder neck.
• Circulatory dysfunction of the proximal urethra, e.g. following an anterior urethroplasty, and if the urethra's corpus spongiosus cannot be mobilized extensively enough.

Special instruments/suture material

• Special retractor (Scott retractor or Bookwalter retractor).
• Curved metal probes and flexible cystoscope.
• Extended nose speculum.
• Microcoagulation set.
• Magnifying glasses and headlight.
• Monofilic, absorbable 3/0 to 5/0 suture material.

Operative technique

Reconstruction of the bulbar urethra

• Post-traumatic strictures of the posterior urethra are broken down into bulbar strictures (anterior strictures) and membranous strictures (posterior strictures).
• Bulbar strictures are usually caused by 'straddle trauma', while membranous strictures are typically the result of urethral disruption due to a pelvic fracture.
• The anterior and posterior strictures are usually short, which makes them ideally suited for a stricture resection by means of spatulated end-to-end anastomosis.
• If a stricture is longer than 3 cm, penile curvature or penile shortening usually results. This should be taken into account when choosing this surgical procedure, and the patient should be enlightened as to the complications. The literature [13] describes satisfactory results up to a stricture length of 7 cm; but in our experience, the resultant penile curvatures and penile injuries cause patients to be dissatisfied with the results of the surgery [5].

Stricture resection and bulbar end-to-end anastomosis

• Place the patient in a slightly hyperextended lithotomy position (Fig. 37.3). In our experience, a hyperextended lithotomy position is not necessary.
• We prefer a median perineal incision extending close to the anus (Fig. 37.4). However, a lambdoid cut or perianal incision with extension in the midline of the perineum is also possible.
• The bulbocavernosus muscle is split down the middle (Fig. 37.5) and the urethral bulbus is laid open in the area of the stricture. The stricture may be localized using a 20 Fr curved metal probe or with a flexible cystoscope.
• The urethra is mobilized from the cavernous corpora (Fig. 37.6).

- The stricture is resected into healthy corpus spongiosum, i.e. when blood begins to drip from the urethral stumps (Fig. 37.7). Note that the spongiofibrosis may extend beyond the actual stricture itself, in which case it must also be resected.
- The adequately mobilized urethral stumps are spatulated at 6 and 12 o'clock, to arrive at a sufficiently wide anastomosis later (Fig. 37.8). Remember that the anastomosis will shrink by roughly 20%.
- It should be possible to adapt the mobilized urethral stumps without any tension. First, the posterior wall is sutured with 4–6 single stitches (Fig. 37.9). The stitches are sewn in two layers (mucous layer and corpus spongiosum); however, a single-layer suture that catches all layers of the wall is also possible.
- The same suture technique is used to suture the anterior wall, to arrive at a wide, tension-free anastomosis (Fig. 37.10). To take some of the tension off the anastomosis suture, the urethral stumps may be affixed to the area surrounding the urethra with several single-stitch sutures.
- Finally, the bulbocavernosus muscle is reconstructed over the urethra (Fig. 37.11). If there is enough cavernous tissue, it may be sutured across the anastomosis as a Turner-Warwick roofplasty.
- The wound is drained with suction drainage, and the perineal incision is closed layer by layer.

Reconstruction of the membranous urethra (bulboprostatic anastomosis)

- A combined MCU/retrograde urethrogram, carried out in a 45° Lauenstein position, is the best way to determine the precise length of the urethral stricture (Fig. 37.12). Any additional spongiofibrosis is best detected using a 10 MHz ultrasound probe. Counterindications for bulboprostatic anastomosis are the same as for bulbobulbar anastomosis. The stricture length should not exceed 2–3 cm.
- A reconstruction of the membranous urethra is usually also possible by perineal access (Fig. 37.13). The abdominal or abdominoperineal access is reserved for cases that cannot assume a lithotomy position because of extreme loss of motion, and for rare 6–9 cm defects in the membranous and prostatic urethra, including a demonstrably severe injury to the bladder neck requiring bladder neck reconstruction.
- The central tendon is dissected to expose the prostatic apex, taking care to completely remove all scar tissue that surrounds the stricture. The end of the stricture may be located using a suprapubically inserted curved metal probe or a flexible cystoscope. The scar tissue must be removed down to the healthy tissue of the prostatic apex, which has sufficient blood supply, keeping as much as possible of the intrinsic sphincter structures intact. The distal end of the stricture is easily determined by inserting a transurethral probe, and is cut off in the healthy tissue.
- The posterior urethra is extensively dissected proximally (Fig. 37.15). Here, too, the bulbocavernosus muscle is split

above the urethra, taking advantage of the bulbar and anterior urethra's elasticity to be able to suture a tension-free bulboprostatic anastomosis later.
- A special long nose speculum has been designed (Fig. 37.16), which is long enough to open the apex of the prostate sufficiently.
- A nose speculum is used to hold open the prostatic apex (Fig. 37.17). A circular single-stitch suture (10–12 anastomosis sutures) to the prostatic apex can be easily sewn in full view.
- A bent-open curved needle (e.g. CT-2) is inserted lengthwise in the needle holder and used to pierce the apex from the outside in, including the mucous tissue. Gripping the tip of the needle with the needle holder, the needle is pushed into the bladder, where it may be easily turned and led to the outside without traumatizing the urethral tissue (Fig. 37.18).
- The distal urethral stump is spatulated to approximate the width of the prostatic apex. If the anastomosis cannot be adapted without tension because the urethral stump is too short or inelastic, the path to the apex may be shortened by splitting the corpora cavernosa down the midline (Fig. 37.19). This may shorten the distance to the apex by 1–2 cm.
- A similar result may be achieved by detaching one crus of the corpora cavernosa (Fig. 37.20). This, too, may help to reduce the tension on the anastomosis by reducing the distance between the apex and the urethral stump by another 1–2 cm.
- Sometimes it is necessary to partially resect the symphysis to shorten the distance (Fig. 37.21). The resection is carried out at the lower edge of the symphysis using a bone chisel and does not impact on pelvic stability. A complete resection of the symphysis, as in abdominoperineal surgery, is only very rarely necessary.
- The shortening of the way from the anterior short urethra to the apex of the prostate is evident (Fig. 37.22).
- As in bulbobulbar anastomosis, the anastomosis is sewn with 10–12 single-stitch sutures throughout all layers using 3/0 monofilic absorbable suture material. The wound is also drained and closed as in the bulbobulbar anastomosis technique.

Tips

- Use a reliable retractor (Scott or Bookwalter) to expose the surgical field sufficiently.
- Stay near the midline during surgery.
- Remove all scarred tissue around the stricture.
- Look out for the sphincter structure and the erectile nerves.
- Create a wide, tension-free anastomosis.
- Remove the indwelling catheter early when the MCU shows a watertight anastomosis.

Complications

The surgery bears the risk of additional loss of erection. There may also be postoperative incontinence due to surgery-related

damage to the intrinsic sphincter organ when the bladder neck is incompetent, i.e. when the bladder neck is involved in the primary trauma or after a TURP. Our institution has carried out 63 cases of bulboprostatic anastomosis following a complete urethral disruption:
• Thirty patients (48%) were rendered impotent by the primary trauma.
• Four patients became impotent as a result of the operation.
• Three patients experienced postoperative stress-related incontinence.

Alternative procedures to bulboprostatic anastomosis

Because there is a duty to inform patients about these consequences of the surgery, younger patients who continue to be potent after the pelvic trauma will usually refrain from a bulboprostatic anastomosis. We recommend that these patients undergo a suprapubic urinary diversion, e.g. a Mitroffanof procedure, which is carried out in most cases.

In cases of incomplete membranous stricture (e.g. membranous catheter strictures, incomplete urethral ruptures, etc.), the stricture can be split exactly down the midline with buccal mucosa onlay plasty, inner prepucial patch, or two-stage mesh graft plasty. Dissecting strictly down the midline ensures that tissue that is important for erectile function and urethral bloodflow is not severed.

Results

Stricture resection and anastomotic repair in bulbar stricture

At our institute, 42 patients with bulbar stricture were treated with stricture resection and end-to-end anastomosis. In only one case (2.4%) did a stricture relapse, requiring another surgical intervention. None of the patients suffered incontinence as a result of the surgery.

Five patients (11.9%) already had erectile dysfunction prior to the operation. No additional impotence was observed following the surgery.

Therefore, bulbar stricture resection with end-to-end anastomosis is the safest known procedure, with excellent long-term results.

Stricture resection and anastomotic repair in membranous strictures

In these usually complex strictures, stricture resection and bulboprostatic anastomosis yielded good results. Because these strictures are usually the result of severe pelvic trauma in which the urethra is disrupted from the pelvic floor, and during which the neurovascular bundles that are essential to erection are torn, 30–50% [2] of the patients already have erectile dysfunction prior to the bulboprostatic anastomosis.

Buccal mucosa onlay plasty (Fig. 37.23)

The long-term results our institution has seen from this surgical procedure are also satisfactory. We have carried out buccal mucosa patch plasties in 22 cases and saw three relapsed strictures over a period of 7 years.

All the methods described in this chapter are equally suited for reconstructing the posterior urethra, but today the use of buccal mucosa is preferred because of its simple harvesting, the specific tissue characteristics, and the excellent possible immunologic benefits.

Two-stage mesh graft urethroplasty (Fig. 37.24)

Similarly satisfactory results were achieved in similar cases using one-stage penile flap urethroplasty in 18 cases, and two-stage posterior mesh graft urethroplasty in 14 cases.

Remarks

End-to-end anastomosis of the bulbar urethra and bulboprostatic anastomosis to reconstruct a short bulbar and complex membranous urethral stricture are excellent methods for keeping the posterior urethra open in the long term. Surgery is usually possible via a perineal approach. The complication rates are low and the rate of success lies at over 95%. To avoid serious complications, such as postoperative impotence, the alternative techniques described in this chapter should be used for young, potent men.

References

1 Carr LK, Webster GD. Posterior urethral reconstruction. Atlas Urol Clin N Am 1997;5(1):125–37.
2 Corrier JN, Rundy DC, Benson GS et al. Voiding and erectile function after delayed one-stage repair of posterior urethral disruptions in 50 men with a fractured pelvis. J Trauma 1994; 37(4):587–90.
3 Jordan GH. Wide mobilisation of the urethra. J Urol 1988;139:332.
4 Jordan GH. End-zu-end Harnröhrenanastomose bei post-traumatischen Harnröhrenstrikturen. Akt Urol 1999;30:275–86.
5 Kessler TM, Fisch M, Heitz M, Olianas R, Schreiter F. Patients' satisfaction with the outcome of surgery for urethral strictures. J Urol 2002;167:2507–11.
6 Kessler TM, Schreiter F, Kralidis G, Heitz M, Olianas R, Fisch M. Long-term results of surgery for urethral stricture: a statistical analysis. J Urol 2003;170:840–4.
7 Koraitim MM. Experience with 170 cases of posterior urethral strictures during 7 years. J Urol 1985;133:408.
8 Koraitim MM. Pelvic fracture urethral injuries: evaluation of various methods of management. J Urol 1996;156:1288–91.
9 Morey AF, McAninch JW. Reconstruction of posterior urethral disruption injuries: outcome analysis in 82 patients. J Urol 1997; 157(2):506–10.
10 Mundy AR. Reconstruction of posterior urethral distraction defects. Atlas Urol Clin N Am 1997;5(1):139–74.

11 Schreiter F. Die zweizeitige Urethaoplastik. Urologe A 1998;37: 42–50.

12 Schreiter F, Noll F. Mesh-graft urethroplasty using split-thickness skingraft or foreskin. J Urol 1989;142:1223.

13 Webster GD, Ramon J. Repair of pelvic fracture posterior urethral defects using an elaborated perineal approach: experience with 74 cases. J Urol 1999;145:535.

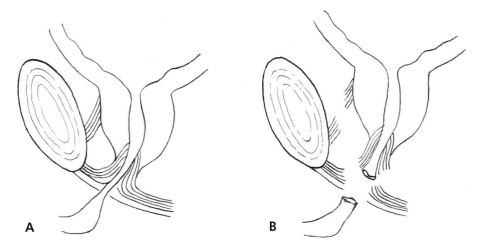

Figure 37.1 The mechanism of membranous urethral disruption.

A

B

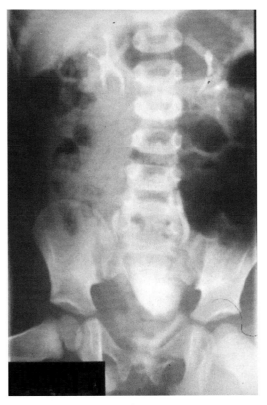

Figure 37.2 'Pie in the sky bladder'.

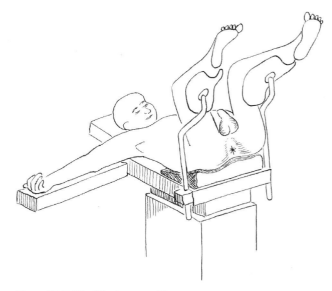

Figure 37.3 The lithotomy position.

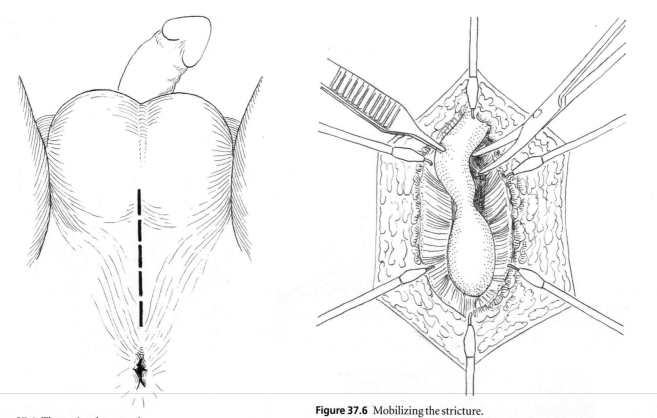

Figure 37.4 The perineal approach.

Figure 37.6 Mobilizing the stricture.

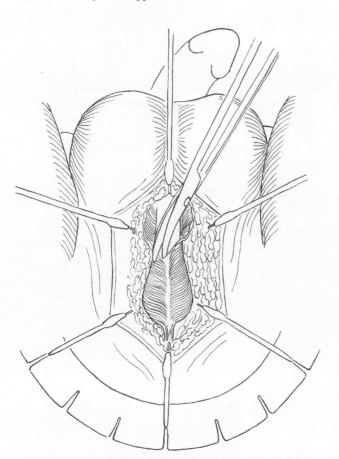

Figure 37.5 Incising the bulbocavernosus muscle.

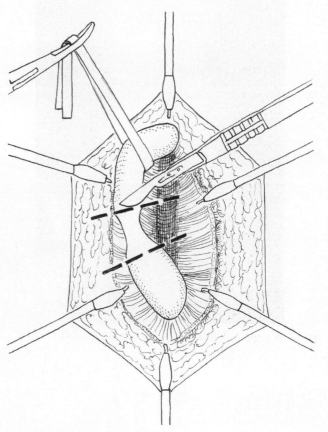

Figure 37.7 Resecting the stricture.

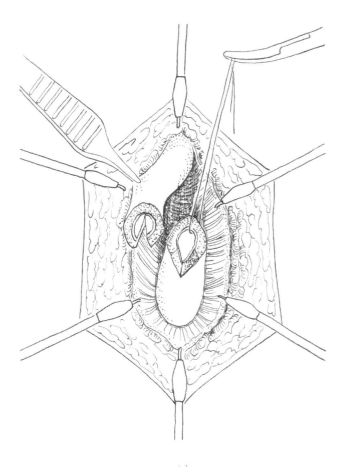

Figure 37.8 Spatulating the urethral stumps.

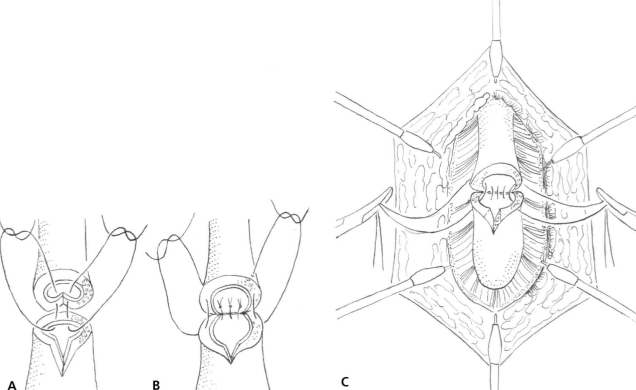

A   B   C

Figure 37.9 Suturing the posterior wall.

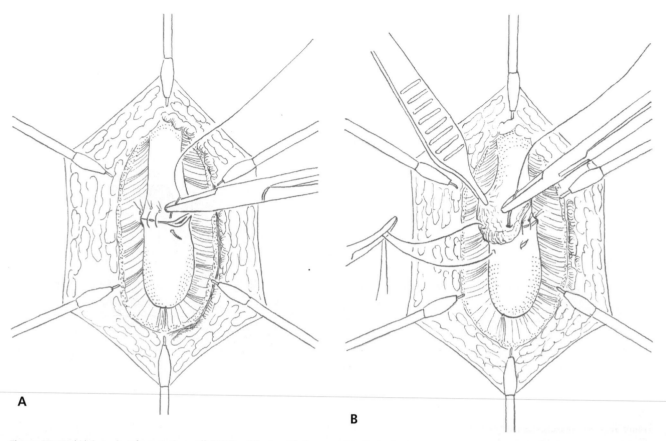

Figure 37.10 (A) Suturing the anterior wall. (B) Roofplasty with the corpora cavernosum.

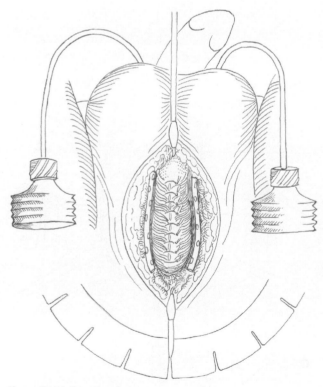

Figure 37.11 Suturing the cavernous muscle.

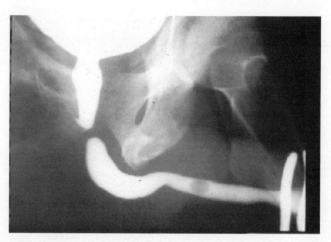

Figure 37.12 A combined urethrogram and MCU.

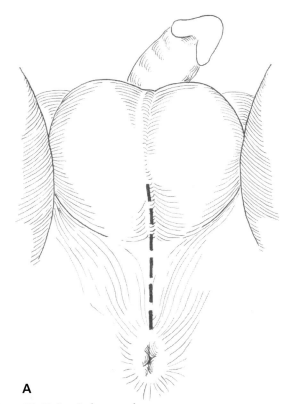

A

Figure 37.13 Surgical approach.

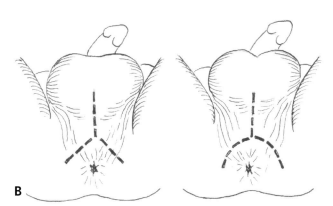

B

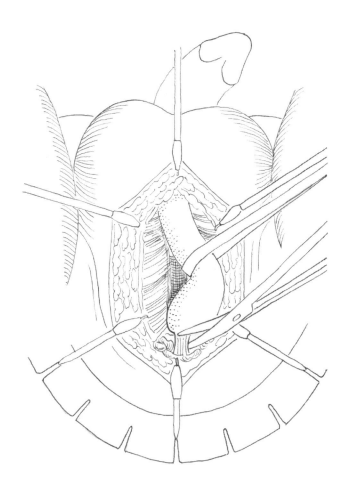

Figure 37.14 Preparing the central tendon.

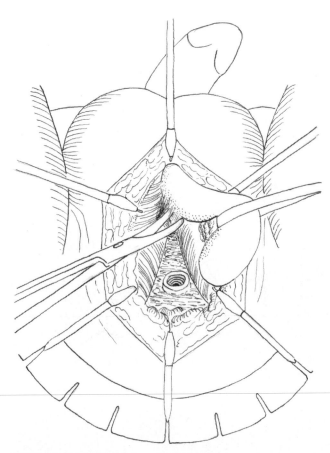

Figure 37.15 Mobilizing the posterior urethra.

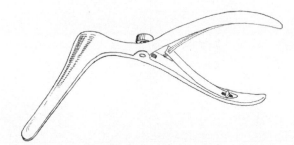

Figure 37.16 The special speculum.

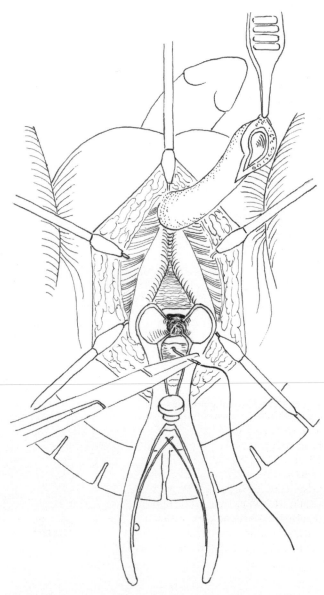

Figure 37.17 Using the speculum to open the prostatic apex.

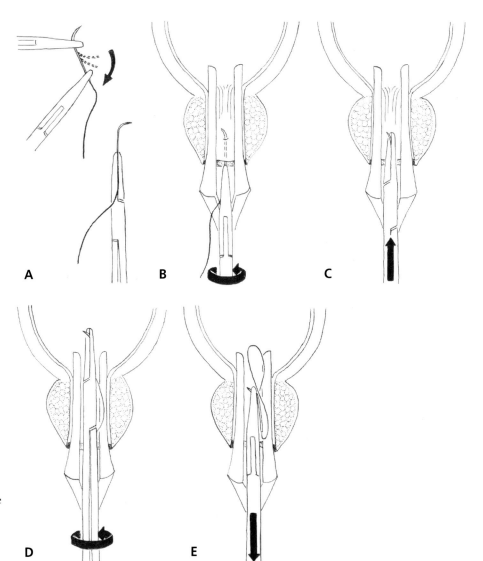

Figure 37.18 The stitch technique using curved and straight needles. (A) Bending open the curved needle. (B) The speculum is held open in the apex of the prostate, allowing a single stitch to be placed. (C) Gripping the tip of the needle. (D) The needle is pushed into the bladder. (E) The needle is turned and led to the outside without traumatizing the prostate tissue.

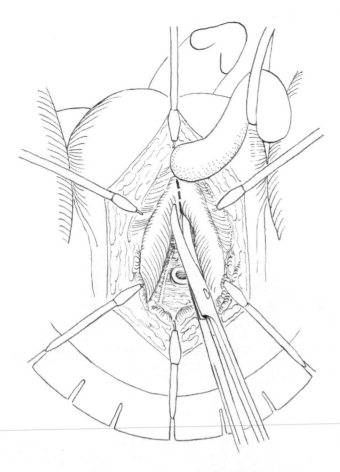

Figure 37.19 The procedure for a short distal urethra.

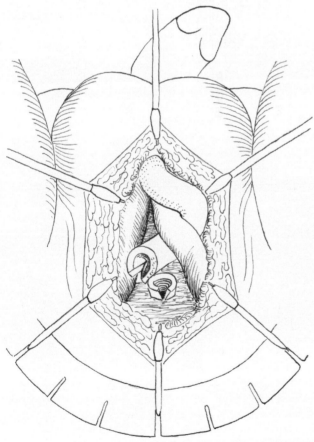

Figure 37.20 Rerouting the mobilized urethra behind the circumferentially dissected corporal body on one side.

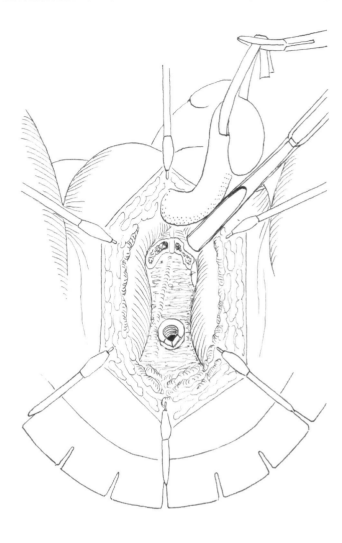

Figure 37.21 Excising the lower limb of the pubis bone under the exposed corporal bodies.

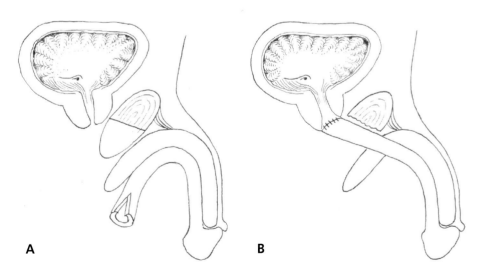

Figure 37.22 Shortening the way to the apex of the prostate.

A   **B**

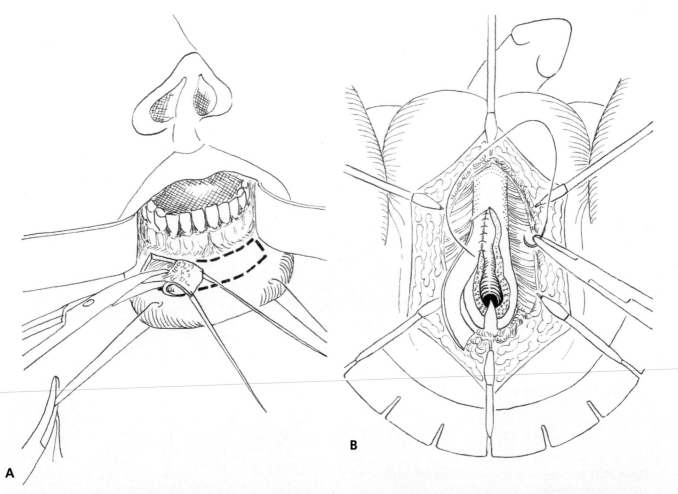

Figure 37.23 Buccal mucosa onlay plasty. (A) Harvesting the buccal mucosa. (B) The flap is turned to the rim of the spatulated urethra.

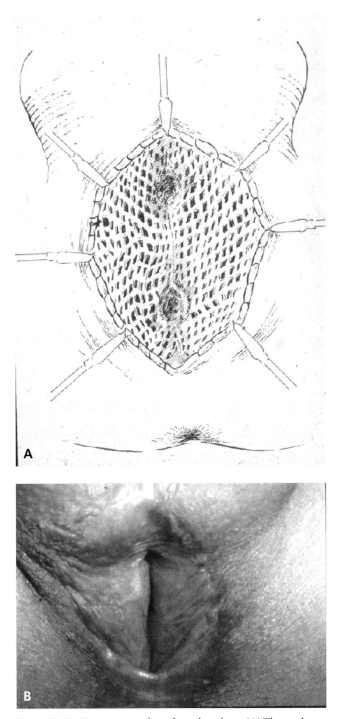

Figure 37.24 Two-stage mesh graft urethroplasty. (A) The mesh graft covers the defect of the urethra. (B) The healed transplant.

Chapter 38
Two-Stage Mesh Graft Urethroplasty

F. Schreiter

Introduction

Most uncomplicated strictures of the anterior and posterior urethra are successfully treated with a one-stage procedure. Among these procedures are stricture resection and consecutive end-to-end anastomosis or contemporary methods of tissue transfer, such as flap procedures. However, complex strictures with significant scar tissue formation of the urethra, strictures that have undergone prior repeated surgery, and urethra malformations found in patients with hypospadia continue to present a challenge for surgery. The problems arise from a lack of healthy elastic tissue needed to reconstruct the urethra. This applies in particular for long strictures that involve the entire length of the urethra.

The classic two-stage methods developed in the 1950s, represented here by the Bengt-Johanson procedure, were based on marsupialization of the strictured urethra, followed by a second operative stage after healing of the first stage. All these methods used scrotal or perineal skin for reconstructing the urethra. Bengt-Johanson's great achievement was the development of a reconstructive surgical urethral treatment that is suitable for all types of strictures. However, the drawback of this method was that hair growth occurred due to the use of scrotal and perineal skin, which could lead to chronic urinary tract infection, abscesses, calculus, and fistulas. Scrotal skin, which is extremely elastic, often resulted in the formation of diverticula and sacculations in the neourethra.

Consequently, the author investigated the use of a mesh graft procedure in an effort to become independent of scrotal or perineal skin by using hairless skin, which is transplanted free in a two-stage procedure. The high contraction and stricture recurrence rate when penile hairless skin was used in a single-stage procedure precluded us from applying our technique as a single-stage procedure.

Although the two-stage mesh graft procedure is a safe operation that can be used for every type of stricture, its real advantage is apparent when used for complex strictures, especially when there is severe scar tissue formation and the absence of healthy penile skin for reconstruction of the neourethra.

Basic considerations in complex urethral strictures

The surgical principle is the free transfer of full-thickness skin (the inner layer of the foreskin or distal penile skin) or very thin split-skin grafts in circumcised patients. A mesh graft dermatome is used to process the loose grafts into a mesh. This mesh graft is transplanted to the location of the exposed and marsupialized urethra. After the complete epithelialization of the free transplanted mesh graft, there will be an ample amount of hairless, vital, and soft tissue that can be used to reconstruct the new urethra in a second surgical stage.

To improve surgical results, three important principles should be taken into account when performing surgery on complex urethral strictures:
- The tissue required to easily shape a new urethra, that is wide enough and free from tension, can be created through loose transplants of full-thickness skin (the inner layer of the foreskin has proven best for this purpose), or distal penile shaft skin, or — in most cases of long and complicated strictures — split-skin grafts.
- This results in a neourethra that is free from hair, thereby preventing chronic infection, calculus formation, restructuring, and sacculation.
- The free grafts should heal in an open and dry environment. This requires a two-stage surgical procedure. Therefore, for reasons of dependability and security, very complex strictures should be treated with a two-stage surgical procedure.

Two-stage mesh graft urethroplasty meets these requirements of treating complex urethral strictures.

Pathophysiology

Extended and complex urethral strictures are either iatrogenic, as the result of a traumatic insertion of endoscopic instruments (catheter, cystoscope, resectoscope) or the result of a urethritis caused by prolonged indwelling catheter application. This especially occurs with long-term indwelling catheter treatment in patients with cardiac or post-traumatic shock, through pressure necrosis and hypotension. Secretion of mucous and infection along the catheter, in conjunction with pressure damage caused by the foreign body (catheter), promote the formation of periurethral infiltrates. The infection then leads to the formation of scarred bridges between opposite regions of mucous membranes, and above all to a cicatricial contraction of the corpus spongiosum urethrae (spongiofibrosis). Postoperative infections, calculus formation, and reoccurrence caused by repeated operations on a urethral stricture, especially when scrotal skin was used to reconstruct the urethra, result in an extended and complex stricture, often affecting the meatus of the urethra. The more pronounced the scarring, the greater the urethra's tendency to shrink and the more extensively the urethral stricture will manifest.

Preoperative management

The patient's genital area is shaved, including the perineal region. The bowels are thoroughly emptied prior to surgery. Complete bowel preparation is performed using laxatives.

Special instruments/suture material

- Compressed air or electrically driven split-skin dermatome for harvesting the split-thickness skin graft.
- A mesh graft dermatome to prepare the mesh (e.g. E Zimmer width 1×1.5).
- One or two $1:1.5$ ratio mesher sheets.
- A set of Benique-sounds, knob-sounds, and bipolar pickups for electrocoagulation.
- Metzenbaum scissors.

Surgical approach

In anterior urethral stricture cases, the patient can be bedded in a supine position. The lithotomy position is used in cases of posterior or extended strictures.

Operative technique

Anterior urethroplasty
- In uncircumcised patients, the foreskin is used, as this tissue is best suited for full-thickness skin grafts. First, perform an extended circumcision (Fig. 38.1).
- Stretch the 50–60 cm^2 of foreskin obtained in this way onto the cork board, carefully and completely remove the subcutaneous tissue using the scissors. The fatty tissue has been completely removed when no larger vessels are visible on the full-thickness skin graft any more. This is necessary to achieve rapid revascularization of the free graft from the nutritive base (Fig. 38.2).
- If no foreskin is available, thin split-skin grafts may be used. Here, skin from the inside thigh, the groin above the hairline,

and buttocks is an obvious choice due to the lithotomy position of the patient undergoing urethral surgery (Fig. 38.3).
- To remove the split skin, use an electric or compressed air-driven split-skin dermatome with adjustable incision width and size.
- Using a mesh graft dermatome, the foreskin or shaft skin is processed to a mesh, in a $1:1.5$ ratio (Fig. 38.4).
- The skin on the penile shaft is incised in the raphe along the length of the stricture (Fig. 38.5).
- The stricture is cut open along its length with a knife or scissors (Fig. 38.6).
- The stricture must be laid open down to the healthy urethral tissue, where no spongiofibrosis is evident along the spongy body of the urethra.

The free meshed graft is sewn into the edge of the marsupialized urethra and the edge of the penile skin. As there is a certain shrinking tendency during the healing process, the sewn-in grafts should be as wide as possible. The graft is fixed in place by means of an interrupted running absorbable suture (Fig. 38.7).
- After 1–2 weeks, the graft has healed and the epithelialization is complete (Fig. 38.8).
- After 8–12 weeks, the graft has stabilized to such an extent that the second stage of the surgery, shaping the new urethra, can be carried out.

Second stage

The second stage is performed after complete epithelialization of the graft. The reconstruction of the neourethra should not be performed before 8 weeks. The longer the time between the first and the second step of the operation, the better the quality of the tissue that is used for the reconstruction of the urethra.
- A sufficiently wide circumferential incision of the graft is made (Fig. 38.9).
- Mobilization of the transplanted penile skin has to be directed laterally, not mobilizing the transplant tissue, which is used for the reconstruction of the neourethra.
- A 24 Fr catheter is used to close the graft, which is elastic, supple, has good circulation, and tends to roll up, with an interrupted running suture using absorbable monofilament thread. Pick a suture technique whereby an inverting, interrupted suture occurs on the outside of the cutting edge of the graft, so no epithelium is left outside, thus preventing later fistula formation (Fig. 38.10).
- To cover the skin defect, the penile shaft skin must now be completely mobilized (Fig. 38.11).
- Use the scissors to remove the epithelium from the edges of the glans; this will form the back wall of the meatus to be created.
- To begin, form an asymmetric advancement flap according to Marberger and Byars. To perform this, the outer penile skin has to be incised dorsally.

- On the dorsal side of the penis, connect the skin of the penile shaft to the edge of the inner foreskin layer on the glans with single stitches.
- The top of the flap of penile shaft skin, which has been rotated to the front, is sewn to the edges of the glans, from which all epithelium has been removed, to form the front wall of the passage to be formed. This puts the meatus nearly at the tip of the glans.

The asymmetric rotation flap is put on the penile shaft in such a way that the suture line of the newly formed neourethra is covered.

The Marberger–Byars sliding flap technique completes the stricture repair (Fig. 38.12).

A loose circular pressure bandage ensures good hemostasis. Thin suction drainage may be used.

Posterior urethroplasty with partial replacement of the urethra

- The back section of the urethra is nearly always easily accessed via a midline perineal incision. Other access paths to the rear of the urethra, involving the formation of a broad-based perineal flap, are usually unnecessary and are only required if there is extreme scarring in the perineal raphe.
- The completely obliterated urethra is laid open and resected, exposing the proximal and distal healthy urethra (Fig. 38.13).
- The resultant urethral defect is lined with a mesh graft and fixed at the edge of the perineal skin and at the rim of the urethral stumps with 5/0 monofilament suture (Fig. 38.14).
- After healing of the transplant the reconstruction of the urethra is made analogously to the anterior urethroplasty.

Complex strictures along the entire length of the urethra

- In complex strictures that run the length of the urethra, the stricture is best opened by dividing the scrotum. Therefore, the skin incision runs through the raphe of penis, scrotum, and perineum (Fig. 38.15).

After splitting the bulbocavernosus muscle, the urethral stricture is cut open lengthwise with the scissors as far as the healthy urethral tissue.

- To reduce the resultant graft surface, the side of the scrotum is stitched up above the testicles (Fig. 38.16).
- To have a sufficient amount of transplantable tissue, it is necessary to resort to a split-skin graft at this point. If foreskin is available, it is best used for the penile part of the urethra (Fig. 38.17).
- After the healing of the graft, it is peritomized, as in the treatment of anterior strictures. The lateral scrotum sutures are opened in order to restore the anatomy of the scrotum after the urethra has been reconstructed. When circumcising the graft, special attention should be paid to ensure that the graft is well

separated in the bulbous part and is not cut too widely, in order to prevent pouch-like diverticulation at this location (Fig. 38.18).

- After healing of the graft, a sufficient peritomy is performed to create the neourethra (Fig. 38.19).
- The neourethra is closed using the method given for the anterior stricture, using inverted running stitches, as an interrupted running suture using 4/0 monofilament absorbable material (Fig. 38.20).
- After the reconstruction of the neourethra, the penile shaft skin is once again sewn across the neourethra's suture row as an asymmetric sliding flap (Figs 38.21, 38.22).

Dressing technique

The technique used to dress the area is of extreme importance. This is particularly true for dressing after the first stage. Movements between the mesh graft and the underlying surface, as well as contact with the opposite mesh graft planes, must be avoided under all circumstances.

To achieve this, fatty gauze is used to cover the whole wound area. Additionally, an edge of a strip of the fatty gauze is inserted into the proximal and distal ends of the urethra, because here the contact of the opposite mesh graft planes is likely (Fig. 38.23).

Absorbent gauze soaks up the wound secretions, whose production is increased during the first postoperative days. The gauze keeps the wound bed dry and supports healing (Fig. 38.24).

To apply gentle pressure to the mesh graft and to enhance contact to the underlying surface, an elastic bandage fixes the layers of dressing (Fig. 38.25).

The first change of the dressing should not be done until a period of 5–7 days has elapsed. In this period the revascularization of the graft takes place, and this phase of revascularization should not be interrupted by an early change of the dressing.

Tips

Mesh graft urethroplasty is not suited for primary hypospadia repair. The mesh graft should not be placed directly on the spongy body of the penis' 'naked' tunica albuginea once the chorda has been removed. This is because there would be an interaction between the split skin mesh graft transplant and the tunica albuginea, causing the graft to form scarification, resulting in another cord-like scar and a bent penis.

However, two-stage mesh graft urethroplasty is a good choice for reconstructing the urethra in patients with hypospadia. Once the scar tissue has been removed, these patients, who have typically undergone several prior operations, usually have enough soft subcutaneous tissue that can serve as a nutritive base for the mesh graft transplant, as does the tunica dartos of the scrotum. To have a nutritive tissue sheet between the tunica albuginea of the penis and the transplant is of extreme importance for the soft and scarless healing of the transplanted graft.

Because split-skin grafts tend to shrink and form scars, it is important to ensure that the grafts are not cut too thick when taking a split-skin graft. The grafts should be so thin that they are translucent and that writing on the base underneath the transplant remains legible through it.

When using the foreskin as a full-thickness skin graft, extreme care must be taken to completely remove the layer of fat from the underside of the graft, to allow for rapid immigration of capillary blood vessels into the graft. In full-thickness skin grafts, revascularization always takes a bit longer than in split-thickness skin grafts, and the danger of transplant rejection is greater in full-thickness skin grafts. Any remaining subcutaneous fat prevents the rapid revascularzation of the full-thickness skin grafts.

Postoperative care

Postoperatively, bowel movement should be avoided for at least 5–7 days. This can be managed by the use of tinctura opii or other bowel movement stopping drugs. This stopping of bowel movement is especially important in long or posterior strictures, because fecal contamination is likely due to the extent of the incision. These patients are kept on bed rest for 7 days and are not allowed to go home for another week.

References

1 Blandy JP, Singh M, Tresidder GC. Urethroplasty by scrotal flap for long urethral strictures. Br J Urol 1968;40:261.
2 Byars LT. A technique for consistently satisfactory repair of hypospadias. Surg Gynecol Obstet 1995;100:184.
3 Devine PC, Horton CE, Devins CJ, Sr, Devine CJ, Jr, Crawfort, HH, Adamson JE. Use of full thickness skin grafts in repair of urethral strictures. J Urol 1963;90:67.
4 Johanson B. Reconstruction of the male urethra in strictures. Application of the buried intact epithelium tube. Acta Chir Scand 1953;167(Suppl):1.
5 Marberger H, Bantlow KH. Ergebnisse der Harnröhrenplastik nach Johanson. Urologe A 1976;15:269.
6 Schreiter F, Koncz PM. Traitement des stenoses uretrales compliquees par suture uretrale bout-a-bout et uretrplastie par greffe libre de prepuce. Les implants cutanes dans la reparation des stenoses uretrales. J Urol, Necker Masson, Paris, 1983;34–41.
7 Schreiter, F, Noll F. Meshgraft urethroplasty. World J Urol 1987;5:41.

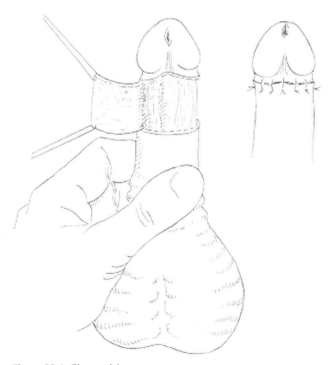

Figure 38.1 Circumcision.

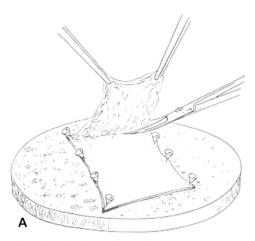
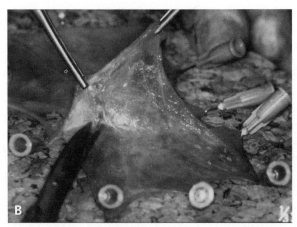

Figure 38.2 Defatting the graft.

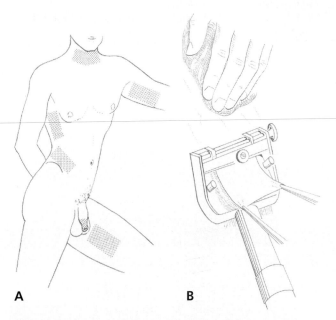

Figure 38.3 Harvesting the mesh graft: (A) possible sites on the body, and (B) the split-skin dermatome.

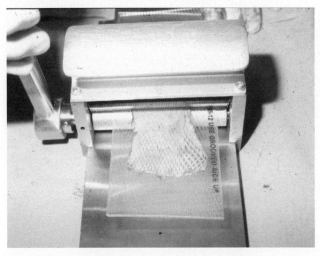

Figure 38.4 Meshing the graft (mesh graft dermatome).

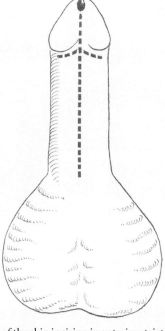

Figure 38.5 Line of the skin incision in anterior strictures.

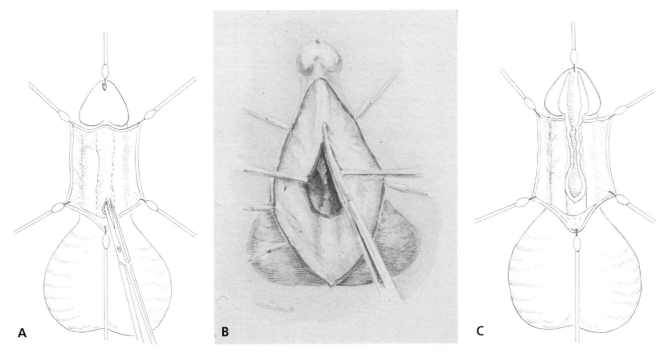

Figure 38.6 Marsupialization of the strictured urethra.

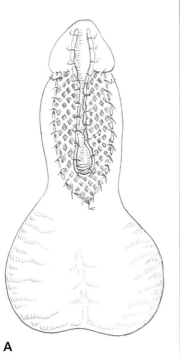

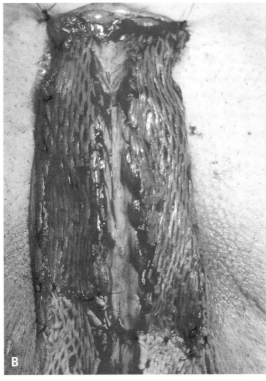

Figure 38.7 Mesh graft transplant, sutured in place.

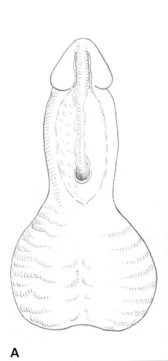

A

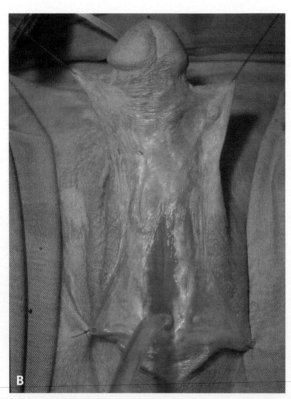

B

Figure 38.8 Healed transplant.

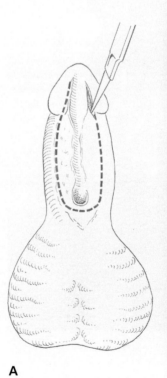

A

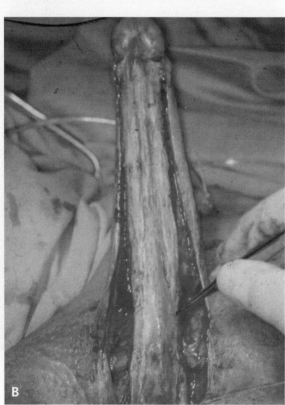

B

Figure 38.9 Peritomy of the healed transplant.

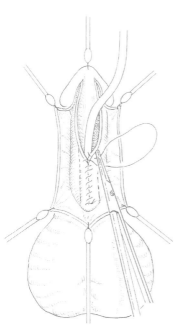
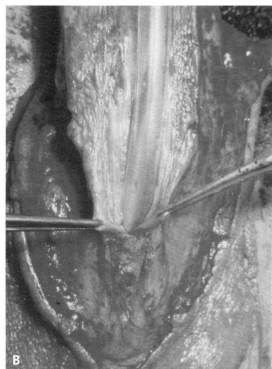

Figure 38.10 Suturing the neourethra (stitch technique). **A**

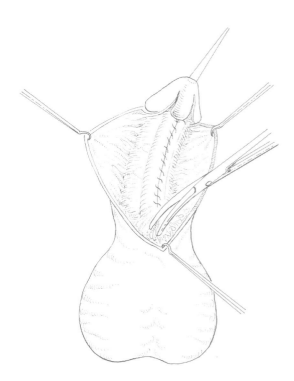

Figure 38.11 Mobilizing the penile skin.

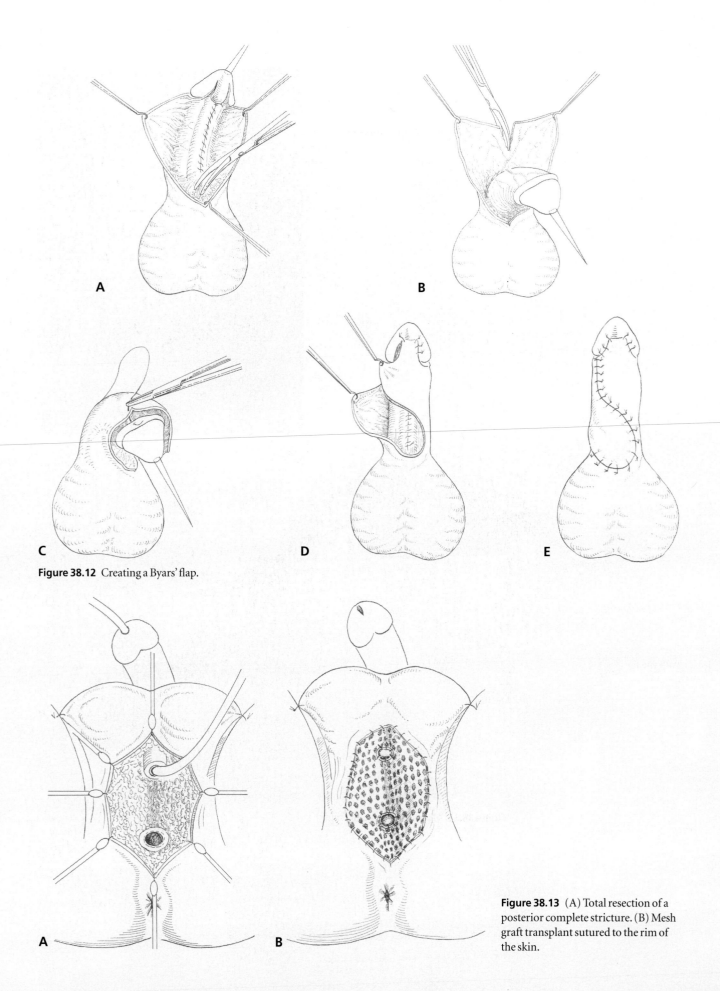

Figure 38.12 Creating a Byars' flap.

Figure 38.13 (A) Total resection of a posterior complete stricture. (B) Mesh graft transplant sutured to the rim of the skin.

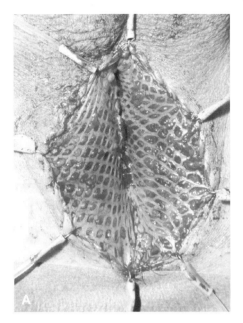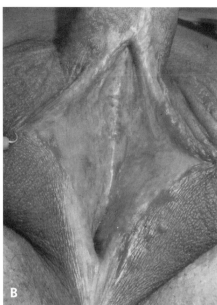

Figure 38.14 (A) Covering the wound with mesh graft. (B) The healed transplant.

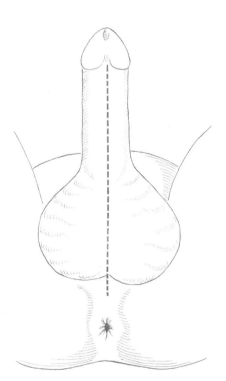

Figure 38.15 Incision of a total stricture of the urethra.

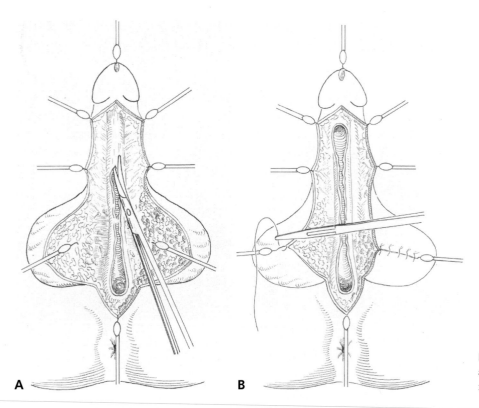

Figure 38.16 Division of the scrotum and marsupialization of the urethra to narrow the transplant surface.

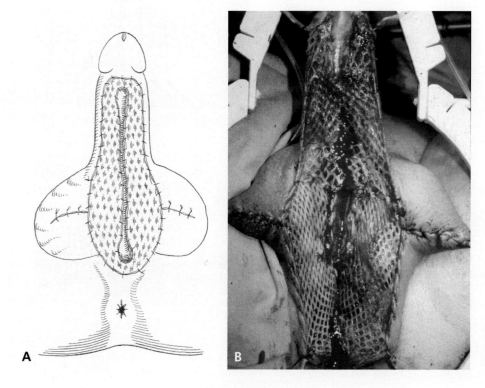

Figure 38.17 The transplanted mesh graft.

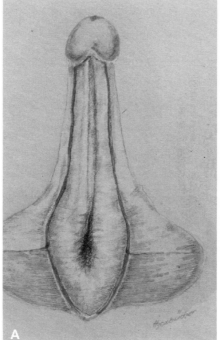

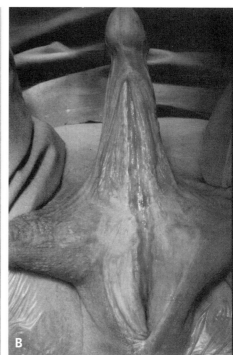

Figure 38.18 The healed mesh graft transplant.

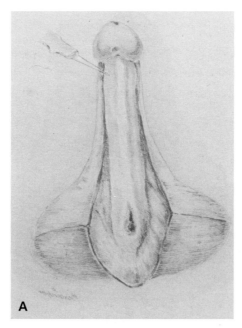

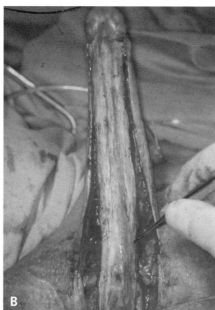

Figure 38.19 Peritomy of the healed transplant and the cutting lines to reconstruct the scrotum.

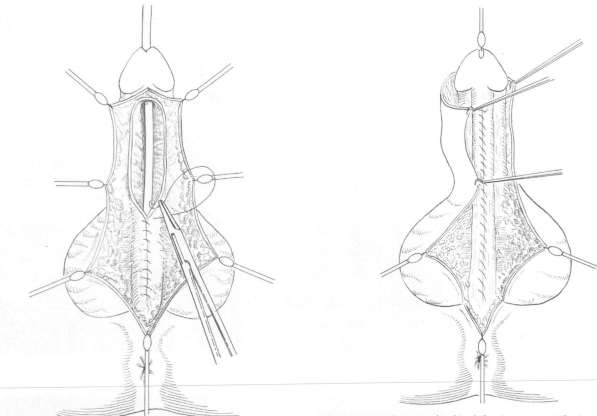

Figure 38.20 Suturing the neourethra.

Figure 38.21 Covering the skin defect (asymmetric flap) and reconstruction of the scrotum.

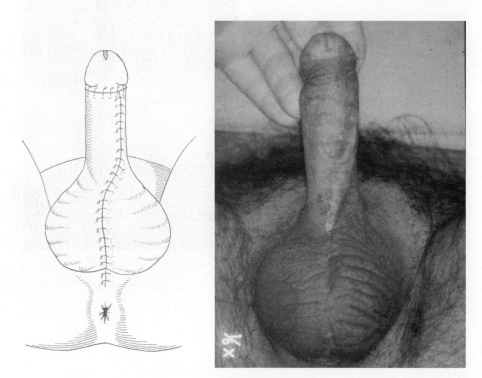

Figure 38.22 The completed reconstruction.

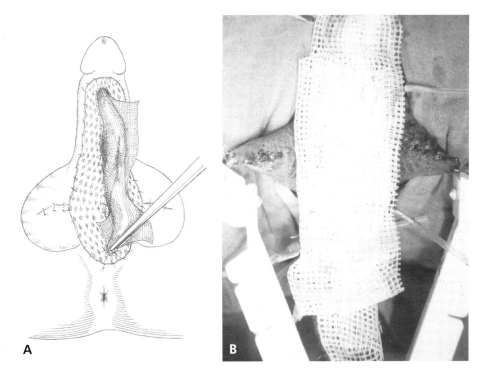

Figure 38.23 Fatty gauze is inserted into the proximal and distal urethra to prevent stenosis.

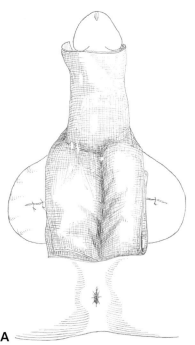

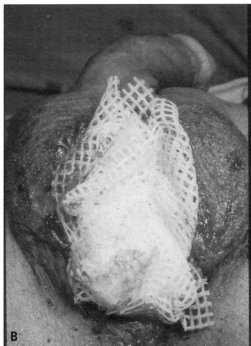

Figure 38.24 Fatty gauze is placed between the two transplanted surfaces to prevent bridging and adhesion.

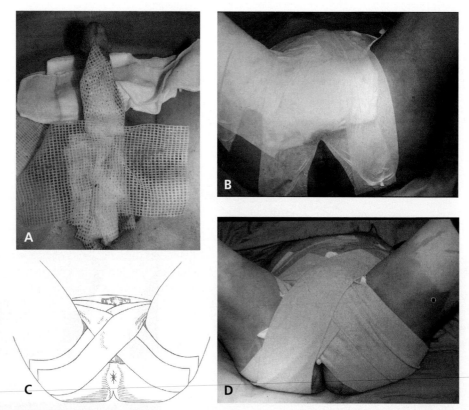

Figure 38.25 An elastic bandage fixes the dressing over the graft.

Chapter 39
Artificial Urinary Sphincter: Bladder Neck, Bulbar, Membranous, and Double Cuff Implantation

F. Schreiter

Introduction

For more than 30 years, complicated cases of urinary incontinence have been successfully treated by implanting an artificial sphincter (AS). The current model, AS 800, is the culmination of a successful development process. It is technologically mature, leaves hardly any room for improvement, and rarely experiences mechanical defects.

Depending on the indication, the AS 800 can be used at the bladder neck in males and females, at the bulbar urethra, at the membranous urethra, and as a double cuff implantation at the bulbus.

In complex cases of urinary incontinence (recurring female incontinence, neurogenic urinary incontinence, congenital or traumatically induced sphincter lesions, urinary incontinence following radical prostatectomy) artificial sphincters are the safest and most successful way to treat urinary incontinence, with success rates exceeding 90%. Today, urinary incontinence following radical prostatectomy accounts for more than 80–90% of all cases of sphincter implantation.

Functional principle of the artificial sphincter

The AS 800 (American Medical Systems, Minnetonka, MI, USA) is made of silicone rubber and consists of three parts (Fig. 39.1):
- A pressure-regulating reservoir, with varying pressure gradients between 50 and 90 cmH$_2$O water column, in 10 cm increments (51–60 cm, 61–70 cm, etc.); this is available in stores.
- An inflatable cuff that fits around the urethra and closes it when inflated.
- A pump that controls and regulates the transfer of liquid from the cuff to the pressure-regulating balloon.

The device works hydraulically, which is why it is filled with a blood-isotone liquid (NaCl or a mixture of X-ray dye and sterilized water).

When at rest, the cuff is inflated and holds the urethra closed. The pressure gradient of the pressure-regulating balloon determines the closing pressure of the urethra. The urethra's closing pressure is approximately 20–25 cmH$_2$O lower than that of the pressure-regulating balloon, and needs to be only slightly higher than the bladder's pressure at rest. Thus, in our experience, a pressure-regulating balloon of 61–70 cmH$_2$O is enough to create approximately 40 cmH$_2$O closing pressure at the urethra. This also ensures continence during sneezing, coughing, and strong physical activity.

The liquid is transported from the cuff to the pressure-regulating balloon using the pump; as the cuff empties, the urethra opens and the bladder can be emptied.

The pump's control assembly contains a resistor that delays the liquid's return transport to the cuff by 2–3 min, leaving enough time for passing water/urinating while the urethra is open. Once the cuff has been automatically reinflated, the urethra is closed again and urine can collect in the bladder.

A deactivation button on the pump controls can be used to stop the backflow from the pressure-regulating balloon when the cuff is deflated, causing the cuff to remain empty. This is called 'deactivating the sphincter'. Pressing the button again will reactivate the cuff's closing function. This is called 'activating the sphincter'.

Indications

All forms of urinary incontinence caused by weaknesses of the natural sphincter vesicae. These include:
- Post-prostatectomy incontinence.
- Stress-related urinary incontinence in women (primary hypotonic urethra, afunctional urethra following failed anti-incontinence surgery).
- Neurogenic urinary incontinence (with a stable detrusor).
- Congenital sphincter defects (epispadia, extrophia).
- Traumatic sphincter lesions.

Special indications

In cases of urodynamically proven hyperactivity of the detrusor or a low-compliance bladder, an artificial sphincter may only be implanted if you succeed in immobilizing the detrusor with medication or improving the bladder capacity. If drug treatment fails, the detrusor must be surgically augmented, with isolated and detubularized bowel segments.

In cases of reflux to the upper urinary tract, an antireflux procedure is recommended.

Patient selection

- Bladder capacity over 200 cm^3.
- Urodynamic findings (normally active or hypoactive detrusor; normal or elevated compliance).
- No obstruction (residual urine less than 50 cm^3).
- No reflux.
- Sufficient manual dexterity.
- Patient should be motivated.
- Children under the age of 10 years should not be operated on if possible.
- Normal intelligence levels (for understanding the system's function and handling).

Contraindications

See the criteria for patient selection.

Anesthesia

Spinal, peridural, or general anesthesia.

Special instruments/suture material

- Scott retractor.
- Right-angled dissection clamps (Overholt).
- Six covered mosquito clamps.
- Large curved blunt-tip forceps.
- AS preparation package.
- Connector clamp.
- Three pots of differing sizes.
- Satinsky scissors.
- Two tubing passers.
- Usual instruments for bladder operations.
- Sutures: 2/0 and 4/0 absorbable, monophile.

Surgical approach

- Median episiotomy and pararectal for bulbar, membranous, and double cuff implants.
- Cherney's incision (transverse hypogastric) for bladder neck implants.

Bulbar implantation in males

Implanting a single cuff at the urethral bulbus only leads to complete continence in rare cases (approximately 4% [1]). That is why we gave up using this implantation technique in the 1970s and adjusted the surgical procedure so that the cuff is implanted at the site of the natural sphincter. This results in the advantage of improved continence and lower rates of erosion. Bulbar implantation using a perineal incision is currently being recommended with the argument that the procedure is simple enough for ambulatory treatment. However, it has the same disadvantages as the original bulbar implantation technique used by Brandley Scott. The procedure currently being recommended places the pressure-regulating balloon in an extraperitoneal position next to the bladder instead of in an intraperitoneal position. The importance of keeping the balloon inside the peritoneum has been repeatedly emphasized by Scott and the author of this chapter. If the balloon is implanted extraperitoneally, a fibrous membrane forms around the pressure-regulating balloon, causing it to shrink and raise the pressure in the system. This pressure increase may cause damage to the urethra. Therefore, this implantation technique is not recommended.

Operative technique

- Lithotomy position with the option of lowering the legs if necessary.
- Perineal incision in the midline.
- Split the bulbocavernosus muscle.
- Mobilize approximately 2–3 cm along the urethra.
- The further course of the surgery is the same as in the membranous implantation technique (see below).

Membranous implantation in males
Operative technique

- Place the patient in the lithotomy position.
- Make a median or star-shaped incision in the perineal raphe.
- Expose the crura of the corpora cavernosa from the bifurcation up to the insertion of the os ischium.
- Incise the ligamentum triangulare below the bifurcation of the crura and next to the urethra.
- Expose and transect the central tendons and dissect the bulborectal musculature below the bulbous and the membranous part of the urethra.
- Prepare the area behind the ligamentum triangulare below and adjacent to the symphysis.
- Insert the cuff sizer and determine the length of the cuff by circular measurement.

- Insert the proper length cuff over the cuff sizer. The sizer is removed afterwards.
- Lower the legs.
- Make a pararectal incision above the inguinal canal, on the side of the cuff tubing.
- Open up the peritoneum.
- Implant the pressure-regulating balloon inside the peritoneum, and close up the peritoneum.
- Fill the pressure-regulating balloon with 22 cm³ of blood-isotone liquid.
- Prepare a scrotal pouch starting from the pararectal incision above the abdominal fascia and precisely in the layer between the scrotum's tunica dartos and tunica vaginalis of the testes.
- Fixate the pump in the scrotum from the outside using a Babcock clamp.
- Run the cuff tubing above the symphysis using the tubing passer.
- Connect the tubing within the pararectal incision using a straight connector to the reservoir and a right-angled connector to the pump.
- Close both incisions layer by layer without drainage.
- Deactivate the sphincter for 4–6 weeks.
- Place a 12 Fr indwelling catheter for 2 days.

Double cuff implantation

In approximately 15% of cases, there will be a recurrence of urinary incontinence following a sphincter implantation. Usually, the cause is tissue atrophy of the urethra underneath the cuff, which reduces the urethra's closing pressure. Theoretically, the lowered closing pressure could be remedied by reimplanting a pressure-regulating balloon with a higher pressure. But this would mean a considerably higher risk of erosion for the urethral tissue.

However, the urethra's closing pressure may also be increased—without risk of erosion—by enlarging the cuff's compression area according to the formula:

Urethral resistance = pressure × area

Two side-by-side cuffs on the urethra will increase the urethra's closing pressure without risk, with 90–95% security of continence.

Indications

- Tissue atrophy.
- Status after sphincter explantation, e.g. due to an infection on the plastic material.
- Status after erosion of a single cuff.
- Status after radiation to the bladder neck region (e.g. following radical prostatectomy).

Advantages

At this point in time, the double cuff implantation is the most common technique for implanting an artificial sphincter. It is an easier technique than membranous implantation and results in a high continence rate. This is why many surgeons routinely use it today, e.g. in patients with urinary incontinence after radical prostatectomy (P. Althaus, Berlin, pers. comm.).

The advantages are obvious; its sole disadvantage is the additional cost for the second cuff.

Surgical technique

- Place the patient in the lithotomy position.
- Make a perineal incision in the middle of the perineum.
- Split the bulbocavernosus muscle.
- Prepare a 5 cm long section of the bulbar urethra.
- Insert two 4.5 cm long cuffs side by side.
- Close the bulbocavernosus muscle over the implanted cuffs.
- Guide both cuff tubes into the pararectal incision above the symphysis.
- Fill the balloon with 22 + 2 cm³ (second cuff) of blood-isotone liquid.
- Connect all tube connections to the implanted pump using a Y-connector and to the pressure-regulating balloon using a straight quick connector.
- Continue as in membranous implantation technique above.

Bladder neck implantation

The quality of continence is higher in bladder neck implants than in all forms of bulbar and membranous implants. Therefore, we use this method whenever possible. It is possible in neurogenic urinary incontinence (meningomyelocele), female incontinence, congenital and traumatic sphincter defects, and in cases of incontinence following transurethral resection of the prostate (TURP). However, because 80–90% of patients with urinary incontinence come for treatment following a radical prostatectomy, the bulbar techniques are used increasingly often.

Operative technique in males

- Place the patient in a lithotomy position with the legs down.
- Insert a 16 Fr balloon catheter and empty the bladder.
- Make a Cherney's incision (transverse) and blunt dissect the cavum rezii.
- Incise the fascia endopelvina next to the prostate.
- Locate the bladder neck by pulling on the catheter.
- Blunt dissect with the thumb and index finger placed precisely at the bladder neck around the prostate.

- Pass a right-angle clamp under the prostate and use it to perforate Denonvilliers' fascia below the prostate.
- Insert the cuff sizer and measure the length of the cuff.
- Insert the cuff while the cuff sizer is still in place, using the right-angle clamp.
- Close the cuff using the latch and position it correctly.
- Open the peritoneum and insert a pressure-regulating balloon, usually with a routine pressure of 61–70 cmH$_2$O. Close up the peritoneum.
- Pass the cuff and balloon tubing through using a tubing passer.
- Prepare the scrotal pouch precisely between the tunica dartos and the tunica vaginale scrotalis.
- Insert the pump into the scrotal pouch.
- Fill the pressure-regulating balloon with 22 cm^3 of blood-isotone liquid.
- Pass the tubes through above the inguinal canal using the tubing passer. Use straight quick connectors to connect the tubes.
- Close the incision layer by layer without drainage.
- Deactivate the cuff for approximately 5 days.
- Drain the urine via the urethra for 2–3 days using a 12 Fr indwelling catheter.

Operative technique in females

- The bladder is routinely opened at the vertex.
- Pack the vagina to fully extend it.
- Under visual control, prepare the vaginal urethral septum under the bladder neck while controlling the dissection with the left index finger in the vagina. Use Satinsky scissors.
- The rest of the implantation technique is as in males, above.
- Maintain catheter drainage for approximately 7 days (bladder suture).
- Suction drainage into the cavum rezii.

Tips

- Extremely careful asepsis before and during surgery (beware of infection on the plastic surfaces).
- Bloodless preparation during surgery to prevent hema-

tomas (danger of infection) and to avoid drainage (gateway for infection).
- Avoid at all costs any intraoperative damage to the urethra, rectum, and vagina.
- In women, ensure a watertight bladder suture with a continuous two-layer suture (monophile, absorbable).
- Use precise cuff sizing.
- Select a pressure-regulating balloon in the 61–70 cmH$_2$O range, but never above 80 cmH$_2$O because of the danger of pressure necrosis in the urethra and high pressure atrophy.
- Routine postoperative deactivation of the device.

Postoperative care

- Reposition the pump in the first 2 days after surgery to prevent a malpositioning of the pump.
- Give perioperative prophylactic antibiotics for 5 days, beginning on the day before the surgery.
- In bladder neck implants, activate the sphincter on the sixth day after surgery.
- Activate the sphincter at the bulbar or membranous urethra after 4–6 weeks.
- Give intensive postoperative training to patients in handling the device.

References

1 Montague DK, Angermeier KW, Paolone DR. Long-term continence and patient satisfaction after artificial sphincter implantation for urinary incontinence after prostatectomy. J Urol 2001; 166(2):547–9.
2 Schreiter F, Noll F. Bulbar artificial sphincter. Eur Urol 1985; 11:294–9.
3 Schreiter F, Noll F. The artificial sphincter AS 800. In: Urinary Incontinence (Steg A, ed.). Churchill Livingstone, London, 1993: 241–57.
4 Schreiter F, Noll F. Artificial sphincter in the female. In: Female Urology (Kursch EDE, McGuire G, eds). J.B. Lippincott, Philadelphia, 1994:259–65.
5 Scott FBW, Bradley E, Timm GW. Treatment of urinary incontinence by an implantable prosthetic sphincter. Urology 1973;1: 252–4.

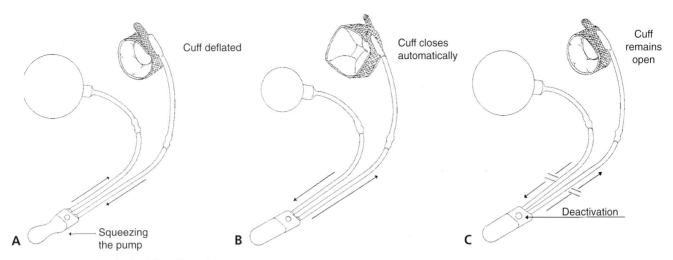

Cuff deflated

Cuff closes automatically

Cuff remains open

Deactivation

A   ← Squeezing the pump   B   C

Figure 39.1 Functional principles of the AS 800.

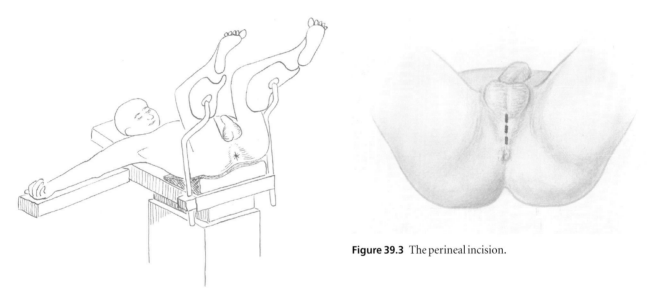

Figure 39.2 The lithotomy position.

Figure 39.3 The perineal incision.

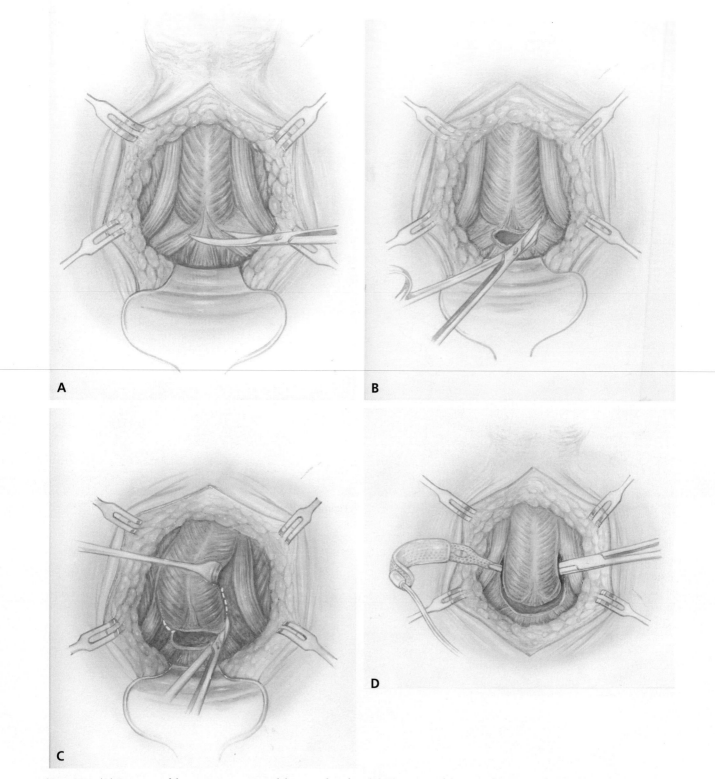

Figure 39.4 (A) Exposure of the crura cavernosa and the central tendon. (B) Dissection of the central tendon and the bulbourethral musculature. (C) Exposure of the ligamentum triangulare. (D) Incision of the ligamentum triangulare and insertion of the cuff behind the ligamentum triangulare using a right-angle clamp.

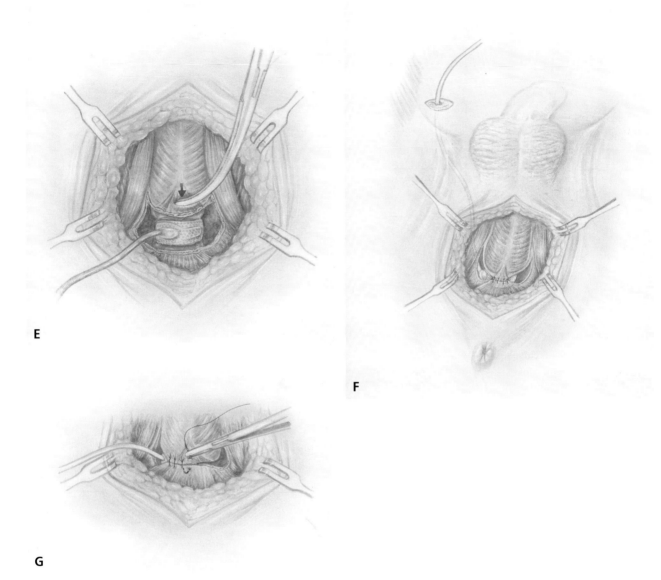

Figure 39.4 *Continued.* (E) Position of the cuff at the membranous urethra. (F) Reconstruction of the central tendon. (G) The cuff migrates down to, and is placed at, the membranous urethra.

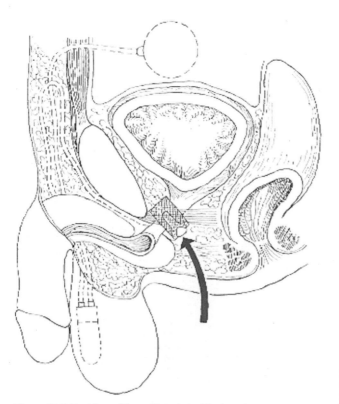

Figure 39.5 Position of the cuff partly inside the pelvis.

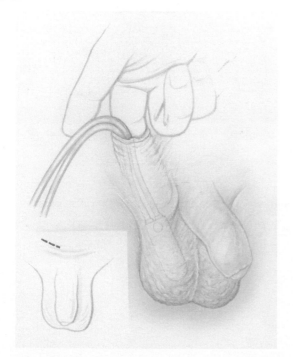

Figure 39.6 The pump and pressure-regulation balloon are implanted from the pararectal incision.

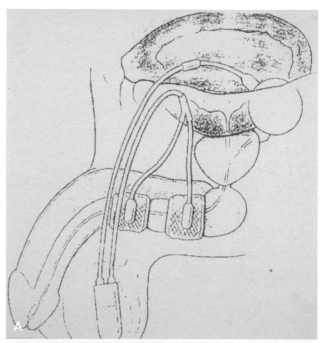

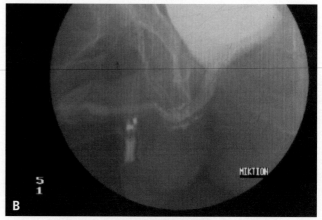

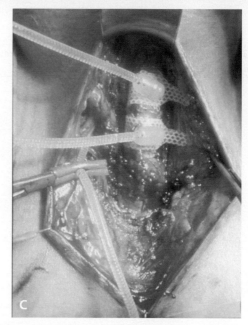

Figure 39.7 (A) Double cuff implantation using a Y-connector. (B) Micturating cystourethrogram showing the placement of the double cuff. (C) The double cuff *in situ* at the bulbar urethra.

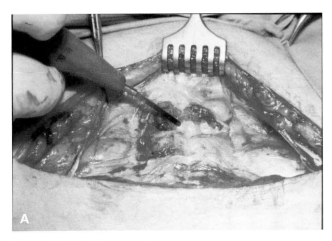 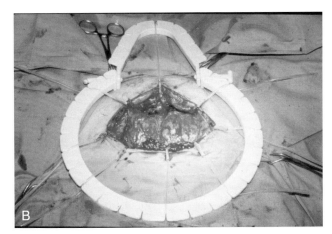

Figure 39.8 The Cherney incision.

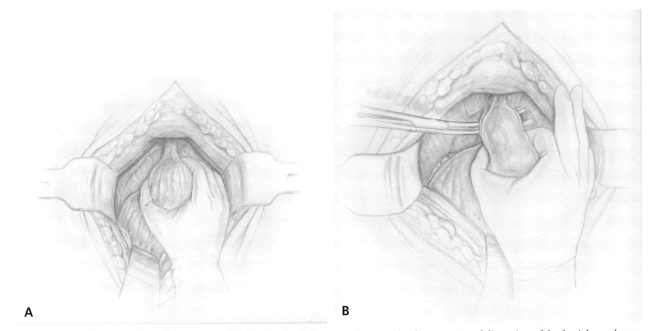

A   **B**

Figure 39.9 (A) Blunt dissection of the prostate. (B) Passing the right-angle clamp under the prostate and dissection of the fascial membrane.

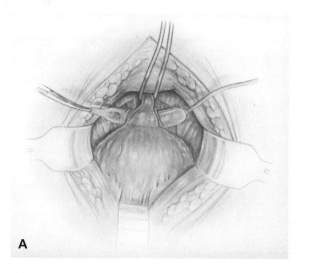

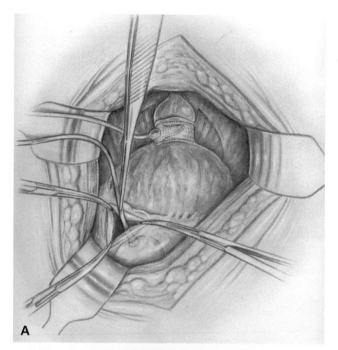

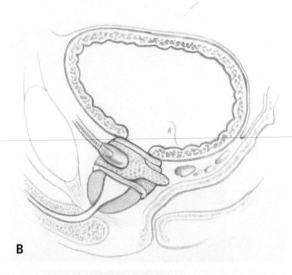

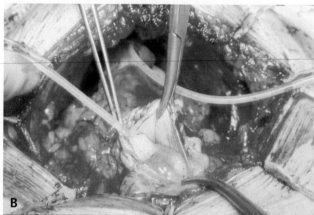

Figure 39.11 Implantation of the pressure-regulating balloon intraperitoneally.

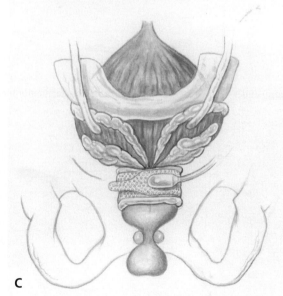

Figure 39.10 (A) Insertion of the cuff. (B) Position of the cuff at the bladder neck. (C) The cuff in relation to the seminal vesicles.

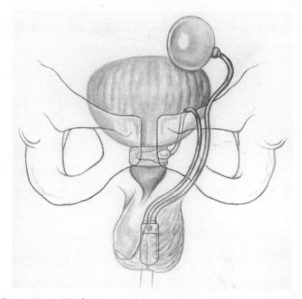

Figure 39.12 Final position of the whole device.

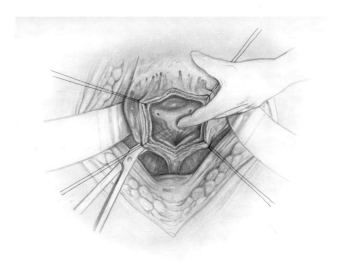

Figure 39.13 The bladder is routinely opened at the vertex for better visual implantation control.

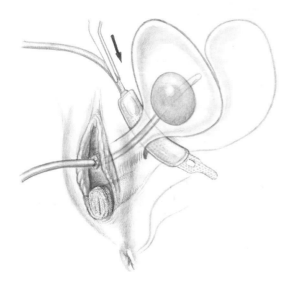

Figure 39.15 Implantation of the cuff.

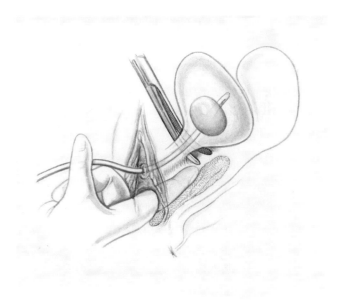

Figure 39.14 The vagina is packed for proper extension. The left index finger controls the vagina during dissection.

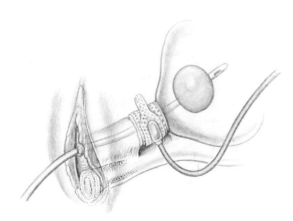

Figure 39.16 Position of the cuff at the bladder neck.

Section 6
Female Urology

Introduction

A. Fischer

It is not easy to select the ingredients for a section called 'Female Urology' as, with the arrival of the last millenium's end, we have reached a point where a lot of things have started to change in female urology or urogynecology (as it is most commonly referred to):

- understanding of the pelvic floor function;
- surgical strategies deriving therefrom; and
- the possibility of using different forms of implants for reconstructive surgical attempts.

In understanding the pelvic floor function, the Integral Theory developed by Peter P. Petros and Ulf Ulmsten in the late 1980s and first published in 1990, was the background for a change in the treatment of incontinence and prolapse. This theory emphasizes the role of pelvic ligaments and fascia in the structure and function of the pelvic floor. A key concept of this theory is that even minor degrees of ligamentous laxity have the potential to cause quite major pelvic floor symptoms and that these are potentially curable by reinforcing pelvic ligaments using tapes or by restoring the fascial integrity using implants. Therefore, the reader will find conventional approaches to incontinence and prolapse surgery as well as those deriving from the Integral Theory. *The basic concept here is that three muscle forces acting in different directions* (pubococcygeus muscle (PCM), levator plate (LP), and longitudinal muscle from the levator ani to the anus (LMA)) *together with the main pelvic floor ligaments* (pubourethral ligament (PUL), uterosacral ligaments (USL), and arcus tendineous of the endopelvic fascia attached to the arcus tendineus of the levator ani muscle (ATFP)) *transmit their forces to the relevant structures* (i.e. the bladder neck opening and closing mechanism, anal opening and closing mechanism) *by those ligaments with the help of a well-attached and normally mobile and elastic vagina.*

The minimalist, surgical, tension-free approach and the excellent results obtained have unleashed a rapid evolution in the surgical technique (not to mention a plethora of different tapes, meshes, and delivery instruments). An extensive discussion arose long before the surgical concepts were properly evaluated and those working on the pelvic floor had

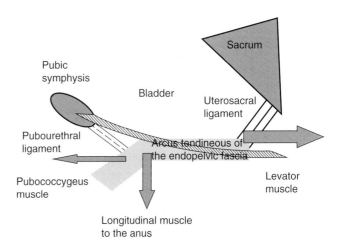

established solid concepts applicable to most of the cases they encountered. Instead of 'think and watch—rethink and do—observe and rethink and perhaps then adjust your own strategy', many started doing things without watching closely, without thinking properly, and without observing thoroughly. This will probably end up in bad results and unhappy patients (at the least) and may wrongly discredit a theory and its derived surgical approaches.

In the developement of implants in particular, over the last years we have not always followed straight paths; some ended early (e.g. the first generation meshes), some were even dead-ended (e.g. microporous multifilament tapes). But there has been, and still is, an incredible forward pushing force in all those workgroups developing new concepts so that innovations and improvements rapidly arise from their predecesor's ashes.

We now have established certain basic standards in this new field:

- the use of macroporous monofilament meshes made of polypropylene;
- the use of tension-free techniques; and
- the use of the obturator hole as a surgical passway.

This is the basis for the forward movement of this ongoing process and there will still be lots of changes, developments, and adjustments.

But there are still a lot of techniques covered in this section that have not changed much over the last years: Burch colposuspension, fistula repair, abdominal sacrocolpopexy, etc. We all know that the multitude of different procedures coming under the same name do not necessarily produce the same results. So the aim here is to show a generally acceptable standard for these procedures and to elaborate the reasons for their choice in each chapter.

I think this is the place to commemorate Professor Ulf Ulmsten of Uppsala University, Sweden who recently died. We are grateful for his understanding of the Integral Theory and for the help he gave to Professor Peter P. Petros—the man who tripped loose this avalanche of innovations by developing the Integral Theory—to publish it together with him. Out of this understanding for developing the first technique and device he helped to completely change the approach to the surgical cure of female urinary stress incontinence.

This is also the place to thank Professor Hohenfellner, and G. Müller, who had to adjust his drawings several times to fit our needs. During the period of working on this section, I have admired Professor Hohenfellner's open-minded approach to the new techniques we wanted to include in this book to give this section a special topicality. Last, but not least, I want to thank him for the honor of being asked to edit this section—being a gynecologist. I think this is the future of female urology and urogynecology—joint efforts of all those working on the improvement of women's quality of life, so heavily disturbed or even destroyed by pelvic floor disorders. May the result of our small workgroup's joint efforts be helpful to the reader on the everyday battlefield of female urology, to the benefit of women suffering in this field.

I would like to dedicate this chapter to my wife and children with gratitude for their love and for their understanding of how important my work in urogynecology is to me.

Dr. med. Armin Fischer
Section editor

Part 6.1
Female Urinary Stress Incontinence

Introduction to the Surgical Treatment of Stress Urinary Incontinence

A. Fischer

General remarks

Surgery is never the first-line treatment of female urinary stress incontinence: estrogens, pelvic floor muscle exercise, exclusion of motor urge, pessaries, or electrophysiotherapy, where necessary, have to precede the surgical efforts to cure or improve the symptoms. In some cases Duloxetin as a serotonin/noradrenaline reuptake inhibitor may be a good choice of treatment, at least for some time.

The reasons for becoming stress incontinent are numerous, as are the defects that may occur, but not all defects are revealed to or detected by the investigator even in a very thoroughly executed investigation.

The patient has to be aware that success in incontinence surgery does not necessarily mean achievement of complete continence. Improvement is also a success, especially if the onset of urge symptoms as a side effect can be avoided.

After unsuccessful conservative treatment, as well as in cases of insufficient effect of conservative treatment, surgery may be desired by the patient. Preoperative evaluation of severity, previous surgical and conservative therapeutic efforts, urological, gynecological, and other physical disorders or accompanying conditions including the daily or irregular pharmaceutical treatment of concomitant diseases, may influence the advice given to the patient. In particular, look for the following:

- A sufficient estrogen effect on the urethra and vagina (proliferation index of cells: 3–4) (e.g. 0.5 mg estriol locally twice a week).
- No urinary tract infection.
- Colpitis has to be excluded.
- No inflammatory skin diseases in the region of the pubis.
- Use perineal/introitus ultrasound to check anatomy; X-ray or MRI are rarely necessary.
- Exclude gynecological malignoma.
- Check that the indications for colporrhaphy and hysterectomy are coexisting (see Table 5).

The administration of a cephalosporine (third generation) is recommended before starting the procedure. No anti-coagulation treatment should be given before or shortly after the surgery.

In mixed incontinence all causes for urge symptoms have to be checked first; pharmaceutical treatment (trial) of urge symptoms is advisable. Is there an anatomical defect that could explain the onset of urge symptoms?

This leads directly to the question of preoperative urodynamics. Standards all over the world, as well as the possibility of getting a urodynamic study before operating on an incontinent woman, vary a lot and local medicolegal protocols should be respected in order to avoid trouble with rightfully pressed charges by unsatisfied patients. Urodynamics are uncomfortable but do not harm a patient, unlike the wrong choice of treatment.

Recommendations

- Urodynamic studies using cystomanometry are advisable for the exclusion of urge incontinence; in some countries they are considered a must (if only for medicolegal reasons).
- The resting and stress profiles of the urethra make postoperative monitoring easier; the Valsalva leak point pressure may also be useful.
- Inspection and palpation of the vagina and pelvic floor, including a stress test (the examination has to be performed with a full bladder).
- Ultrasound of the kidneys, abdomen, and perineum to examine bladder neck mobility, position, and funnelling. Pelvic floor reaction to stress and squeezing maneuvers.
- Videourodynamics are not available everywhere and therefore cannot become a general standard in the diagnostics of urinary stress incontinence before surgery. In many cases, however, thorough conventional urodynamics and a good standard in perineal ultrasound (or lateral cystography) will be sufficient.
- MRI studies are sophisticated but expensive. They should therefore be restricted to cases where the decision for a procedure depends on the MRI findings. Again, thorough clinical

and sonographic examination should be sufficient in most cases.

- *Anesthesia.* Try to develop a standard approach with the anesthesist. Retropubic (and transobturator) slings can be done under local anesthesia, especially if a cough test is desired. Otherwise, spinal/epidural or general anesthesia both work. For transobturator incontinence procedures with a mean duration of 6–8 min (in an experienced surgeon's hands), spinal/epidural anesthesia may be more than is needed—analgesic sedation should be sufficient. For the Burch procedure and fascial slings both methods may be used; the anesthesist should therefore counsult the patient if the surgeon is happy with either type of anesthesia being used.
- Adequate (local) estrogenization must be maintained for the patient's lifetime. Local application of estriol (2 × 0.5 g/week) is also possible in most patients with a history of mammarian cancer.
- *Postoperative treatment.* If there is drainage in Retzius' space or vaginal packing it is usually removed on the second day (after 24 h). Start micturition on day 3–5, keeping to the protocol, and remove the (suprapubic) catheter when the post voiding residual is below 50 cm^3. A kidney ultrasound should be performed before the patient is dismissed. Antibiotics should be given according to clinical standards.
- Postoperatively, the patient should avoid heavy lifting and strenuous work for at least 6 weeks. There should be no intercourse for approximately 2–4 weeks, depending on vaginal healing status.
- One to 2 weeks after a transvaginal sling (TVS) operation, the patient can resume all other normal activities (except for lifting and straining).
- In allergic patients, consider the season.

Urethral mobility, prolapse, and incontinence procedures

The most difficult problem to be solved when surgical treatment for urinary incontinence is needed is which method to choose. The right choice of method often determines the success or failure, as well as the side effects, of the procedure.

In surgical incontinence treatment the most important factors that have to be considered are:
- Urethral and bladder neck mobility: defect of paraurethral fixation.
- Simultaneous vaginal descent/prolapse:
  - anterior midline defect;
  - anterior lateral defect;
  - central defect;
  - posterior defect.
- Intrinsic sphincter deficiency.
- Funneling of the bladder neck.
- Laxity of the suburethral vagina (hammock).
- Previous operations for incontinence.
- Previous gynecological surgery.
- The patient's desires.

The following tables and algorithms have been designed to help in the complexity of finding the right procedure, even in primary cases, and to show the interdependence between prolapse and incontinence treatment.

Urethral and bladder neck mobility are definitely the most important conditions that have to be evaluated before surgery in order to make the right choice and to keep side effects (obstruction, retention, urge) low.

Imaging is very useful in the decision-making process. Perineal ultrasound or a lateral cystogram (or even dynamic MRI) will provide a good assessment of bladder neck mobility and the movement of the bladder base when straining.

Table 1 summarizes the order in which different therapies are considered, as seen in current practice in patients with recurrence. At the moment there is no established rule as to the correct sequence of therapies. For each treatment, the whole algorithm (cf. Tables 2 and 3) has to be applied as other factors that have an impact on continence have to be taken into account, and the surgical concept has to be chosen accordingly. Even though this is a surgical manual, the right way to approach female incontinence is to start any treatment with prevention before or during the first pregnancy. By following this advice, hopefully, the use of an artificial sphincter and urinary deviation will remain the very last options to finally get a patient dry.

Figures 1 and 2 evaluate the importance of urethral kinking in incontinence procedures, and how to evaluate this risk using clinical examination and ultrasound or MRI.

Tables 2–4 give practical help in selecting the right treatment, depending on the preoperative findings. There are many causes of a defect that influences continence and there is not (yet) one treatment to fit them all. Urogynecology probably has to be considered to be more of an art than of a science at the moment.

Table 5 discusses the indications of the most commonly used surgical procedures, as well as their relation with additional conditions or previous therapies.

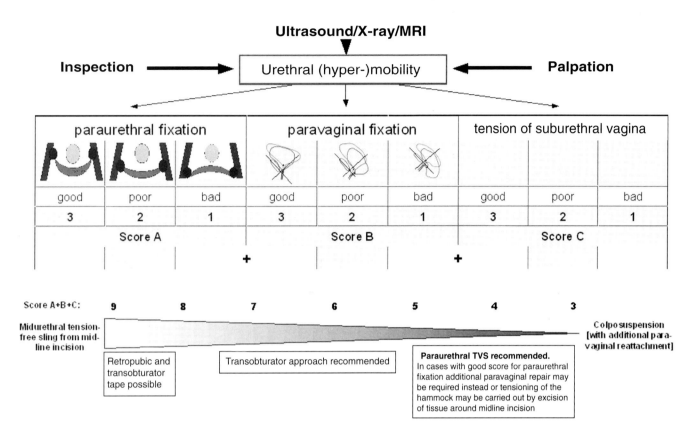

Figure 1 Evaluation of the risk of urethral kinking with midurethral slings, depending on the paraurethral tissue's fixation and laxity. As the risk of kinking increases, simple midurethral slings should be used with increasing caution or not used at all.

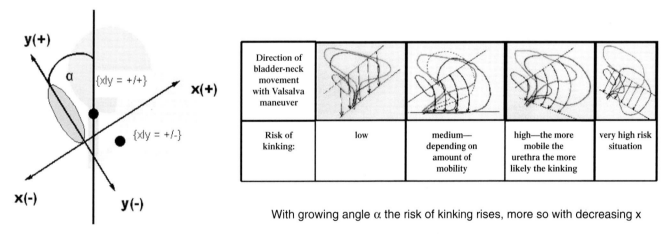

With growing angle α the risk of kinking rises, more so with decreasing x

Figure 2 Evaluation of the risk of urethral kinking with midurethral slings depending on bladder neck movement with increased abdominal pressure. With a coordinate system the movement of the bladder neck can be described better than with just the use of angle α. A growing angle and decreasing values for *x* and *y* with Valsalva maneuver represent a high-risk situation.

Table 1. The dilemma of 'what to do when' in current practice leads to a multitude of protocols, reflecting the uncertainty in choosing a method.

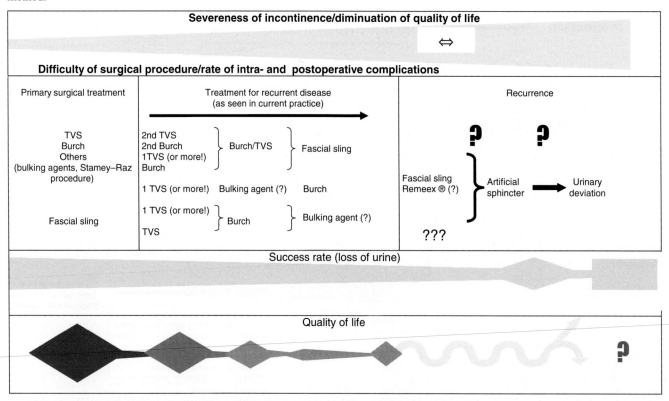

Table 2. Surgical procedures for stress urinary incontinence. Algorith for the use of tension-free midurethral slings (TVS).

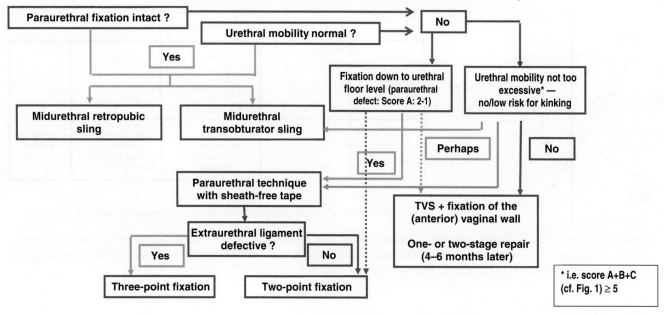

Table 3. Surgical procedures for stress urinary incontinence. Algorithm for the use of conventional surgical procedures for female stress incontinence. ISD, intrinsic sphincter deficiency.

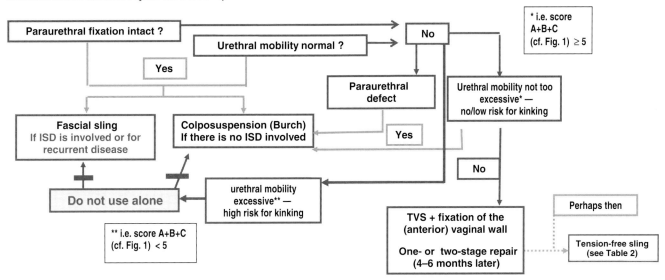

Table 4. Synopsis of the patient's morphology and defects needed to select an adequate procedure.

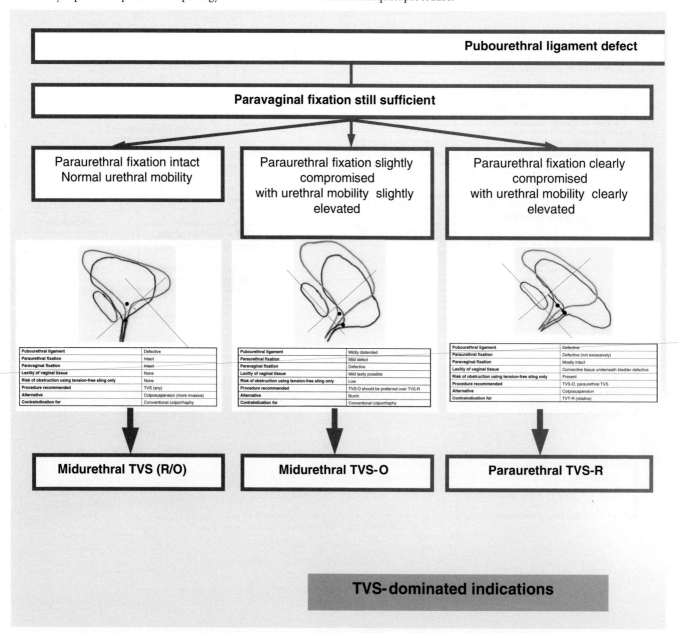

ATOM, anterior transobturator mesh (see Chapter 45); SUI, stress urinary incontinence; TVS-O, transobturator transvaginal sling (see Chapter 43); TVS-R, retropubic transvaginal sling (see Chapter 42).

Table 4. *Continued*

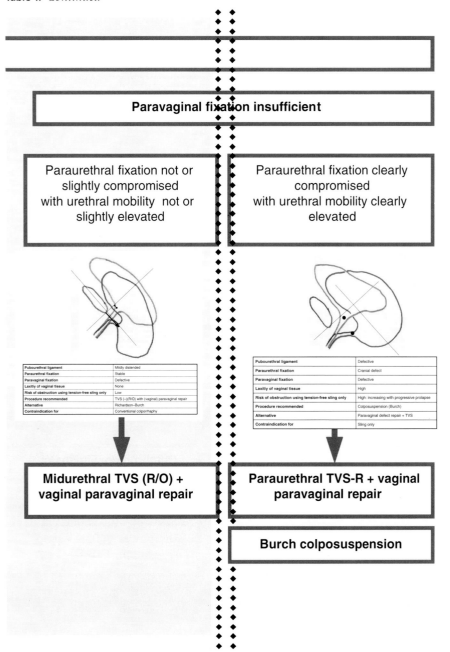

Paravaginal fixation insufficient

| Paraurethral fixation not or slightly compromised with urethral mobility not or slightly elevated | Paraurethral fixation clearly compromised with urethral mobility clearly elevated |

Pubourethral ligament	Mildly distended
Paraurethral fixation	Stable
Paravaginal fixation	Defective
Laxity of vaginal tissue	None
Risk of obstruction using tension-free sling only	Low
Procedure recommended	TVS (–)(R/O) with (vaginal) paravaginal repair
Alternative	Richardson–Burch
Contraindication for	Conventional colporrhaphy

Pubourethral ligament	Defective
Paraurethral fixation	Cranial defect
Paravaginal fixation	Defective
Laxity of vaginal tissue	High
Risk of obstruction using tension-free sling only	High: increasing with progressive prolapse
Procedure recommended	Colposuspension (Burch)
Alternative	Paravaginal defect repair + TVS
Contraindication for	Sling only

Midurethral TVS (R/O) + vaginal paravaginal repair

Paraurethral TVS-R + vaginal paravaginal repair

Burch colposuspension

Table 4 continued on next page

Table 4. *Continued*

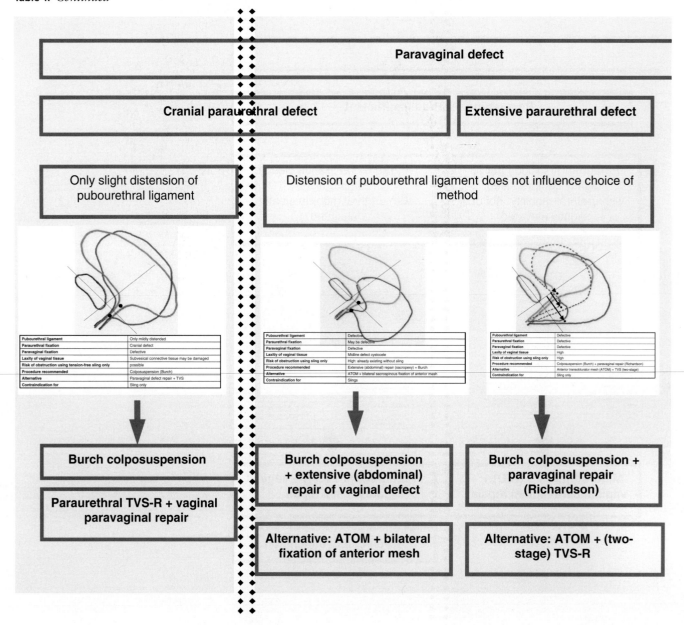

Paravaginal defect		
Cranial paraurethral defect		**Extensive paraurethral defect**
Only slight distension of pubourethral ligament	Distension of pubourethral ligament does not influence choice of method	

Pubourethral ligament	Only mildly distended
Paraurethral fixation	Cranial defect
Paravaginal fixation	Defective
Laxitiy of vaginal tissue	Subvesical connective tissue may be damaged
Risk of obstruction using tension-free sling only	possible
Procedure recommended	Colposuspension (Burch)
Alternative	Paravaginal defect repair + TVS
Contraindication for	Sling only

Pubourethral ligament	Defective
Paraurethral fixation	May be defective
Paravaginal fixation	Defective
Laxitiy of vaginal tissue	Midline defect cystocele
Risk of obstruction using sling only	High: already existing without sling
Procedure recommended	Extensive (abdominal) repair (sacropexy) + Burch
Alternative	ATOM + bilateral sacrospinous fixation of anterior mesh
Contraindication for	Slings

Pubourethral ligament	Defective
Paraurethral fixation	Defective
Paravaginal fixation	Defective
Laxitiy of vaginal tissue	High
Risk of obstruction using sling only	High
Procedure recommended	Colposuspension (Burch) + paravaginal repair (Richardson)
Alternative	Anterior transobturator mesh (ATOM) + TVS (two-stage)
Contraindication for	Sling only

Burch colposuspension	**Burch colposuspension + extensive (abdominal) repair of vaginal defect**	**Burch colposuspension + paravaginal repair (Richardson)**
Paraurethral TVS-R + vaginal paravaginal repair	**Alternative: ATOM + bilateral fixation of anterior mesh**	**Alternative: ATOM + (two-stage) TVS-R**

Table 4. *Continued*

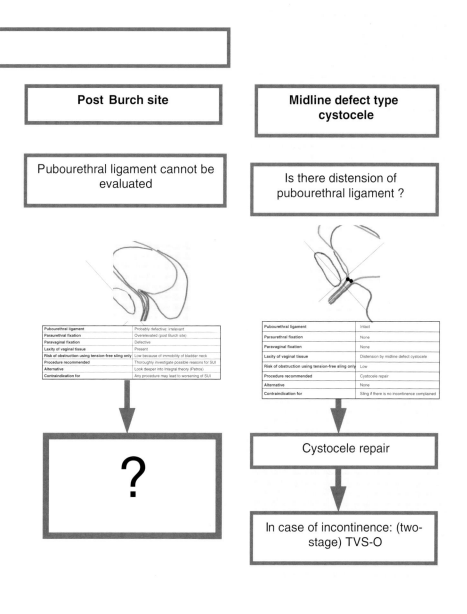

Table 5 Indications of the most common surgical procedures for stress urinary incontinence and conditions with an influence on their outcome.

	Use as *primary* surgical treatment …	… if	In cases with ISD	Indication for simultaneous hysterectomy**	Possible after failed Burch	Possible after failed fascial sling	In presence of midline-defect cystocele	In presence of lateral defect cystocele	In presence of rectocele	In presence of vault prolapse
Burch (modifications): see Chapter 41	Yes*	(Former) golden standard—for some indications still best option*	Worse results than obtained with fascial slings	**No**	–	Possible but rarely reasonable	Do cystocele repair vaginally first, resect vaginal skin moderately and **then** do colposuspension otherwise kinking may occur	Do Richardson procedure at the same time (see Chapter 46) otherwise kinking will occur	Induces rectocele Existing rectocele will grow Stabilization is recommended	Beware of possible existing or induced kinking Mind the fact that instability of vault fixation may by itself induce incontinence Simultaneous vault fixation is often recommended Because
Fascial sling: see Chapter 42	Yes	Intrinsic sphincter deficiency (ISD) is diagnosed	Former treatment of choice with ISD		**Yes**, as long as more obstruction can be tolerated/ overcome by detrusor (onset of urgency)	–	Do cystocele repair vaginally first, resect vaginal skin moderately and **then** do sling **before** closing vaginal incision otherwise kinking may occur	Do vaginal paravaginal repair at the same time (see Chapter 46) otherwise kinking will occur	Induces rectocele Existing rectocele will grow Stabilization is recommended	
Retropubic tape TVT® type: see Chapter 43		Inclusion criteria apply Differentiation in use of the three different types of midurethral tension-free slings is explained in the two algorithms and the following figures	Results seem to indicate fairly good results with TVS (being a sling after all) with less invasivity and complications than known using fascial slings		**Yes**, but mobility of bladder neck and suburethral vagina is crucial for success	Possible but rarely reasonable, high risk of obstruction and urge – in some cases (urge, tethered vagina syndrome) **after** dissection of fascial sling better than before dissection	Mind dislocation of sling in combined cases Beware of possible kinking	Do vaginal paravaginal repair at the same time (see Chapter 46) – look out for paraurethral defect and choose right sling procedure (see Table 2) Beware of possible kinking	No problem if rectocele itself does not pose problems	a loose vault may be responsible for incontinence, think about correction of incontinence in a second operation using a tension-free transobturator or retropubic system
Paraurethral tape: see Chapter 43							Dislocation (towards) bladder neck still **may** occur in combined surgery Beware of possible kinking		No problem if rectocele itself does not pose problems	
Transobturator tape: see Chapter 44	Yes*						Safest technique when it comes to dislocation in combined surgery Beware of possible kinking		No problem if rectocele itself does not pose problems	

*Differentiation in the use of the different types of midurethral tension-free, Burch, and fascial slings is explained in the two algorithms (Table 2 and 3) and Figs 1 and 2.

**Hysterectomy is indicated in prolapse repair when the family plan is fulfilled; or if the uterus itself is involved in the descent (the uterine fixation itself is defective) or if the likelihood of a stable reconstruction is reduced by leaving the uterus in place. It should also be removed in cases of uterine or cervical pathology (dysplasia, fibroids, bleeding disorders, etc.).

Chapter 40
Burch Colposuspension

U. H. Fr. Witzsch, R. A. Bürger, S. C. Müller, and R. Hohenfellner

Introduction

Burch described colposuspension as a modification of the Marshall–Marchetti–Kranz procedure (the periosteum is more vulnerable than Cooper's ligament, and there is no periostitis). It is not always necessary to tie the vaginal fascia directly to the ligament (Fig. 40.5A); instead, the suture became a loop—this is called Cowan's modification and it is the most common technique (Fig. 40.5B)

The surgical principle is the re-elevation of the bladder neck into the abdominal pressure zone so there is equal transmission of intra-abdominal pressure to the bladder neck, which closes off the urethra (transmission theory by Enhörning).

Patient counseling and consent

Healing attempts include improvement, not just complete cure, and it should be remembered that urge may occur even with normal cystometry. Self-catheterization is very rarely needed but may be necessary in some cases (usually temporarily). Preoperative information about side effects should be emphasized.

Indications

Stress urinary incontinence with primary or secondary insufficiency (or rejection) of conservative treatment, and descended bladder neck due to sphincteric incompetence (see Tables 1 and 3, pp. 268 and 269).

Limitations and risks

Intrinsic sphincter deficiency (ISD) is defined by a UCP_{max} level of ≤ 20 cmH$_2$O or a Valsalva leak point pressure (VLPP) of <60 (40) cmH$_2$O [4]. ISD leads to a reduction of success rate (by 20%!), although the use of slings in these cases seems to result in better cure rates. Too much elevation of the bladder neck leads to voiding difficulties. Depending on the degree of overcorrection, the patient will most likely first suffer from retention (residual volume), then lose the feeling to void, then the feeling for the amount of urine stored in the bladder combined with retention, and finally the ability to empty the bladder at all. These conditions should be resolved by loosening the elevation even if it means another laparotomy.

Contraindications

- General contraindications against surgery.
- Immobile suburethral vagina and bladder neck above the sacrococcygeal inferior pubic point line.
- Urge incontinence (especially when anticholinergics do not improve the patient's situation).

Preoperative management

See introduction to Part 6.1.

Anesthesia

See introduction to Part 6.1.

Special instruments/suture material

An abdominal retractor may be helpful in some cases; use either mono- or multifilament nonabsorbable sutures (1/0 or 0/0) with a round body needle (i.e. MO-6).

Operative technique

- Place the patient in a modified lithotomy position.
- Disinfect and place a sterile draping, leaving access to the vagina (also disinfected).
- Use a 18–20 Fr Foley catheter.
- Make a blunt dissection of Retzius' space (Fig. 40.1).
- There is no need to dissect the urethra, bladder neck, or bladder base—just free the vaginal fascia periurethrally from the fat and connective tissue using a swab and by lifting the

blader neck area of the vagina with two left-hand fingers in the vagina (for right-handed surgeon).

• Only use scissors for dissection when blunt dissection cannot be achieved because of scars from previous operations.

• Assess the mobility of the bladder neck and proximal urethra.

• Venous bleeding might need suturing.

• Visualize Cooper's ligament on both sides.

• Two (or three) sutures will be needed on both sides. Start with the first suture at the level of the bladder neck 0.8–1 cm lateral to the urethra (Fig. 40.2). Choose a helix-like stitch technique (Fig. 40.3) to anchor the suture nicely in the vaginal fascia and to minimize bleeding.

• Do the next suture 0.8–1 cm cranial and lateral to the first in the same way. In some cases it may seem sensible to do another caudally to the first suture (in fragile tissue).

• Each of the sutures has to be anchored in Cooper's ligament. Start with the first suture approximately 1 cm away from its insertion near the symphysis and do the next anchoring 0.6–0.8 cm lateral to the first (avoid getting too close to the big veins crossing the backside of the pubic bone a little bit further laterally, or the obturator nerve).

• Do the same on the other side.

• Elevate the vagina.

• Keep your left index and middle fingers in the vagina and let the assistant tie the sutures. Tell the assistant when to stop pulling on the knot. The vagina is supported by the suture, not by the finger anymore, and after having tied all the sutures the part of the catheter block close to the urethra should rest behind the symphysis leaving enough space between the urethra and symphysis to put in the index finger (Fig. 40.4)

• The urethra should rest on a hammock [3] (Fig. 40.5B) rather than squeezed between the vaginal fascia and symphysis due to tight sutures (Fig. 40.5A).

• Make sure there is no bleeding. If the area is not completely dry use a drainage—but only then.

• Put in a suprapubic catheter and close the abdomen.

Tips

• It is sometimes easier to dissect the bladder from the vagina with 50 or 100 cm^3 of water or urine in the bladder, because the bladder's boundaries are easier to recognize.

• If you cannot decide on the right tissue layer to put the suture through, then in selected cases cystotomy may be an option.

• Try to avoid the large veins running on top of the vaginal fascia. If you accidentally puncture one, do not remove the suture—go around the vein with a second stitch and tie the suture before passing it through Cooper's ligament.

• Most of the bleedings stop as soon as the sutures are tied by elevating the vagina.

• Avoid placing sutures too far cranially or medially. These might ligate the ureter.

Postoperative care

See introduction to Part 6.1.

Complications

• Wound complications = 5.5%:
  • infection, hematoma = 3.4%;
  • hernia, wound dehiscence = 1.8%;
  • others = 0.3%.
• Urinary tract infection = 3.9%.
• Ostitis pubis = 2.5%.
• Bladder lesions = 1.6%.
• Urethral obstruction = 0.7% (to 1.5%).
• Transvesical/transurethral sutures = 0.3%.
• Transureteral sutures or obstruction = 0.1%.
• Fistulas = 0.3%.
• Exitus letalis = 0.2%.

Troubleshooting

• The more procedures that are included in the same surgery, the more difficult the correct adjustment of the sutures becomes. It is worth discussing with the patient how many procedures to perform at any one time.

• Avoid the veins on the back of the pubic bone lateral to the attachment points for the colposuspension sutures.

• It may be useful, but generally it is not necessary, to visualize the external iliac vessels and obturator nerve. But beware—they are close.

Remarks

Reasonably set up multicenter studies show an equal efficacy of the Burch colposuspension technique compared with tension-free midurethral slings. Preoperatively choosing one of these methods, taking into account additional pathology, seems to be a wise thing to do.

• Consider the abdominal approach to cure concomitant prolapse.

• A paraurethral or paravaginal defect may jeopardize the success of a tension-free sling because of too much urethral rotation.

• A previous, correctly placed, midurethral tension-free sling may still be ineffecective, even with no other vaginal pathology that could explain the failure (according to the integral theory).

To do

• Make sure the vaginal fascia (white) is exposed before placing the sutures, to avoid bladder injury.

• Let the assistant tie the sutures while the surgeon's left hand remains intravaginally to control the 'tension' of the sutures, or vice versa.

- A suprapubic catheter with a protocol of residuals is good to have, but remove the catheter as soon as residuals are under 50 cm^3, but not earlier than 5 days.

Not to do

- Excessive mobilization causes denervation.
- Sutures tied too tightly cause urge and residual urine.

References

1 Burch JC. Urethrovaginal fixation to Cooper's ligament for correction of stress incontinence, cystocele and prolapse. Am J Obstet Gynecol 1961;81:281–90.
2 Burch JC. Cooper's ligament urethrovesical suspension for stress incontinence. Am J Obstet Gynecol 1968;100:764–74.
3 Cowan W, Morgan HR. A simplified retropubic urethropexy in the treatment of primary and recurrent urinary stress incontinence in the female. Am J Obstet Gynecol 1979;133:295–301.
4 McGuire E. 1: Urinary incontinence clinical correlations. AUA Update Ser 1990;01.IX:Lesson 37.
5 Tanagho EA. Colpocystourethropexy. In: Female Urology, Vol. 15 (Raz, ed.). W.B. Saunders, Philadelphia, 1983:252.
6 Tanagho EA. Colpocystourethropexy: the way we do it. In: Current Operative Urology, Vol. 5 (Whitehead, ed.). J.B. Lippincott, Philadelphia, 1990:73.
7 Operationen bei Belastungs- (Streß-) Inkontinenz: In: Atlas der Gynäkologischen Operationen, Vol. 21 (Käser, Ikle, Hirsch, eds). Thieme Verlag, 1983:21.1.
8 Walters MD, Karram MM. Clinical Urogynecology. Mosby-Year Book, St Louis.
9 Witzsch U. Operationen zur weiblichen Inkontinenz (Teil 1): Kolposuspension nach Burch und Faszienzügelplastiken. In: Ausgenühlte Urologische Op-Techniken Step by Step (Hohenfellner R, ed.). Thieme, Stuttgart, 1997.

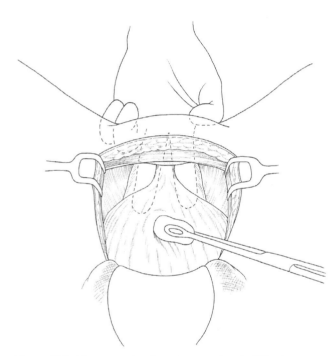

Figure 40.1 After separating the rectus muscles, start blunt dissection of Retzius' space with the help of two intravaginal fingers (use the left hand for a right-handed surgeon and vice versa).

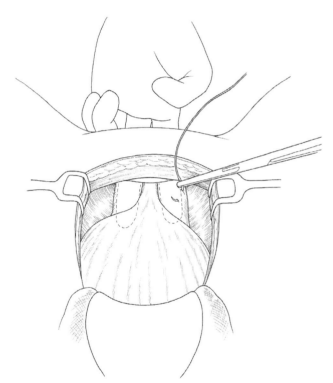

Figure 40.2 Put the first suture in at the level of the bladder neck 0.8–1 cm lateral to the urethra. Do not penetrate into the vagina with the needle. This is done after dissecting off all bladder tissue from the (white and smooth-surfaced) vagina with the help of some pressure from the intravaginal fingers.

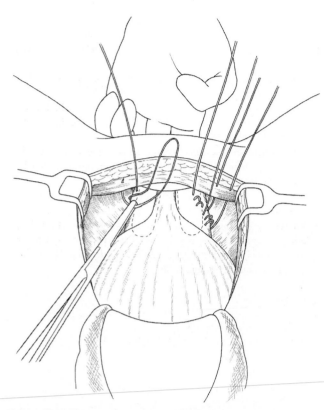

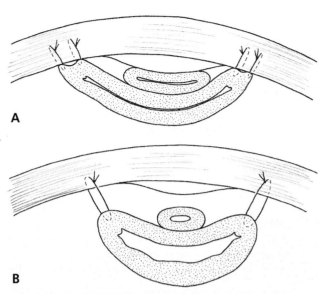

Figure 40.5 (A) Sutures tied so that the vaginal fascia comes into contact with Cooper's ligament is called a Burch colposuspension. (B) Sutures tied so that the urethra rests on a hammock, leaving the sutures as slings on both sides, is called Cowan's modification of the Burch colposuspension. This is the technique most frequently used.

Figure 40.3 Choose a helix-like stitch technique to anchor the suture nicely in the vaginal fascia and to minimize bleeding. In most cases another suture 0.8–1 cm cranial and lateral to the first will be sufficient.

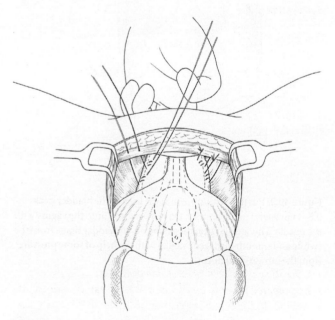

Figure 40.4 Once the sutures are tied make sure that the part of the catheter block closest to the urethra rests behind the symphysis, leaving enough space between the urethra and symphysis to put in the index finger.

Chapter 41
Fascial Sling Plasty for Female Urinary Stress Incontinence

U. H. Fr. Witzsch, R. A. Bürger, S. C. Müller, M. Höckel, and R. Hohenfellner

Introduction

This technique has been successfully used for many years, and was introduced in 1962 by Narik and Palmrich [8]. It increases the urethral closure pressure and elevates the urethrovesical junction. Using autologous fascia, various techniques have been described to perform the sling, which can be formed from the rectus fascia, fascia lata, or the aponeurosis of the external oblique muscle. The inguinovaginal sling procedure uses the aponeurosis of the external oblique muscle. Native, cadaveric, and synthetic materials have been used, but foreign material can no longer be used.

There is low morbidity and good functional results, although the original method has some disadvantages: extended Pfannenstiel incision, hematomas, prolonged postoperative pain, and nonaesthetic scar formation. The minimally invasive modifications that have been introduced (open surgery, laparoscopic approach) should show good long-term results, without the need for synthetic slings or allografts.

Patient counseling and consent

- Paravesical bleeding/hematoma.
- Lesions of the bladder, ureter, and urethra.
- Fistula formation.
- Abdominal wall hernias.
- Retention and voiding difficulties.
- Self-catheterization or permanent suprapubic cystotomy.
- Urgency.
- Dyspareunia.

Indications

- Second to third degree primary stress urinary incontinence.
- Recurrent incontinence after previous surgery.
- First to second degree additional cystocele that can be corrected vaginally at the same time.

Limitations and risks

Abdominal and vaginal scarring due to previous operations can make the procedure very difficult or even impossible, or means modifications have to be made to the procedure [11]. Previous surgery will also make complications (e.g. lesions, fistula) and side effects (e.g. urgency) more likely to occur.

Contraindications

- Previous Pfannenstiel laparotomy.
- Previous hernia repair using the aponeurosis to cover the hernia.
- Reduced hip joint mobility.
- Prolapse that needs abdominal repair.

Preoperative management

See introduction to Part 6.1.

Anesthesia

See introduction to Part 6.1.

Special instruments/suture material

- Standard instruments for the abdominal approach.
- Satinsky scissors
- Breisky specula.
- 16–18 Fr laparoscope or urethroscope.
- 24 Fr resectoscope.
- Additional equipment for balloon dissection.
- Suprapubic catheter.

Operative technique

Open technique

- Place the patient in the lithotomy position.
- Be prepared for both an abdominal and a vaginal approach.
- A wide skin incision is performed that ends medial to the superior anterior iliac spine on each side.
- Following dissection of the subcutaneous tissue, a dissection of the fascial strip from the aponeurosis of the external oblique muscle is performed (12 cm long and 2–3 cm wide) (Fig. 41.1).

- Prepare the retropubic tunnel (Fig. 41.2), with the entrance between the rectus and oblique muscles.
- Perform a colpotomy and vaginal dissection to the endopelvic fascia (Fig. 41.3).
- The fascial strips are blindly pulled through the pelvic fascia (Fig. 41.4).
- Approximate the fascial strips with single interrupted sutures, beginning distally, until the stress test becomes negative (Figs 41.5–41.7).
- Close the colpotomy.
- The transurethral and suprapubic catheters are inserted.
- The fascial gap on both sides is closed with interrupted sutures.
- Subcutaneous suction drains are used and the skin incision is closed.

Pelviscopic technique
Abdominal phase
- Place the patient in a lithotomy position.
- Use an 18 Fr Foley catheter.
- A 1.5 cm skin incision is made symmetrically on each side of the midline, approximately 3 cm above the pubic bone within the previously shaved hairy area.
- The subcutaneous fatty tissue is dissected bluntly and lifted up with a long specula to clear and identify the aponeurosis of the external oblique muscle.
- A laparoscope is inserted and two parallel incisions of the fascia are performed with the scissors under vision.
- The incisions are 2–3 cm apart and 12 cm in length. The transverse incision of the cranial end is performed with Satinsky scissors.
- Once connected with the pubic bone, the fascial strip is then pulled out. The same procedure is performed contralaterally (Fig. 41.8).
- The retropubic space is opened with an incision in the muscle-free triangular area above the pubic tubercle.
- A laparoscope armed with an inflatable balloon is inserted into the paravesical space and the balloon is blown up. Consecutively, the bladder is transposed medially and the pelvic floor is exposed.

Vaginal phase
- A median incision is made 1 cm below the external urethral meatus.
- Incise the urethrovaginal septum and dissect the paravesical space bluntly with the tip of the finger. Palpating the pubic bone, the dissection is performed until the illuminated balloon is seen through the endopelvic fascia.
- Incise the endopelvic fascia.
- A pull-through maneuver of the two fascial slings is carried out with a flat Overholt clamp (Fig. 41.4.).
- Both fascial strips are connected with interrupted 5/0 Maxon sutures to create the dorsal plate of the V-shaped sling below the urethra (Figs 41.5–41.6).

- The gap between the sling and the midurethra is narrowed so that the tip of the finger can just be inserted.
- Fill the bladder with 300 cm^3 of saline and remove the Foley catheter.
- Perform a stress test: ask the patient to cough or, alternatively, if the patient was under general anesthesia, perform a series of short pushes upon the bladder (Fig. 41.7).
- If there is still a loss of a few drops of urine, additional sutures should be placed to further elevate the urethra. The stress test is repeated if necessary.
- If the patient is dry, close the colpotomy with interrupted sutures. The retropubic incisions are closed after placing one subcutaneous suction drainage on each side.
- A control cystoscopy is then performed to exclude bladder injury. During cystoscopy a suprapubic tube is inserted under vision, and after cystoscopy a Foley catheter is inserted into the bladder.

Tips

When bleeding occurs from the paravesical veins, fill the bladder with 300 cm^3 of saline for 5–10 min. The bleeding should then stop — if not, insert drainage with suction.

Postoperative care

See introduction to Part 6.1.

Complications

Bladder lesions may occur when penetrating the endopelvic fascia with an instrument. After the use of the Overholt clamp, no sutures are necessary. After passage of the entire sling, a two-layer closure of the defect is necessary. Perform cystoscopy afterwards.

Bleeding may occur from the paravesical veins.

Results

Open technique
- Bladder injury occurred intraoperatively in 3.1% of 180 patients. All were repaired immediately.
- Postoperatively, wound infection or hematoma was seen in 1.8%.
- Forty-eight per cent had a prolonged interval with the cystostomy tube. However, after 6 months, 98% were able to void spontaneously and without residual urine.
- The mean hospital stay was 11.5 days.
- Follow-up was available in 111 patients for a mean of 8.9 years (range 6 months to 30 years) after surgery.
- Urinary tract infections without residual urine occurred in 14% of patients and urge symptoms in 29%. Both were treated conservatively.
- Dyspareunia was reported in 5% of patients but disappeared in all but two under estrogen substitution. The latter two patients had scars at the area of the anterior colpotomy.

• In 2% of patients, clean intermittent catheterization was initially necessary, but could be terminated within 12 months.
• The stress urinary incontinence cure rate was 78% in patients without previous incontinence operations.
• Patients undergoing surgery for recurrent incontinence following previous repair without the use of foreign materials were continent in 59% of cases. The continence rate was 25% in patients in whom synthetic or cadaveric slings had been used previously.

Pelviscopic technique

• In 15 patients using the minimally invasive method, no intra- or postoperative complications were observed.
• The patients could be discharged on the second or third postoperative day. Further treatment was continued in an outpatient setting.
• Mean operating time was 75 min (range, 55–100 min) and showed a decrease with growing experience.
• The mean follow-up period was 7 months (range, 2–10 months) and all 15 patients were able to void spontaneously without residual urine after 4 weeks. Also, complete continence was achieved in all patients after the operation.

References

1 Chaikin DC, Rosenthal J, Bhivais JG. Pubovaginal fascial sling for all types of stress urinary incontinence: long-term analysis. J Urol 1998;160:1312–16.
2 Cross CA, Cespedes RD, McGuire EJ. Our experience with pubovaginal slings in patients with stress urinary incontinence. J Urol 1998;159:1195–8.
3 Haab F, Trockmann BA, Zimmern PE, Leach GE. Results of pubovaginal sling for the treatment of intrinsic sphincteric deficiency determined by questionnaire analysis. J Urol 1997;158:1738–41.
4 Handa VL, Stone A. Erosion of a fascial sling into the urethra. Urology 1999;54:923.
5 Hohenfellner R, Petri E. Sling procedures. In: Surgery of Female Incontinence, Vol. 6 (Stanton SL, Tanagho EA, eds). Springer Verlag, Berlin, 1986:69–76.
6 McGuire E. 1: Urinary incontinence clinical correlations. AUA Update Ser 1990;01.IX:Lesson 37.
7 Müller SC, Steinbach F, Maurer FM, Melchior SW, Stein R, Hohenfellner R. Long-term results of fascial sling procedure. Int Urogynecol J Pelvic Floor Dysfunct 1993;4:199–203.
8 Narick G, Palmrich AH. A simplified sling operation suitable for routine use. Am J Obst Gynecol 1962;84(3):400–5.
9 Norris JP, Breslin DS, Staskin DR. Use of synthetic materials in sling surgery: a minimally invasive approach. J Endourol 1996; 10:227–31.
10 Witzsch U, Bürger RA, Müller SC, Hohenfellner R. Operationen zur weiblichen Inkontinenz (Teil 1): Kolposuspension nach Burch und Faszienzügelplastik. Akt Urol 1991;22:I–XII.
11 Witzsch U, Bürger RA, Fisch M, Hohenfellner R. Operationen zur weiblichen Inkontinenz (Teil 2): Kombination von Faszienzügelplastiken und Kolposuspension, asymetrischen Zögel. In: Ausgenühlte Urologische Op-Techniken Step by Step (Hohenfellner R, ed.). Thieme, Stuttgart, 1997.

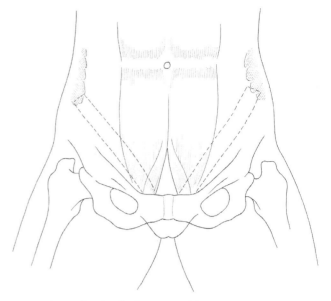

Figure 41.1 Following the dissection of the subcutaneous tissue, the fascial strip is dissected from the aponeurosis of the external oblique muscle (12 cm long and 2–3 cm wide).

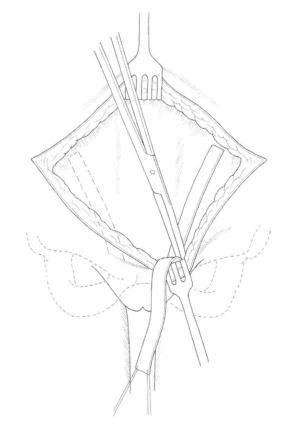

Figure 41.2 The abdominal entrance of the retropubic tunnel, used to pass the fascial sling, is now prepared before changing to the vaginal site.

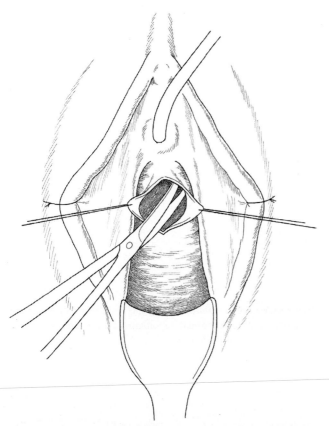

Figure 41.3 Perform a colpotomy and use Metzenbaum scissors to dissect the endopelvic fascia off the vaginal skin's fascia to create the vaginal part of the sling's tunnel.

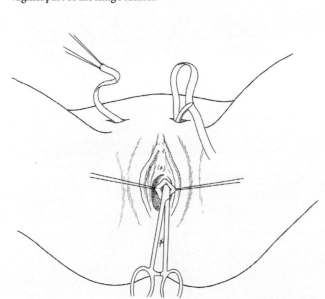

Figure 41.4 Penetrate the arcus tendineous of the endopelvic fascia using a blunt instrument (an Overholt clamp of appropriate size) and make the instrument exit the dissected abdominal aperture of the tunnel.

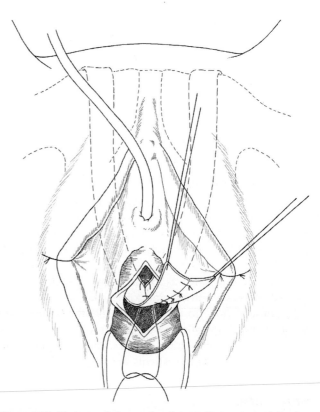

Figure 41.5 Underneath the urethra the two slings are now joined together using interrupted sutures. Start with the posterior row of sutures using suprapubic abdominal pressure on the filled bladder to decide how many stitches are needed to achieve continence (assessed by the amount of leakage).

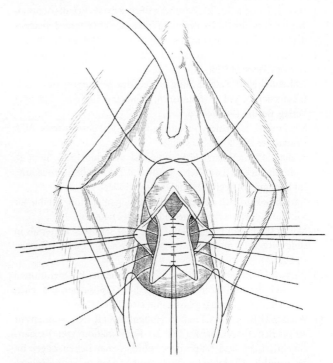

Figure 41.6 Continue with the anterior row of sutures for exact positioning and tension.

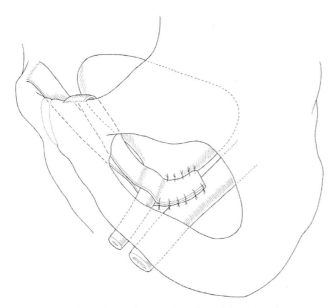

Figure 41.7 After joining the anterior edges of the slings, the stress test should be negative.

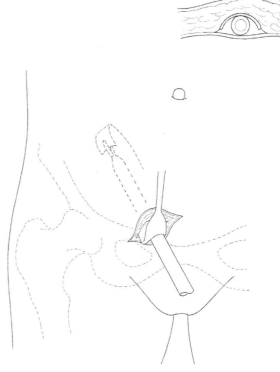

Figure 41.8 After the suprapubic incision is made, the same kind of fascial sling is dissected after insufflation and dissection of the fat tissue. After a transverse cut with Satinsky scissors, the mobile sling is pulled out in the midline and positioned (with a suture attached).

Chapter 42
Transvaginal Tension-Free Sling Operations for the Treatment of Female Stress Incontinence (TVS Operations)

A. Fischer

Introduction

This technique is based on the Integral Theory by Petros and Ulmsten in 1990 [6]. The mechanism of action differs from that of conventional sling operations as the bladder neck is not displaced backwards into 'abdominopelvic equilibrium'. The defective pubourethral ligaments are replaced, and, in addition, the defective connection between the urethra and vagina is restored (see below).

Patient counseling and consent

See introduction to Part 6.1.

Indications

- Genuine stress urinary incontinence.
- Mixed incontinence, if:
  - the urge component can be successfully suppressed medically (e.g. with anticholinergic drugs);
  - the urge component is (probably) caused by insufficiency of the periurethral ligamentous structures (pubourethral ligaments) or defective sacrouterine ligament fixation of the vagina, which may be reflected on imaging by a funnel appearance of the bladder neck.
- Urge incontinence, which is produced by insufficiency of the periurethral ligamentous structures (pubourethral ligaments) or defective uterosacral ligament fixation of the vagina, which is reflected on imaging by a funnel appearance of the bladder neck.
- Masked stress urinary incontinence occurring after prolapse surgery, in individual cases at the same session or ideally in two stages.

Limitations and risks

- The surgeon should be familiar with the surgical technique of bladder neck suspension.

- The mesh implant (e.g. with TVT®) must not come into contact with forceps, clamps, or clips.
- Since this is a technique whose effect is based on the function of the pelvic floor muscles, their voluntary (and involuntary) activity is essential for the success of the technique.
- See also introduction to Part 6.1.

Contraindications

This procedure is relatively contraindicated in pregnancy, in adolescents, or if pregnancy is planned or desired in the future. General contraindications to operative procedures (coagulation disorders, local, or generalized infections, etc.) also apply.

Preoperative management

See introduction to Part 6.1.

Anesthesia

Before inserting the two needles, give a further 20–60 mg propofol. The patient will then have had secure analgesia for insertion and cystoscopy and will be fully awake again and responsive for the cough test. See also introduction to Part 6.1.

Special instruments/suture material

- Standard instruments for vaginal operations.
- TVT® introducer instrument.
- TVT® metal catheter guide.
- TVT® implant set or similar commercially available set for transvaginal tension-free midurethral slings (see Plate A1 between pp. 112 and 113.).

Operative technique
Midline operation
- Use suprapubic and vaginal local anesthesia, a transurethral Foley catheter (18 Fr), and ensure an empty bladder.

- Make a midline incision under the midurethra (Fig. 42.1).
- Dissect both sides, creating a tunnel wide enough for the tape to pass through and perforation of the endopelvic fascia with the tip of the scissors (Fig. 42.2).
- Insert the tunneling instrument into the vaginal incision and, having passed the endopelvic fascia, make contact with the pubic bone (Fig. 42.3). Stay in close contact and make the tip of the needle gently slide up the pubic bone until the tip penetrates the muscle fascia, subcutaneous fat, and skin (Fig. 42.4).
- Fill the bladder with $300\,cm^3$ of saline and perform a thorough cystoscopy with the needle still in place (Fig. 42.5).
- Pull out the needle and some of the tape; cut the needle and secure the tape with a Kocher clamp (Fig. 42.6).
- Repeat the maneuver on the other side.
- Place the tape in a tension-free way under the midurethra and pull out both sheaths using a pair of scissors or an Overholt clamp to prevent the tape from tensioning while pulling the sheaths out (Fig. 42.7).
- Close the incisions and empty the bladder again.

Paraurethral fixation

- Make two paraurethral incisions in the area of the (missing or fading) paraurethral sulcus starting approximately 1 cm off the external meatus and ending in the bladder neck area (vaginal epithelium and fascia) (Fig. 42.8).
- Create a tunnel under the midurethra (Fig. 42.9).
- Make the needles pass through Retzius' space on both sides and perform a cystoscopy (Fig. 42.10). Pass the tape through the tunnel created earlier (Fig. 42.11) or first pass the tape through and then the needles.
- Pass the tape through Retzius' space using the instruments and system you have selected (Fig. 42.12).
- Now reattach the vaginal skin to the pelvic floor muscle by using a U-shaped suture running from the vaginal skin through the pubococcygeus muscle and back. *The distance you choose between the points of entry or exit for the needle in the vaginal skin (between those points and between them and the incision) will later decide the tension you can give the suburethral vagina, as well as by tying the suture.* First close the incision and repeat the procedure on the other side before tensioning the tape and tying the sutures (Fig. 42.13).
- Insert the Hegar dilator or tunneling instrument, pull on the tape to get it into contact with the urethra, and then push it down a little to make sure it is tension-free. Then gently tie the sutures to approximate the vagina to the muscle, not tightening the hammock (suburethral vagina) too much (Fig. 42.14).

Tips

- Marking the exit site (target area) is helpful.
- Maintain close contact with the bone.

- Hold the handle (parallel to the floor) and the needle (parallel to the axis of the urethra) correctly.
- Make sure the patient is correctly positioned—steep angulation of the legs leads to contusion of the pelvic organs so the pelvic wall vessels come close to the operation field.
- Stick to the technique described.
- Look for a training site to see and feel the procedure.
- A midurethral tape in women with a paraurethral defect with a loose hammock may lead to overcorrection (especially with the cough test) or persistence of incontinence. Choose the best procedure before you start operating (see Table 2, p. 268).

Postoperative care

- A temporary local irritation of the wound or a foreign body reaction can occur. This can lead to extrusion, erosion, fistula formation, or inflammation. Injuries of the intestine (or bladder) should always be considered in such cases.
- Temporary or permanent stenosis of the urinary tract can occur in cases of overcorrection. This sometimes necessitates secondary procedures.
- All other risks and side effects of surgical procedures, which the patient must be informed of before giving informed consent, can occur, so the patient must be appropriately monitored postoperatively.
- Further treatment in the narrower sense is not necessary.
- Because of detrusor activation or sensory urge symptoms (especially in patients with a low bladder capacity preoperatively due to incontinence) it may be necessary to treat with an anticholinergic drug for a certain period (e.g. 6 weeks) to relieve the patient's symptoms.

Complications

Intraoperative phase

- *Bladder perforation* (maximum 4%):
  - always perform a cystoscopy; be thorough and put in enough saline ($300\,cm^3$);
  - remove the needle and do the procedure again; if cystoscopy is done after removal of the needles and perforation occurs, remove the tape and do the procedure again;
  - leave the Foley catheter for 24 h per bladder perforation (for perforation on both sides, leave the Foley catheter for 48 h);
  - videocystoscopy makes the detection of perforations easier.
- *Hemorrhage* (about 2%; surgical revison about 0.5%):
  - big vessels are only endangered by the wrong technique;
  - if there is bleeding after dissection of the tunnel, 2–5 min of compression should be sufficient;
  - postoperative hematomas do not necessarily cause symptoms;
  - high residual volumes post voiding should raise suspicion;

• a transurethral or suprapubic catheter may be necessary;
• the development of hematomas should be documented;
• in cases of circulatory effects and large dimensions, abdominal revision of Retzius' space should be considered;
• if there are no symptoms no action is needed.

Intermediate phase

• *Infections* (rare):
  • cystitis may occur;
  • there are practically no reported cases of infections with macroporous monofilament tapes.
• *Intolerance* (extremely rare): no intolerance of the implant has been identified hitherto.
• *Micturition disorders* (more frequent); these are due to:
  • overcorrection;
  • urethral hypermobility in association with prolapse of the anterior vaginal wall (pinchcock mechanism with kinking);
  • temporary urethral or periurethral swelling;
  • periurethral hematomas or hematomas around the bladder neck; these are usually small in size (between 3 and 5 cm), leading to compression (larger hematomas cause pain and a drop in hemoglobin).

Long-term phase

• *Secondary obstructive abnormalities of micturition*:
  • onset of prolapse;
  • constriction by shrinking or excessive fibrosis.
• *Urge symptoms*; these can be due to:
  • shifting of the tape out of the midurethra (after combined surgery for anterior prolapse (colporrhaphy);
  • shrinking;
  • development of prolapse/worsening of a prolapse;
  • perforation of the bladder wall;
  • the tape was accidentally put in the detrusor muscle (pointed needle);
  • tension;
  • bad pelvic floor muscles;
  • neurologic disorder.
• *Rare problems*:
  • retropubic pain because of irritation of the detrusor or periosteum;
  • recurrence (check this is really recurrence, or is another defect responsible?);
  • primary ineffectiveness (wrong choice of treatment according to the Integral Theory);
  • loose uterosacral ligaments;
  • loose hammock;
  • tethered vagina;
  • function of the pelvic floor muscles is insufficient.

Troubleshooting

• In the case of 'overcorrection' with increased residual urine levels or other signs of subvesical obstruction, either make an early revision (open up the colpotomy, loosen the tape with scissors, and close again) or put in a suprapubic catheter while waiting for the tape to heal. It can then (after approx. 6 weeks) usually be cut in two suburethrally in the midline without difficulty (under local anesthesia). Loss of continence should be expected in only a few cases.
• A febrile postoperative course, intestinal atony, and gas coming from the skin puncture sites, especially with a corresponding odur or a rapid worsening in condition, should lead to a suspicion of bowel injury and lead to rapid investigation and treatment.
• Submucous implantation of the tape can lead to its secondary migration as a result of necrosis or lysis due to inflammation. Consider it in postoperative cases of urinary tract infection, urge, and hematuria.
• Placement of the tape in the detrusor muscle is also conceivable. This can lead to bladder malfunction, e.g. dysuria or urgency. In this case resection of the tape-bearing segment of the detrusor should be considered if the diagnosis is confirmed (MRI or surgical exploration of Retzius' space may be necessary).
• Ureter injuries, shifting or distortion, or outflow obstruction as a result of subtrigonal hematomas should be considered.

Results

The long-term results of the Scandinavian working groups and an article from Italy were published in 2001 in a supplement to the *International Urogynecology Journal* under the title 'Tension-free vaginal tape—a minimally invasive surgical procedure for treatment of female urinary incontinence' edited by Stuart Stanton [8]. Overall, there is a cure rate of 85–90% reported, especially in first-line treatment; a cure rate of about 65% should be achieved in secondary surgical treatment.

Be wary of results showing a cure rate over 90%, as this can only be achieved by trading the disappearance of stress incontinence against symptoms of irritation/obstruction, such as urge and retention, which will go up in number.

Colposuspension and fascial slings are not superior to this technique, especially in cases where no paraurethral or paravaginal defect exists. The paraurethral technique reduces side effects and improves the outcome in patients with no such defects.

Remarks

Only do this kind of procedure if you have sufficient experience in pelvic floor and bladder neck surgery. Stay away from the big vessels.

To do

Differentiate between: (i) simple pubourethral defects with intact paraurethral attachment of the vagina to the pubococcygeus muscle via the endopelvic fascia, and (ii) combined defects that need, in addition to a midurethral tape, the restoration of the paraurethral fixation of the 'hammock' — the suburethral vagina (see Table 2, p. 268).

The correct technique prevents puncture of the bladder, especially during the insertion of tension-free vaginal tape when the needles remain in close contact with the periosteum while being guided retropubically. An exit site is selected approximately 2 cm lateral to the midline and about 1 cm above the upper border of the pubic bone.

Not to do

If you have any doubts that what you are going to do might not be the right technique for the patient (or for you), do not use this kind of procedure.

References

1 Falconer C, Ekman-Ordeberg G, Malström A, Ulmsten U. Clinical outcome and changes in connective tissue metabolism after intravaginal slingplasty in stress incontinent women. Int Urogynecol J 1996;7:133–7.

2 Fischer A, Arnold B, Meghil S, Hoffmann G. Probleme nach TVT-implantation. Gynäkol Prax 2001;25:67–82.

3 Fischer A, Arnold B, Scheler P, Hoffmann G. Sensorische Drangsymptomatik nach TVT — Ergebnisanalyse einer Subpopulation. Aktuel Urol 2002;33:129–35.

4 Fischer A, Dodidou-Najm A, Hoffmann G. TVT-Durchtrennung bei obstruktiver Miktionsstörung und Drangsymptomatik. Aktuel Urol 2002;33:523–30.

5 Fischer A, Hoffmann G. TVT (tension-free vaginal tape) — ein neues Implantat zur Behandlung der weiblichen Harninkontinenz. Gynäkol Prax 1999;23:281–97.

6 Petros P, Ulmsten U. An integral theory and its method for the diagnosis and the management of female urinary incontinence. Scand J Urol Nephrol Suppl 1993;153:1–93.

7 Petros P, Ulmsten U. An integral theory of female urinary incontinence. Experimental and clinical considerations. Acta Obstet Gynecol Scand Suppl 1990;153:69.

8 Stanton S (ed.). Tension-free vaginal tape — a minimally invasive surgical procedure for treatment of female urinary incontinence. Int Urogynecol J 2001;12(Suppl. 2).

9 Ulmsten U, Henriksson L, Johnson P, Varhos G. An ambulatory surgical procedure under local anesthesia for treatment of female urinary incontinence. Int Urogynecol J 1996;7:81–6.

10 Ulmsten U, Hilton P, Ferrari A, Fischer W, Jacquetin B. Tension-free vaginal tape procedure: a microinvasive surgical technique for GSI. Abstracts of the 22nd Annual Meeting of the International Urogynaecology Association (IUGA). Int Urogynecol J 1997;8(1).

11 Zacharin RF. The suspensory mechanism of the female urethra. J Anat 1963;97:423–7.

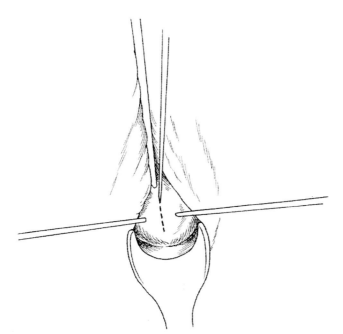

Figure 42.1 Perform a midline incision under the midurethra using the external meatus and catheter cuff-marked bladder neck for orientation.

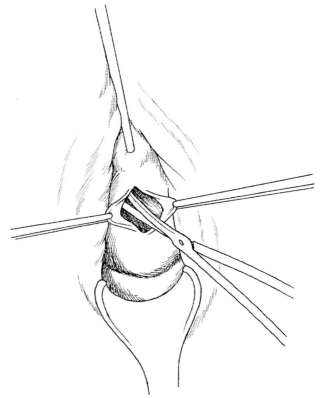

Figure 42.2 Dissection to both sides creates a tunnel wide enough for the tape to pass through. The perforation of the endopelvic fascia with the tip of the scissors makes entering the retropubic space with the tunneling instrument easier.

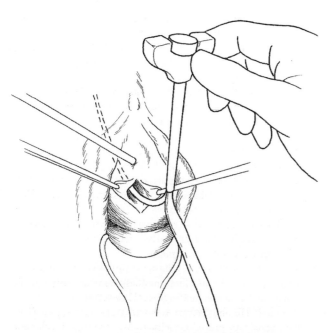

Figure 42.3 Insert the tunneling instrument into the vaginal incision and, having passed the endopelvic fascia, make contact with the pubic bone.

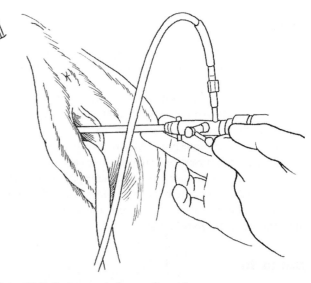

Figure 42.5 Cystoscopy is then performed.

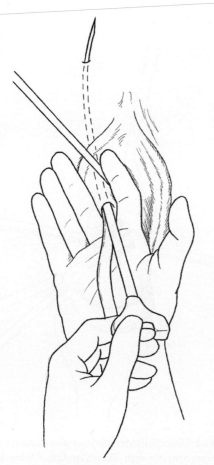

Figure 42.4 Stay in close contact and make the tip of the needle gently slide up the pubic bone until the tip penetrates the muscle fascia, subcutaneous fat, and skin.

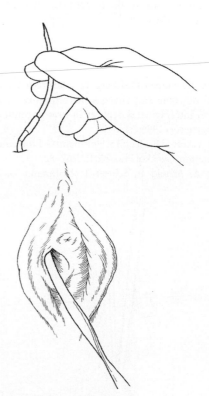

Figure 42.6 Pull out the needle and some of the tape, cut the needle, and secure the tape with a Kocher clamp.

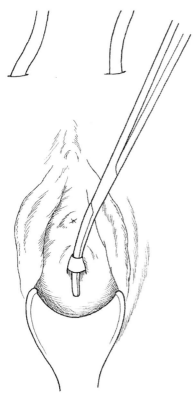

Figure 42.7 Place the tape in a tension-free way under the midurethra. If tape with plastic sheaths is used, then pull out both sheaths now using a pair of scissors or a clamp to prevent the tape from tensioning while pulling.

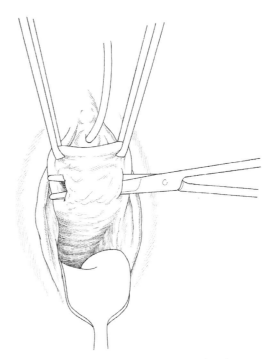

Figure 42.9 Create a tunnel under the midurethra using Metzenbaum scissors.

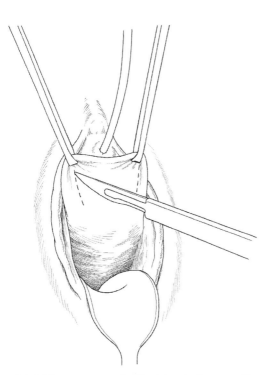

Figure 42.8 Make two paraurethral incisions in the area of the (missing or fading) paraurethral sulcus starting approximately 1 cm off the external meatus and ending in the bladder neck area (vaginal epithelium and fascia).

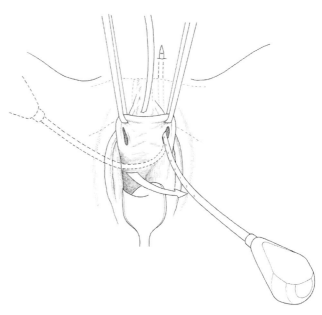

Figure 42.10 Make the needles pass through Retzius' space on both sides and perform a cystoscopy.

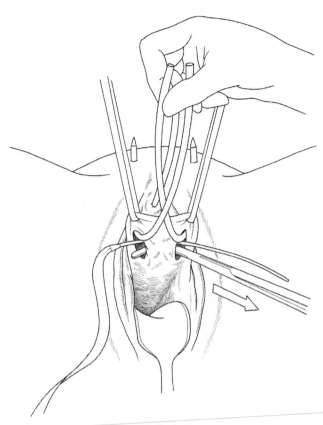

Figure 42.11 First make the tape pass through the tunnel (it is advisable to use a nonprotected monofilament macroporous tape for this procedure, e.g. Serasis® tape, Serag-Wiessner, Germany).

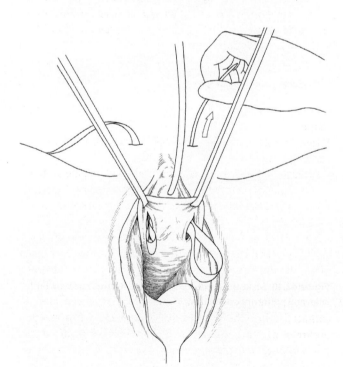

Figure 42.12 Make the tape pass through Retzius' space on both sides and pull on the ends to bring the tape into loose contact with the urethra.

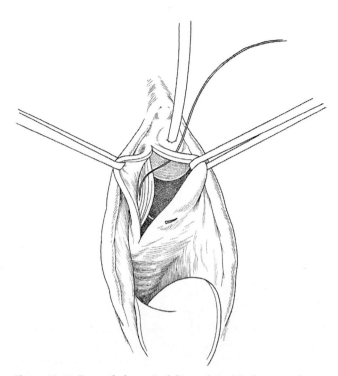

Figure 42.13 Reattach the vaginal skin to the pelvic floor muscle using a U-shaped suture running from the vaginal skin through the pubococcygeus muscle, and back.

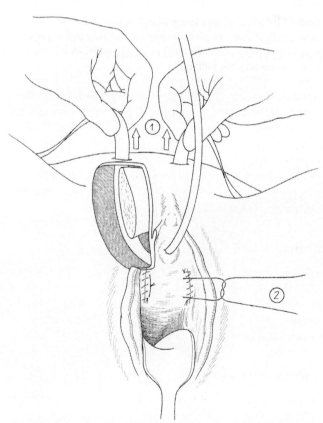

Figure 42.14 Insert a Hegar dilator or tunneling instrument, pull on the tape to get it into contact with the urethra, and then push it down a little to make sure it is tension-free. Gently tie the sutures to approximate the vagina to the muscle, not tightening the hammock (suburethral vagina) too much.

Chapter 43

Transobturator Tension-Free Sling Operations for the Treatment of Female Stress Incontinence (TOS Operations)

A. Fischer

Introduction

Transobturator tension-free slings were developed at the end of the 20th century and the first data on Uratape® (Porgès, France) were published in 2001. This way of introducing a tension-free midurethral sling was mainly developed with the aim of reducing the side effects of retropubic slings like TVT® and SPARC®. It was hypothesized that there would be no difference in the outcome between the retropubic and transobturator approaches.

Patient counseling and consent

Even though there are no large studies available to prove the equal efficacy of transobturator slings compared with those introduced retropubically, it seems to be safe to say that no large numbers of bladder perforations and no vessel or nerve lesions have occurred, and that there seems to be an advantage in not passing too closely to the bladder and the unknown veins in Retzius' space. Patients with (multiple) previous retropubic surgery should be informed that this approach exists and minimizes the risk of complications.

Indications

These are same as for the retropubic technique (see Chapter 42)—that is, the procedure is suitable for patients without a paraurethral fixation defect, or with only a minor defect. In severe cases we still prefer the paraurethral technique as shown in Chapter 42.

Limitations and risks

See introduction to Part 6.1 and Chapter 42.

Contraindications

See Chapter 42.

Preoperative management

See introduction to Part 6.1.

Anesthesia

See introduction to Part 6.1.

Special instruments/suture material

The standard instruments for vaginal operations are needed. A TOT (transobturator tape) introducer instrument/TOT implant set or a similar commercially available set for transobturator tension-free midurethral slings is also required (see Plate A2 between pp. 112 and 113.).

Operative technique

- Put the patient in the Trendelenburg position, disinfect and drape.
- Insert a Foley catheter with block ($10\,\text{cm}^3$) and look out for the bladder neck area.
- Make an incision over the midurethra and palpate on both sides for the obturator hole. Incise on both sides near the pubic bone a little above the middle of the anterior line of the foramen (cf. Fig. 43.2).
- With Metzenbaum scissors, dissect a tunnel on both sides staying underneath the vaginal fascia until the inferior ramus of the pubic bone is reached (Fig. 43.1). It is recommended, especially initially, to create a tunnel wide enough to be able to insert the index finger so that the tip of the finger can later on contact the tip of the instrument the moment it perforates the obturator membrane (*with some experience it is as safe to just put your finger into the paraurethral sulcus to palpate the tip of the instrument through the vaginal skin*) (Fig. 43.2).
- Insert the helix-shaped instrument into the skin incision and push it through the leg's fascia (*depending on the qualitiy of the patient's connective tissue this may need some effort*). The in-

strument's axis should be approximately 45° to the vertical (Fig. 43.3).

- After this first loss of resistence you will notice the instrument rotate around the pubic bone. Gently push on to overcome a second (and perhaps third) resistance—from the obturator membrane. Get into (direct) contact with the tip of the instrument and guide it to exit through the vaginal incision (Fig. 43.4). This is the only time the instrument's axis is adjusted because the paraurethral sulcus must be overcome without penetrating it. Otherwise the instrument's movement is a rotational one only.
- Now attach the tape to the instrument and reverse the movement just made to make the tape pass the tunnel (Fig. 43.5).
- Do the same on the other side. A cystoscopy can then be performed if suitable.
- Adjust the tape's tension, pull out the sheaths (if there are any), and close the incisions (the external incisions do not necessarily need suturing) (Fig. 43.6).

Tips

- It is not necessary to create a tunnel so large that the surgeon's finger can go in and all the way to the pubic bone. In the simple cases, a restricted dissection leads to less bleeding and a more stable position of the tape.
- Keep the index finger inside the vagina to control gliding of the instrument from the bone to the incision; it should feel as if the instrument is gliding on the finger to avoid penetrating a wrong tissue layer, the urethra, or the vagina.

Postoperative care

- Watch for voiding 2–3 h after the surgery.
- Antiphlogistics or pain medication are recommended once only after the procedure; after that only a few patients require medication.
- The patient can be discharged after residual-free voiding has occurred twice.

Complications

Being a sling procedure, all the complications mentioned in Chapter 42 can occur. Bladder lesions are extremely rare, and bleeding has not yet been reported to be a problem. The obturator vessels and nerves are sufficiently far away to be unharmed. Urgency and retention, resulting from overcorrection (a problem with using nontension-free tape) can be avoided by not using the cough test and putting the tape in really loosely. This may end up in a lower cure rate (remember that overcorrections are dry and therefore 'cured'), but considering the problems that result from overcorrection it is well worth it.

Troubleshooting

Always use monofilament macroporous tape to ensure proper healing and to avoid inflammatory reactions (as seen with IVS® tape).

Results

Even though no long-term results on the cure rate are published yet, there seems to be little doubt that the method should be as effective as the retropubic procedure. The only thing remaining to be clarified is whether there is a subpopulation of stress incontinent women that should get one specific procedure to improve their outcome. There is definitely a lower risk of bladder perforation and a practically nonexistent risk of bleeding.

Remarks

Be very careful in patients with paravaginal defects. By turning the instrument around the pubic bone, there is a slight risk of bladder base injury quite close to the ureter ostium. This is because the bladder base is no longer resting on the endopelvic fascia attached to the arcus tendineous of the levator ani muscle.

To do

- Whenever you are not sure about the bladder's integrity, do a cystoscopy.
- Be as cautious with transobturator systems as you would be with retropubic systems.
- If you think you will have to do an anterior colporrhaphy at the same time, use a transobturator system; this cannot shift towards the bladder neck because of its different fixations on both sides.

Not to do

- Do not apply tension to the tape.
- Do not use a hook-shaped instrument to go from the inside out—you may lose your way and end up in the obturator vessels.

References

1 Dargent D, Bretones S, Georges R et al. Insertion of a suburethral sling through the obturator membrane in the treatment of female urinary incontinence. Gynecol Obstet Fertil 2002;30:576–82.

2 Delorme E. Transobturator urethral suspension: mini-invasive procedure in the treatment of stress urinary incontinence in women. Prog Urol 2001;11:1306–13.

3 Fischer A, Fink T, Zachmann S. Transobturatorielle Schlingensysteme (Monarc®, Serasis®TO): ein erster Erfahrungsbericht von 150 Fällen. J Urol Uriogynäkol 2005;12:15–21.

4 Herrmann V, Palma PCR, Riccetto CLZ *et al.* Minimally invasive surgical treatment for stress urinary incontinence — preliminary results with Monarc®. Abstract Meeting of the International Urogynaecology Association, Argentina, 2003. Int Urogynecol J 2003;14(1).

5 Karram MM, Segal JL, Vassallo BJ *et al.* Complications and untoward effects of the tension-free vaginal tape procedure. Obstet Gynecol 2003;101:929–32.

6 Pelosi, Marco A. II and III: The new transobturator sling reduces

the risk of injury during surgery for stress urinary incontinence. O B G Management 2003;July:17–20, 30–8.

7 Peyrat L, Boutin JM, Bruyere F *et al.* Intestinal perforation is a complication of TVT procedure for UI. Eur Urol 2001;39:603–5.

8 Walters MD, Tulikangas PR, LaSala C *et al.* Vascular injury during tension-free vaginal tape procedure for stress urinary incontinence. Obstet Gynecol 2001;98:957–9.

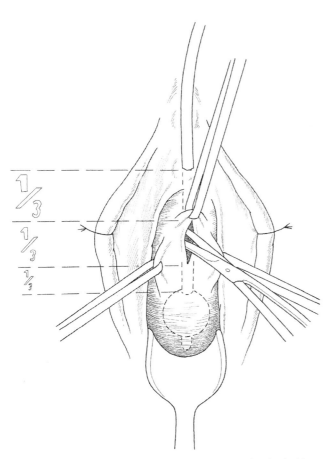

Figure 43.1 From a midline incision, dissect a tunnel on both sides staying underneath the vaginal fascia until the inferior ramus of the pubic bone is reached, using Metzenbaum scissors.

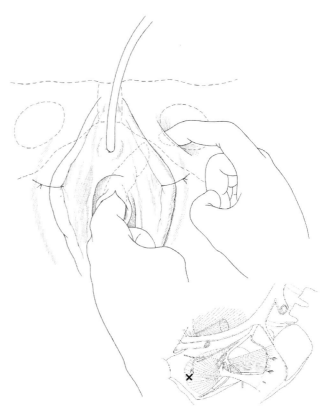

Figure 43.2 Create a tunnel wide enough to insert the index finger so that the tip of the finger can later on contact the tip of the instrument the moment it perforates the obturator membrane. The level of the skin incision on both sides is near the pubic bone, a little above the middle of the anterior line of the foramen. Inset: the anatomy of the pelvic wall as seen from the inside. The cross marks the point of penetration with the instrument.

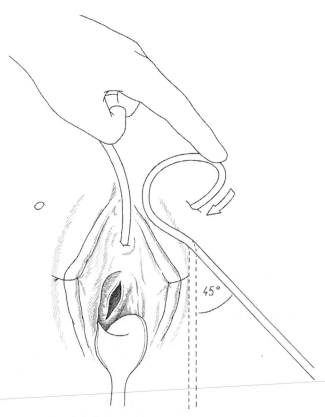

Figure 43.3 Insert the helix-shaped instrument into the skin incision and push it through the leg's fascia. The instrument's axis should be approximately 45° to the vertical.

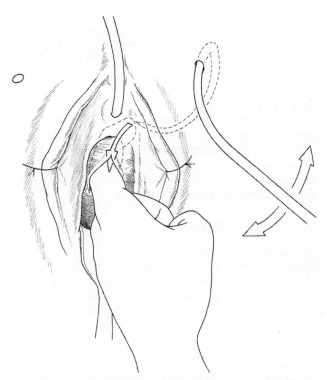

Figure 43.4 After penetrating the obturator membrane, get into (direct) contact with the tip of the instrument and guide it to exit through the vaginal incision.

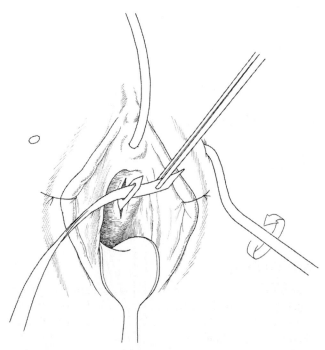

Figure 43.5 According to the product chosen for the procedure, now attach the tape to the instrument and reverse the movement just made to make the tape pass through the tunnel (in this figure the reusable Serasis TO® instrument is shown with an eye to pass the tape through).

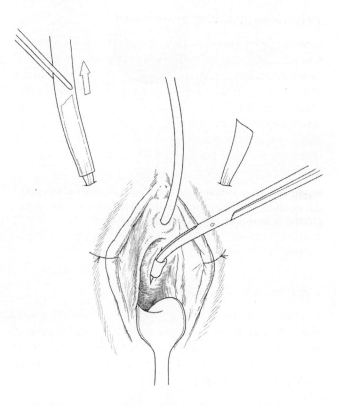

Figure 43.6 Adjust the tape's tension, pull out the sheaths (if there are any), and close the vaginal incision.

Chapter 44
Urethrolysis for Retention and Obstruction after Incontinence Surgery

H. M. Scarpero and V. W. Nitti

Introduction

Intervention for iatrogenic obstruction is required in approximately 1–3% of patients after sling procedures. The obstruction may be due to misplaced sutures or slings that were placed too medially (leading to urethral deviation, kinking, or scarring) or too distally (leading to kinking or obstruction). The most common technical error causing obstruction in sling surgery is hypersuspension of the bladder neck and proximal urethra by excessive tension.

Patient counseling and consent

Obstructive symptoms include: an inability to void, intermittent retention, slow or interrupted stream, straining to void, urinary frequency, urinary urgency, and urge incontinence. The patient should be warned that symptoms may persist after urethrolysis. Additionally, incontinence may be worse than before, or absolute incontinence may result. The rate of recurrent stress urinary incontinence is 0–19% after urethrolysis without concomitant resuspension.

Indications

Urethrolysis is indicated if bothersome obstructive and/or irritative symptoms persist beyond 3 months after incontinence surgery and do not respond to conservative measures.

Limitations and risks

Preoperatively evaluate the probable benefit for the patient and the risk of the procedure, in correlation with the patient's symptoms and degree of bother. If the estimated benefit exceeds the possible damage, then it is suggested that the patient undergoes the procedure.

Contraindications

In the case of erosion, the eroded material should be excised fully and the urethra allowed to heal. Urethrolysis may be safer as a second procedure.

Preoperative management

• All patients require a focused history and physical. Key elements in the history are the patient's preoperative voiding status and the temporal relationship of the lower urinary tract symptoms to the surgery.
• Urodynamics, radiographic, and endoscopic studies are performed in select cases.

Anesthesia

General or regional anesthesia.

Special instruments/suture material

• Instruments needed for pubovaginal sling procedures.
• Rigid cystoscope.
• Weighted vaginal speculum.
• Debakey and Boney forceps.
• Metzenbaum scissors.
• Right-angle clamp.
• Self-retaining retractor for an abdominal approach (Balfour or Bookwalter retractor).

Operative technique
Retropubic urethrolysis

• Make a Pfannenstiel or low midline incision.
• Expose the retropubic space, and release all prevesical and retropubic adhesions to restore complete mobility. The vesicourethral unit should be freely moveable.
• Dissect the urethra and urethrovesical junction off the pubic bone without separating them from the anterior vaginal wall. Lateral dissection (sometimes as far as the ischial tuberosities) depends on the degree of scarring. In most cases a paravaginal defect results from this dissection.

- Close the paravaginal defect by reapproximating the paravaginal and internal obturator fascia along the arcus tendineous (cf. Fig. 46.12). Use nonabsorbable 2/0 sutures, and do not tie them yet.
- Open the peritoneum and mobilize the omentum; create a pedicle omental flap to place between the urethra and bone. Secure with 2/0 polyglycolic acid (PGA) sutures against the bone.
- Tie the paravaginal sutures.
- Perform a cystoscopy (efflux of indigo carmine from the ureteral orifices and inspection for urethral injury).
- If no efflux is blue, thread an open-ended catheter and confirm ureteral patency before closing the abdomen.

Transvaginal urethrolysis

- Make a 3 cm long inverted, U-shaped incision with its apex half way between the bladder neck and urethral meatus.
- Laterally dissect along the periurethral fascia to the pubic bone.
- Perforate the attachment of the endopelvic fascia to the obturator fascia to enter the retropubic space (Fig. 44.1).
- Open the retropubic space on both sides and dissect the urethra from the undersurface of the pubic bone to free it completely proximal to the bladder neck (the index finger can be placed between the urethra and bone) (Fig. 44.2).
- In cases of extremely difficult dissection between the urethra and bone, use a suprameatal incision for urethrolysis.
- Sometimes after recurrent transvaginal urethrolysis (after failed prior urethrolysis), interposition of a Martius labial fat pad flap between the urethra and pubic bone may be desirable.
- Perform cystoscopy (efflux of indigo carmine from the ureteral orifices and inspection for urethral injury).
- Close the vaginal incision with 2/0 PGA sutures.

Suprameatal urethrolysis

- Make an inverted, U-shaped incision on the anterior vaginal wall and around the urethral meatus (1 cm distant) between the 3 and 9 o'clock positions (Fig. 44.3).
- Develop a plane above the urethra, and facilitate dissection by traction on the vaginal flap with an Allis clamp.
- Perform further blunt dissection using the index finger.
- Dissection of the lateral wings of the pubovaginal sling or suspension sutures may be necessary (Fig. 44.4).
- Place a Martius flap if desired.
- Perform cystoscopy.

Sling incision

- Make an inverted U- or midline incision to expose the bladder neck and proximal urethra.
- Expose the sling (the more tension there is, the more difficult this becomes) (Fig. 44.5).
- Separate the sling from the periurethral fascia below—this may be facilitated by traction on both sides using Allis clamps.

A right-angle clamp above the sling helps when cutting it in the midline.
- Mobilize edges of the sling unless they snap back into the retropubic space (Fig. 44.6).
- Excise synthetic material, and leave the auto- or allograft ends.
- Perform cystoscopy and close the vaginal incision.

Tips

- Keep the tips of the scissors against the pubic symphysis during sharp dissection.
- Identify the boundaries of the vagina and urethrovesical junction by placing a nondominant finger into the vagina.
- Resupport of the urethrovesical junction after urethrolysis may be desirable in select cases: where there is extensive mobilization or stress incontinence coexisting with obstruction.
- For the incision of a very tight sling, it may be advisable to insert a cystoscope into the urethra to isolate the sling.
- If the sling cannot be clearly identified at sling lysis, then formal transvaginal urethrolysis should be performed.

Postoperative care

A Foley catheter can be left in for 2–3 days—or longer if bladder or urethral injury has occurred—after urethrolysis and vaginal packing for 24 h. Prophylactic antibiotics should be given for up to 2 days after removal of the catheter. A post void residual urine estimation should be made by bladder scan and uninstrumented uroflow on the first postoperative visit. Oral pain medication may be needed.

Complications

- Lesions of the bladder and urethra, secondary necrosis, and abscesses.
- Bleeding from bladder vessels, vessels running with the arcus tendineus of the endopelvic fascia (paracolpium), and retropubic vessels.
- Ligature or kinking of the ureter after hemostasis of severe (arterial) bleeding.
- Complications resulting from gaining an omental flap or Martius flap.

Troubleshooting

- Urodynamics do not correlate with symptoms—they have no predictive value for the cure rate (relief of obstruction). The postoperative voiding status (compared with preoperative voiding) is more reliable.
- Obstructive uroflowmetry with high detrusor pressure and a steep rise of pressure in the urethra closing pressure profile over the sling/scar area are indicators that back up clinical symptoms, but are far from consistent.

• Failure may be due to persistent or recurrent obstruction, detrusor instability, impaired detrusor contractility, or learned voiding dysfunctions.

• Recurrent obstruction may be caused by periurethral fibrosis/scarring or intrinsic damage to the urethra as a result of urethrolysis.

Results

Reported success rates range from 50 to 93%; most publications include cases with multiple previous operations, and only two citations are based on pubovaginal slings (50 and 66% success rates). In our own institution, the success rate is about 65%.

Sling lysis seems to be more successful, at a rate of 84%. Failure to void properly was seen in 16%, but irritative symptoms improved in these patients. Stress incontinence occurred in 17%, in most cases soon after surgery.

Remarks

The authors of this chapter prefer a transvaginal approach as the primary operation (it is easier, with reduced morbidity and fast recovery), but use the retropubic approach as a secondary operation after a failed transvaginal procedure or primarily in cases with unfavorable vaginal anatomy, after reports of injuries or fistulas, or other complications after previous surgical treatment. Removal of synthetic slings is done retropubically.

The only parameter that is predictive of success seems to be that there should have been *no prior urethrolysis*.

To do

• Try the vaginal route as the primary surgical approach for obstruction after a sling procedure.

• Using polypropylene slings and simple dissection is, in most cases, sufficient to treat obstruction. Excessive dissection is only necessary if there are additional symptoms to voiding difficulties (e.g. urgency).

• Use local estrogens to improve healing of vaginal tissue, to smooth scars, and to get better mobility of the urethra.

Not to do

After abdominal dissection of polypropylene sling material, do not pull on the sling to extract it, even with the suburethral part dissected. The adhesion to the periurethral tissue may damage the urethra (tear, rupture). A vaginal dissection of the sling, up to its penetration of the endopelvic fascia, is advisable before removing the supradiaphragmal part through a small laparotomy. This is only necessary if it is suspected that there is tape running through the detrusor muscle (severe urge incontinence is often a symptom).

References

1 Amundsen CL, Guralnick ML, Webster GD. Variations in strategy for the treatment of urethral obstruction after a pubovaginal sling procedure. J Urol 2000;164:434–7.

2 Bass JS, Leach GE. Bladder outlet obstruction in women. Problems Urol 1991;5:141–54.

3 Carr LK, Webster GD. Voiding dysfunction following incontinence surgery: diagnosis and treatment with retropubic or vaginal urethrolysis. J Urol 1997;157:821–3.

4 Cross CA, Cespedes RD, English SF *et al.* Transvaginal urethrolysis for urethral obstruction after anti-incontinence surgery. J Urol 1998;159:1199–201.

5 Foster HE, McGuire EJ. Management of urethral obstruction with transvaginal urethrolysis. J Urol 1993;150:1448–51.

6 Ghoniem GM, Eigmasy AN. Simplified surgical approach to bladder outlet obstruction following pubovaginal sling. J Urol 1995;154:181–3.

7 Goldman RB, Rackley RR, Appell, RA. The efficacy of urethrolysis without resuspension for iatrogenic urethral obstruction. J Urol 1999;161:196–8.

8 Nitti VW, Raz S. Obstruction following anti-incontinence procedures: diagnosis and treatment with transvaginal urethrolysis. J Urol 1994;152:93–8.

9 Nitti VW, Carlson KV, Blaivas JG *et al.* Pubovaginal sling lysis by midline incision. Urology 2002;59(1):47–51.

10 Nitti VW, Raz S. Urinary retention. In: Female Urology, 2nd edn (Raz S, ed.). W.B. Saunders, Philadelphia, 1996:197–213.

11 Petros PE, Ulmsten U. The free graft procedure for cure of the tethered vagina syndrome. Scand J Urol Nephrol Suppl 1993;153:85–7.

12 Petros PE, Ulmsten U. The tethered vagina syndrome, post surgical incontinence and I-plasty operation for cure. Acta Obstet Gynaecol Scand Suppl 1990;153(69):63–7.

13 Petrou SP, Brown JA, Blaivas JG. Suprameatal transvaginal urethrolysis. J Urol 1999;161:1268–71.

14 Webster GD, Kreder KJ. Voiding dysfunction following cystourethropexy: its evaluation and management. J Urol 1990;144:670–3.

15 Zimmern PE, Hadley HR, Leach GE, Raz S. Female urethral obstruction after Marshall–Marchetti–Krantz operation. J Urol 1987;138:517–20.

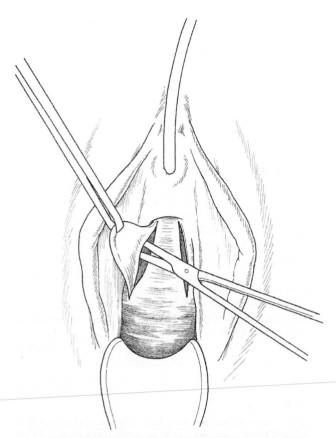

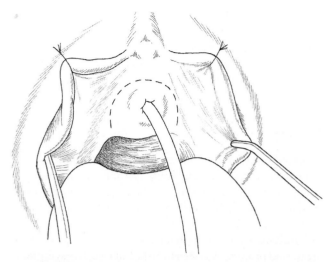

Figure 44.3 Make an inverted, U-shaped incision on the anterior vaginal wall and around the urethral meatus (1 cm distant) between the 3 and 9 o'clock positions.

Figure 44.1 Perforate the attachment of the endopelvic fascia to the obturator fascia to enter the retropubic space after a vaginal incision.

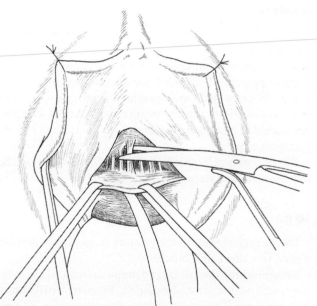

Figure 44.4 A possible dissection of the lateral wings of the pubovaginal sling or suspension sutures may be necessary.

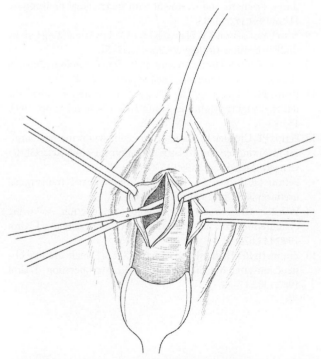

Figure 44.2 Open the retropubic space on both sides and dissect the urethra from the undersurface of the pubic bone to free it completely proximal to the bladder neck.

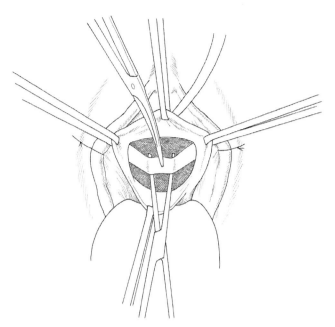

Figure 44.5 Expose the sling (the more tension there is, the more difficult this becomes).

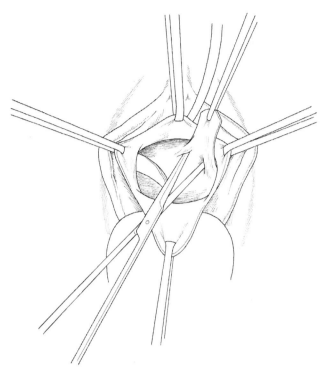

Figure 44.6 Mobilize the edges of the sling laterally unless they snap back into the retropubic space.

Part 6.2
Other Procedures in Female Urology

Chapter 45
Prolapse Repair

A. Fischer

Introduction

Prolapse or descent of the pelvic floor ligaments may occur, with or without muscular deficiencies. To stabilize the organs' position in the pelvis there are:
- muscular contraction;
- fixation by ligaments; and
- the mass of the levator muscle as a mechanical pressure barrier.

There are three main types of defect: anterior (midline or lateral), central, or posterior.
- *Anterior defect*:
  - midline defect: a tear in the pubocervical layer of the endopelvic fascia;
  - lateral defect: a detachment of the vagina's connection to the pelvic floor muscle between the arcus tendineus of the endopelvic fascia and that of the levator muscle.
- *Posterior defect*: in a rectocele, the vaginal wall protrusion contains the extended ampoule of the rectum. A defect of the rectovaginal layer of the endopelvic fascia can be located in the midline, laterally, or transversally near the vaginal entry.
- *Central defect*: the enterocele contains a protrusion of the peritoneum containing parts of the small intestine in most cases. Rectoceles and enteroceles often appear combined. Protrusion of the small intestine may also appear in the upper part of the anterior vaginal wall, camouflaged as a cystocele (this is an anterior upper enterocele).

Patient counseling and consent

The understanding of patients about the relationship between prolapse and incontinence/constipation often seems limited. When explaining the disease and the cure, always stress that:
- the present problems may not be cured;
- the present problems may become worse;
- new problems can occur;
- recurrence is possible or even likely;
- previously nonexisting incontinence may afterwards be the most annoying problem and cannot always be cured, especially if it is urge incontinence.

You should also mention the possibility of fistula formation.

Indications

The procedure is indicated in symptomatic prolapse where there is:
- urinary retention with recurrent urinary tract infections;
- outlet problems and constipation;
- rubbing, chafing, excoriation, or the feeling of a foreign body in the vagina or between the legs;
- other complaints (such as dyspareunia).

Limitations and risks

- Multiple previous operations (this increases the risk of intraoperative complications and the formation of lesions of the bladder and/or rectum and small intestine). These risks should be discussed with the patient prior to surgery.
- Destruction of the levator plate by, for example, forceps extraction. Therefore use an implant to stabilize the posterior wall defect (anchoring it may be tricky).
- A short vagina may be difficult to anchor vaginally because the sacrospinous ligaments are too far away; sometimes the abdominal approach seems the better choice if the use of posterior tape (see below) is not an option.
- Tissue that is highly scarred may cause problems with continence when it is stretched and attached to some distant structure (Integral Theory by Petros and Ulmsten [30]). Always try to work without tension.

Contraindications

- Temporary contraindications: local infections, bad estrogen status.
- General contraindications: as for general surgery.

- Relative contraindication: bad ratio between benefits and side effects.

Preoperative management

Pelvic floor exercises should have been performed regularly. Sometimes it is not possible to decide whether a repair can be done without foreign material, especially in recurrence—if you cannot get the patient's consent on the use of mesh or other materials do not operate. See also introduction to Section 6.

Anesthesia

See introduction to Part 6.1.

Special instruments/suture material

- Instruments for vaginal surgery.
- Breisky's specula.
- Langenbeck's specula.
- Deschamps' needle (for sacrospinous fixation).
- Suture material: in most cases PGA sutures will do; for mesh anchoring PDS (2/0) may be helpful. For sacrospinous fixation on one side (right) we use PDS 1/0 with a CT-1 or CT-2 needle depending on how much space there is to maneuver. For fixations on both sides (where a sling has to be used, as in colposuspension, in order not to obliterate the rectum between the sutures) we use Ethibond® with an MO-6 needle.
- For implant use: the biomaterials needed include Pelvisoft® (Bard Ltd, UK)—a porcine dermal collagen—and InteXen® (AMS, USA)—also of porcine dermal origin—or Stratasis® (Cook, Ireland)—of porcine intestinal origin (mucosa of small bowel). Even though there is written denial of the possibility of prionic contamination of the product by the industry in acellular matrix, the patient should be advised of the material's origin. Good results have been obtained using meshes designed for use in gynecological surgery.
- Synthetic material: mono- or oligofilament meshes; macroporous (70 μm). They should be made out of polypropylene and their weight should not exceed 50 g of fibers per m².
- Some products get sharp edges when cut into shape and size, which may cause erosions. The chosen mesh should have smooth edges when cut.
- See Plages A1 and A2, between pp. 112 and 113.

Operative technique

Anterior vaginal repair (with/without implant) for midline defect

- Perform an anterior midline colpotomy from the bladder neck to the apex.

- Dissect the cystocele up to the lateral attachment of the anterior vaginal wall on both sides (with thorough hemostasis).

Without implant (Fig. 45.1)

- Look out for the dissected tissue layer underneath the detrusor muscle (this is the endopelvic fascia—the urogenital diaphragm) after performing the midline colpotomy.
- Dissect the vaginal fascia from the endopelvic fascia using the avascular layer between both.
- Use U-shaped sutures to bring the tissue together under the midline where the defect has occurred.
- Starting at the bladder neck, usually 3–5 sutures will be necessary to double the tissue layer.
- Excess vaginal skin is resected (very cautiously).
- Adapt the skin with running sutures (2/0 or 3/0 PGA).

With implant (Fig. 45.2)

- The implant patch (which is cut prior to its fixation, according to the size needed—tension-free!) is sutured to the junction of the fascias (bladder and vagina), staying away from the patch edge by 4–5 mm, with 0/0 or 1/0 PGA or 2/0 PDS.
- Place one suture underneath the urethra in the midline and one on either side underneath the bladder base to keep the implant in the right position.
- Use a running suture to close up the vaginal incision after moderate resection of surplus vaginal wall tissue.
- Use vaginal packing for 24 h and an indwelling bladder catheter for the same amount of time. Give a single-shot antibiotic treatment prior to the surgery.

Anterior vaginal repair for lateral defect with implant and transobturator tape for reinforcement (ATOM) with or without the uterus in place
Without the uterus in place (Fig. 45.3)

- Start with a posterior colpotomy. If there is need for posterior repair as well do it longitudinally; if not a horizontal incision should be sufficient.
- Dissect the tissue to get down to the sacrospinous or sacrotuberal ligament (depending on length of the vagina—in most cases one would look for the sacrotuberal ligament on both sides).
- Put in a single nonabsorbable suture, taking a good grip of the sacrotuberal (or sacrospinal) ligament; cut off the needle and attach the suture to a clamp; let it rest for now. Repeat procedure on the other side.

With or without the uterus in place (Fig. 45.4)

- Perform an anterior midline colpotomy from the bladder neck to the apex.
- Dissect the cystocele up to the lateral attachment of the anterior vaginal wall on both sides (with thorough hemostasis).
- Where the tissues of the vaginal wall, the endopelvic fascia layer, and the tendinous arc of the levator muscle meet they are now recognized to be either distended or torn.

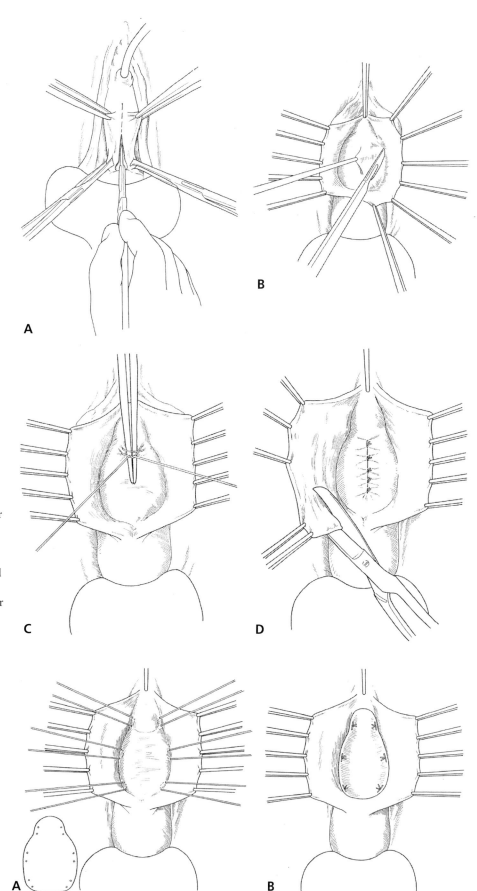

Figure 45.1 Anterior vaginal repair for a midline defect without an implant. (A) Perform a midline colpotomy looking out for the urogenital diaphragm. (B) Dissect the vaginal and endopelvic fascia. (C) U-shaped sutures bring the tissues together under the midline. (D) Cautiously resect the excess vaginal skin.

Figure 45.2 Anterior vaginal repair for a midline defect with an implant. (A) Put in sutures (about three on each side) through the bladder's fascia at the point where it joins the vaginal skin's fascial layer. (B) Attach the implant to these sutures before closing the colpotomy.

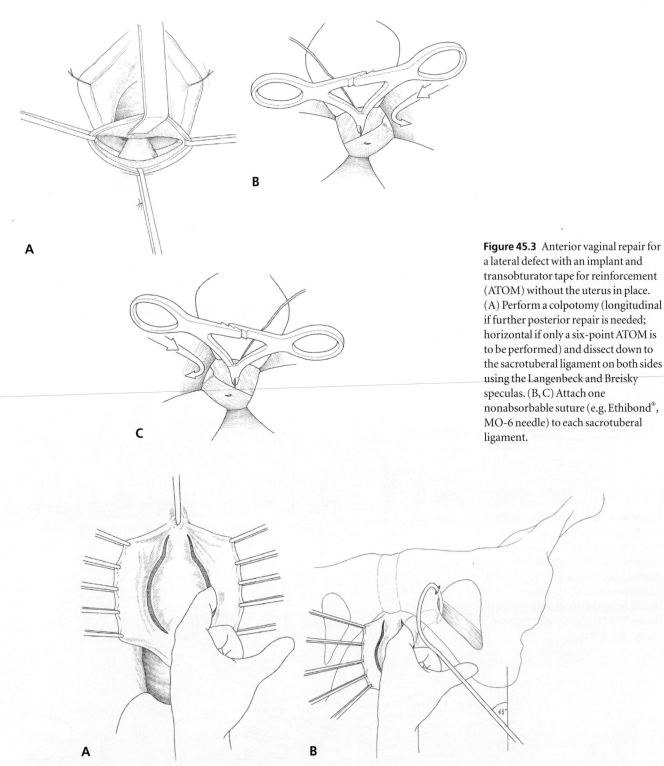

Figure 45.3 Anterior vaginal repair for a lateral defect with an implant and transobturator tape for reinforcement (ATOM) without the uterus in place. (A) Perform a colpotomy (longitudinal if further posterior repair is needed; horizontal if only a six-point ATOM is to be performed) and dissect down to the sacrotuberal ligament on both sides using the Langenbeck and Breisky speculas. (B, C) Attach one nonabsorbable suture (e.g. Ethibond®, MO-6 needle) to each sacrotuberal ligament.

Figure 45.4 ATOM with and without the uterus in place. For both the ATOM proceduces, (A) dissect the cystocele up to the lateral attachment of the anterior vaginal wall on both sides (the arcus tendineous will either be torn or only distended there). (B) Introduce the helix-shaped instrument through the obturator hole to get the anterior sling positioned underneath the trigone (angle approximately 45°).

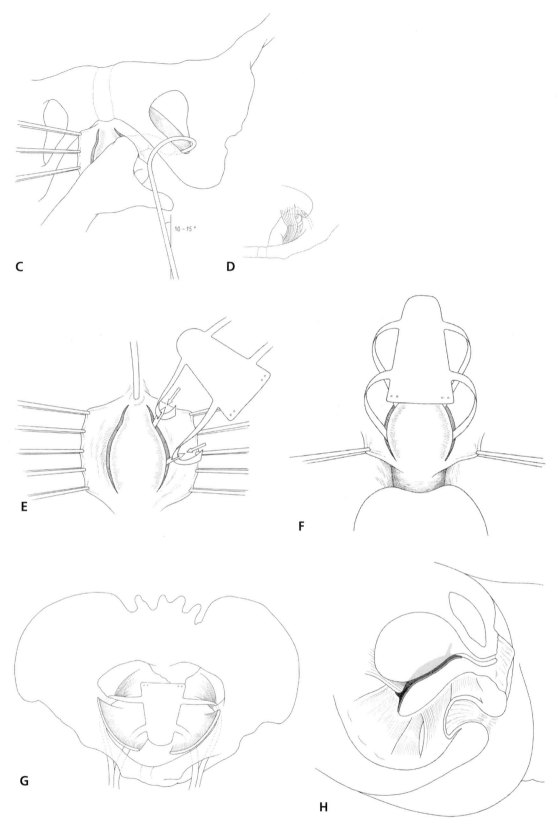

Figure 45.4 *Continued.* (C) In a second attempt on the same side penetrate the obturator membrane at the base of the obturator hole in the lower anterior angle (axis of the instrument approximately 15°). (D) Circumvent the levator and obturator muscles with the instrument to arrive at their posterior edge approximately one finger width above the ischial spine. This is facilitated by pulling the muscle's edge towards you using the index finger already introduced to palpate the spine. (E) Do one side first. Attach the tape to the instrument and make it run through the tissue after each insertion of the instrument. (F) Repeat the procedure on the other side. (G) Put the implant in the right position—it forms a hammock for the bladder extending between the pelvic floor walls. (H) The implant enables the bladder (and anterior enterocele in a six-point ATOM procedure) to rest on the newly created hammock.

• First introduce the helix-shaped instrument through the obturator hole to get the anterior sling positioned underneath the trigone. Do one side first. Attach the tape to the instrument and make it run through the tissue.

• In a second attempt on the same side, penetrate the obturator membrane at the basis of the obturator hole in the lower anterior angle.

• Circumvent the levator and obturator muscles to arrive at their posterior edge approximately one finger width above the ischial spine.

• Pull through the second (posterior) tape.

• Repeat the procedure on the other side.

• Put the implant into the right position using two atraumatic forceps; resect excess vaginal skin.

• Put in one to three 3/0 PDS sutures to attach the anterior transobturator mesh (ATOM) to the bladder neck area.

• If the uterus is in place, attach the posterior end of the mesh with three more stitches to the cervix (Fig. 45.5).

• If the uterus is not in place, use the appropriate instrument (Deschamps modification) and introduce it through the posterior incision to make it run up laterally on both sides, through the lateral defect or through the endopelvic fascia, so that the suture attached to the sacrotuberal (sacrospinal) ligament and fixed to the instrument can be pulled out there (Fig. 45.6). Take the sutures and pull them through so that they can be attached to the posterior corners of the mesh implant. Tie the sutures to the mesh so that it can be spread in a tension-free way underneath the bladder base.

• In either situation, then close the vagina on top of the implant without tension.

Lower posterior vaginal repair of a midline defect (without/with implant)

• Perform a posterior midline colpotomy.

• Dissect the rectocele.

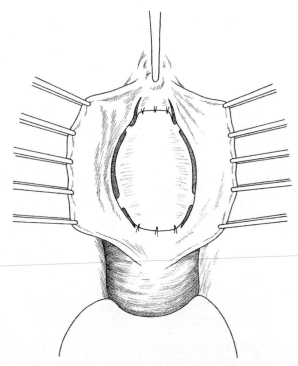

Figure 45.5 ATOM with the uterus in place. Three 3/0 PDS sutures are used to attach the mesh to the bladder neck area, and three more stitches to attach the posterior end of the mesh to the cervix in a four-point ATOM case.

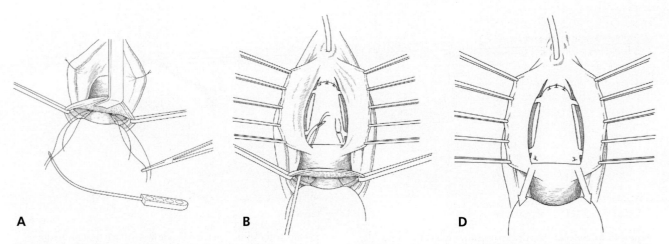

A   **B**   **D**

Figure 45.6 ATOM without the uterus in place. (A) Make the sacrotuberal sutures run through the Deschamps modification (e.g. Serasis V® instrument). (B) The instrument, with the suture, penetrates the endopelvic fascia laterally (or goes through the defect in the arcus tendineous) in order to make the suture appear next to the implant's posterior edge, where it is attached. (C) The sutures are gently tied so that the implant is stretched and the vector forces of the suture pull the posterior edge of the implant down towards the sacrotuberal ligaments.

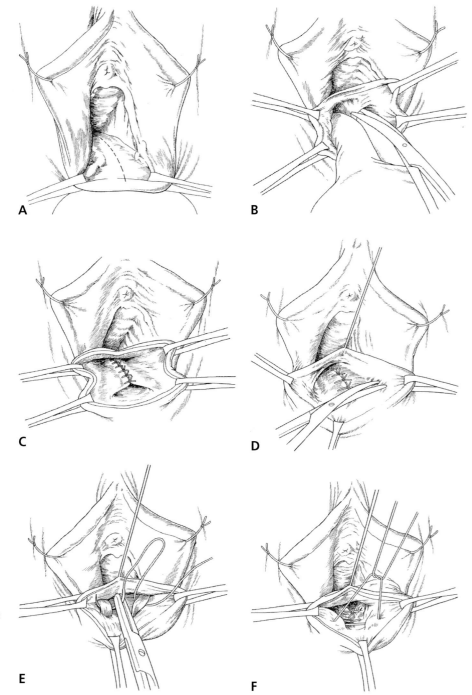

Figure 45.7 Lower posterior vaginal repair of a midline defect without an implant. (A) Perform a midline colpotomy. (B) Dissect the rectocele. (C) Plicate the perirectal connective tissue with 3–5 interrupted sutures. (D) Incise the insertion of the rectovaginal lamina of the endopelvic fascia on both sides to gain access to the levator muscle. (E) A good bite of muscle is taken on both sides, protecting the rectum, to bring out the lower portions of the levator ani muscle. (F) Tie the cranial suture to make suturing easier and finish restoring the perineal body before closing the colpotomy.

Without implant (Fig. 45.7)

- Perform a midline colpotomy.
- Dissect the rectocele with Metzenbaum scissors, using blunt dissection when possible (blunt dissection only works when the right tissue layer has been opened up).
- Plicate the perirectal connective tissue with 3–5 interrupted sutures.
- Incise the insertion of the rectovaginal lamina of the endopelvic fascia on both sides to gain access to the levator muscle.
- The dissection here should not be too excessive in order not to disturb the innervation of the levator running on its surface.
- Using 1/0 PGA sutures (with a CT-1 needle), a good bite of muscle is taken on both sides, protecting the rectum, which is close, by using a Breisky speculum to push it to the opposite side.

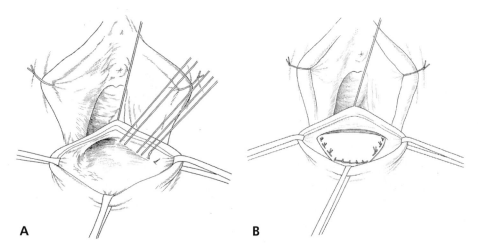

Figure 45.8 Lower posterior vaginal repair of a midline defect with an implant. (A) Sutures are put into the endopelvic fascia or to the pelvic wall just underneath the vagina's lateral attachment—the upper suture close to the levator muscle's cranial edge. (B) Prepare the sutures, then introduce the patch into the prepared cavity, and tie the sutures. The lower end is transversally sutured to the perineal body's connective tissue before closing the colpotomy.

- Tie the cranial suture to bring out the lower portions and to make suturing easier.
- By opening up the space on top of the external anal sphincter in the direction of the ischiorectal fossa, access to the often retracted bulbocavernous muscle is gained with a large enough needle (CT-1). The remnants of this muscle are often torn or cut during delivery when the baby's head penetrates the pelvic floor; they should be joined again in the midline to form a solid perineal body in order to prevent stool outlet problems after surgery.
- Use good hemostasis.
- The vaginal skin and perineum are closed with a running 2/0 or 3/0 PGA suture.
- The vagina is packed for 24 h.
- No antibiotics are needed in cases without implant use.

With implant (Fig. 45.8)

- The lateral attachment of the posterior layer of the endopelvic fascia to the vaginal wall and levator muscle is the limit for the dissection (only used in large protruding rectoceles where the fascia is torn on one or both sides).
- In midline tears (the average case), keep dissection to a minimum. Cranial dissection for lower posterior defects should not exceed 6 cm (from the vaginal entrance) because if the defect goes further up additional fixation is needed.
- Prepare the sutures, then introduce the patch into the prepared cavity.
- Suture the patch to the endopelvic fascia or to the pelvic wall just underneath the vagina's lateral attachment (in cases of more excessive lateral dissection).
- The patch's upper end is sutured to the vaginal wall in its vicinity to make sure that all three layers interconnect properly.
- The lower end is transversally sutured to the perineal body's connective tissue using a small but sharp needle (V-7) with a 2/0 PGA suture.
- By opening up the space on top of the external anal sphincter in the direction of the ischiorectal fossa, access to the often re-tracted bulbocavernous muscle is gained with a large enough needle (CT-1). The remnants of this muscle are often torn or cut during delivery when the baby's head penetrates the pelvic floor; they should be joined again in the midline to form a solid perineal body in order to prevent stool outlet problems after surgery.
- Use a running suture to close up the vaginal incision after moderate resection of surplus vaginal wall tissue.
- Use vaginal packing for 24 hours and an indwelling bladder catheter for the same time.
- Single-shot antibiotic treatment is given before the operation starts.

Upper posterior vaginal repair (combined with sacrospinous/sacrotuberal fixation of the vagina's apex) (Fig. 45.9)

- Perform a posterior midline colpotomy.
- Dissect the rectocele and the vagina's lateral connective tissue to get to the levator muscle on both sides.
- Penetration of the perirectal connective tissue gives way to either the sacrospinous or sacrotuberal ligament.
- This operation can be performed unilaterally or bilaterally. If deviation of the vagina's axis is to be avoided and the patient already complains about a certain amount of dyspareunia before the operation, tension-free bilateral fixation should be preferred.
- According to the length of the vagina, the appropriate ligament is chosen and three absorbable sutures (sharp CT-1 needle, 1/0 PDS) are passed through if fixation is only planned on one side. Keep a distance of at least 1.5 cm from the ischiadic spine to avoid lesions to the pudendal vessels or nerve, and keep the rectum out of the way using a Breisky's speculum.
- All six ends of the sutures are passed through the vaginal wall (from inside out) but are not tied yet for a unilateral procedure.
- For a bilateral fixation, a nonabsorbable suture is chosen because the vagina cannot be directly attached to the ligament

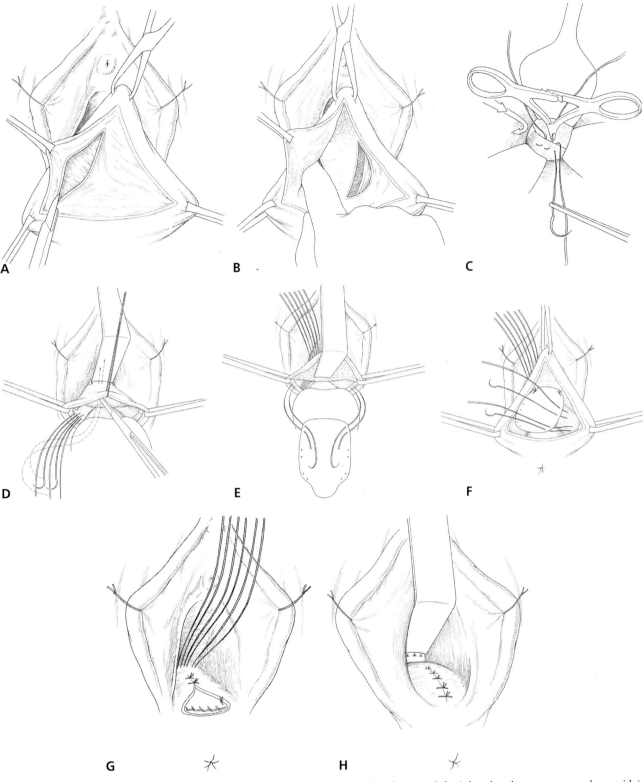

Figure 45.9 Upper posterior vaginal repair combined with sacrospinous/sacrotuberal fixation of the vagina's apex. (A) Perform a posterior midline colpotomy and dissect the rectocele and the vagina's lateral connective tissue to get to the levator muscle on both sides. (B) Penetration of the perirectal connective tissue gives way to either the sacrospinous or sacrotuberal ligament. (C) Attach the sutures to the ligament. (D) The ends of the sutures are passed through the vaginal wall (from inside out) but are not tied yet in case of unilateral fixation (in cases of bilateral fixation the sutures are attached to the vagina's fascia but they do not appear on the outside). (E) A 2/0 PDS suture is put into the upper edge of both levator muscles at the point where the levator and coccygeus muscles meet together in cases of combination with posterior mesh-supported repair. (F) Then one side of the patch after the other is sutured to the levator muscle. (G) The patch is then is attached to the perineal body tissue. (H) After resection of the overlapping vaginal wall tissue, the vaginal incision can be closed down to the vaginal entrance. The sutures are then tied in cases with unilateral fixation.

as obliteration of the rectum would result if this was done on both sides. Use two sutures per side. Attach the suture to the vaginal fascia. The suture must not penetrate the vaginal epithelium and the security of the knots must be good (0/0 or 1/0 Ethibond® with a MO-6 or CT-1 needle).

With implant
- A 2/0 PDS suture is placed in the upper edge of both levator muscles at the point where the levator and coccygeus muscles meet.
- An implant of appropriate size can now be attached by its corners to those sutures. As the knot is tied, the implant approaches the muscle.
- One side of the patch after the other is sutured to the levator muscle using two or three PDS interrupted sutures.
- Tie the sacrotuberal/sacrospinous fixation sutures in a bilateral fixation.
- Close to the vaginal entrance, two levator and one or two bulbocavernous sutures are needed to reconstruct the perineal body.
- The patch then is attached to the perineal body tissue using a 2/0 Vicryl running suture with an SH needle.

Without implant
- Alternatively, a conventional posterior repair, as shown in Fig. 45.7A–F, may be performed.

With or without implant
- After the resection of the overlapping vaginal wall tissue, the vaginal incision can be closed down to the vaginal entrance.
- The sacrotuberal/sacrospinous fixation sutures can now be tied in a unilateral fixation.
- If necessary, more of the bulbocavernous muscle can be put together in the midline before closing the perineal skin defect.
- Rectal palpation at this point of the operation is absolutely necessary as is thorough hemostasis during the whole procedure.
- There is no need for drainage, but before putting a catheter into the patient's bladder we put a package into the vagina, leaving it for 24–48 h.
- A single-shot antibiotic treatment (second generation cephalosporine) is given before the operation starts.

Infracoccygeal sacropexy (ICS) with posterior tape-supported vault fixation (Fig. 45.10)
- Make a horizontal incision of the vault or beneath the cervix.
- Dissect the enterocele away from the vault.
- Look for remnants of the uterosacral ligaments.
- Incise the endopelvic fascia laterally and below the ligaments to gain access to the spine and posterior edge of the levator muscle using the index finger.
- Incise both buttocks 2 cm laterally and 3 cm below the anal equator.

- Insert the tunneler instrument and push it forward to the level of the anal equator, then enter the ischiorectal fossa.
- Go up all the way lateral to the levator muscle to reach the tip of the finger that rests on the levator's edge some 1 cm above the ischial spine.
- Circumvent the levator muscle and make the instrument exit; introduce the tape and repeat the procedure on the other side, making the tape go inside out again.
- Fix the tape to the remnants of the uterosacral ligaments (using 0/0 PGA, CT-2 needle).
- Close the vaginal incision with a running suture of 2/0 PGA.
- Note that if the ICS is to be combined with a posterior mesh repair, a SerATOM® implant can be used (Fig. 45.10H). Cut off the anterior tapes ('arms') and leave the posterior ones to be used as described above. There is no more need for further fixation of the cranial part of the implant. We only use two sutures on both sides to attach the middle and the lower part of the implant before suturing it to the perineal body.

Vaginal repair of a lateral defect (Fig. 45.11)
- Marking sutures are placed at the level of the urethrovesical junction and vaginal apex.
- Perform a vaginal hysterectomy if required; otherwise make a vertical incision.
- The vaginal epithelium is dissected off the pubocervical fascia from the cut edge of the epithelium to the urethrovesical junction. A classic anterior colporrhaphy can then be performed if there is a midline defect or if the fascial tissue seems to be rarified due to distension.
- The dissection is continued laterally until the index finger can be passed between the vaginal epithelium and the pubocervical fascia into the retropubic space anterior to the ischial spine.
- With the finger in the retropubic space, the dissection is continued anteriorly along the inferior ramus of the pubis and medially to the symphysis pubis, revealing the whole of the white line.
- The first suture is placed 2 cm anterior to the ischial spine and a further 4–6 sutures are placed running from here to the attachment of the white line near the pubic bone, leaving each needle attached.
- The final suture is now brought to penetrate the lateral edge of the periurethral pubocervical fascia.
- The second suture penetrates the pubocervical fascia and the undersurface of the vaginal epithelium near the urethrovesical junction at the level of the marker stitch.
- Continue working back proximally until the suture near the ischial spine is used to secure the most cephalad portion of the pubocervical fascia to the undersurface of the epithelium near the vaginal apex.
- Tie the sutures sequentially, beginning periurethrally, and close the vagina as usual.

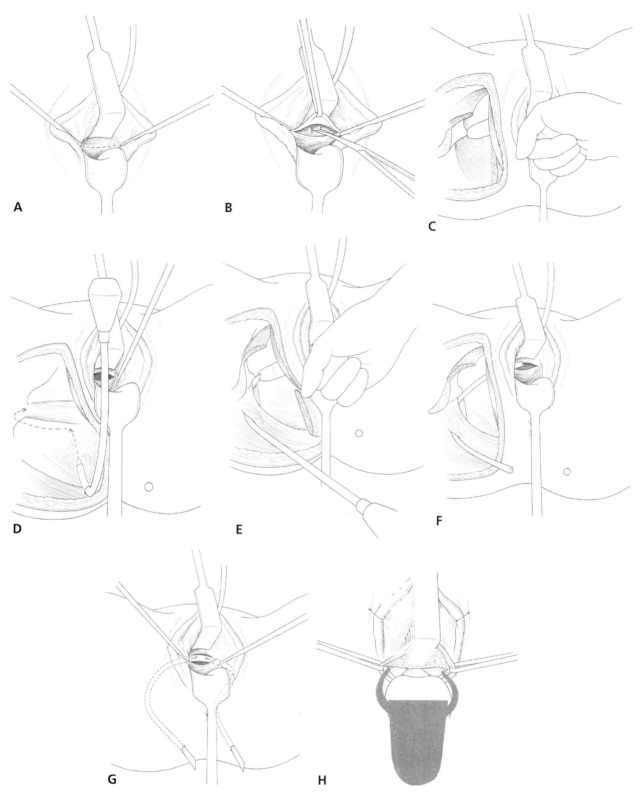

Figure 45.10 Infracoccygeal sacropexy (ICS) with posterior tape-supported vault fixation. (A) A horizontal incision is made of the vault or beneath the cervix. (B) Dissect the enterocele away from the vault and look for remnants of the uterosacral ligaments. (C) Incise the endopelvic fascia using the index finger. (D) Insert the tunneler instrument and push it forward to the level of the anal equator, then enter the ischiorectal fossa. (E) Go up all the way lateral to the levator muscle to reach the tip of the finger that rests on the levator's edge some 1 cm above the ischial spine. (F) Circumvent the levator muscle and make the instrument exit, introduce the tape and make it run through. (G) Fix the tape to the remnants of the uterosacral ligaments or the lateral vagina fascia. (H) If ICS is to be combined with a posterior mesh repair, a SerATOM® implant can be used.

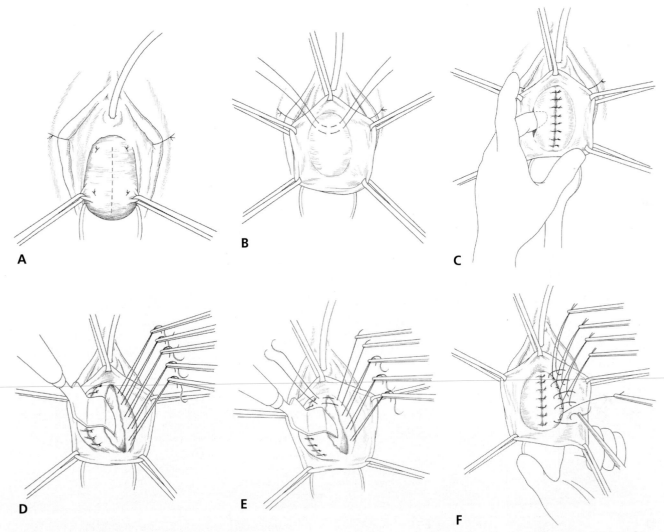

Figure 45.11 Vaginal repair of a lateral defect. (A) The vertical incision. (B) A classic anterior colporrhaphy can be performed if there is a midline defect or if the fascial tissue seems to be rarified due to distension. (C) With the finger in the retropubic space, the dissection is continued to reveal the whole of the white line. (D) The

sutures are run through the attachment of the white line near the pubic bone, leaving each needle attached. (E, F) The sutures then penetrate the pubocervical fascia and then the undersurface of the vaginal epithelium from the bladder neck-marking stitch to the ischial spine level.

Abdominal repair of a lateral defect (Fig. 45.12)

• Perform a hysterectomy if required (uterosacral plication) using a permanent suture material.

• Enter the space of Retzius and retract the bladder medially and insert the left forefinger into the vagina to expose the defect and edges of the fascial tear.

• Place the first stitch opposite the bladder neck in the anterolateral vaginal sulcus. Use a running suture or interrupted sutures.

• Pass the needle through the arcus tendineus 1.5–2 cm below the obturator foramen. Place a further 2–4 sutures more distally and one or two more proximally. Additionally, the sutures can be anchored in Cooper's ligament. Tie all the sutures at the same time.

Abdominal approach of a central defect

The open approach is very similar to laparoscopic colpopromontofixation (see Chapter 46) and is therefore not discussed here.

Tips

• When doing a combined repair start with the anterior wall. Put in a midurethral tape if needed but do not decide on its 'tension' until the posterior repair is completed.

• Always do a clear dissection of the sacrospinous ligament complex to avoid bleeding and pudendal nerve lesions.

• Be generous in the primary use of suprapubic catheters (it is nicer for the patient to already have it in when coming out of the anesthesia), especially in recurrent cases.

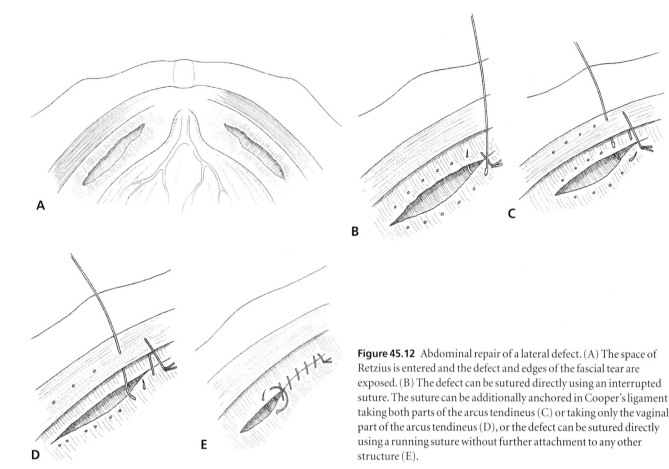

Figure 45.12 Abdominal repair of a lateral defect. (A) The space of Retzius is entered and the defect and edges of the fascial tear are exposed. (B) The defect can be sutured directly using an interrupted suture. The suture can be additionally anchored in Cooper's ligament taking both parts of the arcus tendineus (C) or taking only the vaginal part of the arcus tendineus (D), or the defect can be sutured directly using a running suture without further attachment to any other structure (E).

Postoperative care

- Give the patient perioperative antibiotics.
- Use a vaginal pack for 24–48 h (with mesh, for 48 h).
- A suprapubic catheter is not necessary with tension-free anterior mesh repair; but it is nice to have one with conventional anterior colporrhaphy and it is very helpful with sacrospinous/sacrotuberal fixation.
- Start micturition between day 3 and 5, depending on the extent of surgery and the patient's well being.
- An estriol suppository and vaginal disinfection every 2 days for 2 weeks is helpful to reduce the smell of the discharge and to facilitate the healing process.

Complications

- Lesions of the bladder, rectum, small bowel, ureter, urethra, and pudendal and obturator nerves.
- Bleeding, abscess, hematoma, and ileus.
- Healing problems.
- Rejection of the implants.
- Recurrence.

- Incontinence (urinary, stool), urge, and constipation.
- All other surgery-associated complications (e.g. thrombosis, embolism).

Troubleshooting

- Do not do too much at a time (to spare the patient another hospital stay or another surgery); do one thing at a time (as a general principle).
- Be careful combining prolapse and incontinence procedures—a lot of experience is needed here. Most of the patients understand the problem of overcorrection and are willing to come for a second, small procedure.
- Evacuate hematoma in patients with mesh implants in order to save the implant. Secondary infection of the hematoma and surrounding tissue often means loss of the implant.

Results

Anterior repair

Considering the long history and wide adoption of this procedure there have been few studies published on its effectiveness for anterior vaginal prolapse. Definitions of recurrence vary between authors and numbers lost to follow-up is often not stated.

Author	Recurrence	Follow-up (years)
Goff 1933	4/86 (4.6%)	1–8
Moore 1955	0/9	0.5–1.5
Friedman 1970	0/4	2–4
Stanton et al. 1982 [38]	8/54 (15%)	2
Macer 1978	22/109 (20%)	5–20
Walter 1982	0/86	1–2.5
Porges 1994	10/388 (3%)	1–20

Posterior repair

Author	Recurrence/cure rate	Follow-up (months)
Cundiff et al. 1998 [8]	Recurrence 18%	12
Kenton et al. 1999 [21]	Cure rates: 90% for protrusion and dyspareunia, 54% for difficult defecation, 43% for constipation, and 36% for manual evacuation	12
Karram et al. 2001 [19]	Recurrence >5.5%	6–36
Sze & Karram 1997 (review) [40]	Recurrence 11%	12–120
Porter et al. 1999 [31]	Cure rates: 55% for defecation, 73% for pain/pressure, 74% for vaginal mass, and 65% for splinting Recurrence approximately 18%	≥6
Meschia et al. 1999 [25]	Recurrence 6%	Unknown

Paravaginal repair

There are few large, long-term series, but success rates seem to be high for the repair of prolapse. In correctly selected patients, results can be favorable (150 patients, 97% success rate, with a follow-up of 60% at 30 months and 50% at 48 months).

Author	Recurrence	Follow-up (years)
Goetsch 1954	1/7 (15%)	2
Richardson et al. 1976 [33]	2/60 (3%)	1.7
Shull & Baden 1989 [35]	8/149 (5%)	0.5–4
Richardson et al. 1981 [32]	10/213 (5%)	2–8
Shull et al. 1994 [36]	4/56 (7%)	0.1–5.6

Infracoccygeal sacropexy (ICS)

Except for data from the originating workgroup (Australian Association of Vaginal Incontinence Surgeons) there is only one report, published on 21 patients with prolapse and urge, with a 76% cure rate for urge and a 100% cure rate for prolapse. The editors' own data suggest that ICS is safe and effective but not in cases with a vaginal length that exceeds the depth of the levator muscle by much. In those cases an anterior enterocele is likely to occur (soon). We therefore use this technique only in patients with a vagina shorter or as long as the levator reaches into the depth of the pelvis. In all other cases we prefer a sacrotuberal fixation (Amreich procedure).

Remarks

This surgical procedure needs an experienced surgeon. If you wish to start using these procedures, get some hands-on training first, with supervision of the first procedures you do on your own.

To do

• In posterior repair the reconstruction of the perineal body is essential for proper functioning of the rectum; outlet obstruction may result from poor surgical technique.
• Continue estrogen treatment after surgery.
• Continue pelvic floor exercises for 4–6 weeks, depending on the extent of the surgery.
• Make sure the patient returns if incontinence occurs (onset after discharge).

Not to do

• Do not treat an asymptomatic prolapse or talk a patient into prolapse repair.
• Do not promise good cure rates and that any problems can be completely cured.
• Do not use tension. If tension is applied the patient will end up with voiding difficulties, retention, urgency, or pain.
• Do not use mesh if the rectum has been injured or sutured as the risk of infection is too high.
• Do not use multifilament microporous tapes or meshes as the risk of trouble is enormous (chronic infections, healing difficulties, erosions, abscesses—just to name a few).

References

1 Anthuber C, Schüssler B, Hepp H. Die operative Therapie des Scheidenblindsackvorfalls. Die abdominale Sakrokolpopexie. Gynäkologe 1996;29:652–8.
2 Baden WB, Walker T. Surgical Repair of Vaginal Defects. J.E. Lippincott, Philadelphia, 1992.
3 Beck RP, McCormick S. Treatment of urinary stress incontinence with anterior colporrhaphy. Obstet Gynecol 1982;59:269.

4 Colombo M, Milani R, Vitobello D, Maggioni A. A randomized comparison of Burch colposuspension and abdominal paravaginal defect repair for female stress urinary incontinence. Am J Obstet Gynecol 1996;175:78–84.

5 Cross CA, Cespedes RD, English SF, McGuire EJ. Paravaginal vault suspension for the treatment of vaginal and uterovaginal prolapse. J Pelvic Surg 1997;3:81–5.

6 Cruikshank SH, Muniz M. Outcomes study: a comparison of cure rates in 695 patients undergoing sacrospinous ligament fixation alone and with other site-specific procedures—a 16-year study. Am J Obstet Gynecol 2003;188(6):1509–12; discussion 1512–15.

7 Cumberland VH. A preliminary report on the use of prefabricated nylon weave in the repair of ventral hernia. Med J Aust 1952;1:143–4.

8 Cundiff GW, Weidner AC, Visco AG, Addison WA, Bump RC. An anatomic and functional assessment of the discrete defect rectocele repair. Am J Obstet Gynecol 1998;179(6):1451–6; discussion 1456–7.

9 DeLancey JO. Anatomic aspects of vaginal eversion after hysterectomy. Am J Obstet Gynecol 1992;166:1717–28.

10 Farnsworth BN. Posterior intravaginal slingplasty (infracoccygeal sacropexy) for severe posthysterectomy vaginal vault prolapse—a preliminary report on efficacy and safety. Int Urogenecol J 2002;13:4–8.

11 Francis WJA, Jeffcoate TNA. Dyspareunia following vaginal operations. Br J Obstet Gynaecol 1961;68:1.

12 Gardy M, Kozminski M, DeLancey J et al. Stress incontinence and cystoceles. J Urol 1991;145:1211.

13 Haase P, Skibsted L. Influence of operations for stress incontinence and for genital descensus on sexual life. Acta Obstet Gynecol Scand 1988;67:659.

14 Hardiman PJ, Drutz HP. Sacrospinous vault suspension and abdominal colposacropexy: success rates and complications. Am J Obstet Gynecol 1996;175:612–16.

15 Harper C, Permacol TM. Clinical experience with a new biomaterial. Hospital Medicine 2001;62:90–5.

16 Iglesia CB, Fenner DE, Brubaker L. The use of mesh in gynecologic surgery. Int Urogynecol J Pelvic Floor Dysfunct 1997;8:105–15.

17 Jackson SR, Avery NC, Tariton JF, Eckford SD, Abrams P, Bailey AJ. Changes in metabolism of collagen in genitourinary prolapse. Lancet 1996;347:1658–61.

18 Kahn MA, Stanton SL. Posterior colporrhaphy: its effects on bowel and sexual function. Br J Obstet Gynaecol 1997;104:82–6.

19 Karram M, Goldwasser S, Kleeman S, Steele A, Vassallo B, Walsh P. High uterosacral vaginal vault suspension with fascial reconstruction for vaginal repair of enterocele and vaginal vault prolapse. Am J Obstet Gynecol 2001;185(6):1339–42; discussion 1342–3.

20 Kaum H-J, Wolff F (eds). Die vaginale sakrospinale/sakrotuberale Scheidenstumpffixation. Geschichte, Grundlagen, Technik und Ergebnisse. Steinkopff Verlag, Darmstadt, 2002.

21 Kenton K, Shott S, Brubaker L. Outcome after rectovaginal fascia reattachment for rectocele repair. Am J Obstet Gynecol 1999; 181(6):1360–3; discussion 1363–4.

22 Lambrou NC, Buller JL, Thompson JR, Cundiff GW, Chou B, Montz FJ. Prevalence of perioperative complications among women undergoing reconstructive pelvic surgery. Am J Obstet Gynecol 2000;183:1355–80.

23 Makinen J, Kahari VM, Soderstrom KO, Vuorio E, Hirvonen T. Collagen synthesis in the vaginal connective tissue of patients with and without uterine prolapse. Eur J Obstet Gynecol Reprod Biol 1987;24:319–25.

24 McCall ML. Posterior culdeplasty. Obstet Gynecol 1957;10: 595.

25 Meschia M, Bruschi F, Amicarelli F, Pifarotti P, Marchini M, Crosignani PG. The sacrospinous vaginal vault suspension: critical analysis of outcomes. Int Urogynecol J Pelvic Floor Dysfunct 1999;10(3):155–9.

26 Mouchel T, Wurst C, Mouchel J. Faut-il encore faire des myorraphies des releveurs? In: La Perineologie: Comprendre un Equilibre et le Preserver. Groupement Europeen de Perineologie (Beco J, Mouchel J, Nelissen G, eds). Maison d'Edition, Verviers, Belgium, 1998.

27 Niesel A, Neeb U. First experience with infracoccygeal sacropexy according to Petros in vaginal prolapse and urinary urge incontinence. Geburtsh Frauenheilk 2003;63:870–4.

28 Petros PE. Vault prolapse I: dynamic supports of the vagina. Int Urogynecol J Pelvic Floor Dysfunct 2001;12(5):292–5.

29 Petros PE. Vault prolapse II: restoration of dynamic vaginal supports by infracoccygeal sacropexy, an axial day-case vaginal procedure. Int Urogynecol J Pelvic Floor Dysfunct 2001;12:296–303.

30 Petros PE, Ulmsten U. An anatomical classification—a new paradigm for management of urinary dysfunction in the female. Int J Urogynecol Pelvic Floor Dysfunct 1999;10:29–35.

31 Porter WE, Steele A, Walsh P, Kohli N, Karram MM. The anatomic and functional outcomes of defect-specific rectocele repairs. Am J Obstet Gynecol 1999;181(6):1353–8; discussion 1358–9.

32 Richardson AC, Edmonds PB, Williams NL. Treatment of stress urinary incontinence due to paravaginal fascial defect. Obstet Gynecol 1981;57:357–62.

33 Richardson AC, Lyon JE, Williams NL. A new look at pelvic relaxation. Am J Obstet Gynecol 1976;126:568–73.

34 Shull BL. Equilibrium. Am J Obstet Gynecol 2002;187(6):1431–3.

35 Shull BL, Baden WF. A six-year experience with paravaginal defect repair for stress urinary incontinence. Am J Obstet Gynecol 1989;160:1432–5.

36 Shull BL, Benn SJ, Kuehl TJ. Surgical management of prolapse of the anterior vaginal segment: an analysis of support defects, operative morbidity, and anatomic outcome. Am J Obstet Gynecol 1994;171:1429–39.

37 Shull BL, Capen CV, Riggs MW, Kuehl TJ. Preoperative and postoperative analysis of site-specific pelvic support defects in 81 women treated with sacrospinous ligament suspension and pelvic reconstruction. J Obstet Gynecol 1992;166:1764–71.

38 Stanton SL, Norton C, Cardozo L. Clinical and urodynamic effects of anterior colporrhaphy and vaginal hysterectomy for prolapse with and without incontinence. Br J Obstet Gynaecol 1982;89:459.

39 Symmonds RE, Williams TJ, Lee RA et al. Posthysterectomy enterocele and vaginal vault prolapse. Am J Obstet Gynecol 1981;140:852.

40 Sze EH, Karram MM. Transvaginal repair of vault prolapse: a review. Obstet Gynecol 1997;89(3):466–75.

41 Van Geelen JM, Theeuwes AG, Eskes TK et al. The clinical and

urodynamic effects of anterior vaginal repair and Burch colposuspension. Am J Obstet Gynecol 1988;159:137.

42 Virtanen H, Hirvonen T, Mäkinen J, Kiilholma P. Outcome of thirty patients who underwent repair of posthysterectomy prolapse of the vaginal vault with abdominal sacral colpopexy. J Am Coll Surg 1994;178:283–7.

43 White GR. An anatomic operation for the cure of cystocele. Am J Obstet Dis Women Child 1912;65:286–90.

44 White GR. Cystocele: a radical cure by suturing lateral sulci of vagina to white line of pelvic fascia. J Am Med Assoc 1909;853: 1707–10.

Chapter 46
Laparoscopic Colpopromontofixation

A. Mottrie, P. Martens, R. Bollens, P. Dekuyper, Chr. Assenmacher, M. Fillet, R. Van Velthoven, and H. Nicolas

Introduction

This is the authors' method of choice; it is reproducible, quick, and relatively easy to perform. There is a short learning curve ($\pm$ 20 cases) and excellent short- and long-term results. In case of stress incontinence, the procedure should be combined with a transvaginal urethral sling.

Patient counseling and consent

The patient should be warned of classic possible complications of laparoscopic surgery with the implantation of prosthetic tissue (such as bowel lesions, bleeding, and the infection of prosthetic materials).

Indications

This procedure is indicated where there is descent of at least one of the three compartments of the vagina (anterior cystocele, posterior rectocele, and/or dome (uterine descent and/or enterocele)). If there is stress incontinence, combine the procedure with a transvaginal urethral sling.

Limitations and risks

The limitations include chronic pulmonary obstructive disease (COPD) and cardiac insufficiency, as well as a history of multiple operations in the small pelvis.

Contraindications

Extreme COPD or cardiac insufficiency.

Preoperative management

- Bowel preparation (Prepacol®).
- Exclude urinary infection.
- Perioperative broad-spectrum antibiotics for 24 h.

Anesthesia

General anesthesia.

Special instruments/suture material

- Classic laparoscopic materials: 3 × 5 mm port, 1 × 10 mm port, endoscopic grasping forceps, bipolar forceps (Microfrance®), monopolar scissors, and two needle holders.
- Multifilament polyester mesh (Parietex®).
- Suture material: 2/0 Ethibond® for fixation of the prosthesis to the elevator muscles and anterior vaginal wall, 2/0 Vicryl® for a McCall culdoplasty and closure of the peritoneum, and 0/0 Pro-Tack® or Ethibond® for fixation of both meshes to the promontorium.

Operative technique

- Patient positioning and operating room configuration are very important (Fig. 46.1). The surgeon is positioned at the left side of the patient, with the first assistant at the contralateral side. A videoscreen is placed at the foot of the bed.
- The necessary implants are prepared (Fig. 46.2).
- Insufflation of the abdomen is done through a Veress needle, up to 15 mmHg.
- The 'diamond' configuration is used for trocar placement. The umbilical port is placed blindly, the latter three are placed under direct vision after introducing a 0° lens through the umbilical port.
- Trendelenburg positioning up to 30° allows the bowel to fall away out of the small pelvis (Fig. 46.1).
- Intra-abdominal adhesions are taken down, the sigmoid is held to the left and the peritoneum is incised at the level of the promontory.
- The anterior longitudinal ligament is freed, taking care especially of the left common iliac vein. The median sacral vein and artery running over the ligament can be spared or, alternatively, coagulated with a bipolar forceps. The pararectal peritoneal fold is opened down to the uterosacral ligament in

order to be able to retroperitonize both prostheses at the end.
- If the uterus is in place, it is fixed at the abdominal wall with a transcutaneous stitch using a straight needle. Alternatively, a laparoscopic subtotal hysterectomy may be performed if indicated.
- For placement of the posterior mesh, the Douglas pouch is opened and the posterior vaginal wall is freed as well as the pararectal levator muscles (Fig. 46.3). In order to avoid bleeding from hemorrhoidal vessels and possible denervation through excessive dissection of the rectum, stick to the laterodorsal side of the vaginal wall.
- A culdoplasty according to McCall is then performed (Fig. 46.4). The circumferential suture approximates both uterosacral ligaments, so reinforcing the Douglas pouch. This restores the normal anatomical relationship between the rectum and vagina.
- A right-angled retractor is placed on the anterior lip of the vagina in order to stretch the anterior vaginal wall. The bladder is filled with 100–200 mL of saline water in order to improve bladder definition.
- The peritoneal fold is opened and the vesicovaginal space is entered.
- The anterior vaginal wall is freed bluntly up to the urethrovesical junction, but not beyond in order not to disturb innervation of the bladder. This is manually controlled with a finger put inside the vagina.
- Small bleeders are coagulated with the bipolar forceps. The second mesh is put inside and fixed on the anterior vaginal wall with two running sutures of 2/0 Ethibond® (Fig. 46.5).
- When the uterus is still in place, the running sutures end at the level of the cervix.
- The end of the mesh is now put to the back of the uterus through a hole in the right broad uteral ligament. Alternatively, it can be cut into two strips that can be pulled through bilaterally.
- The promontofixation is then performed (Fig. 46.6). The already freed promontory is exposed.
- The Pro-Tack® is introduced through the medial suprapubic trocar. This tacking device utilizes a helical coil of 3.9 mm diameter to achieve secure fixation. The forceps grasps the posterior mesh, which is tightened over the promontory and fixed on the promontory with two tacks. Now the anterior mesh is grasped and pulled over the promontory.
- Several tacks are inserted through the mesh into the periosteum and the anterior longitudinal ligament. The excess mesh is cut away and removed.
- As an alternative to the tacker, both meshes can be fixed using a nonabsorbable suture.
- Finally, retroperitonealization is performed with a 2/0 Vicryl® running suture (Fig. 46.7).

Tips
- Watch out for the right ureter while doing the McCall culdoplasty.
- Dissection of the anterior vaginal wall should be up to the urethrovesical junction, but not beyond in order to avoid instability of the bladder.
- The depth of dissection or degree of tension can be controlled manually through a finger in the vagina.
- Meshes and needles are put intra-abdominally through the umbilical 10 mm port.

Postoperative care
Drink and food can be consumed on the first postoperative day. The catheter is removed on the second postoperative day.

Complications
Complications are rare.
- If there is bladder perforation, close with 2/0 Vicryl® and leave the bladder catheter in for 4 days.
- If there is vaginal perforation, close the lesion in two rows to secure a watertight repair and give broadspectrum antibiotics for 48 h.
- If there is bowel perforation, close the perforation with 3/0 Vicryl® and stop the procedure.

Results
There are excellent anatomical results (>95% have no recurrence). As to functional results, the stress incontinence rate depends on whether it is combined with a transvaginal urethral sling. If there is no sling, *de novo* stress incontinence is estimated to be 20%, and is easily solved by putting a transvaginal urethral sling in. Bladder instability improves or disappears in 60%.

To do
- If there is a problem with insufflation through the Veress needle or when intra-abdominal adhesions are expected, do not hesitate to use an open introduction using the Hasson technique.
- Retroperitonealization should be done with care to avoid postoperative bowel adhesions.
- Avoid manual contact with the vagina to avoid infection of the meshes. If contact is made (e.g. during a check of the depth of the vaginal dissection), change gloves.

Not to do
- Avoid excessive dissection of the rectum (denervation).
- Do not put too much tension on the meshes (perineal pain, *de novo* stress incontinence, etc.).

References

1 Deval B, Fauconnier A, Repiquet D *et al.* Surgical treatment of genitourinary prolapse by the abdominal approach. Apropos of a series of 232 cases. Ann Chir 1997;51(3):256–65.
2 Reddy K, Malik TG. Short-term and long-term follow-up of abdominal sacrocolpopexy for vaginal vault prolapse: initial experience in a district general hospital. J Obstet Gynaecol 2002;22(5):532–6.
3 von Theobald P. Laparoscopic promontofixation. J Chir (Paris) 2001;138(6):353–7.
4 Wattiez A, Canis M, Mage G, Pouly JL, Bruhat MA. Promontofixation for the treatment of prolapse. Urol Clin North Am 2001; 28(1):151–7.

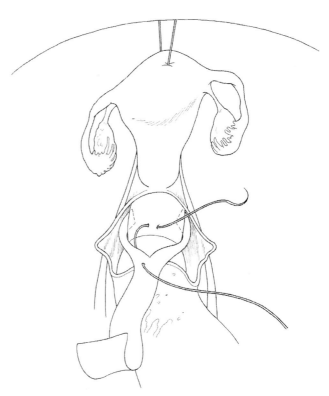

Figure 46.3 For the placement of the posterior mesh, the Douglas pouch is opened and the posterior vaginal wall is freed as well as the pararectal levator muscles.

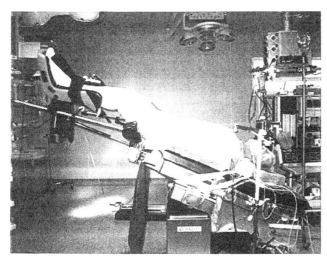

Figure 46.1 The patient's position.

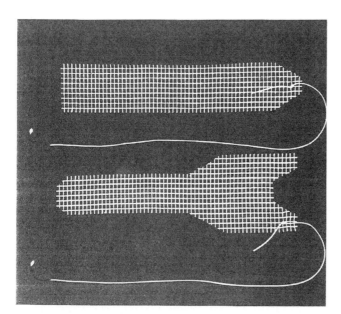

Figure 46.2 The prepared implants.

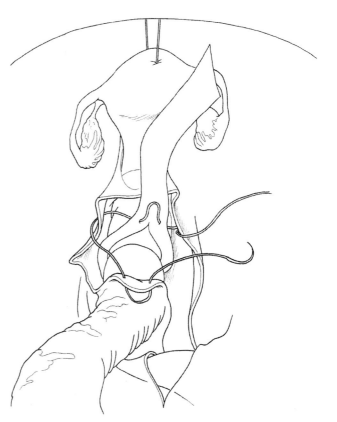

Figure 46.4 The McCall culdoplasty is performed.

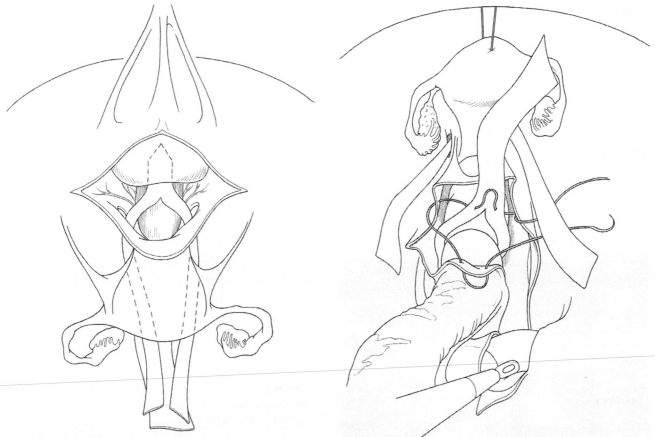

Figure 46.5 The second mesh is put inside and fixed on the anterior vaginal wall with two running sutures of 2/0 Ethibond®.

Figure 46.6 The promontofixation is then performed.

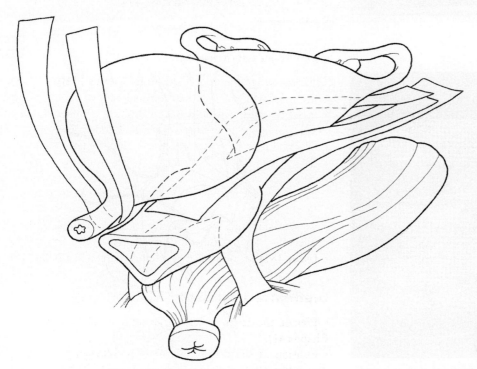

Figure 46.7 Retroperitonealization is performed with a 2/0 Vicryl® running suture.

Chapter 47
Diverticula of the Female Urethra: Urethral Reconstruction

J. Steffens, P. H. Langen, and R. Hohenfellner

Introduction

A rare, noncongenital disease, with 2% incidence between 30 and 70 years, may follow infection of the paraurethral glands in the distal infrasphincteric segment of the urethra. The size of the diverticulum varies between 1 and 10 cm; sometimes there is more than one diverticulum in the urethrovaginal septum.

Patient counseling and consent

The patient should be warned that suburethral swelling between the bladder neck and external meatus with urethral discharge (that can be obtained by massaging the anterior vaginal wall) may be combined with symptoms:
- Acute: fever, dysuria, reduced flow, or retention.
- Chronic: frequency, urgency, hematuria, dyspareunia, and dribbling of urine.

Indications

The procedure is indicated in patients with symptomatic diverticula. The reconstruction technique described can also be used for urethal defects of other origins and after the excision of foreign bodies, intraurethral tapes, sutures, and bulking agents (e.g. Teflon®).

Limitations and risks

Risks include fistulas, scars with stenosis (strictures), and the onset of stress incontinence.

Contraindications

General contraindications against surgery.

Preoperative management

- Transvaginal ultrasound.
- MRI (gadolinium).
- Dynamic cysturethrogram with postmicturition X-rays.
- Urethroscopy/diverticuloscopy with flexible instrument.

Anesthesia

Spinal, epidural, and general anesthesia.

Special instruments/suture material

- 12–14 Fr urethroscope.
- Instruments for vaginal surgery.
- Diathermic needle.
- Small retractors.
- For reconstruction, in addition: instruments for the fascial sling and instruments allowing the harvesting of peritoneum or oral mucosa.

Operative technique

Marsupialization (according to H. Spence [11])
- Perform a urethroscopy and diverticuloscopy.
- Incise the meatus towards the protruding vagina with the cystoscope inside the urethra or diverticulum.
- Dissect the caudal wall of the diverticulum (Fig. 47.1).
- Incise the vagina according to the position of the diverticulum.
- Perform an excision of the lateral walls of the diverticulum (Fig. 47.2).
- Suture the joining wall of the diverticulum and that of the vagina (4/0 PGA) creating a hypospadia (Fig. 47.3).
- Use an 18 Fr Foley catheter for a few days (Figs 47.4, 47.5).

Urethral reconstruction (Figs 47.6–47.14)

- Prepare the 15 cm fascial slings, with a pubic basis (see Chapter 41).
- Excision of the defect (Fig. 47.7) is followed by lateral

mobilization of the vaginal skin, dissecting it from the urethral tissue layer (Fig. 47.8).

- Close the urethral defect with 3/0Maxon® interrupted sutures (Fig. 47.9).
- If the results will be too narrow, prepare the oral mucosa for interposition (4/0 Monocryl® running suture) (Fig. 47.10).
- Cover the first suture with the Martius flap from the labia maiora (Fig. 47.11) and the free peritoneal tissue transplant (harvested while dissecting the fascial strips for the fascia sling procedure) (Fig. 47.12).
- Perform a pull-through maneuver of the fascial slings (Fig. 47.13).
- The suburethral joining of the sling is done using 3/0 Maxon® interrupted sutures. Start with the posterior suture row and use the provocation test in between sutures (Fig. 47.13).
- For the anterior row, use the same suture material.
- Close the colpotomy (Fig. 47.14).
- Perform a suprapubic cystotomy.

Tips

Use a lithotomy position, and fixation of the labia on both sides with sutures.

Postoperative care

Use sitzbaths after removal of the catheter, and uroflowmetry and a postmicturition residual volume test.

Complications

- Fistulas.
- Stenosis.
- Incontinence.

Troubleshooting

Fistulas often occur when surgery of a diverticulum and primary reconstruction are combined.

Remarks

- Use marsupialization first, and let the result heal completely.
- Micturition with artificial hypospadia does not pose a problem.

- Complicated reconstruction procedures are often due to an insufficient surgical technique for the cure of the diverticula with resulting large defects and incontinence.

To do

- Make sure there is a very thorough dissection between the vagina and urethra after a sufficiently wide excision of the scar.
- Covering the first row of sutures is an absolute must.
- A fascial sling is the incontinence procedure of choice.
- Use provocation to judge the amount of bladder neck elevation with 300 cm^3 of saline in the bladder.

References

1 Blavais GJ, Heritz DM. Vaginal flap reconstruction of the urethra and vesical neck in women: a report of 49 cases. J Urol 1996;155:1014–17.
2 Davis BL, Robinson DG. Diverticula of the female urethra: assay of 120 cases. J Urol 1970;104:850–4.
3 Davis HJ, Telinde RW. Urethral diverticula: an assay of 121 cases. J Urol 1958;80:34–9.
4 Ganabathi K, Leach GE, Zimmern PE et al. Experience with management of urethral diverticulum in 63 women. J Urol 1994;152:1445–52.
5 Hirsch HA, Käser O, Ikle FA. Fisteln der unteren Harnwege. Atlas der gynäkologischen Operationen 6. Auflage, Kapitel 20. Thieme, Stuttgart, 1999:588–93.
6 Khati NK, Javitt MC, Schwartz AM et al. MR imaging diagnosis of a urethral diverticulum. Radiographies 1998;18:517–20.
7 Leach GE. Urethrovaginal fistula repair with Martius labial fat pad graft. Urol Clin North Am 1991;18:409–13.
8 Leng WW, McGuire EJ. Management of female urethral diverticula: a new classification. J Urol 1998;160:1297–300.
9 Moore TD. Diverticulum of female urethra: an improved technique of surgical excision. J Urol 1952;68:611–15.
10 Romanzi LJ, Groutz A, Blavais JG. Urethral diverticulum in women: diverse presentations resulting in diagnostic delay and mismanagement. J Urol 2000;164:428–33.
11 Spence HM, Duckett JW. Diverticulum of the female urethra: clinical aspects and presentation of a simple operative technique for cure. J Urol 1970;104:432–6.
12 Witzsch U, Bürger RA, Fisch M, Hohenfellner R. Operationen zur weiblichen Inkontinenz: Kolposuspension nach Burch und Faszienzügelplastik. In: Ausgewählte Urologische OP-Techniken (Hohenfellner R, ed.). Georg Thieme Verlag, Stuttgart, 1997: 327–30.

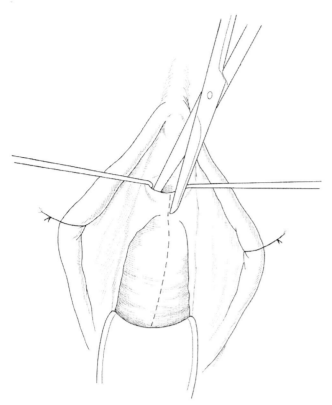

Figure 47.1 Dissection of the proximal urethra and cutting open of the diverticulum.

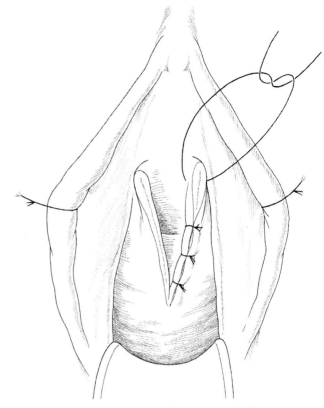

Figure 47.3 Interrupted sutures adapting the wall of the diverticulum to the vaginal wall.

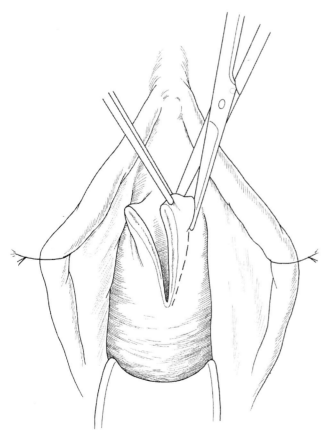

Figure 47.2 Excision of the walls of the diverticulum.

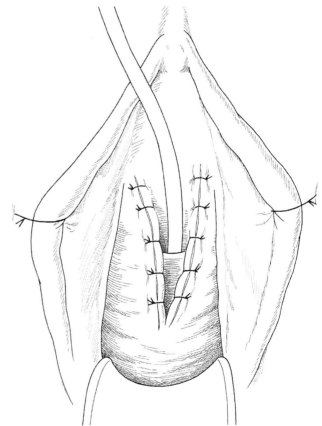

Figure 47.4 A 14 Fr Foley catheter in the urethra with a created 'hypospadia'.

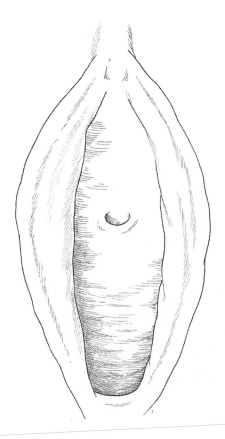

Figure 47.5 The situation after completion of the healing process (cf. Fig. 47.3).

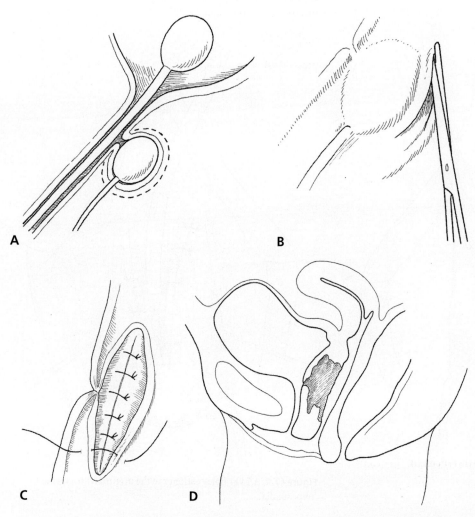

Figure 47.6 Development of urethral defects after surgery for diverticula (cf. Fig. 47.7): (A) preoperative; (B,C) intraoperative; and (D) postoperative.

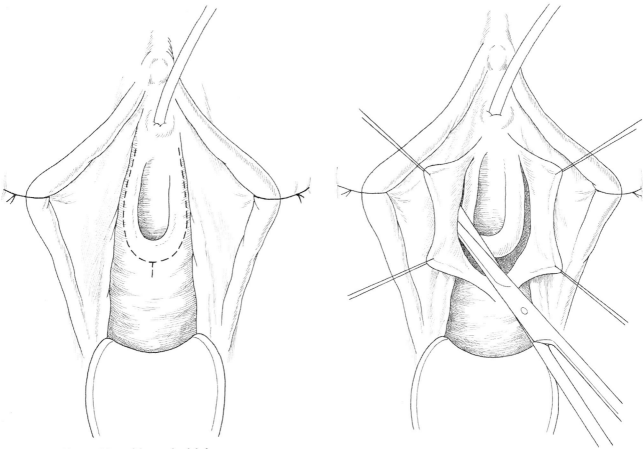

Figure 47.7 Circumcision of the urethral defect.

Figure 47.8 Mobilization laterally as far as possible.

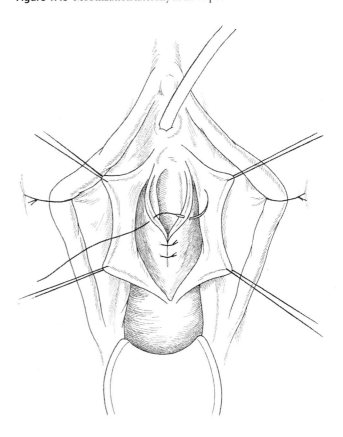

Figure 47.9 Closing of the urethral defect (sparing the mucosa) over an 18 Fr Foley catheter.

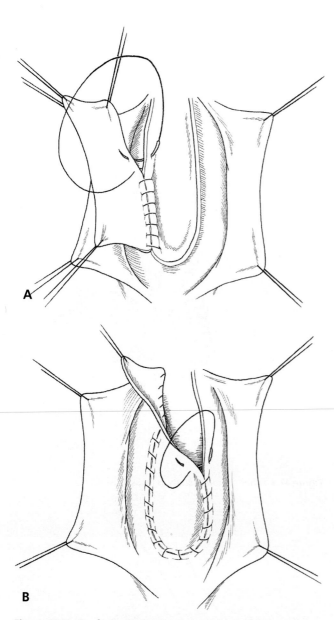

Figure 47.10 An alternative is to use interposition of the buccal mucosa.

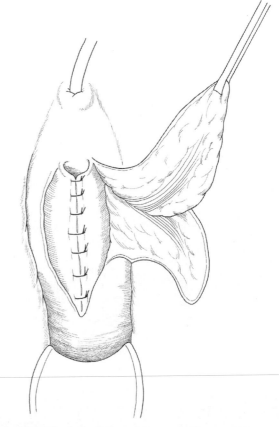

Figure 47.11 Cover the first row of sutures with a Martius flap.

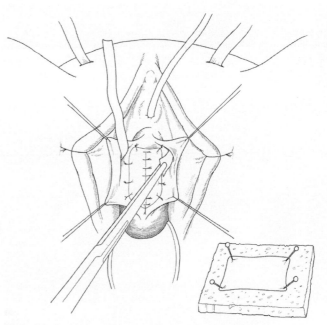

Figure 47.12 Alternatively, use a free peritoneal transplant harvested when dissecting the fascial slings: the pull-through maneuver of the fascial slings.

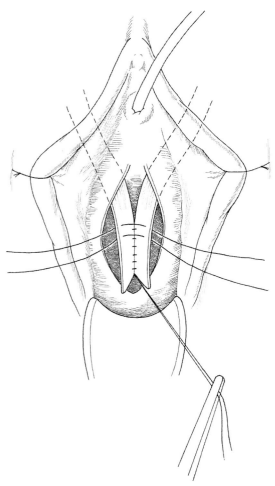

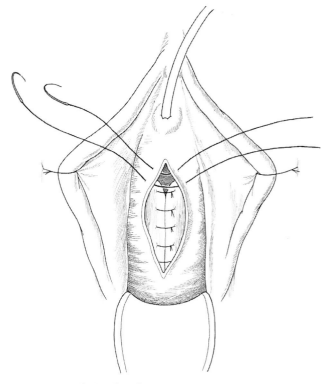

Figure 47.14 Closing the colpotomy.

Figure 47.13 Suture together the fascial slings of both sides starting with the backside. The provocation test uses $300\,\text{cm}^3$ saline inside the bladder.

Chapter 48
Vesicovaginal Fistulas: Vaginal Approach

R. Hohenfellner

Introduction

The vaginal approach is mainly used by gynecologists; it is less invasive and is used especially in the obese, elderly, and sexually inactive as the vagina becomes shorter postoperatively.

Patient counseling and consent

Estrogen treatment is given locally in preparation for the operation (4–6 weeks minimum) and should be continued postoperatively to counteract shortening by scar tissue contraction.

Indications

This procedure is indicated in small fistulas, postirradiation, and if the vagina is not too narrow.

Limitations and risks

There is a risk to the trigone and bladder neck as they are close to the site of surgery.

Preoperative management

• Check if the marked Trendelenburg lithotomy knee–chest position is possible because it is mandatory.
• Condom cystoscopy: to measure bladder capacity in irradiated patients.
• Are the ureter orifices close to the fistula?
• Methylene blue IV: used to exclude combined tangential ureterovesico-vaginal fistulas.
• If the orifices are borderline, insert 6 or 8 Fr splints or stents.

Anesthesia

General anesthesia.

Special instruments/suture material

• Standard vaginal set.
• Long fine instruments.
• Fine Zadinsky scissors.
• Cystostomy set.
• 8 and 20 Fr Foley catheters.
• Bipolar coagulation.
• Magnification lens system and headlight.
• Suture material: 4/0 and 5/0 Monocryl and Maxon, and PDS.

Operative technique

• Insert the 8 Fr Foley catheter in the fistula. Place four stay sutures (Fig. 48.1).
• Incise the fistula circumferentially (3–4 cm margin) and divide it into four segments using a fine long scalpel (Fig. 48.2).
• The anterior scarred vaginal epithelium is dissected carefully, segment by segment (the injection of NaCl is helpful), just as much as is necessary to find the cleavage plan (the septum vesicovaginale). There is further delicate separation for 1 cm.
• Pull on the Foley catheter and resect the everted mucosa of the fistula channel (0.2 cm) in order to 'freshen' the margin.
• Remove the Foley so the fistula channel will invert spontaneously.
• Modification is required for larger defects, or defects that occurred during preparation and under tension. A free buccal mucosa graft is taken from the lip, is thinned, and with the mucosa inside is sutured as a patch with 5/0 Monocryl around the fistula margin (see Chapter 47).
• Adapt the detrusor transversally 'broad surface to broad surface' with 4/0 PDS sutures. Carefully avoid placing stitches through the bladder mucosa (Figs 48.3, 48.4).
• Incise the labium (Fig. 48.5) and prepare a small, well-vascularized, medial pedicel, subcutaneous fatty tissue flap. An eyelid retractor is helpful!

• Turn the flap 180° inside to cover the suture line and fix the edges with 5/0 Monocryl (Fig. 48.6).
• The healthy tissue flap interposition is completed by partial colpocleisis with 4/0 PDS sutures (Fig. 48.7).
• The vagina is packed for 48 h.
• A cystostomy, in addition to the 20 Fr Foley, is placed for perfect bladder drainage.

Postoperative care

Give antibiotics until the catheter is removed. The patient is mobilized the next day. Remove the splints, if inserted, on day 8 to 10 and the Foley catheter on day 12 to 14. Remove the cystostomy when there is residual free voiding the next day. (Otherwise wait until the bladder can be emptied spontaneously and the residual urine is not more than 50 mL.)

Complications

• If the Foley cathther is blocked but the cystostomy is working, wait and see—do not irrigate!
• If there is flank pain, use ultrasound. If the pelvis is dilated insert a nephrostomy immediately.
• In irradiated cases the vaginal wound healing may be delayed.

Results

For small, even postirradiation fistulas, the success rate is up to 90%.

References

1 Birkhoff JD, Wechsler M, Romas NA. Urinary fistulas: vaginal repair using a labial fat pad. J Urol (Baltimore) 1977;117:595.
2 Carl P, Praetorius M. Der transvesikale Verschluss von Blasenscheidenfisteln. Geburtsh Frauenheilk 1974;34:699.
3 Döderlein D. Die 'Einroll-Plastik' zum Verschluss großer Blasendefekte am blinden Ende der Scheide. Zbl Gynäk 1955;77:93.
4 Eisen M, Jurkovic K, Altwein JE, Schreiter F, Hohenfellner R. Management of vesicovaginal fistulas with peritoneal flap interposition. J Urol (Baltimore) 1974;112:195.
5 Füth H. Zur Operation der Mastdarm-Scheidenfisteln. Zbl Gynäk 1930;54:2882.
6 Hartl H. Reconstruction of the urethra. In: Gynecological Urology (Youssef AF, ed.). C.C. Thomas, Springfield, IL, 1960.
7 Ingelman-Sundberg A. Pathogenesis and operative treatment of urinary fistulae in irradiated tissue. In: Gynecological Urology (Youssef AF, ed.). C.C. Thomas, Springfield, IL, 1960.
8 Keettel WC, Sehring FG, DeProsse CA, Scott JR. Surgical management of urethrovaginal and vesicovaginal fistulas. Am J Obstet Gynecol 1978;131:425.
9 Kiricuta J, Goldstein AMB. The repair of extensive vesicovaginal fistulas with pedicled omentum: a review of 27 cases. J Urol (Baltimore) 1972;108:724.
10 Latzko W. Behandlung hochsitzender Blasen- und Mastdarmscheidenfisteln nach Uterusexstirpation mit hohem Scheidenverschluß. Zbl Gynäk 1914;38:906.
11 Latzko W. Postoperative vesicovaginal fistulas. Am J Surg 1942;58:211.
12 Lawson JB. Vesical fistulae into the vaginal vault. Br J Urol 1972;44:623.
13 Lawson JB, Hudson CN. The management of vesicovaginal and urethral fistulae. In: Surgery of Female Incontinence (Stanton SL, Tanagho EA, eds). Springer Verlag, Berlin, 1986:193.
14 Lufuma. Considérations sur les facteurs de pronostic dans la cure de fistules vesico-vaginales obstétricales. Apropos de 64 cas. Act Urol Belg 1977;45:332.
15 Mahfouz N. Genitourinary fistulae. In: Gynecological Urology (Youssef AF, ed.). C.C. Thomas, Springfield, IL, 1960.
16 Malloy TR, Wein AJ, Carpinello VL. Transpubic urethroplasty for prostatomembranous urethral disruption. J Urol (Baltimore) 1980;124:359.
17 Martius H. Die gynäkologischen Operationen, 7. Thieme, Stuttgart, 1954.
18 Mattingly RF. TeLinde's Operative Gynecology, 5th edn. Lippincott, Philadelphia, 1977.
19 Mayer HGK, Pauli HK. Der Verschluss der Vesicovaginalfistel nach Latzko. Geburtsh Frauenheilk 1970;30:403.
20 O'Connor V, Jr, Sokol JK, Bulkley GJ, Nanninga JB. Suprapubic closure of vesicovaginal fistula. J Urol (Baltimore) 1973;109:51.
21 Osterhage HR. Therapie und Ergebnisse urologischer Komplikationen nach gynäkologischen Operationen. Geburtsh Frauenheilk 1977;37:857.
22 Parsons L. Urologic complications following gynecological surgery. In: Progress in Gynecology, Vol. V (Meigs JV, Sturgis H, eds). Grune & Stratton, New York, 1970.
23 Pechersdorfer M. Peritoneal-Fettlappen-Plastik zum Verschluss der Blasenscheidenfistel. Geburtsh Frauenheilk 1964;24:1079.
24 Pratt JH. Lesions of the female urethra. Clin Obstet Gynecol 1967;10:227.
25 Rader ES. Post-hysterectomy vesicovaginal fistula: treatment by partial colpocleisis. J Urol (Baltimore) 1975;114:389.
26 Russell CS. The management of vesicovaginal fistulae (excluding those resulting from radiation damage). J Int Fed Gynaecol Obstet 1970;8:1.
27 Stoeckel W. Gynäkologische Urologie. In: Handbuch der Gynäkologie (Veit J, Stoeckel W, eds). Thieme, Leipzig, 1938.
28 Symmonds RE. Loss of the urethral floor with total urinary incontinence. Am J Obstet Gynecol 1969;103:665.
29 Tanagho EA. Neourethra: rationale, surgical technique, and indications. In: Surgery of Female Incontinence (Stanton SL, Tanagho EA, eds). Springer Verlag, Berlin, 1980.
30 Thüroff JW, Hutschenreiter G, Frohneberg D, Hohenfellner R. Das freie Peritoneallappentransplantat in der Chirurgie des Nierenbeckens und Ureters. Akt Urol 1980;11:189.
31 Trotnow S. Früh- und Spätergebnisse bei der Behandlung von Blasen-Scheiden-Fisteln durch vaginale Operationsverfahren. Urologe A 1977;16:267.
32 Turner-Warwick R. The use of the omental pedicle graft in urinary tract reconstruction. J Urol (Baltimore) 1976;116:241.
33 Williams DL, Snyder H. Anterior detrusor tube repair for urinary incontinence in children. Br J Urol 1977;48:671.

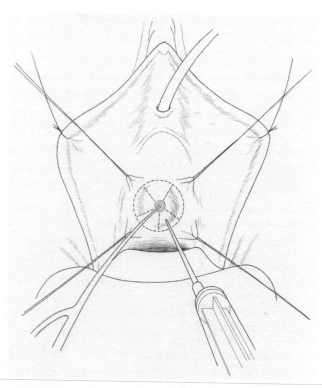

Figure 48.1 Insert an 8 Fr Foley catheter in the fistula and place four stay sutures.

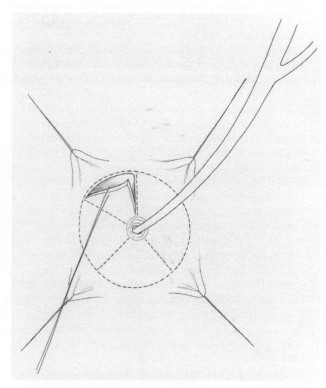

Figure 48.2 Incise the fistula 3–4 cm circumferentially and divide it into four segments using a fine long scalpel.

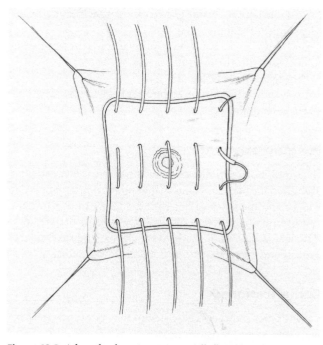

Figure 48.3 Adapt the detrusor transversally 'broad surface to broad surface' with 4/0 PDS sutures. Avoid placing stitches through the bladder mucosa.

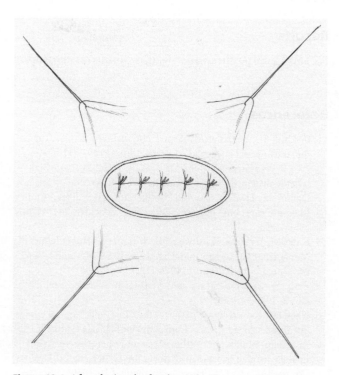

Figure 48.4 After closing the first layer, the tissue needed to cover these sutures has to be harvested.

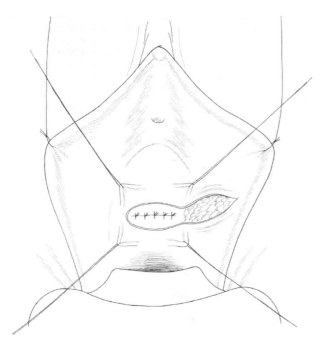

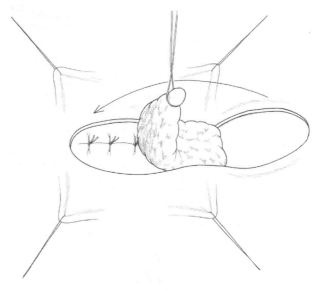

Figure 48.6 Turn the flap 180° inside to cover the suture line and fix the edges with 5/0 Monocryl.

Figure 48.5 The labium is incised and a small, well-vascularized, medial pedicel, subcutaneous fatty tissue flap is prepared.

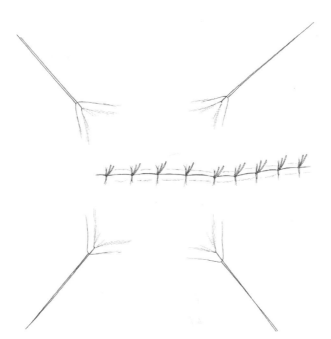

Figure 48.7 The healthy tissue flap interposition is completed by partial colpocleisis with 4/0 PDS sutures.

Chapter 49

Urinary Diversion in Complicated Cases: Conversion of a Colon Conduit to a Mainz Pouch II with Simultaneous Formation of a Neovagina

J. Leissner, G. D'Elia, M. Fisch, and R. Hohenfellner

Introduction

In patients with multiple malformations of the urinary tract and reproductive system, the first step of reconstructive surgery is often to create an incontinent urinary diversion. When the patient is growing, the question of quality of life arises and patients ask for continent urinary diversion and normal sexual activities. In these cases, reconstructive surgery is highly sophisticated and a challenge for each surgeon, especially after previous failed operations. The operative strategy has to be adapted individually to each patient.

Here we present a surgical strategy in a patient with congenital malformation of the genitourinary tract and status post incontinent urinary diversion and failed previous operative attempts.

There is a three-pronged strategy for this procedure:
• To construct a rectal reservoir with incorporation of the conduit.
• To build a neovagina out of the ileocecal region of the intestine.
• To treat any gynecological malformations.

Patient counseling and consent

Counseling should be given according to the individual situation and the needs of the patient. In the case report, the procedure was advised for the following problems: urogenital sinus, single kidney, multiple previous operations, colon conduit, and a rudimentary vagina that developed a hematometra during puberty with a need for surgical reintervention.

Indications

The procedure is needed for different reasons, such as complications or secondary development. In the case report, the patient wanted to get rid of her stoma so the colon conduit had to be converted into a sigma rectum pouch. The cecum there-fore had to be used to create a neovagina (good vascularization, good mobility) in order to create a tension-free anastomosis between the cecum and the vaginal vault (3 cm in this case).

Limitations and risks

These vary according to the individual situation to be treated.

Contraindications

These are according to the generally applicable rules for surgical treatment.

Preoperative management

Preoperative management is adapted to the planned procedure.

Anesthesia

General anesthesia.

Problems in presented case and strategy

• The patient's wish for continent urinary deviation.
• The patient's wish to be able to have intercourse.
• Multiple previous surgeries.
• The loss of the right kidney and a lesion of the left ureter with psoas hitch reconstruction as a child.
• Colon conduit with antirefluxing implantation of the left ureter because of persisting incontinence.
• Choice between one long or two shorter procedures, considering previous problems of adhesions after past surgeries.

Operative technique

• Perform a midline laparotomy.

• Dissect the adhesions.
• Mobilize the cecum up to the hepatic flexure of the colon and incise the mesentery (Fig. 49.1).
• Mobilize the rectum and sigmoid colon up to splenic flexure of the colon.
• The gynecologist should perform a hysterectomy and ovarectomy on the left side.
• Exclude 12 cm of cecum for the formation of the neovagina and end-to-end anastomosis of the terminal ileum and ascending colon (Fig. 49.2).
• Close the aboral end of the cecal segment using an interrupted seromuscular suture (Fig. 49.2).
• Perform an appendectomy in the appendicular region, incise the vaginal vault, and use end-to-end anastomosis with interrupted sutures (tension-free) after bringing down the cecum into the pelvis (Fig. 49.3).
• Explant the conduit from the skin and fascia, resect 2 cm (Fig. 49.4), and make a 3 cm antimesenterial incision (Fig. 49.5).
• V-shaped positioning of the sigma and antimesenterial incision over approximately 10 cm; with a continuous suture of the medial edges to form a 'pouch plate' that is sutured to the promontory with nonabsorbable sutures (Fig. 49.6).
• Perform an anastomosis of the lateral edges of the pouch with the opened-up conduit (Fig. 49.7).
• The pouch is retroperitonealized and the pelvis is sealed with omentum.

• Place the ureter splint, rectal tube, wound drainages, and vaginal glass-plug.
• Close the abdomen.

Postoperative care

Care is the same as for a Mainz pouch II procedure. The neovagina should be dilated frequently until the patient is regularly having intercourse.

Results

The case report patient is continent with a good life quality and good functioning of her remaining kidney.

References

1 Bürger RA, Stein R, Bauer H, Witzsch U, Hohenfellner R. Neovagina. In: Ausgewählte Urologische OP-Techniken (Hohenfellner R, ed.). Thieme, Stuttgart, 1997:5.87.
2 Fisch M, Hohenfellner R. Konversion: Inkorporation eines Kolon-Conduits in eine kontinente Harnableitung (Mainz Pouch I und II). In: Ausgewählte Urologische OP-Techniken (Hohenfellner R, ed.). Thieme, Stuttgart, 1997:6.135.
3 Leißner J, Stein R, Fisch M, Fichtner J, Bürger RA, Hohenellner R. Die Zäkumscheide. In: Plastisch-rekonstruktive Chirurgie in der Urologie (Schreiter F, ed.). Thieme, Stuttgart, 1999:403–7.

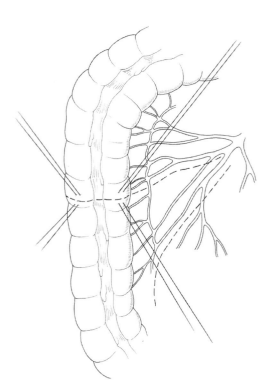

Figure 49.1 Mobilization of the cecum up to the hepatic flexure of the colon and incision of the mesentery.

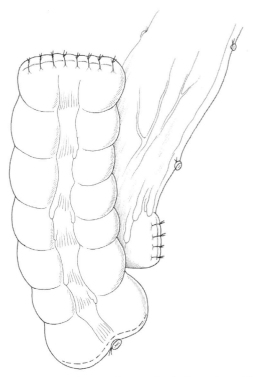

Figure 49.2 Exclusion of 12 cm of cecum for the formation of the neovagina and end-to-end anastomosis of the terminal ileum and ascending colon; closure of the aboral end of the cecal segment with an interrupted seromuscular suture.

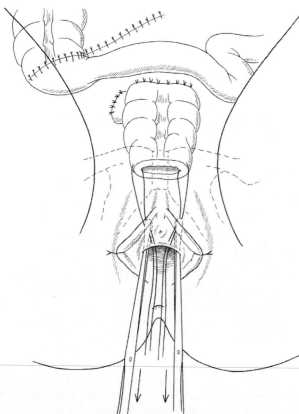

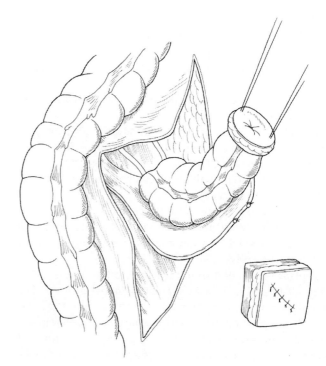

Figure 49.5 Make a 3 cm antimesenterial incision.

Figure 49.3 Typhlotomy in the appendicular region, incision of the vaginal vault, and end-to-end anastomosis with interrupted sutures (tension-free) after bringing down the cecum into the pelvis.

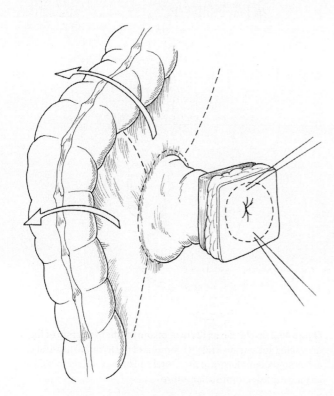

Figure 49.4 Explantation of the conduit from skin and fascia, with resection of 2 cm of the distal end of the conduit.

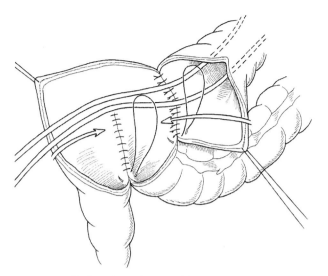

Figure 49.6 V-shaped positioning of the sigma and antimesenterial incision over approximately 10 cm, with a continuous suture of the medial edges to form a 'pouch-plate'.

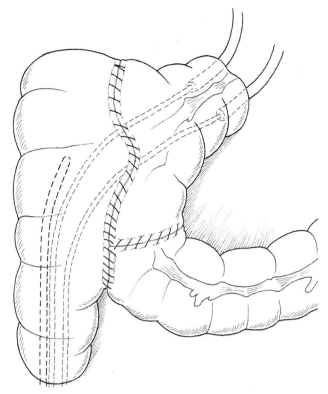

Figure 49.7. Anastomosis of the lateral edges of the pouch with the opened-up conduit.

Chapter 50
Surgical Management of the Congenital Adrenal Hyperplasia Syndrome

D. Filipas

Introduction

The androgenital syndrome, congenital adrenal hyperplasia (CAH), is the main cause for increased virilization of the external female genitalia. It is caused by a 21-hydroxylase defect of the adrenal gland leading to increased synthesis of androgens, which results in intrauterine (17–19 weeks of gestation) fusion of the urogenital sinus and clitoral hypertrophy.

Indications

The type of reconstruction required depends on the anatomical location of the vaginal entrance into the common urogenital sinus. The classification is performed according to Prader—with grade II to IV requiring surgical correction. The surgical procedure is divided into three steps according to the grade of malformation: clitoral recession, flap vaginoplasty (YV-plasty), and labioplasty. These procedures can be applied for all grade of sinus confluence; however it should be understood that they do not change the confluence, but open the sinus. The differentiation between salt-waster's and nonsalt-waster's CAH has a very important impact on perioperative management.

Preoperative management

- Urinalysis, complete blood count, and serum creatinine.
- Preoperative imaging: ultrasound of the abdomen.
- Genitography can be performed preoperatively or directly before the procedure. It gives exact information about the sinus confluence and determines the Prader grade.
- Salt-wasters need perioperative hydrocortisone substitution, which should be monitored by the pediatric endocrinologist.
- Age of surgery: between 6 and 12 months of age.

Anesthesia

General anesthesia; invasive intraoperative monitoring of the serum electrolytes is required in patients with salt-waster's CAH.

Special instruments/suture material

- Magnification glasses.
- Scott retractor (optional).
- Suture material: 6/0 and 5/0 Monocryl, 2/0, 3/0, and 4/0 Vicryl, and nonresorbable stay sutures (4/0 or 5/0 Prolene).
- Standard instruments for hypospadia surgery.
- Vessel loops.
- 6–12 Fr bladder catheter.

Operative technique

- Place the patient in a supine position.
- Place a stay suture at the clitoris.
- Place a bladder catheter.
- Mark the incision lines: the lines are drawn circumferentially around the corona dorsally and then ventrally (Fig. 50.1). Ventrally, the lines preserve the urethral plate and extend around the sinus meatus. A U-shaped perineal flap is marked extending from each ischial tuberosity with the apex near the meatus. A Y-incision is outlined at the base of each labia majora.
- The clitoris is degloved above Buck's fascia leaving the urethral plate attached to the glans.
- The entire clitoris is exposed.
- The erectile bodies, the neurovascular bundle, and the glans, with the attached urethral plate, are separated (Figs 50.2, 50.3).
- There is complete preparation of the erectile bodies to their bifurcation. Erectile tissue directly at the pubic bone is excised, with care not to injure the neurovascular bundle. The distal end of the erectile tissue is separated from the glans and sutured with 4/0 Vicryl.
- If necessary, tailoring of the glans is performed with ventral and/or medial incision and resection of a triangular tissue portion to preserve sensation.

- The glans is than sewn directly to the pubic bone between the stumps of the corporal bodies (Fig. 50.4).
- The phallic skin is divided in the midline to create the labia minora. The phallic skin should not been divided completely as this allows a more natural clitoral hood.
- The perineal flap for vaginoplasty is incised and mobilized with the underlying fatty tissue.
- The urogenital sinus is opened ventrally in the midline up into the vagina (Fig. 50.5). The incision must be extended until a normal vaginal caliber is reached to prevent stenosis. Once accomplished, 4/0 or 5/0 Vicryl sutures are placed from the flap to the vagina (Fig. 50.6). Intravaginally, 6/0 Monocryl sutures are used.
- Labial reconstruction is performed by the divided phallic skin placed lateral to the vaginal entrance.
- The labia majora are mobilized and placed inferiorly as a YV-plasty to their new location, lateral to the new vaginal introitus (Figs 50.7, 50.8).
- No drain is placed.
- Compression dressings and vaginal tamponade are used.

Postoperative care

- The bladder catheter is removed on the fifth to seventh postoperative day.
- The compression dressing is removed after 48 h.
- The vaginal tamponade is removed after 48 h.
- From the day of catheter removal, sit baths should be taken twice per day.
- Serum electrolyte monitoring is necessary in salt-wasters.

Complications

Hematoma can mainly be managed conservatively, but there may be impairment of clitoral sensation.

Troubleshooting

- *Clitoroplasty*: a primary cosmetic problem is the prominence of the glans clitoris. Tailoring of the glans is performed with ventral and/or medial incision and resection of a triangular tissue portion to preserve sensation. It is also important to completely resect the erectile tissue to the bifurcation and pubic bone, so that the glans clitoris can be sewn directly to the bone.
- *Vaginoplasty*: this involves a deep ventral incision of the urogenital sinus up into the vagina until a normal vaginal caliber is reached. The perineal flap needed for the vaginoplasty is incised and mobilized with the underlying fatty tissue. Both steps prevent vaginal stenosis. However, the majority of children need an introital YV-plasty at puberty for satisfactory coitus.
- Dilatation of the vagina is not recommended.

References

1 Alizai NK, Thomas DFM, Liliford RJ *et al.* Feminizing genitoplasty for congenital adrenal hyperplasia: what happens at puberty. J Urol 1999;161:1588–91.
2 Rink R, Yerkes E. Surgical managment of female genital abnormalities. In: Pediatric Urology (Gerhardt J, Rink R, Mouriquand P, eds). W.B. Saunders, Philadelphia, 2001:659–85.

Figure 50.1 Prader grade III–IV androgenital syndrome. The incision line is marked ventrally to preserve the urethral plate, and in a V-form for vaginoplasty. A stay suture is placed at the glans clitoris.

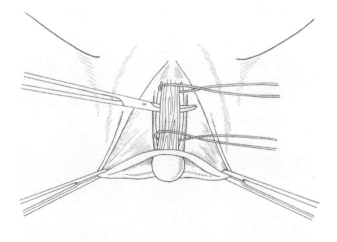

Figure 50.2 The neurovascular bundle is completely separated.

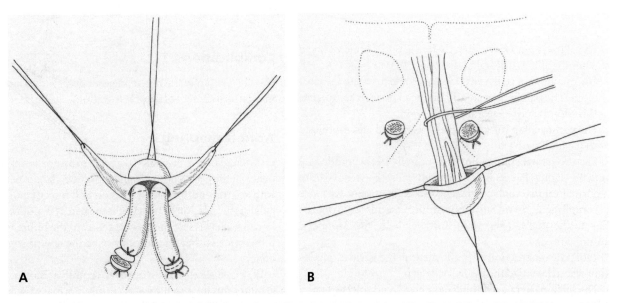

Figure 50.3 (A) Complete preparation of the erectile bodies to their bifurcation. Separation from the clitorial glans with care of the neurovascular bundle. (B) Excision of the erectile bodies directly to the pubic bone and sutured with 4/0 Vicryl.

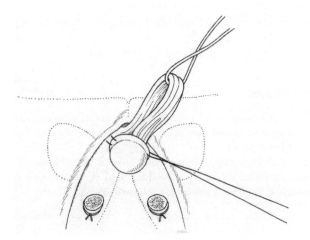

Figure 50.4 Fixation of the clitoral glans to the pubic bone.

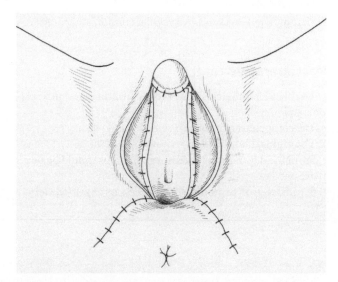

Figure 50.6 The perineal flap is adapted to the entrance of the vagina.

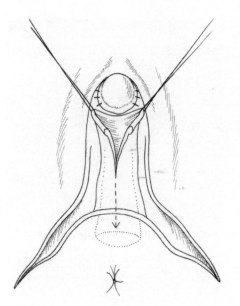

Figure 50.5 The urogenital sinus is opened in the midline up into the vagina.

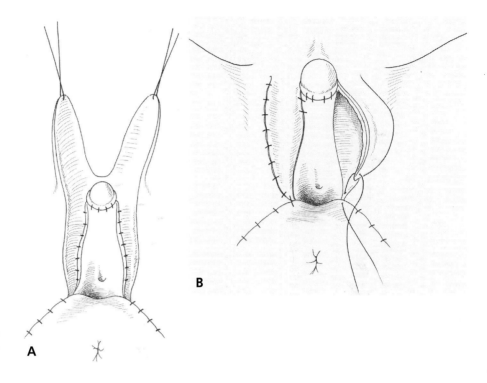

Figure 50.7 (A) The phallic skin is divided in the midline to create the labia minora. (B) Single sutures adapt the previously divided phallic skin laterally to the preserved urethra plate, resulting in reconstruction of the labia minora.

A

B

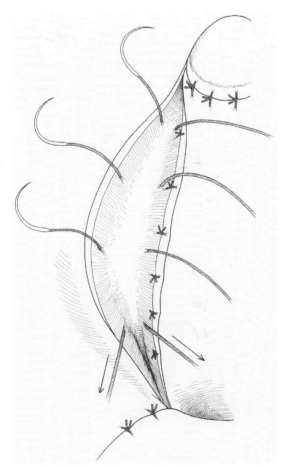

Figure 50.8 The labioplasty is completed with subcutaneous sutures.

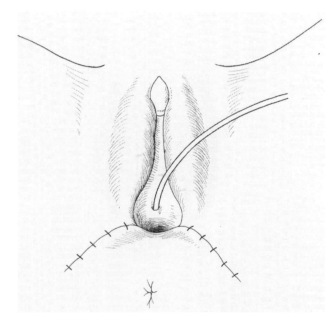

Figure 50.9 The final situation.

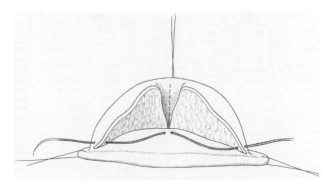

Figure 50.10 Tailoring of the enlarged glans.

Section 7
Radical Pelvic Surgery

Chapter 51
Laterally Extended Endopelvic Resection

M. Höckel and R. Hohenfellner

Introduction

Malignant lower gynecological tract tumors involving the pelvic wall are generally considered to be inoperable. The diagnosis of pelvic side wall involvement is suspected if the tumor mass is fixed to the pelvic wall at palpation. Frequently, one or more symptoms from the 'triad of troubles' are present: hydronephrosis, leg swelling, and pain in the lower back, pelvis, or leg. The diagnosis is confirmed by histopathologic demonstration of neoplastic tissue at the pelvic wall.

For a more accurate description of the location of the tumor at the anatomically complex pelvic side wall a two-dimensional, topographic anatomical classification is proposed, based on its relation to the external/common iliac vessel axis and on the projection (not infiltration) of the tumor on the pelvic girdle. Location of pelvic side wall disease can thus be *peri-iliac* or *infrailiac* in one dimension and *ischiopubic, acetabular,* or *iliosacrococcygeal* in the other dimension.

Peri-iliac tumors can eventually be resected *en bloc* with parts of the related vessels, nerves, and pelvic wall muscles. However, the neurovascular structures vital for leg function (common and external iliac arteries, lumbosacral plexus) should be spared.

Infrailiac pelvic side wall disease (except tumors located at the sciatic foramen) can be treated with the laterally extended endopelvic resection (LEER) procedure. Since the tumors usually do not penetrate the parietal endopelvic fascia, the inclusion of the adjacent striated pelvic wall muscles (obturator internus, pubococcygeus, iliococcygeus, coccygeus), along with the complete urogenital mesentery and internal iliac vessel system, into the pelvic exenteration specimen provides the clear resection margins (R0) necessary for local tumor control. Both abdominal and abdominoperineal exenteration as well as total, anterior, and posterior exenteration can be laterally extended.

Patient counseling and consent

The patient should be counseled about the minimum and maximum extent of resection and reconstructive options.

Indications

Patients with primary and recurrent lower gynecological tract tumors fixed at the pelvic wall below the iliac vessel axis are candidates for treatment with LEER if the following four criteria are met:

- An R0 resection of the tumor is achievable.
- Local tumor control can lead to cure or at least to prolongation of life.
- The patient's general performance status is compatible with the megaoperation and its consequences.
- No or no equally effective alternative treatment is available.

Contraindications

- Tumor location at the sciatic foramen.
- Distant metastases; peritoneal disease; multifocal disease; recurrent tumor > 5 cm in its largest diameter; tumor persistence (or recurrence within 6 months) after completed radiotherapy; or previous intralesional resection.
- Older age (>70 years); significant comorbidity; mental illness; or a patient refusing colostomy.
- Patients with a more than 50% chance of being cured by (chemo)radiation.

Preoperative management

- Mechanical bowel preparation.
- Skin marking of proper stoma sites and eventually landmarks for flap design.
- Broad-spectrum antibiotic combination therapy.

Anesthesia

General anesthesia, invasive monitoring, and postoperative peridural anesthesia.

Special instruments/suture material

- Standard instruments for abdominal and vaginal radical pelvic surgery.
- Bookwalter® retractor (Codman).
- Monopolar and bipolar cautery.
- Ligasure® (Tyco).
- Aortic clamp, vessel tourniquets, and hemoclips (small, medium, and large).
- Cobb periosteal dissectors (small, medium, and large).

Operative technique

- Surgical access is gained through a hypogastric and epigastric midline laparotomy circumventing the umbilicus. For low recurrences, additional perineal incisions at the vaginal introitus (possibly including the anus) are necessary.
- All peritoneal adhesions are lysed and the abdominal and pelvic intraperitoneal compartments are systematically explored by inspection and palpation. Biopsies are taken from all suspicious intraperitoneal sites.
- If intraperitoneal tumor dissemination can be excluded, the retroperitoneal pelvic and midabdominal compartments are opened. On both sides the paracolic and pelvic parietal peritoneum is incised along the psoas muscles and the round ligaments are separated. The peritoneum at the base of the small bowel mesentery is dissected and the duodenum is mobilized against the vena cava and aorta. The small bowel and the right and transverse colon are packed into a bowel bag. The anterior visceral peritoneum of the bladder is incised and the space of Retzius is developed. Both paravesical and pararectal spaces and the presacral space are created. Depending on the location of the recurrent tumor, these spaces may only be partially developed. Intralesional dissection should be strictly avoided. Both ureters are liberated.
- Selective periaortic and pelvic lymph node dissection is performed as dictated by the extent of earlier operations and the intraoperative findings.
- If lymphatic tumor dissemination cannot be demonstrated in frozen sections, LEER is started. A tourniquet is placed around the vena cava inferior at the level of the origin of the inferior mesenteric artery. The aorta abdominalis is mobilized so that it can be easily undermined by a large vessel clamp.
- The infundibulopelvic ligaments are divided and the ureters are cut as low as possible in the pelvis. Biopsies of the distal ureters are examined as frozen sections. Stents are inserted into the ureters.
- The mesosigmoid is skeletized and the blood vessels are ligated at the rectosigmoidal transition. The bowel continuity is interrupted at this site using a gastrointestinal stapler. The sigmoid colon is included in the bowel bag.
- At the tumor-free pelvic wall, the urogenital mesentery containing the visceral branches of the internal iliac vessels, the pelvic autonomic nerve plexus, and the subperitoneal dense connective tissue is completely divided.
- At the tumor-involved side wall the internal iliac artery is ligated and divided where it branches off from the common iliac artery. Thereafter all parietal branches of the iliac vessel system are transected between hemoclips or clamps: the ascending lumbar vein, superior gluteal artery and vein, inferior gluteal artery and vein, and internal pudendal artery and vein. The internal iliac vein can now be divided at its bifurcation as well. The lumbosacral plexus and the piriform muscle are exposed by this maneuver.
- The internal obturator muscle is ventrally incised at the site of the obturator nerve, which is either elevated or divided if it is incorporated in the tumor. The muscle is separated from the acetabulum and the obturator membrane by use of a Cobb periosteal dissector. Below the ischial spine the obturator muscle, which leaves the endopelvis at this point, is divided again, with ligation of the muscle stump. The separated endopelvic part of the obturator muscle in continuity with the attached iliococcygeus and pubococcygeus muscles is retracted medially, exposing the ischiorectal fossa.
- A superficial incision is made caudal to the lumbosacral plexus between the ischial spine and the fourth sacral body, and the coccygeus muscle is elevated from the sacrospinous ligament with a Cobb periosteal dissector.
- At the level of the ischioanal fossa, the lateral vaginal wall is identified and incised. The anterior vaginal wall and urethra are transected. The anal canal is mobilized from the posterior vaginal wall, which is divided after clamping as well. The anorectal transition is separated with an articulated stapling instrument. Now the complete specimen of the laterally extended total exenteration consisting of the urethra, bladder, vagina (uterus and adnexa), and rectum at the tumor side *en bloc* with the complete endopelvic urogenital mesentery, the coccygeus, iliococcygeus, pubococcygeus, and internal obturator muscles, can be removed and examined with multiple frozen sections for tumor margins.
- If necessary the caudal dissection can be shifted further downward to include the vaginal introitus, urethral meatus, and anus—necessitating secondary access from the perineum.
- To improve wound healing, especially in the irradiated pelvis, an omentum majus flap nourished by one gastroepiploic artery is elevated, transposed to the pelvis along the paracolic gutter, and is fixed to the pelvic surface.
- For supravesical urinary diversion either a conduit or a continent pouch is constructed from (nonirradiated) colon segments (see Chapters 54, 57, 59).
- Fecal diversion is accomplished by an end sigmoidostomy if the pelvis has been irradiated.

- The inclusion of the anus and anal canal into the laterally extended pelvic exenteration necessitates the reconstruction of the perineum and pelvic floor. This can be accomplished by the use of a gluteal thigh or a gracilis musculocutaneous flap.
- The laparotomy is closed with a continuous Smead–Jones suture of the musculofascial layers and skin staples.

Postoperative care

- In cases of uneventful course: intensive care for 24 h, total parenteral nutrition for 5 days, and intermediate care (monitoring) and peridural analgesia for 1 week.
- For postoperative management of supravesical urinary diversion, see Chapters 54, 57, 59, 61–63.
- Postoperative pelvic MRI during the third postoperative week.
- Postoperative hospital stay for 4 weeks.

Complications

The most significant complications are intraoperative hemorrhage during dissection of the internal iliac venous system and radiation-related impair of wound healing, which may result in vaginal or rectal stump and laparotomy dehiscence.

In cases of severe intraoperative hemorrhage, the abdominal aorta should be clamped immediately below the origin of the inferior mesenteric artery and the prelaid tourniquet around the vena cava inferior should be closed.

Generally, we do not use irradiated tissue for any reconstructive purpose. Likewise, we avoid anastomoses between two irradiated tissues. Complete covering of the deep endopelvic surface, as well as the vaginal and rectal stump, with an omental flap for therapeutic angiogenesis is essential. The risk of rectal stump dehiscence can be reduced by the creation of a small rectovaginal fistula at the end of the operation. Postoperational pelvic abscesses must be drained and cautiously irrigated.

Results

- 42 patients with recurrent ($n=35$) or primary advanced ($n=7$) gynecological malignancies involving the side wall of the lesser pelvis have undergone LEER since 1996. The majority of the patients suffered from cervical carcinoma ($n=33$) and had received previous pelvic irradiation ($n=30$).
- Tumor-free (R0) lateral margins were obtained in 40 patients.
- Mean operation time was 14 ± 3 h.
- Severe postoperative complications occurred in 16 patients with one treatment-related death.
- Five-year survival probability is 49% for the whole group and 46% for those patients considered only for palliation with current treatment options.
- Most patients without evidence of disease at least 1 year after LEER achieved good quality of life.

References

1 Höckel M. Pelvic recurrences of cervical cancer: relapse pattern, prognostic factors, and the role of extended radical treatment. J Pelvic Surg 1999;5:255–66.
2 Höckel M. Laterally extended endopelvic resection: surgical treatment of infrailiac pelvic wall recurrences of gynecologic malignancies. Am J Obstet Gynecol 1999;180:306–12.
3 Höckel M. Laterally extended endopelvic resection: novel surgical treatment of locally recurrent cervical carcinoma involving the pelvic side wall. Gynecol Oncol 2003;91:369–77.
4 Höckel M, Baußmann E, Mitze M, Knapstein PG. Are pelvic side wall recurrences of cervical cancer biologically different from central relapses? Cancer 1994;74:648–55.

Acknowledgments

The development of LEER has been supported by a grant from Else-Kröner-Fresenius Foundation, Bad Homburg, Germany.

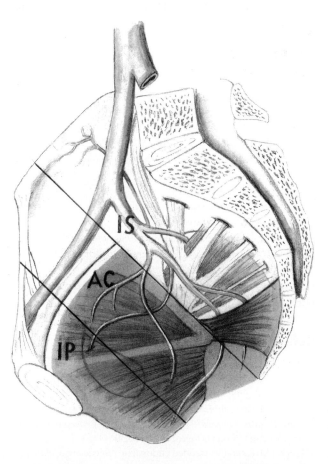

Figure 51.1 The right female pelvic side wall. The shaded zone indicates the location of pelvic side wall tumors that can be treated with LEER. The venous vessels and levator ani muscle have been omitted for clarity. AC, acetabular (middle) part; IP, ischiopubic (anterior) part; IS, iliosacral (posterior) part of the pelvic side wall.

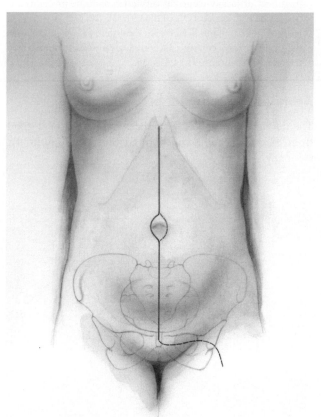

Figure 51.2 In most cases LEER is performed through a hypo- and epigastric midline laparotomy. In very obese patients a modified abdominoinguinal incision can be advantageous.

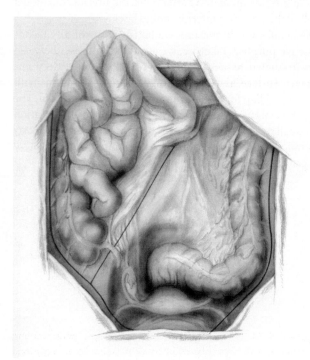

Figure 51.3 Access to the abdominopelvic retroperitoneum.

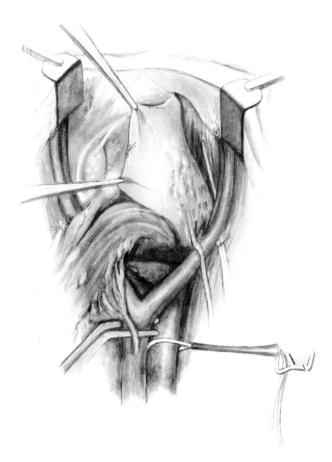

Figure 51.4 After periaortic lymph node dissection, the vena cava inferior and aorta abdominalis are mobilized. Placement of a tourniquet around the vena cava inferior and of a large vessel clamp on the aorta abdominalis at the level below the origin of the inferior mesenteric artery should be made to prepare for temporary large vessel occlusion during later steps of the operation.

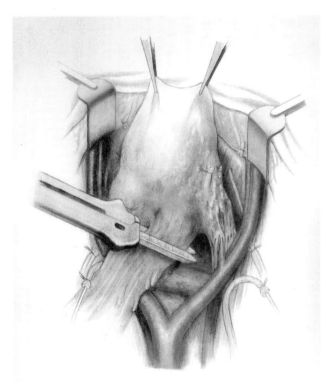

Figure 51.5 After the retroperitoneum is entered, the pararectal and paravesical spaces are completely developed at the tumor-free pelvic side wall (right). These spaces can only be developed in part on the side of the recurrent disease (left). Following selective pelvic lymph node dissection both ureters are transected as deep in the pelvis as possible and are stented. The bowel continuity is interrupted at the rectosigmoid transition.

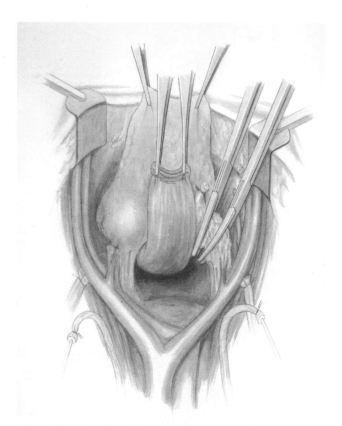

Figure 51.6 Dissection of the tumor-free urogenital mesentery.

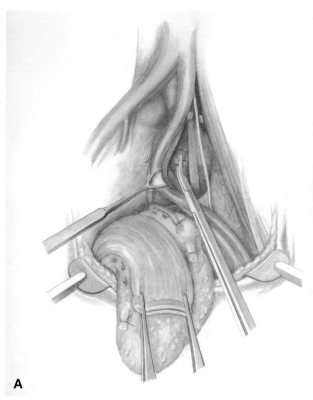

A

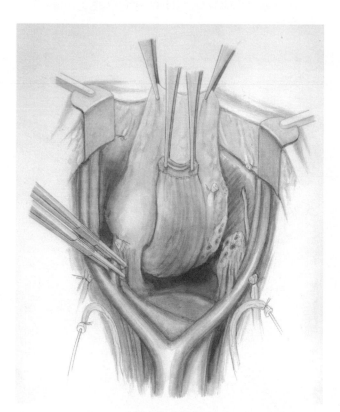

Figure 51.7 Ligation and transection of the internal iliac artery.

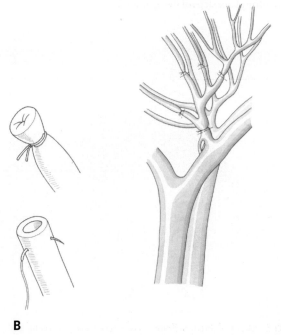

B

Figure 51.8 (A) Transection of the parietal branches of the internal iliac artery and vein after retracting the common/external iliac vessels medially. (B) Depending on the course and diameter of the vessels, hemoclips or stitch-through sutures are administered.

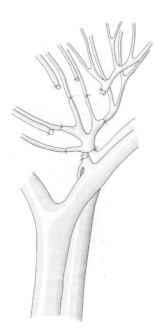

Figure 51.9 After transection of the parietal branches, the internal iliac vein can be ligated and transected to be included into the LEER specimen.

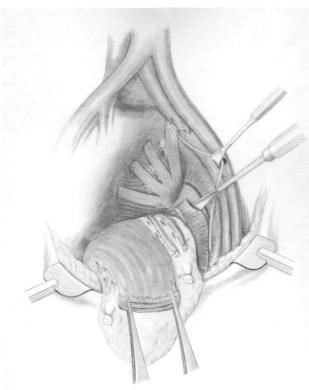

Figure 51.11 Separation of the obturator internus muscle from the acetabulum and obturator membrane with a Cobb periosteal dissector.

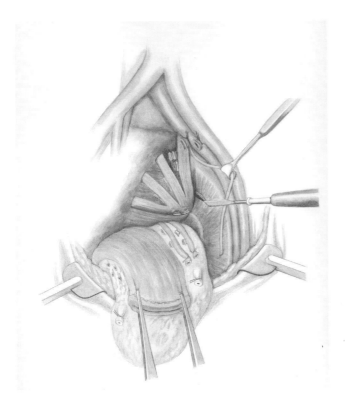

Figure 51.10 Ventral incision of the obturator internus muscle at the site of the obturator nerve, which is retracted.

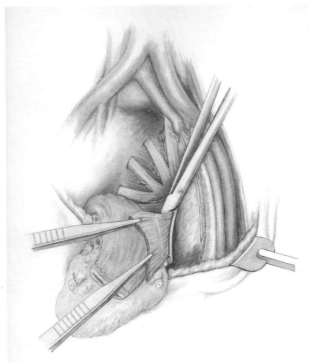

Figure 51.12 The obturator internus muscle is cut after its remaining part has been clamped at the lesser sciatic foramen.

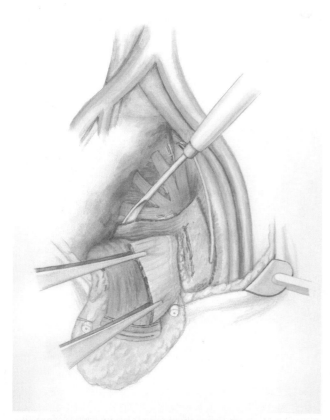

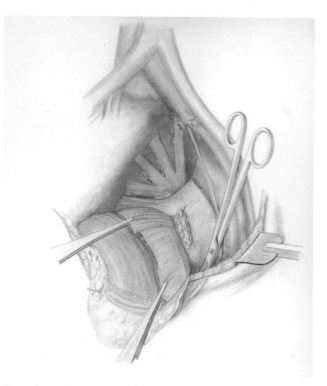

Figure 51.14 Transsection of the proximal urethra, distal vagina, and distal rectum.

Figure 51.13 Elevation of the coccygeus muscle from the sacrospinous ligament with a Cobb periosteal dissector.

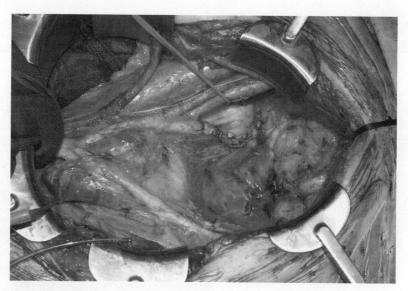

Figure 51.15 The final situation.

Section 8
Urinary Diversion

Chapter 52
Uretero-Ureterocutaneostomy (Wrapped by Omentum)

A. Pycha and M. Lodde

Introduction

Described first in 1967 by A. Roth and modified in 1990, cutaneous ureterostomy by wrapping the ureters with the greater omentum turned out to be quick and easy to learn, demonstrate, and teach.

Patient counseling and consent

The patient has to understand that there is a risk of stoma stenosis followed by hydronephrosis and ore pyelonephritis, with the need for permanent mono-J intubation. The latter would need to be changed every 3–6 months, and stoma correction would also eventually be necessary.

Indications

This is an alternative procedure for permanent incontinent urinary diversion by small or large bowel conduits. It is useful in high-risk patients to shorten the operation time, as well as having low morbidity and mortality.

Limitations and risks

For patients with short ureters following external beam irradiation, change the procedure and perform a transverse conduit (see Chapter 59).

Preoperative management

The bowel should be prepared in case the concept has to be changed and a conduit has to be performed.

Anesthesia

General and epidural anesthesia.

Special instruments

- Fine instruments for ureter preparation.
- Magnification lens system.
- Bipolar coagulation set.
- 5/0 and 6/0 Monocryl suture material.
- 6 or 8 Fr mono-J ureter stents.

Operative technique

- The landmarks include the xyphoid, 12th rib, umbilicus, superior anterior iliac spine, and symphysis.
- Mark the stoma sites between the umbilicus and xyphoid; preferrably on the left pararectal side.
- Carefully prepare bilaterally the ureters, while preserving the arteria testicularis.
- Cross over the right ureter to the left side below the Treitz ligament and above the inferior mesenteric artery, and through a wide vessel-free window of the mesentery behind the colon descendens.
- For the stoma, circular skin excisions are needed according to the ureter diameters but not less then 1.5 cm.
- Excise the fatty subcutaneous tissue to be substituted later on with greater omentum.
- Perform a cross-like incision of the anterior rectus sheet, then blunt separation of the rectus muscle, and a cross-like incision of the dorsal rectus sheet and the peritoneum on the tip of the underlying finger.
- Pull through both ureters at least 1.5 cm above skin level.
- Observe arterial capillary bleeding from both ureter stumps and spontaneous urine ejaculation.
- Split both ureters medially at 3 and 9 o'clock for 1.5 cm.
- Place one 6/0 suture to connect both ureters medially and get a 'fish mouth' stoma.
- Wrap the thinnest part of the far end of the mobilized greater omentum around both ureters like a sheet (without strangulation), and place and fix it subcutaneously.
- Check again the arterial capillary bleeding and spontaneous urine ejaculation.

- Skin stoma: fix the 'fish mouth' ureter with four interrupted 6/0 Monocryl sutures to the epidermis.
- Insert two 6 or 8 Fr mono-J catheters and fix them to the skin. Put a stoma bag in place.

Tips

If the right ureter is short, take the left one to the right side and perform a stoma on the right side.

Postoperative care

Remove the mono-J catheters on day 21 and observe the spontaneous urine ejaculation.

Complications

Reinsert the mono-J catheters in cases of flank symptoms, fever, marked upper tract dilatation found on ultrasound, or an increase of serum creatinine. Ignore mild asymptomatic dilatation.

Troubleshooting

In cases of stoma stenosis, excise the scar tissue surrounding the ureter orifices and substitute it with a buccal mucosa graft taken from the inner surface of the lip. (Free tissue transfer of the buccal mucosa has turned out to be helpful in stoma correction.) See also Chapters 61 and 62.

Remarks

Early postoperative complications following radical pelvic surgery are related closely to the type of urinary diversion. Delayed small bowel function and paralytic ileus was observed in up to 6% of more than 300 small bowel end-to-end anastomoses; this was later accentuated by secondary pulmonary insufficiency, especially in heavy smokers with pulmonary emphysema.

Ureterocutaneostomy, wrapped by the greater omentum, carried out in nonirradiated patients with well-vascularized ureter stumps, turned out to be a well-tolerated alternative procedure for incontinent urinary diversion in high-risk patients. If radical cystectomy has to be carried out (quite often too late) in elderly symptomatic patients with non-organ-confined bladder tumors, ureterocutaneostomy may become the method of choice in the future.

The risks of stoma stenosis may be reduced by the use of the greater omentum wrapped around the ureter and placed between the fascia and the skin [1,5]. In cases of stoma obstruction, mono-J catheters can be reinserted and changed every 6 months without encrustation. Stoma correction can be performed later on using a buccal mucosa graft.

In conclusion, a renaissance of the almost outdated ureterocutaneostomy procedure [6] can be expected in the third millennium as the promise of the ileal conduit procedure has been reduced by the high number of early and late complications [2]. Technical details like the use of the greater omentum may be important, especially in obese patients.

To do

- Check the ureter length following the pull-through maneuver of the ureters.
- Change your approach immediately and perform a colon conduit if the ureter is too short for a tension-free stoma.
- Check arterial capillary bleeding of the ureter stumps.
- Check spontaneous urine ejaculation again after the greater omentum sheet is wrapped around the ureter.
- Only four sutures are necessary to adapt the everted 'fish mouth' ureter stoma to the skin.
- Reinsert the mono-J catheters immediately when the complications mentioned here arise.

Not to do

- Do not connect short, pale ureters to the skin under tension.
- Do not use this technique in patients treated even many years ago by external beam irradiation doses of 45–60 Gy.

References

1 August SF. Cutaneous omento-ureterostomy. J Urol 1967;98: 342.
2 Yoshimura K, Maekawa S, Ichioka K, Terada N, Matsuta Y. Tubeless cutaneous ureterostomy: the Toyoda method revisited. J Urol 2001;165:785–8.
3 Lodde M, Pycha A, Palermo S, Comploj E, Hohenfellner R. Uretero-ureterocutaneostomy (wrapped by omentum). Br J Urol Int 2005;95(3):371–3.
4 Madersbacher S, Schmidt J, Eberle JM *et al.* Long-term outcome of ileal conduit diversion. J Urol 2003;169:985–90.
5 Roth A. Transabdominal transperitoneal bilateral omento-ureterostomy (Exhibit and motion picture). Annual Meeting of the North Central Section, AUA, Cleveland, Ohio, September 27–30, 1967.
6 Winter CC. Cutaneus omento-ureterostomy: clinical application. J Urol 1972;107:233.

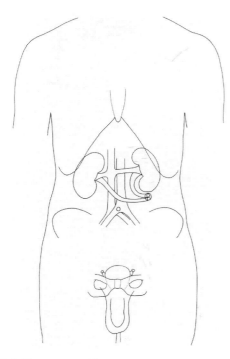

Figure 52.1 The stoma positions.

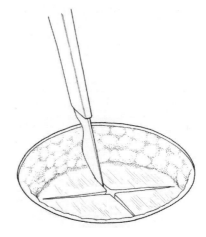

Figure 52.3 Incise the fascia in a cross-like fashion.

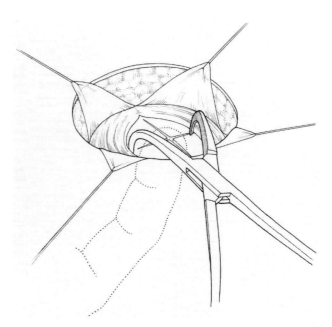

Figure 52.4 Divide rectus muscle bluntly, and incise the dorsal rectus sheet and peritoneum.

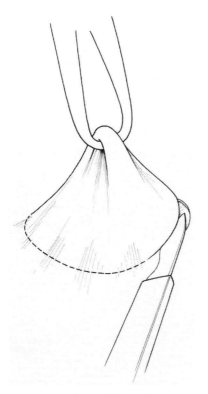

Figure 52.2 Make a 2.5 cm skin excision.

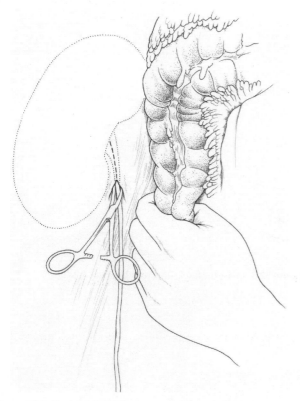

Figure 52.5 Prepare the right ureter pelvic junction.

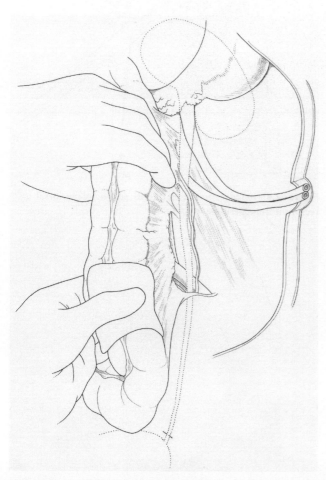

Figure 52.6 The left ureter is prepared and the cross-over maneuver completed.

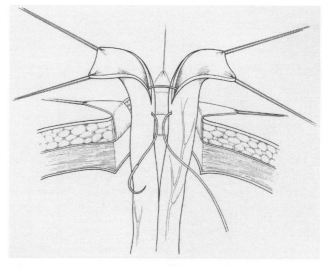

Figure 52.7 Perform the pull-through maneuver with the ureters connected.

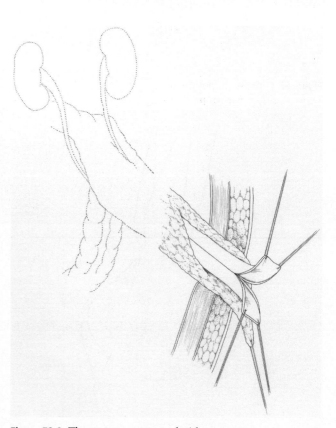

Figure 52.8 The ureters are wrapped with omentum.

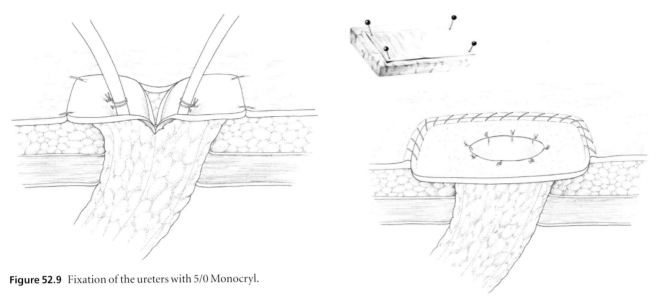

Figure 52.9 Fixation of the ureters with 5/0 Monocryl.

Figure 52.10 Stoma construction with a free buccal mucosa graft.

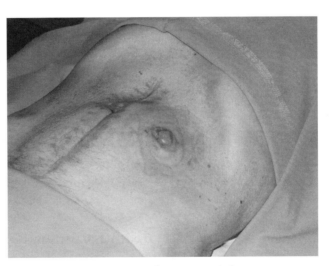

Figure 52.11 The stoma 3 months postoperatively.

Chapter 53
Continent Catheterizable Ileum-based Reservoir

A. Macedo Jr and E. M. Srougi

Introduction

The development of new techniques of bladder augmentation and clean intermittent catheterization (CIC) have changed the prognosis of end-stage bladder disease in children. When both augmentation and suprapubic continent stoma for CIC are required, the classic approach is to create an intestinal reservoir and, additionally, incorporate an efferent tube to it (appendix or Monti tube). We describe a technique in which the conformation of the reservoir includes a tubular, continent outlet for catheterization; therefore the time spent preparing the appendix with its pedicle or making a Monti tube from a second isolated segment of ileum is saved.

Patient counseling and consent

If there is a mean stoma continence of 95%, consider 10–15% surgical revision of the stoma due to stenosis or leakage. Mucus production by the intestinal reservoir, increased risk of urinary stones, and metabolic disorders (acidose) are all possible complications.

Indications

- Neurogenic bladder.
- Bladder exstrophy.
- Posterior urethral valve bladder.
- Whenever a bladder augmentation is needed in association with a Mitrofanoff channel.

Limitations and risks

- Severe urethral incontinence (consider performing a bladder neck procedure as well).
- Social and orthopedic status: ability to perform self-catheterization of the reservoir.
- Compliance to urologic follow-up.

Contraindications

See above.

Preoperative management

Prepare the antegrade bowel with 600–1000 mL of mannitol solution 10%.

Anesthesia

General anesthesia with spinal block for pain control.

Special instruments/suture material

Special instruments are not required, although a Denis-Brown retractor is useful. Intestinal autosutures can be used although they are not necessary.

Operative technique

See Figs 53.1–53.10.

Tips

- Isolate 30 cm of the ileum for augmentations; for bladder substitutions we suggest a further 10 cm for a Studer afferent loop and refluxive ureteral reimplantation (total of 40 cm).
- Open the bladder dome extensively for a wide anastomosis (augmentations).
- The reservoir is created by running 3/0 Vicryl sutures. The valve mechanism is created by 2/0 Prolene interrupted sutures (four to five sutures).
- An infraumbilical pseudoumbilical stoma is preferred in cases of bladder augmentation. The angle of the reservoir anterior wall to the channel is then kept closed, reinforcing the efficiency of the valve. We additionally anchor the reservoir dome to the abdominal wall in order to further increase the resistance of the outlet tube against the abdominal wall. The

distal part of the tube should exit the valve and find the stomal skin without tortuosity to ease the passage of the catheter through it.

• We applied the same principle to the transverse colon in three previously irradiated rhabdomyosarcoma patients with excellent results.

Postoperative care

• The nasogastric tube is removed on day 1 or 2.
• A 12 Fr silicone Foley tube and cystostomy are left in place for 3 weeks. Parents or the patients themselves should clean the reservoir with 20 mL of saline solution daily to prevent mucus occlusion of the urinary tubes.
• Patients are readmitted on day 21 for self-catheterization training by a specialist stoma nurse.

Complications

• Partial dehiscence of the skin closed to the stoma: keep the Foley tube for an additional 1 or 2 weeks.
• Urinary retention due to mucus obstruction: substitute the urethral tube.

Troubleshooting

• Difficulties with the first catheterization of the stoma: do not force, provide an endoscopic evaluation of the outlet channel, place a Foley tube, and wait 4–6 weeks to restart with CIC.

• Stoma stenosis: this can be treated initially by local dilatation under sedation or, if necessary, by reanastomosis of the tube.
• Severe channel stenosis and total incontinence: these are better treated by apendiconeocystostomy.

Results

• $n = 65$.
• Two patients were excluded (undiversion).
• Total continence: 61/63 (after > 4 h).
• Partial continence: 63/63 (after > 2 h).
• Reoperations: 9/63 (14.3%).

To do

• Evaluate the leak point pressure to define urethral resistance (and the necessity of bladder neck repair).
Augmentation: create a pseudoumbilical stoma between the pubis and umbilicus.
• Substitution: place a stoma at the umbilical scar.
• Provide a preoperative nurse interview to explain the care and procedures related to abdominal CIC.

Not to do

• Do not remove the outlet stomal tube before 3 weeks.
• Do not insert a urethral tube with force when resistance is noted during the initial CIC, to avoid perforation of the channel. Check the tube endoscopically.

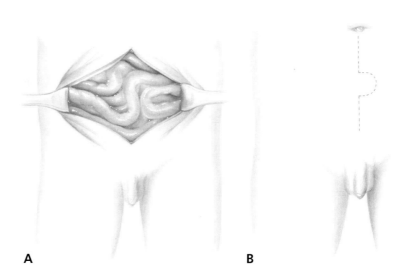

Figure 53.1 A lower midline incision is made with a small left-sided circumferential skin flap for further pseudoumbilical stoma creation.

A   B

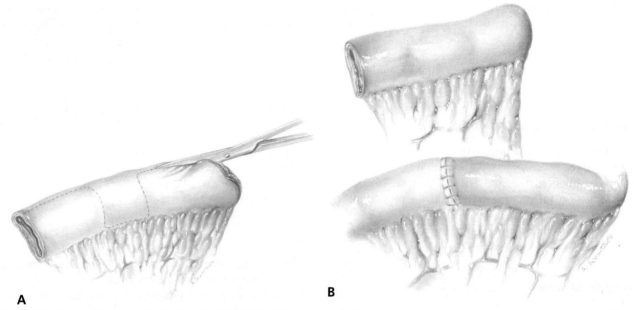

A

B

Figure 53.2 Detubularization of the ileal segment (flap definition).

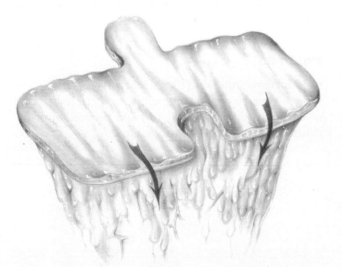

Figure 53.3 Creation of the reservoir plate.

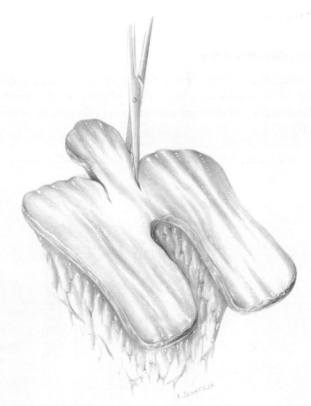

Figure 53.4 The flap can be further incised to produce a longer tube.

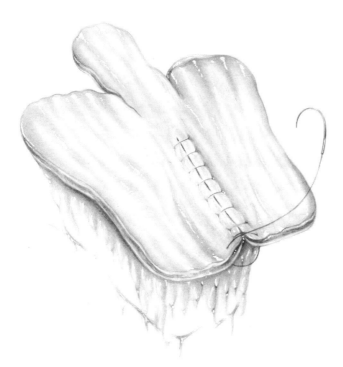

Figure 53.5 Insert a running suture to close the plate of the reservoir.

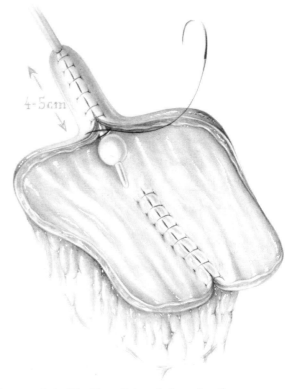

Figure 53.6 A 12 Fr silicone Foley tube is used to allow tubularization of the flap to create an efferent tubular conduit.

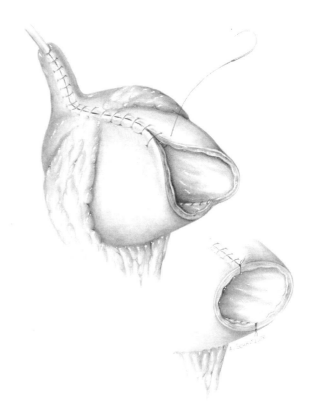

Figure 53.7 The reservoir after anterior wall closure.

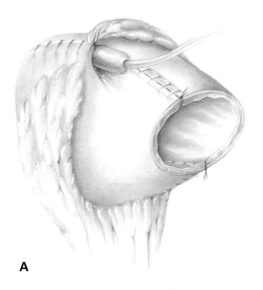

A

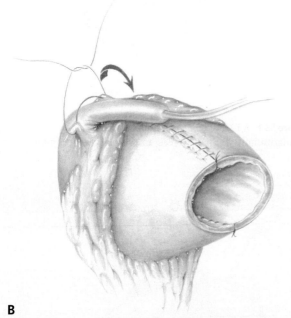

B

Figure 53.8 The tube is embedded to provide continence.

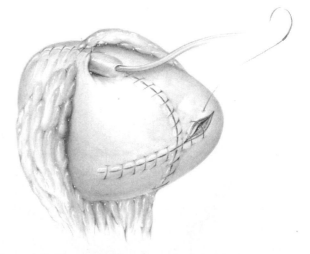

Figure 53.9 The pouch is closed completely for bladder substitution.

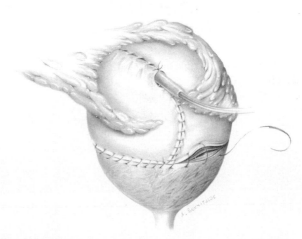

Figure 53.10 The reservoir is anastomosed to the native bladder in cases of augmentation cystoplasty.

Part 8.1
Use of the Large Bowel

Chapter 54
Use of the Large Bowel in Urinary Tract Reconstruction

R. Hohenfellner, M. Fisch, and J. Leissner

Segment selection and large bowel anastomosis

Introduction

In contrast to ileum colon, the large bowel is not used frequently. However, 30–50 cm of healthy bowel, out of 150–200 cm, is available for urinary tract reconstruction. In contrast to using ileum, the advantages are an excellent blood supply and a lesser risk of: ileus, leakage of stool and urine, vitamin B_{12} and magnesium deficiency, and stool frequency. There are excellent long-term results concerning kidney function, and the risk of secondary malignancy is equal to that when using ileum for reconstruction.

Patient counseling and consent

Compliance is mandatory and antiacidotic prophylactic treatment should be given.

Indications

The broad spectrum of indications include bladder augmentation, orthotopic substitution, and urinary diversion in continent or incontinent patients. There is also the option of conversion in a continent sigmorectum pouch or with an umbilical stoma. Unilateral or bilateral ureter substitution and vaginal substitution are also possible. It helps in irradiated patients to select a healthy, previously non-irradiated bowel segment. In cases of repair an extraperitoneal approach from a flank incision is an advantage.

Limitations and risks

- Heavy smokers.
- Neoadjuvant chemotherapy less than 4 weeks before.
- Short and fatty mesentery, 'which does not invite you'.

Contraindications

- History of large bowel malignancy and resection.
- Diverticulosis.
- Crohn's disease.
- Abdominal vascular disease.

Preoperative management

- Bowel enema and X-ray: to check sigma length and for the presence of malignancies.
- Bowel preparation: 6–8 L of Fortran.
- Antibiotics: cephalosporin or metronidazole.

Anesthesia

General and peridural anesthesia.

Special instruments/suture material

- Fine instruments for ureter implant.
- Magnification lens system.
- Bipolar coagulation set; Ligasure.
- Suture material: bowel: 4/0 Maxon, PDS, and RB-1 needle; ureter: 5/0 Monocryl.
- Soft ureter splints, 6 or 8 Fr (Websinger).
- Cold light diaphanoscopy.

Operative technique

- Perform complete large bowel mobilization along the avascular line of Toldt. The hepato-, gastro-, and phrenicocolic ligaments are divided. The greater omentum is mobilized from right to left (preferred) or left to right.
- The ureter is prepared carefully and resected step by step until capillary artery bleeding and spontaneous urine ejaculation are observed.
- Segment selection and ureter cross-over depends on the re-

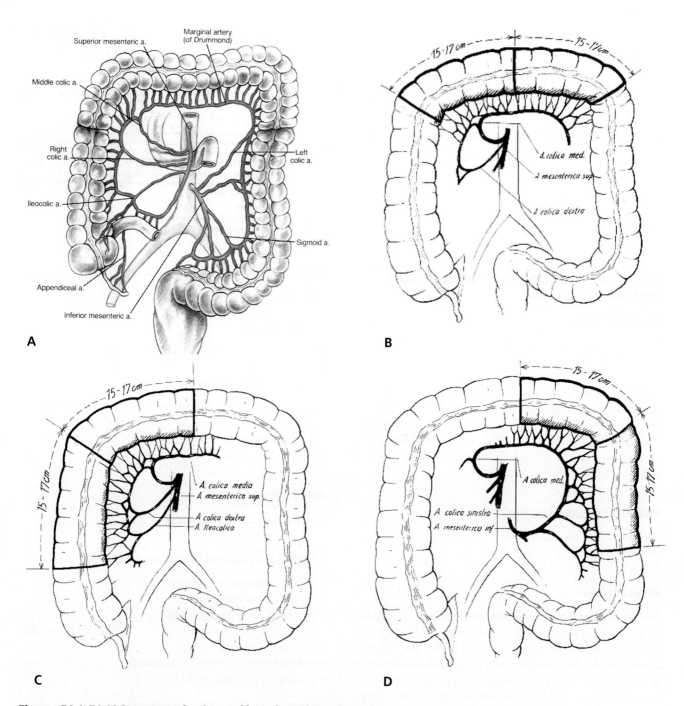

Figures 54.1–54.10 Segment selection and large bowel anastomosis.
Figure 54.1 Segment selection. (A) Main features of the bowel. (B) Short right ureter: use an ascending conduit or transverse ascending pouch. (C) Both ureters short: use a transverse conduit or pyelotransverse pyelocutaneostomy. (D) Short left ureter: use a descending or sigma conduit or transverse descending pouch.

maining length of the ureter stumps. The blood supply of the right ureter is often better than the left one.
• The lateral bowel mesoseparation should be kept to a minimum of about 0.4 cm. Preserve the vasa recta. Use cold light illumination and blunt mesoseparation on the fingertip in order to find the best line of resection; mark with stay sutures.

In an open resection, do not use clamps. Observe capillary artery bleeding from both bowel ends. Clean the separated segment with NaCl.
• Complete a tension-free end-to-end anastomosis with one row of interrupted seromuscular submucosa sutures.
• Remember the 'four 4s': (i) lateral mesoseparation: 0.4 cm;

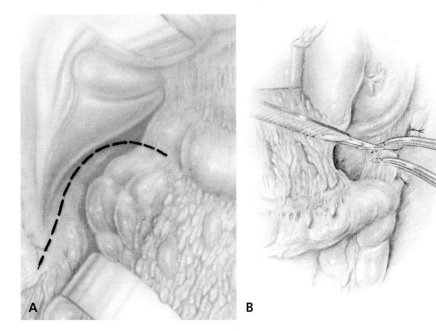

Figure 54.2 Complete large bowel mobilization: (A) the hepatocolic ligament and parts of the gastrocolicum; (B) the phrenicocolic ligament.

A

B

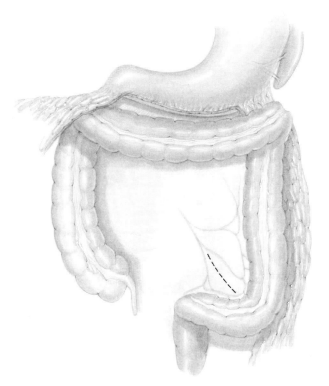

Figure 54.3 Greater omentum separation should be from right to left (preferred) or left to right.

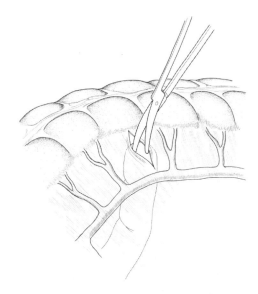

Figure 54.4 Segment separation starts with blunt mesodissection between the two vasa recta over the underlying fingertip.

(ii) stitch distance: four knots; (iii) lateral distance from the bowel margin: 0.4 cm; and (iv) use 4/0 Maxon or PDS.
• Ureter implantation: refluxive in adults and reimplantations; antirefluxive in children.

Tips

• The segment selected will contract when it becomes isolated (use 30–40 cm in adults and 15–20 cm in children). Check there is adequate length before starting the tension-free anastomosis. Remember there is still enough large bowel left to isolate a longer segment!
• In cases of a twisted ureter or bowel, a 90° anastomosis is tolerated but 180° is not!

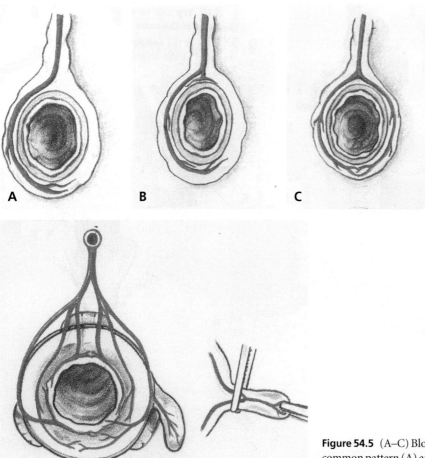

Figure 54.5 (A–C) Blood supply of the ileum showing the most common pattern (A) and rarer arrangements (B, C). (D) Blood supply of the colon. Note that close ligation of the appendix may compromise the bowel blood supply.

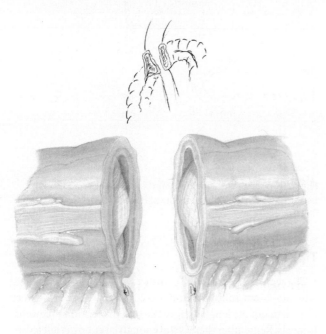

Figure 54.6 Lateral bowel separation should be for a maximum of 0.4 cm. Use open dissection and observe capillary bleeding along the resection line. Use a longitudinal taenia incision to adapt different bowel diameters (inset).

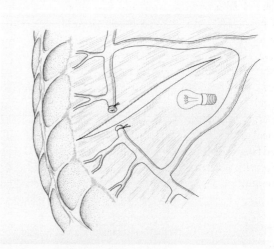

Figure 54.7 Cold light diaphanoscopy is used to continue the mesoincision. It is important to check that there is adequate conduit length before the anastomosis is started.

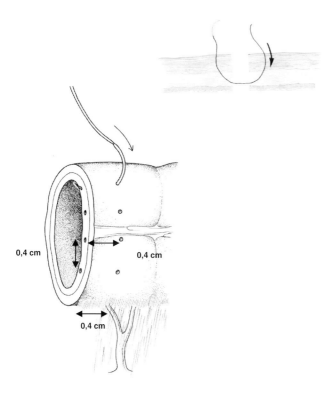

Figure 54.8 The 'four 4s': (i) lateral mesoseparation: 0.4 cm; (ii) stitch distance: four knots; (iii) lateral distance from bowel margin: 0.4 cm; and (iv) single interrupted seromuscular–submucosa suture line using 4/0 Maxon or PDS and an RB-1 needle.

• Clean isolated segments with NaCl solution only (there is a high risk of local allergy and mucosa oedema).
• Check capillary artery bleeding and spontaneous urine ejaculation again before you insert the soft splint. (If not, look for a ureter kink!) Insert the splint up to the first resistance and then withdraw it 1 cm—this is the best position.
• In cases of mesenteric or tunnel hematoma, compress the bowel for 5 min.
• Large mesenteric defects may be covered with free peritoneal grafts taken from the left lateral abdominal wall, covered later on by the colon descendens.
• In critical suture lines, ensure interposition of the greater omentum or a free peritoneal graft between the overlying sutures lines to prevent inner fistula formation (stool into pouch or conduit).
• There is a risk of parastomal hernias at the lateral stoma position.
• Fix the conduit from the inside; if there are problems fix it at 3 o'clock lateral to the abdominal wall. (Beware hernias!)
• Blue stomas are critical stomas. Take a biopsy and observe artery capillary bleeding.
• Perform intracutaneous sutures for stoma fixation.
• Check the conduit is watertight with 75 cm³ of NaCl.
• Check for rectum lesions by filling the empty pelvis with NaCl and insufflate air in the rectal probe. Observe any air bubbles!

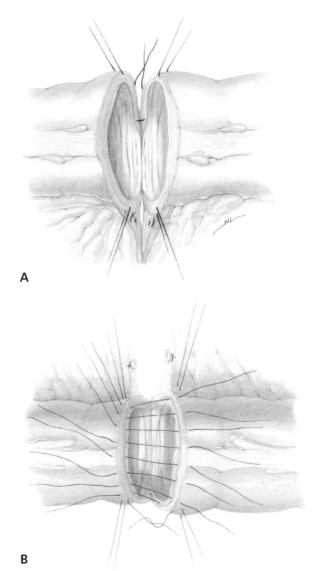

Figure 54.9 Tension-free end-to-end anastomosis, starting at the back (A) and finishing at the front (B).

Postoperative care

Remove the splints on day 8 to 10.

Complications

In nonfunctioning splints where the ultrasound is normal, do not irrigate and wait and see. If the ultrasound shows dilatation, perform a percutaneous nephrostomy.

Troubleshooting

• Diffuse peritonitis: due to stool and/or urine leakage. Revision of the bowel and ureter anastomosis and a right colon transverse anus praeter is needed.

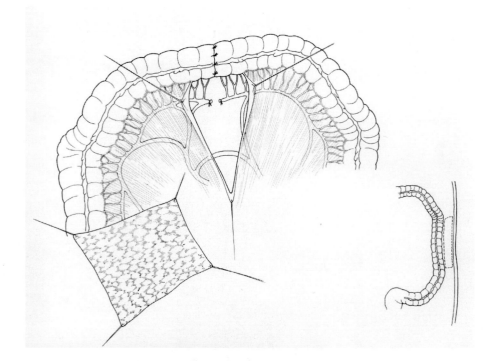

Figure 54.10 Large mesenteric windows may be covered with free peritoneal grafts taken from the left lateral pelvic wall.

• Late ureter obstruction in asymptomatic pelvic malignancy: wait and see; in symptomatic pelvic malignancy, perform a unilateral nephrostomy followed by nephrectomy or embolization. In benign disease, reimplantation is needed.

Results

See Chapters 56, 57, and 59.

Remarks

See Chapters 56, 57, and 59.

To do

• Use well-vascularized ureters and bowel segments that have not been previously irradiated.
• Use tension-free anastomosis.
• Use three layers (multilayer) of interrupted sutures with four knots for 4/0 and five knots for 5/0 material. Use fine ligatures or bipolar coagulation, and omit clips. Start with the posterior wall first and complete the anterior wall anastomosis from each edge.
• Use one layer of seromuscular interrupted sutures.
• Remember the 'four 4s' (see above).
• Avoid twists or kinks, or narrow 'windows'.

• Repeat any part of the procedure if it is not satisfactory before you close the abdomen.
• Use the mobilized greater omentum to fill the empty pelvis.
• Check the abdomen for blood clots and irrigate with distillate water to observe any bleeding.
• Check the epigastric vessels for bleeding when the retractor is removed.

Not to do

If the bowel looks suspect — for example it is short or there is fatty mesentery — change your strategy and use the ileum.

References

1 Hohenfellner R, Black P, Leissner J, Allhoff EP. Refluxing ureterointestinal anastomosis for continent cutaneous urinary diversion. J Urol 2002;168:1013–17.
2 Leissner J, Black P, Fisch M, Höckel M, Hohenfellner R. Colon pouch (Mainz pouch III) for continent urinary diversion after pelvic irradiation. Urology 2000;56(5):798–802.
3 Wammack R, Wricke C, Hohenfellner R. Long-term results of ileocecal continent urinary diversion in patients treated with and without previous pelvic irradiation. J Urol 2002;167:2058–62.

Ureter implantation

See Figs 54.11–54.23.

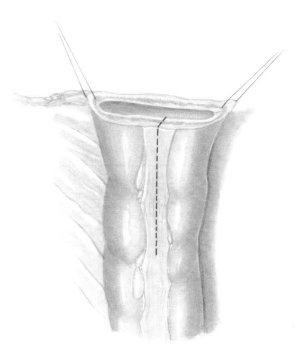

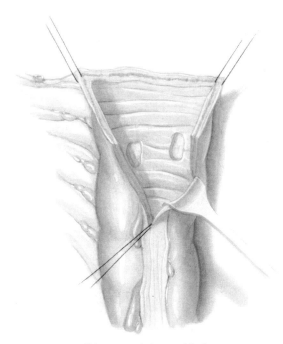

Figure 54.13 An eyelid retractor is inserted for better exposure.

Figures 54.11–54.23 Ureter implantation.
Figure 54.11 An isolated segment is opened along the taenia for 4–5 cm.

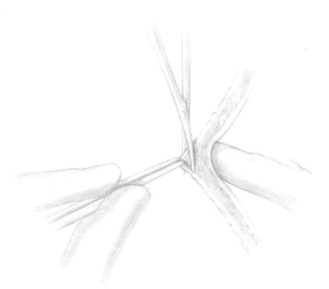

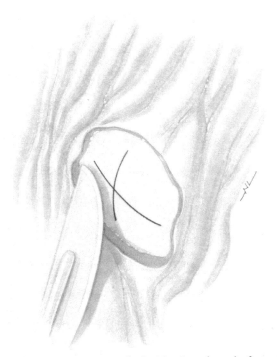

Figure 54.12 The mucosa is excised from the back wall on the tip of the finger.

Figure 54.14 A cross seromuscular incision is made on the fingertip (avoids obstruction).

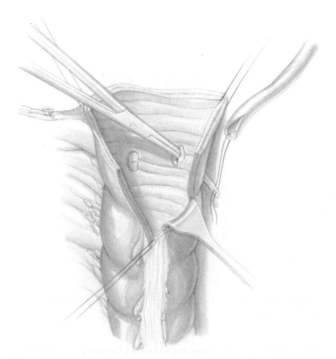

Figure 54.15 Pull-through of the spatulated ureter.

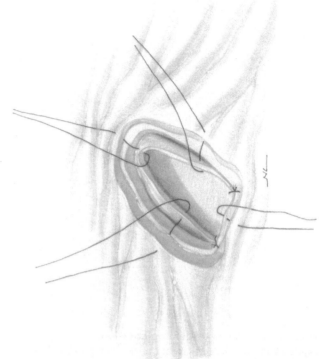

Figure 54.17 Adapt the ureter to the mucosa of the bowel using 5/0 Monocryl and make sure it is watertight.

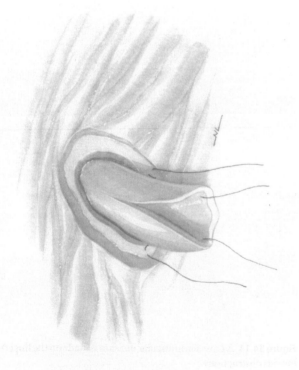

Figure 54.16 Place two seromuscular anchor sutures at 5 and 7 o'clock.

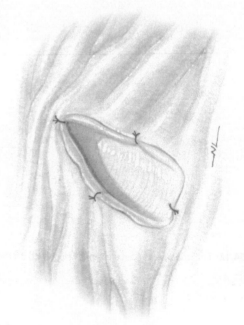

Figure 54.18 Observe spontaneous urine ejaculation in the implanted ureter to make sure there is no kink.

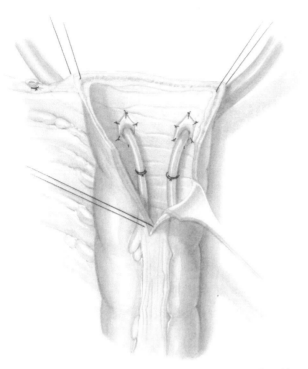

Figure 54.19 The 6 or 8 Fr splints are fixed with 4/0 Vicryl rapid.

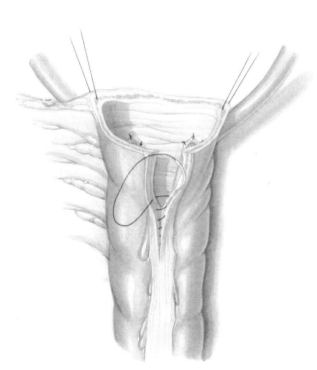

Figure 54.20 Close the incision with a mucosa running suture of 5/0 Monocryl for the first layer.

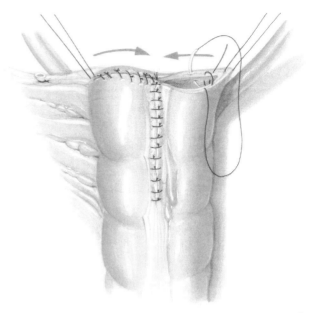

Figure 54.21 Use interrupted seromuscularis 4/0 Maxon sutures for the second layer.

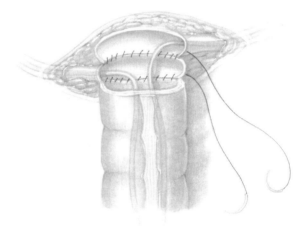

Figure 54.22 Wallace type anastomosis in thick wall dilated ureters.

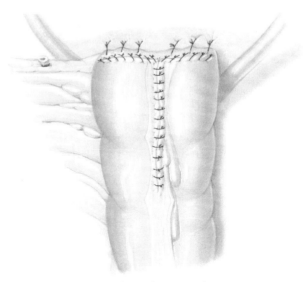

Figure 54.23 Fix the conduit to the retroperitoneum.

Chapter 55
Use of the Greater Omentum in Urinary Tract Reconstruction

R. Hohenfellner, M. Fisch, and J. Leissner

Introduction

The greater omentum with its dense lymphatic network is called the 'policeman' of the abdomen. The rich blood supply comes from the right and left gastroepiploic arteries as well as from branches of the middle colic arteries and the pancreatic artery.

Indications

There is a broad spectrum of indications, for instance:
- substitution of the fat capsule of the kidney;
- to cover peritoneal defects;
- to protect suture lines and to avoid internal fistula formation;
- to fill the empty small pelvis following exenteration.

If the greater omentum is not available, large free parietal peritoneal grafts taken from the lateral border of the abdominal wall can be transferred in order to substitute peritoneal defects or to prevent fistula formation along sutures lines. With the serous surface inside, the greater omentum also works as a matrix to substitute renal pelvic defects.

Limitations and risks

Preservation of the omental blood supply is mandatory to avoid postoperative omental necrosis with fever of unknown origin. Check the blood supply, especially in extended omental mobilization and flap formation. Avoid lesions of the middle colic artery if entering the omental bursa.

Special instruments/suture material

Hemoclips or Ligasure are useful for the division of the omentum from the stomach and the branches of the gastroepiploic vessels.

Tips

In omentum mobilization from right to left (preferred by the authors), the bulk of the omentum fills the empty pelvic cavity and covers the right fossa obturatoria. This prevents small bowel adhesions and ileus developing later on. The left fossa obturatoria is protected by the sigma.

Cold light diaphanoscopy is useful in order to identify the blood vessels of the fatty greater omentum.

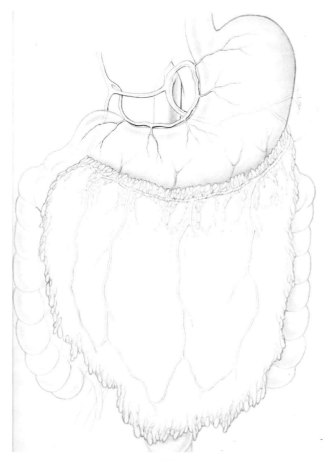

Figure 55.1 The main features of the greater omentum.

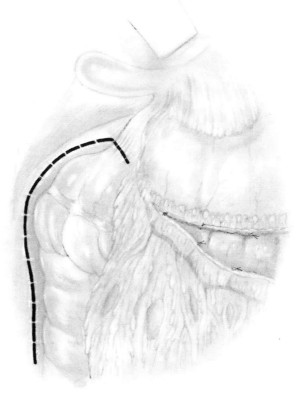

Figure 55.2 Division of the hepatocolic and parts of the gastrocolic ligaments.

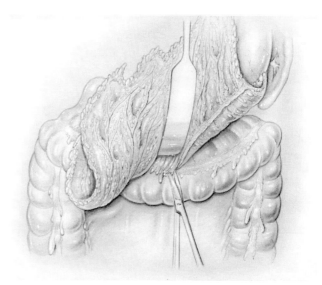

Figure 55.3 Bloodless sharp dissection of the omentum from the transverse colon.

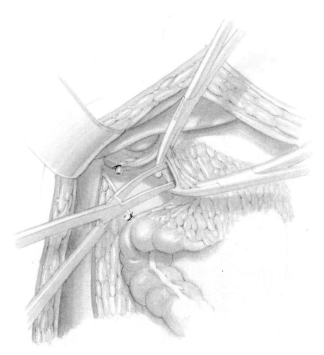

Figure 55.4 The right gastroepiploic vessels are divided.

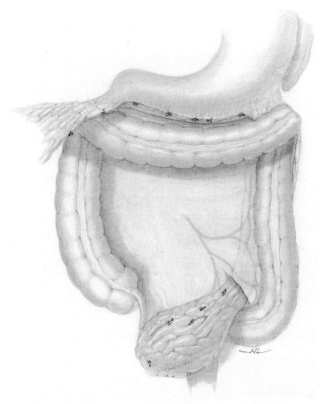

Figure 55.6 The left gastroepiploic vessels are preserved and the omentum is placed retrocolic through an incision of the mesosigma. The omentum fills the empty pelvis.

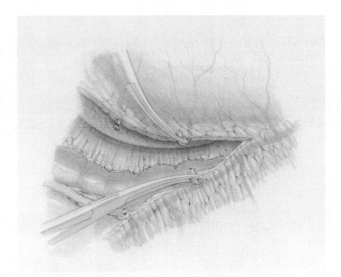

Figure 55.5 The omentum is separated from the stomach.

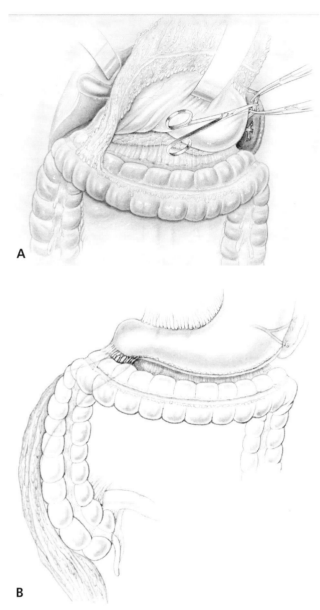

B

Figure 55.7 In left to right mobilization (A), the greater omentum is placed behind the colon and cecum (B).

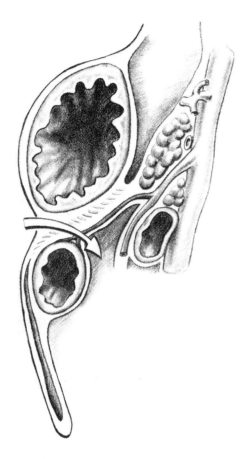

Figure 55.8 Take care to avoid injury to the middle colic artery in inflammatory fixation of the omentum.

Chapter 56
Bladder Substitution with Sigmoid Segments (the Mannheim experience)

M. S. Michel and P. Alken

Introduction

A great variety of different techniques using different parts of bowel have been described since the introduction of surgical bladder substitution. Despite the great range of choice, preference is given to only a few techniques using the small intestine. As in other methods of urinary diversion (pouch/conduit), sigma is seldom used for the formation of neobladders. Bladder substitution with sigma is rather classed as a useful alternative standby that should be familiar to all surgeons and that can be chosen when the use of small intestine is inopportune or even contraindicated, e.g. in metabolic imbalance. The described technique of bladder substitution by a detubularized sigmoid segment is an alternative option in orthotopic bladder replacement [2,4]. Bladder substitution with sigmoid segments can be performed in male as well as in female patients [1,5]. The advantages are the minimal effect on metabolic balance and stool frequency, the anatomical site in the small pelvis, unproblematic anastomosis with the urethra, and uncomplicated implantation of the ureters [3].

Indications

This technique is indicated in orthotopic bladder replacement.

Limitations and contraindications

- General contraindications for orthotopic bladder replacement.
- Pelvic radiation.
- Irritable colon.
- Polypus, tumors, and pronounced diverticulosis of the sigmoid.

Preoperative management

- The usual procedures before urinary diversion are followed.
- A colon contrast enema is performed to exclude diverticula or polypus of the sigma.

- 6–10 L of Ringer's solution is used 1 day before surgery for bowel preparation.
- A rectal tube is inserted preoperatively.

Anesthesia

General anesthesia eventually combined with peridural anesthesia, and invasive intraoperative monitoring (central line, invasive arterial blood pressure monitoring).

Special instruments/suture material

- Standard set for extended abdominal surgery.
- 18 Fr silicon catheter.
- Suture material: 2/0 Vicryl SH; 3/0 and 5/0 Vicryl; 4/0 Safil; 4/0 Maxon; 5/0 Vicryl Rb1; 3/0 Safil Rb1; 3/0 Vicryl Rb1; and 3/0 Dexon II.
- Jackson–Pratt drainage.
- 21 Fr silikon drainage.

Surgical technique

- First perform the cystectomy.
- Then place four 3/0 anastomosis sutures.
- Place the sigmoid section in a U-shape in the small pelvic cavity and check that it is tension-free.
- Place 3/0 stay sutures at the lower site
- Separate a 25 cm long sigmoid loop section with 3/0 Vicryl stay sutures and ligate the mesentery with 3/0 stitches.
- Clean the bowel with nebacetine swabs and rinse with saline solution.
- Perform a sigma end-to-end anastomosis.
- Incise the sigmoid segment antimesenterly.
- Incise the ureters longitudinally, implant the ureters directly, place the anastomosis at the foot end, and place five to six 4/0 stitches along the sides/corner with 5/0 sigmoid mucosa.
- Join the medial edges of the U-shape with continuous 4/0 straight needle stitches. Perform an asymmetric resection at the foot point (anastomosis of the tip of the sigmoid

Table 56.1 Comparison of long-term results in patients with sigmoid versus ileum neobladders.

	Sigmoid neobladder	Ileum neobladder
Patient age (years)	62.6 ± 10.9	66.4 ± 10.2
Follow-up period (years)	8.1 ± 2.1	7.2 ± 1.9
Micturition frequency, day/night	d: 4.3 ± 1.2; n: 1.2 ± 0.3	d: 5.6 ± 1.8; n: 1.5 ± 0.6
Continence, day/night (number)	d: 7/10; n: 6/10	d: 8/10; n: 6/10
Slight incontinence, day/night (number)	d: 3/10; n: 2/10	d: 2/10; n: 3/10
Incontinence, day/night (number)	d: 0/10; n: 2/10	d: 0/10; n: 1/10
Stool frequency per day	1.1 ± 0.2	3.1 ± 1.1
Ureter anastomosis stricture	1	2
Bladder capacity (mL)	621 ± 72	423 ± 51
Flow maximum (mL/s)	20.4 ± 5.2	18.2 ± 6.9
Bladder pressure (cmH_2O)	15 ± 4	18 ± 6
Residual urine (mL)	54 ± 32	43 ± 19

with the urethra) and a buttonhole incision to the urethra anastomosis.

- Place an 18 Fr silicon catheter through the urethra.
- Place the urethra anastomosis with the buttonhole at the sigmoid foot.
- Close the sigmoid neobladder with a continuous 4/0 running suture after the cystostomy is placed and the splints are routed out and fixed using 4/0 Safil.
- Tie the anastomosis suture under traction at the catheter.
- Close the mesenteric slots with 2/0 stitches and serosation of the ureter implantation sites.
- Place the Jackson–Pratt drainage at the ureteric implantation site and a 21 Fr drain on the right paravesical side in the renal pelves.
- Close the wound in layers with abdominal sutures.
- Finish the procedure with skin clamping and a sterile dressing.

Tips

- Check after the cystectomy if the sigma is long enough for tension-free anastomosis with the urethra.
- Perform the sigma anastomosis after removing the fat, especially if the sigma is very fatty.
- Implant the ureters through a tangential tunnel to prevent obstruction.

Postoperative care

Remove the ureteral stents on the 10th (right side) and 11th (left side) postoperative days. The further postoperative course is the same as that for other types of neobladder procedures.

Complications

- *No urine flow through the ureteral splint:* use 2 mL of saline and irrigate the splint in order to remove any blood clots. If the problem recurs perform ultrasound; if the collecting system is dilated place a nephrostomy.
- *Urinary retention after catheter removal:* place a catheter and see if there is mucus; if there is, remove the mucus and catheter. Advise the patient about self-catheterization in order to irrigate the sigma neobladder every 14 days.

Results

For comparison purposes, we selected 20 patients from our own patient population for long-term follow-up and urodynamic evaluation: one group of 10 male patients with an ileum neobladder and a second group of 10 male patients with a sigmoid neobladder. The tumor stage, age, and follow-up period were comparable in all patients. Table 56.1 comprises the most important results.

After a follow-up period of 8 years, almost all patients in both groups were continent during the day or were only slightly stress incontinent. About one-third of both patient groups were slightly incontinent during the night and wore pads at night. Two patients with a sigmoid neobladder and one patient with an ileum neobladder were incontinent at night, where incontinence was defined as at least two nycturia events. The only functional difference revealed by urodynamic evaluation was the larger capacity of the sigmoid neobladder. Stool frequency in patients with an ileum neobladder is three times higher than that in the sigmoid neobladder group.

References

1 Chao R, Lange PH. Sigma-Neoblase. In: Ausgewählte Urologische OP-Techniken (Hohenfellner R, ed.). Georg Thieme Verlag, Stuttgart, 1994:5.89–5.96.

2 Fujisawa M, Gotoh A, Miyazaki S *et al.* Sigmoid neobladder in women after radical cystectomy. J Urol 2000;163(5):1505–9.
3 Fujisawa M, Gotoh A, Nakamura I *et al.* Long-term assessment of serum vitamin B(12) concentrations in patients with various types of orthotopic intestinal neobladder. Urology 2000;56(2): 236–40.

4 Fujisawa M, Isotani S, Gotoh A *et al.* Voiding dysfunction of sigmoid neobladder in women: a comparative study with men. Eur Urol 2001;40(2):191–5.
5 Reddy PK, Lange PH, Fraley EE. Total bladder replacement using detubularized sigmoid colon: technique and results. J Urol 1991;145:51–5.

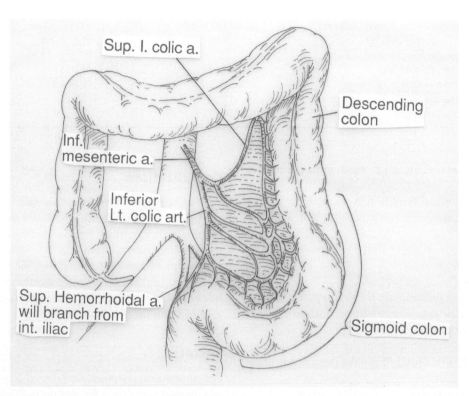

Figure 56.1 Selection of the ideal sigma segment with a good blood supply.

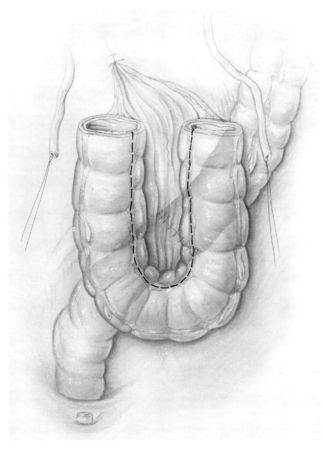

Figure 56.2 Contramesenterical incision of the isolated segment.

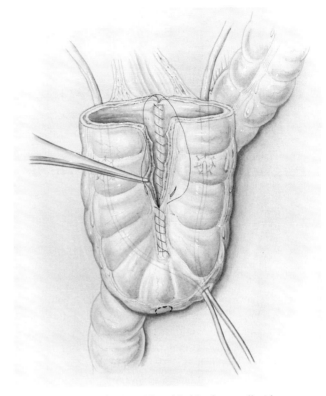

Figure 56. 4 Close the sigmoid neobladder front wall with a continuous 4/0 running double layer suture.

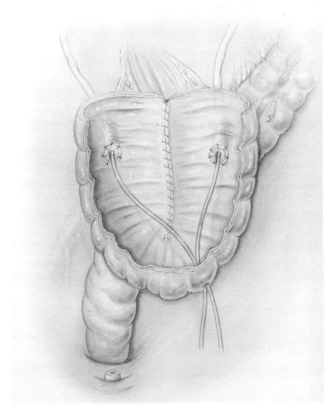

Figure 56.3 Direct ureter implantation.

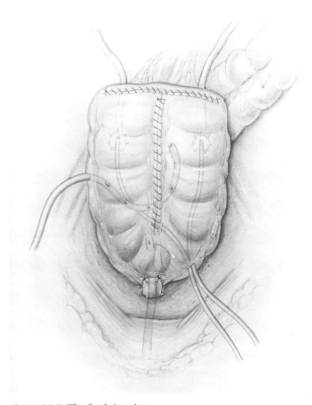

Figure 56.5 The final situation.

Chapter 57

Colon Pouch (Mainz Pouch III) for Continent Urinary Diversion

J. Leissner, M. Fisch, and R. Hohenfellner

Introduction

Urinary diversion in previously irradiated patients has proven to be a challenge that has been addressed with a number of different techniques. A high rate of early and late complications was observed using small bowel segments and ileocecal reservoirs. Based on the high risk for failure of reconstructive surgery in the irradiated field and on the high complication rate after using irradiated tissue for urinary diversion, the 'stay away' principle was adopted with nonirradiated large bowel segments being used for continent urinary diversion [1,4,6].

Here, we describe the technique of the transverse ascending pouch (TAP) and transverse descending pouch (TDP), which was initially introduced in patients with previous pelvic irradiation therapy. The excellent results of TAP and TDP have caused us to contemplate using these techniques not only under special circumstances but as an alternative form of urinary diversion in nonirradiated patients. We have also introduced a direct, refluxing ureterointestinal anastomosis with a very low risk of ureteral obstruction and subsequent deterioration in kidney function.

The advantages of the technique are the preservation of the ileocecal valve, thus limiting adverse effects related to an increased stool frequency. There is no risk of vitamin B_{12} deficiency as it is associated with the use of small bowel segments for urinary diversion [5].

Indications

The technique is indicated in absolute or functional loss of the urinary bladder (patients with muscle-invasive bladder cancer, local tumor recurrence of gynecological malignancies, irreparable vesical fistulas, and neurogenic bladder disorders after failed conservative management). The approach can also be used in patients with complete pelvic exenteration requiring urinary diversion and colostomy.

Limitations and risks

- Patients should understand the problems and risks associated with self-catheterization and should be assessed for their compliance.
- Patient compliance is mandatory for regular postoperative follow-up visits, including measurements of base excess.
- Preoperative existing diarrhea can be worsened by the additional loss of large bowel for the colon pouch.
- Dilatation of the upper urinary tract with normal kidney function is not a contraindication.

Contraindications

- Renal insufficiency with elevated serum creatinine (>2 mg/dL).
- Short bowel syndrome.
- Abnormalities of the colon (diverticula disease, stenosis, tumor).
- Poor compliance.

Preoperative management

- IV pyelogram.
- Renal scintigraphy in cases of upper urinary tract dilatation. Nephrectomy should be considered when the split renal function of one side is less than 20% of the total renal function.
- Contrast enema to exclude diverticular disease or stenosis of the colon. Also estimate the colon length available and decide on a transverse ascending or descending pouch (skin incision circumnavigates the umbilicus on the contralateral side).
- Bowel preparation with mechanical clean-out is needed 1 day preoperatively.

Special instruments/suture material

- Ureteral implantation: 5/0 monofilament sutures (e.g. Monocryl®, Maxon®).

- Pouch wall: 3/0 monofilament sutures (PDS®) with a straight needle.
- Fixation of stents: e.g. 4/0 Vicryl® rapid.
- Umbilical funnel: 3/0 monofilament sutures (e.g. Monocryl®, PDS®).
- Creation of efferent segment: monofilament absorbable sutures for the mucosa (e.g. 5/0 Monocryl®) and nonabsorbable sutures for the seromuscular layer (e.g. 3/0 Prolene®).

Operative technique

- Perform a midline laparotomy from the xiphoid to the pubic symphysis with circumnavigation of the umbilicus on the right side for TDP and on the left side for TAP. This decision is made based on the preoperative enema. In patients who have undergone previous midline laparotomies, the same skin incision should be used to avoid umbilical necrosis and to create a well-vascularized umbilical stoma.
- The small and large bowel are mobilized carefully to avoid serosal lesions and the need for bowel resections.
- The ureters are dissected out of the retroperitoneal tissue where they are often impacted and obstructed in a fibrous mass after irradiation. The ureteral stumps are shortened up to a level at which arterial capillary bleeding, spontaneous peristalsis, and urinary ejaculation are observed.
- The selection of the colon segment depends on the individual length of nonirradiated bowel. Between 35 and 40 cm of transverse colon and either ascending or descending colon are required to create a pouch of adequate capacity (350–400 mL). Complete mobilization of the right or left colic flexure should be performed to gain adequate colon length for the pouch.
- The greater omentum is separated from the transverse colon from right to left in TAP, from left to right in TDP. The blood supply of the colon, which displays some anatomical variability, is identified by transillumination. Resection of the colon is then performed between stay sutures.
- A colo-colostomy is performed with interrupted seromuscular sutures (4/0 monofilament material).
- The colon is detubularized antimesenterically leaving 5–6 cm of the oral or aboral end intact for the creation of the efferent segment.
- This segment is tapered over an 18 Fr silicone catheter. The mucosa is sutured with polyglycol and the seromuscular layer with a nonabsorbable running suture. A pseudoappendix is thus created. Easy catheter gliding is important since a shrinkage rate of up to 30% can be expected.
- A pouch plate is created using a running 4/0 monofilament polyglycol suture on a straight needle.
- Ureteral implantation can be performed with an antirefluxing or refluxing technique.
- *Antirefluxing ureterointestinal anastomosis*: this should be used in children only! A submucosal tunnel of about 2 cm on both sides of the suture link is created between stay sutures.

The ureters are pulled through the tunnel and a neo-ostium is performed with 5/0 absorbable sutures. The ureteral adventitia is fixed at the external pouch wall with two 5/0 sutures.
- *Refluxing ureterointestinal anastomosis*: about 1 cm² of the bowel mucosa is excised on the backside of the pouch plate. The maneuver is facilitated by extension of the pouch wall by a finger placed from the posterior. The seromuscular layer is then incised in the shape of a cross. Care should be taken to observe spontaneous spouting of urine from the ureteral stump in each case following the pull-through maneuver, before the ureter is anchored in the pouch at the 5 and 7 o'clock positions. This is followed by a watertight anastomosis with 5/0 sutures. The ureteral adventitia is fixed at the external pouch wall.
- After performing the ureter–bowel anastomosis, spontaneous urine ejaculation is used as evidence of an unobstructed and torsion-free ureteral course. 6 or 8 Fr smooth ureteral stents are placed and fixed. Along with a 10 Fr pouchostomy, the ureteral stents are led out through the pouch and abdominal wall at separate sites.
- The pouch is closed and the efferent segment is embedded in the anterior suture line of the pouch wall.
- Windows are dissected in the mesentery of the tapered colon between the vessels. The efferent segment is then placed in the suture line and the seromuscular layer of the anterior wall is sutured together through the mesenteric windows using nonabsorbable sutures.
- The anastomosis between the umbilical funnel and the efferent segment is performed at the level of the rectus fascia and the pouch is fixed to the abdominal wall.
- The pouch is fixed at the anterior and lateral abdominal wall with interrupted sutures.
- The omentum is used as a flap to cover the pouch and the bowel.

Postoperative care

- Remove the ureteral stents after 10–14 days.
- Perform an IV pyelogram after removal of the stents.
- Start clean intermittent catheterization after a pouchogram 3 weeks postoperatively.

Results

A continent colon pouch for urinary diversion was performed in 44 female patients following pelvic irradiation [3]. An antirefluxing ureterointestinal anastomosis was performed in 34 patients and a direct refluxing anastomosis in 10 patients [2]. As four nephrectomies were performed, 64 renal units were implanted with an antirefluxing technique and 20 renal units with a direct, refluxing technique.

No early complications related to the pouch procedure were encountered. Intermittent self-catheterization was initiated in all patients according to plan, except in three cases, in which catheter removal was delayed secondary to postoperative bowel dysfunction. Self-catheterization was unproblematic in all patients. A postoperative pouchogram showed reflux in no patients and urodynamic evaluation revealed a median (range) capacity of 480 mL (300–550 mL).

Postoperatively, the upper urinary tract was normal in all preoperatively normal kidneys. In the group of patients with antirefluxing ureterointestinal anastomosis, 28 of 64 renal units were dilated preoperatively. Of the 28 preoperatively dilated kidneys, 23 became normal and five remained dilated. In the group of patients with refluxing anastomosis, eight of 20 renal units were dilated preoperatively. Six of them were normal postoperatively and two showed a persistent grade 1 dilatation.

Follow-up was available in all 44 patients with a mean of 52.2 months (range 13–112 months). All patients with postoperatively dilated renal units were asymptomatic and did not show any deterioration of renal function. Ureteral reimplantation thus did not become necessary.

Pouch-related late complications occurred in eight patients. Two suffered from incontinence of the outlet. Both of these were revised with the creation of a new efferent segment. Stoma stenosis occurred in six patients. Four could be treated by endoscopic incision and two underwent a YV-plasty.

The postoperative stool frequency remained unchanged in all patients. No additional diarrhea or deterioration was reported. As a prophylactic measure, 20 patients used alkalinizing agents when their capillary base excess was less than −2.5 mmol/L.

Remarks

The authors have recently demonstrated the advantage of a refluxing ureterointestinal anastomosis with almost no risk of ureteral obstruction and subsequent deterioration in kidney function, and we are therefore in favor of this technique in normal and dilated ureters [2].

References

1 Hancock KC, Copeland I, Gershenson DM *et al.* Urinary conduits in gynecologic oncology. Obstet Gynecol 1986;67:680–4.

2 Hohenfellner R, Black P, Leissner J, Allhoff EP. Refluxing ureterointestinal anastomosis for continent cutaneous urinary diversion. J Urol 2002;168:1013–17.

3 Leissner J, Black P, Fisch M, Höckel M, Hohenfellner R. Colon pouch (Mainz pouch III) for continent urinary diversion after pelvic irradiation. Urology 2000;56:798–802.

4 Nelson JH. Atlas of Radical Pelvic Surgery. Appleton-Century-Crofts, New York, 1969:181–91.

5 Sagalowsky AI, Frenkel EP. Cobalamin profiles in patients after urinary diversion. J Urol 2002;167:1696–700.

6 Schmidt JD, Buchsbaum HJ, Nachtsheim DA. Long-term follow-up—further experience with and modifications of the transverse colon conduit in urinary diversion. Br J Urol 1985;57:284–8.

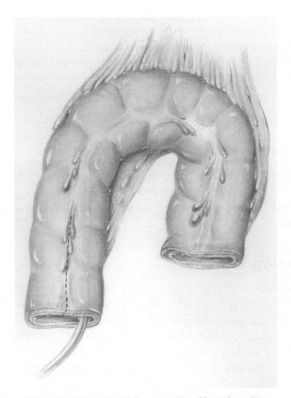

Figure 57.1 About 35–40 cm of nonirradiated large bowel is isolated for pouch formation. The oral end with the indwelling catheter is reserved for the creation of the efferent segment.

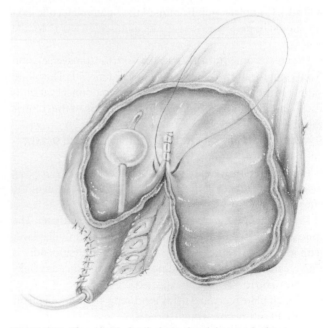

Figure 57.2 The colon is detubularized and the pouch plate is created by running sutures. The aboral end is tapered over an 18 Fr catheter and mesenteric windows are made.

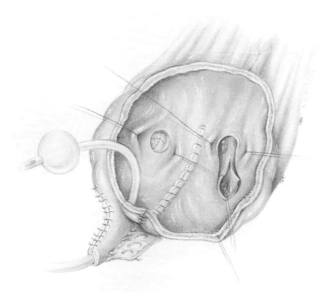

Figure 57.3 Direct ureter implantation.

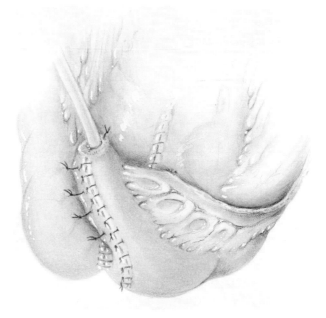

Figure 57.4 The pouch formation is completed. The efferent segment is fixed to the pouch.

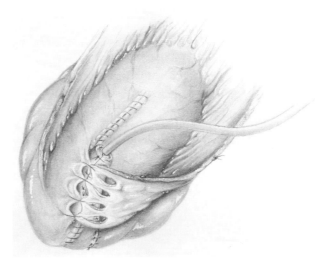

Figure 57.5 The efferent segment is embedded by sutures placed through the mesenteric windows.

Chapter 58
Sigma Conduit

M. Fisch

Indications

The use of a sigma conduit is recommended in children and young adults as an intermediary diversion, with the option of conversion in continent forms of urinary diversion later on. Situations with uncertain outcome (dilated ureters, impaired kidney function) require a temporary zero pressure system (konduit).

Operative technique

• Isolate a 12–15 cm long sigma segment respecting the blood supply.
• Open the isolated segment, longitudinally, for 5 cm instead of the 3 cm used for refluxive implantation.
• Place four stay sutures to mark the tunnel on the back wall on both sides of the mesentery.
• Excise the mucosa.
• Prepare the submucous tunnel 3–4 cm long with small scissors.

• Incise the seromuscular in a cross-like manner on the tip of the underlying finger.
• Pull through the ureter with a flat curved forceps from the retroperitoneum under the serosa of the mesosigmoid inside the bowel.
• Pull through the ureter through the tunnel.
• Observe capillary bleeding and spontaneous urine ejaculation. The ureter has to be resected until capillary arterial bleeding can be demonstrated. No spontaneous urine ejaculation means there is ureter kinking or the tunnel is too narrow (use a magnification lens system to assess).
• Close the oral mucosa window longitudinally with 6/0 Monocryl.
• Incise the ureter at 12 o'clock and shorten the stump to an adequate length.
• Anchor the ureter deep in the seromuscularis with two 5/0 Monocryl sutures at 5 and 7 o'clock.
• Perform an exact mucomucosa anastomosis with 5/0 Monocryl.

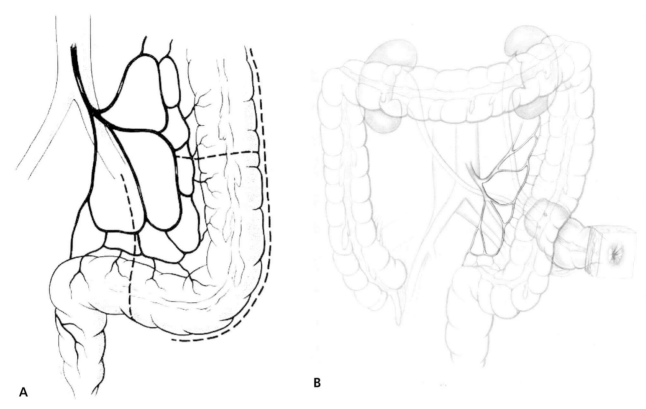

A

B

Figure 58.1 The sigma conduit. (A) Selection of the segment respecting the blood supply. (B) Final view after stoma formation.

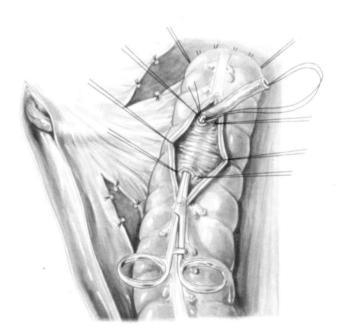

Figure 58.2 The conduit is opened and the right ureter is pulled in submesenterially.

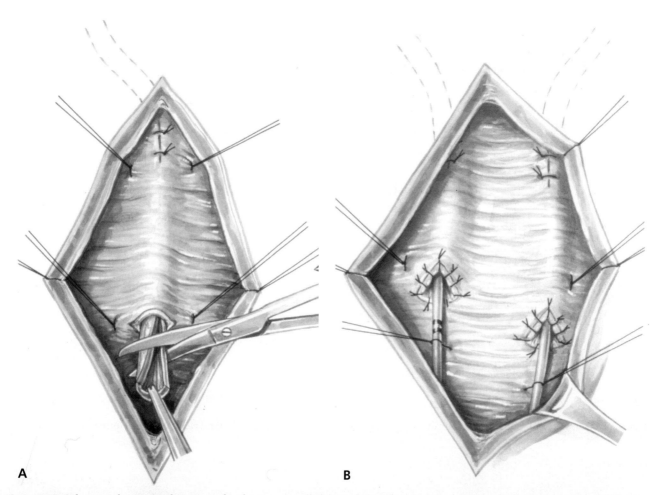

Figure 58.3 Submucosal ureter implantation; after the ureter is pulled through the submucous tunnel, it is cut to its definitive length (A). (B) Completed ureteral implantation.

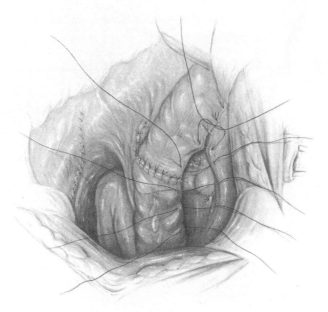

Figure 58.4 The sigma is fixed to retroperitonalize the conduit.

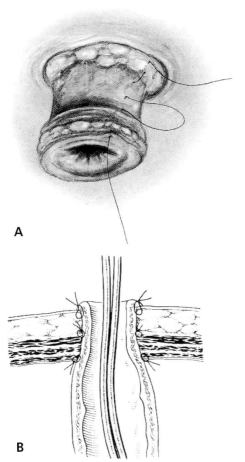

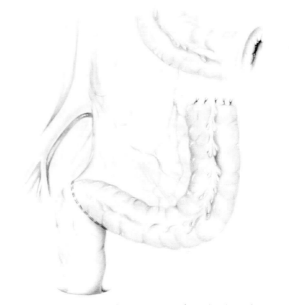

Figure 58.6 The sigma conduit as urinary diversion in vesico-vaginal-rectal fistula (cloaca) with colostomy.

Figure 58.5 Stoma placement. (A) Formation of an everting stoma. (B) Fixation sutures of the stoma.

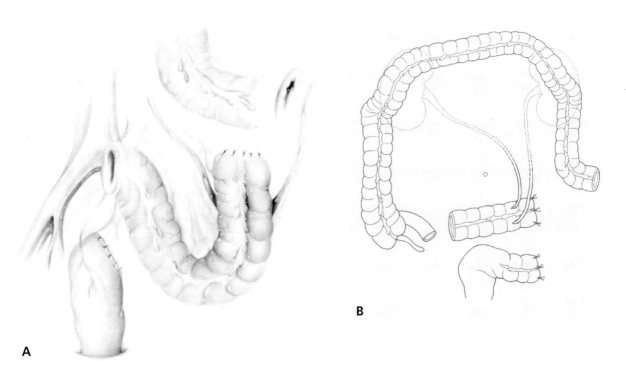

Figure 58.7 The conduit stoma placed on the right side (according to Übelhör): isolation of segment (A). (B) Final view.

Chapter 59
Transverse Conduit

M. Fisch and R. Hohenfellner

Introduction

The transverse conduit is an alternative to the ileal conduit. Its use was first published by Nelson in 1969 [1]. There has been an increase in its use in patients with urologic or gynecological malignoma and adjuvant radiotherapy. Its advantages are many and include the following:

• Cranial position outside the irradiation field so a nonirradiated bowel segment can be used.
• Choice of several segments (ascending, transverse, or descending colon).
• The long mesentery of the transverse colon allows adaptation to each individual situation.
• There is no limitation due to short ureters; adaptation to different lengths of well-vascularized ureteral segments is possible.
• There are various positions for the stomas: either left (use of descending colon) or right (use of ascending colon).
• Isoperistaltic or anisoperistaltic use without consequences.
• Refluxive (adults) and antirefluxive (children) ureteral implantation is possible.
• It is a simple and reproducible technique with a high success rate and a low risk of leakage or bowel obstruction.
• Direct anastomosis to the renal pelvis is possible (pyelo-transverso-pyelocutaneostomy) in patients with a total loss of the ureters after irradiation, in retroperitoneal fibrosis, or in recurrent urothelial tumors in a single kidney ('chimney').
• Access via a supracostal incision is possible in single kidneys.

Indications

• Gynecological/urologic malignomas (also palliative).
• Radiogenic damage of the bowel and distal ureters.
• Incontinence because of radiogenic cystitis.
• Irreparable fistulas (vesicovaginal, recto-vesicovaginal).
• Recurrent retroperitoneal fibrosis/Crohn's disease.
• Unsuccessful high urinary diversion with the need for conversion.
• Recurrent urothelial tumors in a single kidney ('chimney'

with the possibility of direct endoscopic access into the conduit).

Contraindications

• Previous irradiation of the upper abdomen.
• Extensive colon resection.
• Ulcerative colitis.

Limitations and risks

During extensive irradiation, when there is a long mesentery, the ascending, descending, and even transverse colon could be located in the irradiation field.

Operative technique

• Perform a median laparotomy.

Dissection of the ureter

• Identify the ureters at the crossing with the iliac vessels and dissect in the cranial direction.
• Dissect towards the bladder as far as possible.
• The ureters are cut at a level where they show good vascularization (above the the irradiation damage), and there should be bleeding out of the ureteral stump.
• Ligate the stump, and place a stay suture to mark the cranial end.
• Depending on the remaining length of the ureters, it is decided which one can be pulled through retromesenterically to the other side.
• Pull through either the left or right ureter to the opposite side; the retromesenteric entrance should be wide enough and the path of the ureters should be slightly curved in order not to angle or compress it.

Selection of the bowel segment and bowel mobilization

• Select the segment to be used (approximately 15 cm in

length, respecting the course of the vessels), and place stay sutures to outline the segment (Fig. 59.1).
- Mobilize the bowel.
- *Ascending colon*: mobilize the right colonic flexure and separate the greater omentum from the transverse colon over a distance of 10–15 cm, starting on the right side.
- *Descending colon*: mobilize the left colonic flexure and separate the greater omentum from the transverse colon over a distance of 10–15 cm starting on the left side.
- *Transverse colon*: mobilize the right and left colonic flexures and separate the greater omentum from the transverse colon over the whole distance.
- Incise the mesentery lateral to the supplying artery; the arcades are divided between mosquito clamps and are ligated.
- Dissect the fat from the seromuscular layer of the bowel in the area where the segment will be cut; coagulate bleeding vessels.
- Isolate the segment and clean with moist sponges (note that there should be bleeding out of the resection margins).
- Bowel continuity is re-established with a one-layer seromuscular suture (Fig. 59.2).
- Close the mesenteric slit with a running suture.

Ureteral implantation
- Perform a retroperitoneal pull-through of the ureter to the corresponding side (Fig. 59.3).
- The ureter is refluxively implanted (according to Wallace [2]), also in an antidromic manner (Fig. 59.4).
- Position the stoma in the right or left upper abdomen.

Pyelotransverso-pyelocutaneostomy
- Extensive bowel mobilization is needed: the cecum and root of the mesentery are mobilized and Treitz's ligament is dissected.
- The right and left colonic flexures are freed.
- The greater omentum is dissected from the transverse colon and the omental bursa is opened.
- The bowel is exteriorized.
- The ureters are cut at the ureteropelvic junction.
- A 15–30 cm segment of transverse colon is isolated with an adequate blood supply.
- The right renal pelvis is anastomosed end-to-end to the oral end of the conduit by two running sutures (Fig. 59.5); a stent is led out through the conduit before the anastomosis is completed.
- For anastomosis of the left renal pelvis to the conduit, the wall of the conduit is incised at the teniae coli over an adequate length (Fig. 59.6A).
- A stent is inserted into the left kidney; it is then fixed and led out through the conduit.

- End-to-side anastomosis of the renal pelvis and the conduit is achieved with two running sutures (Fig. 59.6B–D).

Positioning and fixation of the conduit
- Fix the conduits retroperitoneally using one or two stitches.
- Close the mesenteric slit with a running suture.
- The colon is fixed from the medial surface to the conduit, thereby ensuring the conduit is extraperitonealized.
- Close the wound.

Tips
- Transilluminating the mesentery with a cold light source reveals the vessels and facilitates the selection of the segment as well as in the preparation of the mesenteric slits.
- When the conduit is positioned on the right side and the left ureter is relatively short, the ureter can be implanted antidromically to the right ureter (like crossed hands of a ballerina). This is applicable for the submucous tunnel technique as well as the Wallace technique.
- The colonic conduit can be peristaltic or antiperistaltic, so the stoma may be positioned in the right or the left upper abdominal quadrant. For anisoperistaltic application, extensive mobilization of Treitz's ligament and the descending part of the duodenum becomes necessary—otherwise, compression of the duodenum by the conduit may result (Fig. 59.7).
- Extraperitonealization of the conduit facilitates revisional surgery as access can be gained by a flank incision starting at the tip of the 11th or 12th rib downwards in a mediocaudal direction. Thus a median laparotomy with extensive bowel mobilization can be avoided. In a single kidney, the primary intervention (creation of the conduit) can be done via a flank incision.

Results
A group of 54 patients with a mean follow-up of 3.3 years (1 month to 10 years) had the following complications:
- Ureteral stenosis: 1.6%.
- Nephrectomy: 3.8%.
- Conduit necrosis: 3.8%.

References
1 Nelson HJ. Atlas of Radical Pelvic Surgery. Appleton-Century-Crofts, New York, 1969.
2 Wallace DM. Ureteric diversion using a conduit: a simplified technique.

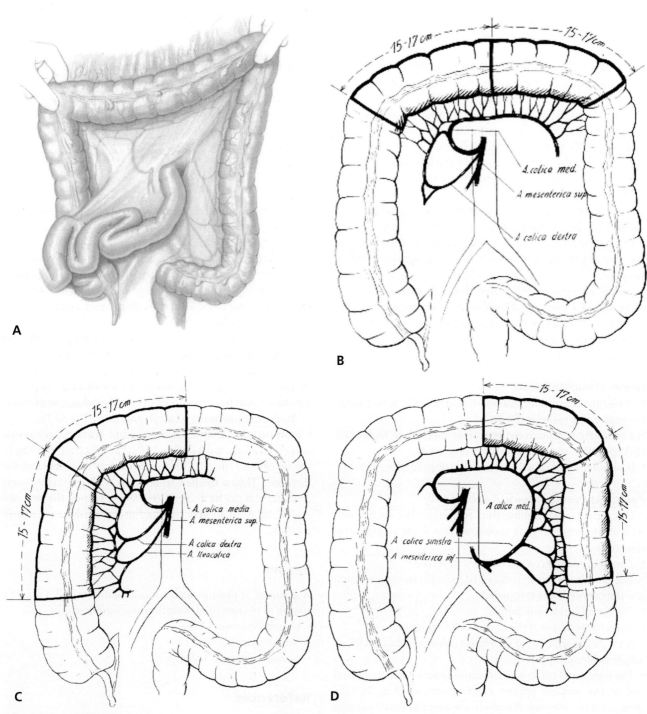

Figure 59.1 Segment selection.

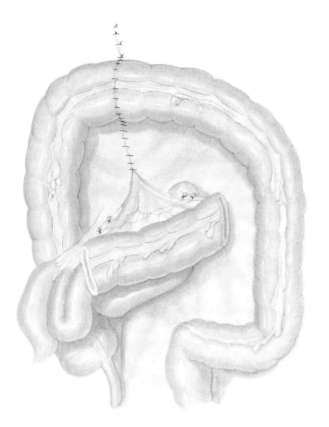

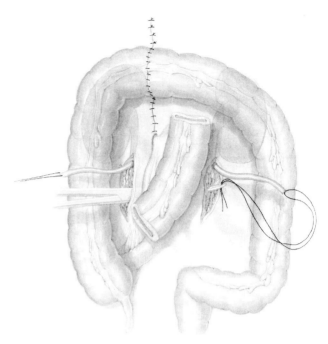

Figure 59.3 The left ureter is brought behind the mesentery to the right side.

Figure 59.2 Bowel continuity is re-established and the mesenteric window is closed.

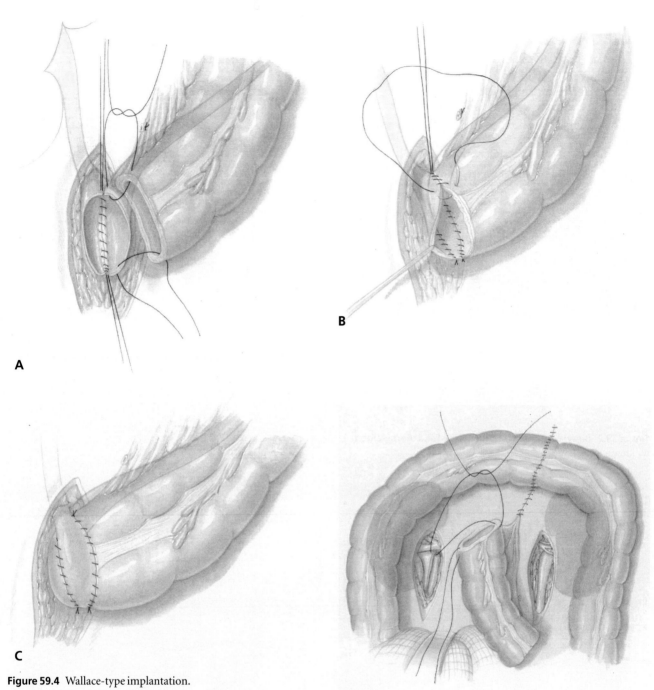

A

B

C

Figure 59.4 Wallace-type implantation.

Figure 59.5 Pyelotransverso-pyelocutaneostomy (right side).

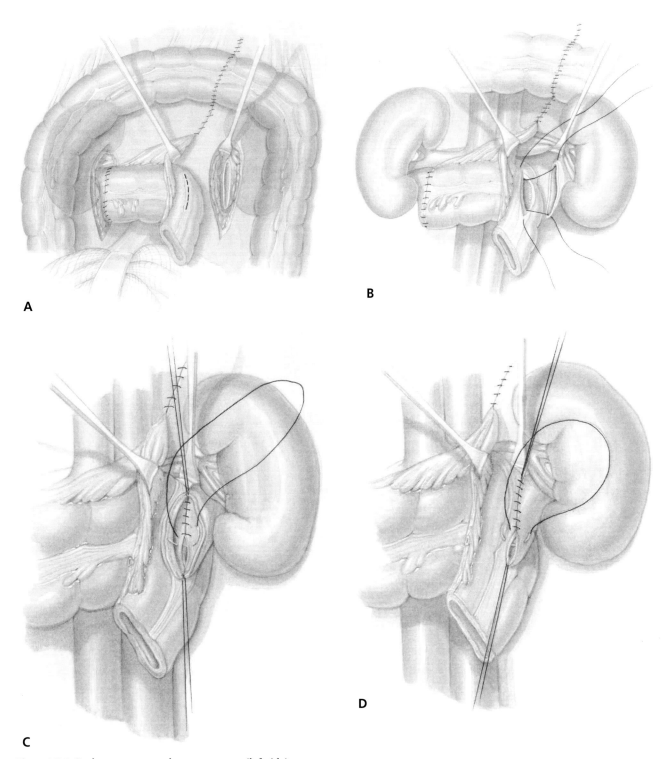

A

B

C

D

Figure 59.6 Pyelotransverso-pyelocutaneostomy (left side).

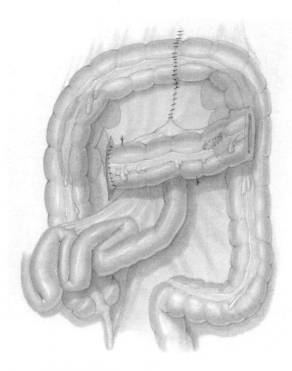

Figure 59.7 The final situation.

Chapter 60
Ureter Substitution

J. Fichtner

Introduction

The author's method of choice in unilateral or bilateral ureter substitution is to use 20–25 cm of colon descendus and sigma in an isoperistaltic 'S-shape' configuration. The technique is easy to perform, demonstrate, and teach. Its advantages include antirefluxive ureter implantation, the terminal ileum is untouched, there is no loop elongation, and there are no nipples.

See Chapter 54 for details of preoperative management, special instruments, operative technique, etc.

Contraindications

- Recurrent panurethelial tumors.
- In fatty immobile mesenterium, change strategy and use small bowel segments instead.

Tips

- Use the retroperitoneal approach; extend the left flank incision in left ureter substitution only.

- In cases of small bladder capacity, combine ureter substitution with bladder augmentation.
- Use antireflux ureter implantation in nondilated ureters and direct refluxive implantation in dilated thick-walled ureters to prevent obstruction.

Postoperative care

Remove the rectal probe on day 5 and the splints on day 8–10. The ureteral catheter should be removed on day 12. Observe residual free voiding before the cystostomy tube is taken out.

Complications

If there is prolonged mucus production, perform intermittent irrigation.

Results

Between 1995 and 2004, in eight patients, unilateral or bilateral ureter substitution was performed successfully. No major complications have been observed.

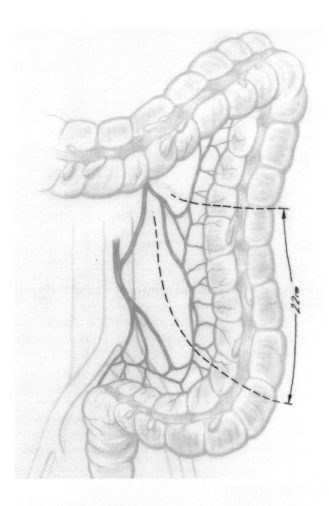

Figure 60.1 The sigma, ascending colon, and splenic flexure are mobilized; 20–25 cm of descending colon are separated; followed by end-to-end anastomosis.

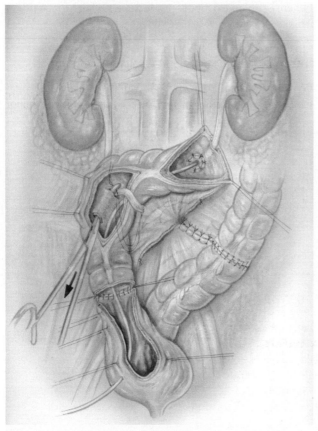

Figure 60.2 The bladder is mobilized and the right-side psoas hitch is completed. An antirefluxive ureter implantation is performed: on the left side using an 'open end' technique and on the right side using the 'buttonhole' technique. Anastomosis of the bowel to the bladder is achieved with interrupted 4/0 Maxon sutures.

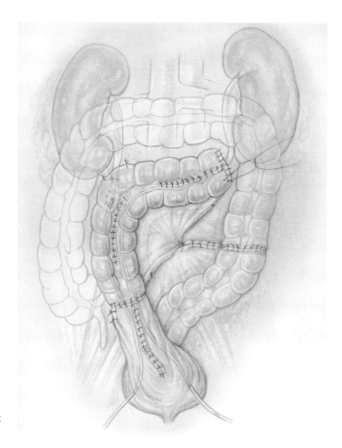

Figure 60.3 The final situation: the segment is fixed retroperitoneally in an S-shaped configuration. The splints and 18 Fr cystostomy are not shown.

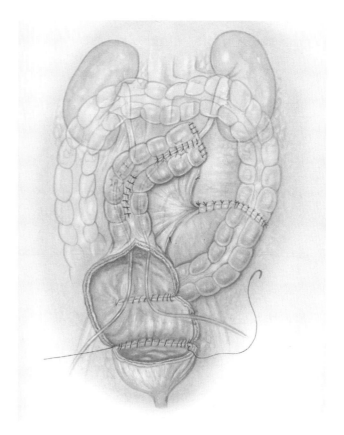

Figure 60.4 Combined ureter substitution and bladder augmentation in a small bladder capacity.

Part 8.2
Stomata in Urology

Chapter 61
Reconstruction of the Umbilicus/Cutaneous Stoma

R. Stein and B. Bräutigam

Introduction

In patients with bladder exstrophy, reconstruction of the umbilicus (e.g. during genital reconstruction or urinary diversion) is a short but, for the patient, important part of the surgery. The reconstructed umbilicus can be used as a continent cutaneous stoma. There are only a few reports in the literature [1–9].

Indications

- Bladder exstrophy.
- Loss of the umbilicus during another operation.
- Continent cutaneous stoma in the lower abdominal wall for catheterization.

Anesthesia

General anesthesia.

Special instruments/suture material

- Eyelid retractor.
- 14–16 Fr Nelaton silicon catheter.
- Suture material: 4/0 to 6/0 Monocryl®.

Operative technique

Reconstruction of the umbilicus

- Mark the position of the umbilicus about a hand's breadth above the line between the spina iliaca anterior and superior, or in small children, 2–3 finger-breadths above this line.
- Make a left semicircular incision of the skin about 2–3 cm from the position of the umbilicue; in patients with adipositis the distance should be longer.
- Use sharp and blunt dissection of the skin flap, leaving a thin layer of subcutaneous tissue intact.
- Insert a 14–16 Fr Nelaton catheter at the 11 o'clock position

into the skin flap and place three or four subcutaneous sutures over the catheter (5/0 Monocryl®).
- Adapt the edges of the skin flap, starting at the deepest point.
- Remove the catheter and fix the deepest point of the skin funnel at the fascia with one or two stitches.
- Close the skin with interrupted sutures (4/0 or 5/0 Monocryl®).

Reconstruction of a continent cutaneous stoma

- After completion of the left semicircular incision, make a cross incision of the fascia and peritoneum.
- Pull through the continence mechanism (e.g. the appendix).
- Insert the catheter in the semicircular skin flap and place three or four subcutaneous sutures over the catheter (5/0 Monocryl®).
- Adapt the edges of the skin flap starting at the deepest point.
- Fix the skin funnel at the continence mechanism with five or six sutures, grasping all layers of the continence mechanism, the fascia, and the skin.
- Close the skin with interrupted sutures (4/0 or 5/0 Monocryl®).

Tips

Careful adaptation of the subcutaneous tissue guarantees a tension-free skin closure with a cosmetically nice scar.

Postoperative care

Remove the dressing on the 3rd postoperative day.

References

1 Cain MP, Rink RC, Yerkes EB, Kaefer M, Casale AJ. Long-term followup and outcome of continent catheterizable vesicostomy using the Rink modification. J Urol 2002;168(6):2583–5.
2 Duckett JW, Lotfi AH. Appendicovesicostomy (and variations) in bladder reconstruction. J Urol 1993;149(3):567–9.

3 Feyaerts A, Mure PY, Jules JA, Morel-Journel N, Mouriquand P. Umbilical reconstruction in patients with exstrophy: the kangaroo pouch technique. J Urol 2001;165(6):2026–7; discussion 2028.

4 Hanna MK, Ansong K. Reconstruction of umbilicus in bladder exstrophy. Urology 1984;24(4):324–6.

5 Hanna MK. Reconstruction of umbilicus during functional closure of bladder exstrophy. Urology 1986;27(4):340–2.

6 Pinto PA, Stock JA, Hanna MK. Results of umbilicoplasty for bladder exstrophy. J Urol 2000;164(6):2055–7.

7 Sozubir S, Ariturk E, Rizalar R, Baris S, Bernay F, Gurses N. A pseudoexstrophy with penile anomaly. Eur J Pediatr Surg 1997;7(1): 55–6.

8 Sumfest JM, Mitchell ME. Reconstruction of the umbilicus in exstrophy. J Urol 1994;151(2):453–4.

9 Tillem SM, Kessler OJ, Hanna MK. Long-term results of lower urinary tract reconstruction with the ceco-appendiceal unit. J Urol 1997;157(4):1429–33.

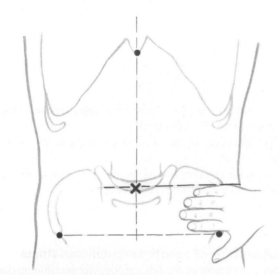

Figure 61.1 Marking the position of the umbilicus.

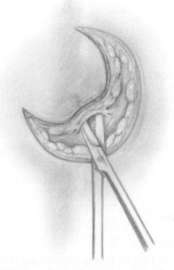

Figure 61.3 Careful sharp/blunt dissection of the skin flap.

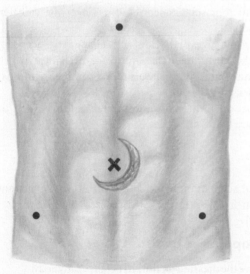

Figure 61.2 Semicircular incision of the skin 2–3 cm away from the marked point.

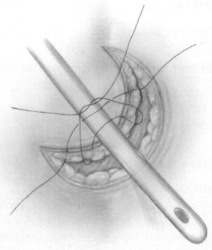

Figure 61.4 Insertion of the Nelaton catheter at the 11 o'clock position.

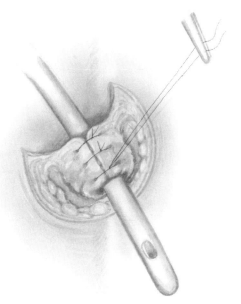

Figure 61.5 Creation of the skin funnel by adaptation of the skin edges starting at the deepest point.

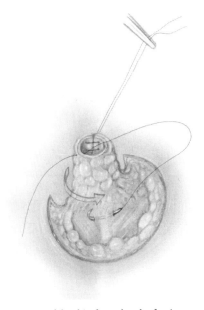

Figure 61.6 Fixation of the skin funnel at the fascia.

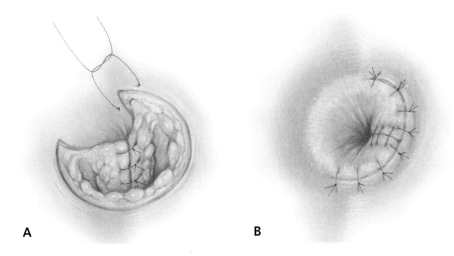

A

B

Figure 61.7 (A) Skin closure with interrupted sutures (4/0 or 5/0 Monocryl®). (B) Final picture.

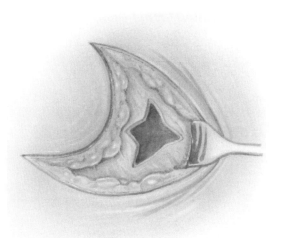

Figure 61.8 Cross-like incision of the fascia and peritoneum.

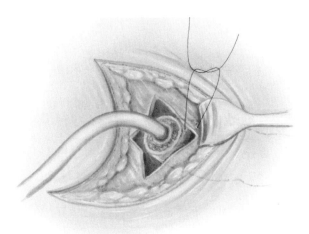

Figure 61.9 Pull through of the continence mechanism and fixation at the fascia.

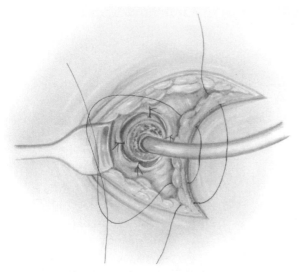

Figure 61.10 Creation of the skin funnel by adaptation of the skin edges, starting at the deepest point.

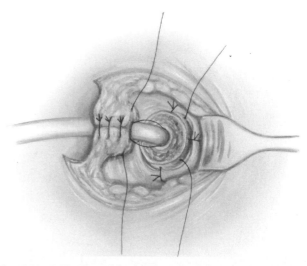

Figure 61.11 Fixation of the skin funnel at the continence mechanism (with 4/0 Monocryl® sutures).

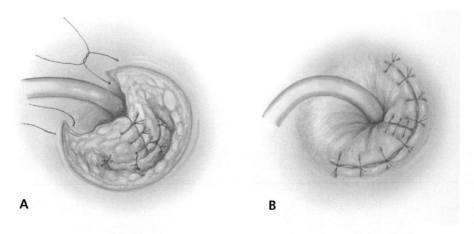

A

B

Figure 61.12 (A) Skin closure with interrupted sutures (4/0 or 5/0 Monocryl®). (B) Final picture.

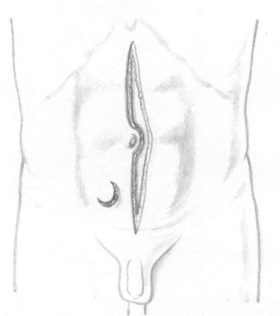

Figure 61.13 Position for a Mitrofanoff stoma.

Chapter 62
Complications of Continent Stomata in Urology

M. Fisch

Introduction

Stoma stenoses occur at different levels. In order to prevent them a vertical 1 cm incision should be made of the umbilical funnel and efferent segment, with subsequent V anastomosis using 4/0 Monocryl (Fig. 62.1).

An open revision is indicated in efferent segment obstruction occurring intraperitoneally (Figs 62.2–62.4). Located at the skin (Fig. 62.5) or at the fascia (Fig. 62.6), a 'Sachse knife incision' will be the first minimal invasive procedure; it is mostly successful and can also be repeated if necessary.

The risk of obstruction increases with the degree of esthetic outcome. An almost invisible stoma located inside the funnel of the umbilicus is at risk of becoming circularly obstructed at skin level. Try treating with a Sachse knife incision first. In recurrent stenoses, a swinging skin flap has turned out to be the method of choice (Figs 62.7–62.10).

Operative technique

- Insert an 8 or 10 Fr Foley catheter.
- Mark the skin incision.
- Incise the scar deep down through the funnel until normal-caliber efferent segment has been reached.
- Mobilize the swinging flap.
- Adapt the tip of the flap on the deepest point of the funnel (using 4/0 or 5/0 Monocryl).
- Change the catheter to a 16 or 18 Fr size.

Tips

- First adapting the flap with untied sutures makes it easier to get the correct position later on.
- The excision of a circular skin strip at the deepest point of the funnel also extends the diameter of the stomal opening.

Postoperative care

The catheter is left in place for 3 weeks until clean intermittent catheterization (CIC) can be started again.

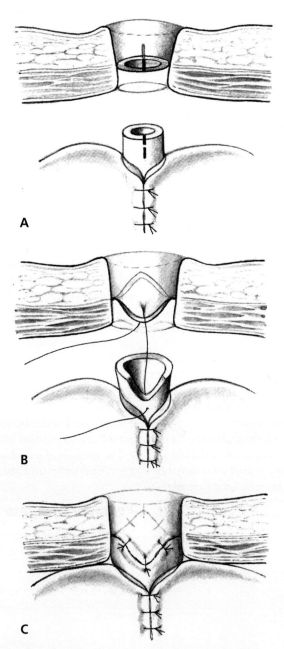

Figure 62.1 To avoid stoma stenosis, a vertical incision of the umbilical funnel (12 o'clock) and efferent segment (6 o'clock) is done (A). Place sutures first (B) and tie later on (C).

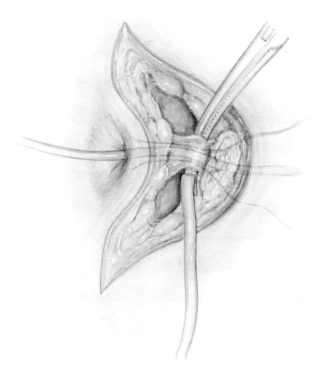

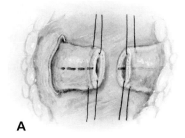

A

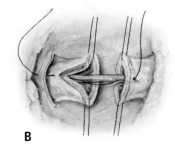

B

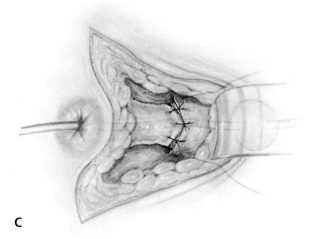

C

Figure 62.2 Circumcision of the umbilicus: arm the efferent segment with a vessel loop.

Figure 62.4 Reanastomosis: the scar is completely excised (A), vertical incisions are made opposite (B) and then tied (C).

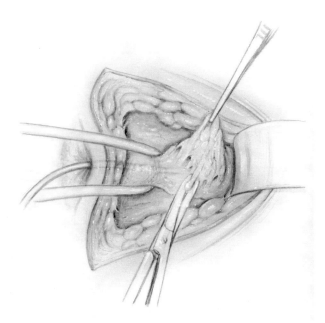

Figure 62.3 The efferent segment is freed from the scar tissue. Be careful of mesenteric vessels.

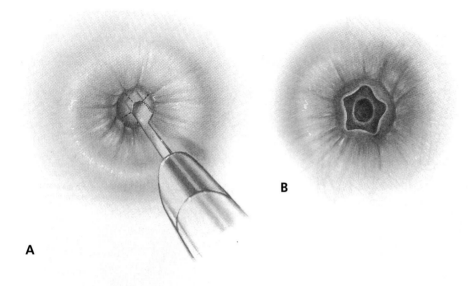

Figure 62.5 Sachse knife incision (A) of the stoma stenosis at the skin level. (B) View after treatment.

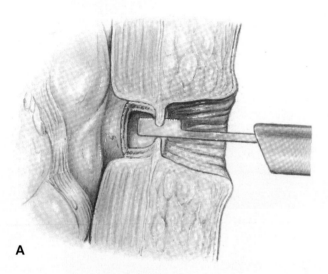

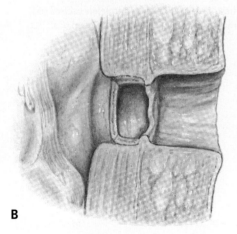

Figure 62.6 Sachse knife incision: lateral view during (A) and after (B) the procedure.

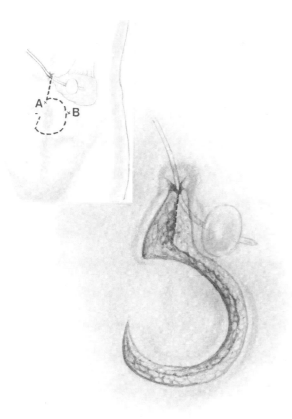

Figure 62.7 Swinging flap: mark the incision line and points A and B before the incision is started.

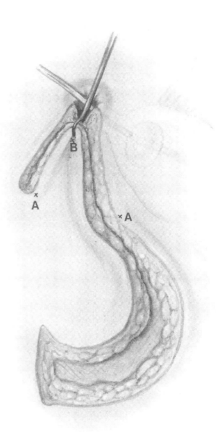

Figure 62.9 Adaptation of swinging flap B to the deepest point of the funnel.

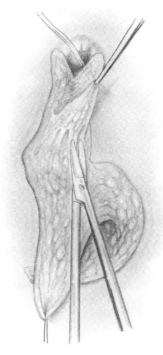

Figure 62.8 Excision of the scar tissue and incision of the funnel. Mobilize the swinging skin flap.

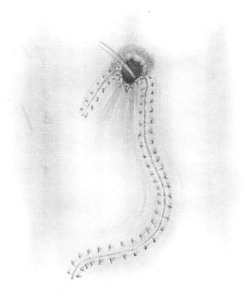

Figure 62.10 Adaptation of the skin with 5/0 Monocryl.

Chapter 63
Complications of Incontinent Stomata in Urology

A. Pycha and M. Lodde

Introduction

Complications are caused by surgical errors and local infections. Common surgical errors include:

- *Stomal location.* Preoperatively, the optimal location should be marked by the stoma therapist (this is especially important in children with neurogenic disorders who will be wheelchair-bound later on). If the stoma is placed too far laterally from the rectus muscle, the abdominal wall innervations (subcostalis, iliohypogastricus, and ilioinguinalis nerves) may be compromised, which results in hernia formation.
- *Stoma construction.* Hernia formation is also observed in extensive separation of the anterior rectus sheet. As the posterior rectus sheet ends above the semilunare line, the lateral fixation of the conduit from inside to the peritoneum becomes important in order to prevent parastomal hernia formation.

A 1.5 cm prominent stoma performed with intracutaneous sutures simplifies postoperative stoma care and avoids 'waterways'.

Loop elongation with kinking of the conduit, residual urine, and upper tract deterioration was first observed in children with ileal conduits. However, long-term observations in adults have demonstrated a similarly high rate of late complications, of up to 80%. Ureterocutaneostomy for palliative urinary diversion may therefore become popular again in the future. For children, young adults, or benign disease, a colon conduit has turned out to be the method of choice.

Local infections, peristomal dermatitis, fistulas, and ulcers with the formation of granulomas may also cause stoma obstruction or retraction later on. Therefore, stoma care by an experienced stoma therapist is as important as stoma construction. The number of early and late complications increases significantly in patients irradiated preoperatively by abdominal external beam (45–65 Gy). It is therefore recommended that bowel segments within the previously irradiated field are avoided.

Indications

- Incarceration of the intestine.
- Problems with urine drainage.
- Limited mobility and quality of life due to dissatisfaction with stoma care.
- Body image problems.

Limitations and risks

- The complexity and length of the operation should not be underestimated.
- Postoperative lung complications often necessitate intensive care supervision.

Preoperative management

- Pulmonary function needs to be optimized, especially in the case of smokers.
- Prepare the intestine with 3–4 L of Endofalk, 1 day prior to surgery.
- The stoma nurse should mark the position of the stoma and possible alternatives.

Special instruments/suture material

- Standard instruments for bowel surgery.
- Supplementary instruments with fine tweezers and scissors.
- Scott retractor.
- Monofilament thread, e.g. 3/0 and 4/0 polyglycolic acid (Maxon).
- 1/0 polytetramethylenadipat (Ethibond).
- Synthetic net, e.g. Ethizip.

Operative technique

Parastomal hernia

- Use a pararectal or flank access.
- Incise the skin, subcutaneous tissue, and fascia. Make sure

there is generous preparation of the fascia from the lateral side to the medial side. Note that the hernia bag filled with the greater omentum or intestine is often situated in the subcutaneous tissue and there is a danger of laceration of the intestine.

- Prepare and separate the hernia bag from the port of entrance; this opens the hernia bag.
- Reposition the contents of the hernia bag (greater omentum, small intestine).
- Resect the hernia bag and close the peritoneum.
- Small defects in the abdominal wall should be closed according to the sandwich technique, following lateral mobilization of the edges:
- perform a running suture of the peritoneum with 4/0 Maxon;
  - position an adapted synthetic net between the peritoneum and the port of entrance surrounding the stoma;
  - close the port of entrance with deep, sweeping, nonabsorbable stitches (1/0 Ethibond);
  - position subcutaneously an adapted synthetic net;
  - close the wound following the positioning of redon drainage.
- Where the defects are larger with no recognizable hernia bag, the stoma should be prepared freely in the form of a half-moon and a synthetic net is inserted into the defect once the lateral cut has been prepared.
- Where the defects are larger and the conduit is sufficiently long, the stoma has to be replaced. A long conduit is a prerequisite in the case of slim patients with large defects. The replacement technique involves:
  - 45° lateral positioning with the flank access extended to the middle and half-moon around the stoma;
  - circular free preparation of the stoma following insertion of a catheter into the conduit (take care not to damage the seromuscularis);
  - spacious preparation of the defect with the opening of the abdominal cavity;
  - adhesiolysis round the conduit and temporary tension-free transfer of the conduit to a cranial or caudal position in respect of the defect;
  - the port of entrance through the rectus muscle must be located at least 6–7 cm away from the defect.
- Once the pulling through of the conduit has been completed, the closure of the defect follows according to the sandwich technique described above.
- Where the conduit is too short, a median laparotomy and repositioning of the conduit is needed.

Stoma prolapse

- Prick through a swab with a two-armed stitch (1/0 Vicryl rapid). The tip of the needle should be protected by the left index fingertip. With this you enter the conduit and once repositioning of the prolapse has been carried out, the outside stitch should be placed out of the area needed for the stoma plate. Repeat the procedure under digital control and knot stitches over a second swab as an abutment.
- After about 2 weeks the stitches will start to be reabsorbed. It is possible for cutaneous stool or urine fistulas to occur as a result but these heal spontaneously.
- In the case of recurrence after the minimally invasive procedure previously outlined or a prolapse and parastomal hernia, open correction is indicated.
- Reposition the prolapse and insert a 20 Fr Foley catheter, blocked with 5–10 mL saline solution.
- Perform circular cutting around the stoma, generous subcutaneous mobilization, and prepare the anterior rectus sheath; the use of a Scott retractor may be helpful.
- Stretching the conduit with stay sutures and the simultaneous pulling of the catheter makes the circular preparation easier. Watch out for lesions of the seromuscular layer and the mesentery of the conduit.
- Position four 3/0 Maxon stitches in a star shape through the seromuscular layer, peritoneum, and posterior rectus sheath; these are finally knotted 'blind'.
- Fix the conduit with 1/0 Ethibond on the anterior rectus sheath. In the case of a conduit being too long, resect up to 3 cm above the level of the skin.
- There should be prominent fixation of the stoma on to the skin with 4/0 Maxon. The stitch should enter subcutaneously to hold the middle part of the seromuscular layer and exit submucously. A stitch through the skin can cause a so-called 'waterway'.
- The Foley catheter should remain unblocked and fixed to the skin for 10 days.

Complications

Intraoperative complications

If there is a bluish color of the conduit, check the following:
- Is the incision of the anterior rectus sheath adequate?
- Is there torsion of the mesentery?
- Is there kinking of the posterior rectus sheath and is the cross-like incision adequate?

Postoperative complications

- *Ischemia and necrosis.* This may result from torsion of the mesentery or port of entrance, or the posterior rectus sheath may be too narrow. If there is limited necrosis, wait and see as there is a chance of spontaneous regeneration from below. If necrosis exceeds the abdominal wall, perform an immediate relaparotomy with new positioning of the stoma.
- *Peristomal infections.* Start with conservative treatment by the stoma therapist. Also consider incision of the abscesses parallel to the adhesive appliance and total excision in cases of phlegmon (with antibiotic protection).
- *Acute intussusception.* The proximal colon may prolapse in the stoma, when there is a risk of incarceration. Manual repositioning often works but is only successful in the short term.

Reintervention is mandatory to resect the hypermobile part of the conduit and to replace the stoma.

References

1 Benson MC, Olsson CA. Cutaneous continent urinary diversion.
In: Campell's Urology, 8th edn, Vol. 4. W.B. Saunders, Philadelphia, 2002:3789–834.

2 Soeder M, Steinbach F, Hohenfellner R. Grundlagen der Stomaversorgung. In: Ausgewählte Urologische OP-Techniken (Hohenfellner R, ed.). Georg Thieme Verlag, Stuttgart, 1997:6.49–6.56.

3 Stomata in der urologie: technik und komplikationen. Akt Urol 2002;33:397–404.

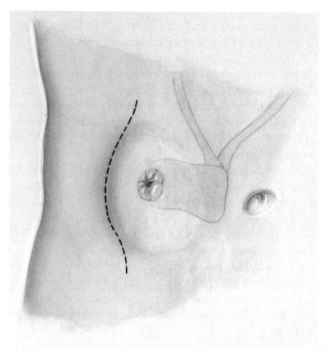

Figure 63.1 Parastomal hernia: pararectal access.

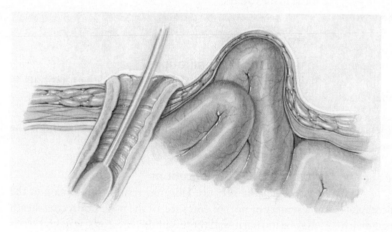

Figure 63.2 Balloon catheter (20 Fr) blocked with 5–10 mL saline solution.

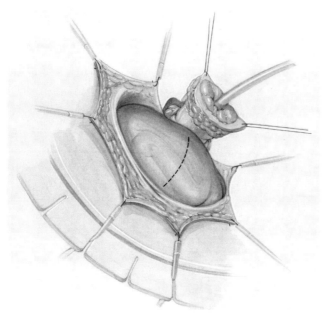

Figure 63.3 Preparation of the hernia bag.

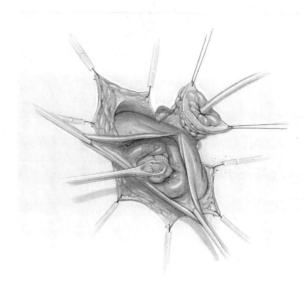

Figure 63.4 Opening of the hernia bag, repositioning of the intestine, and resection of the hernia bag.

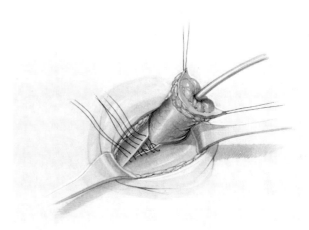

Figure 63.5 After suturing the hernia bag and inner fixation of the conduit, close the anterior rectus sheet with 1/0 Ethibond.

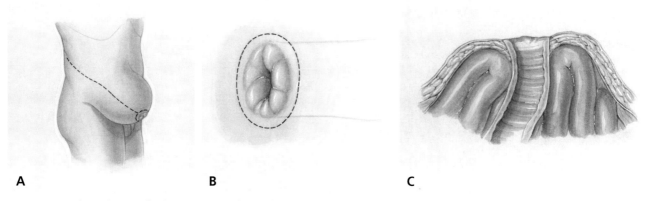

A   B   C

Figure 63.6 In larger hernias, flank access is extended medially, right up to the incision around the stoma.

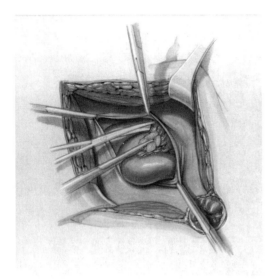

Figure 63.7 Preparation of the hernia bag and opening.

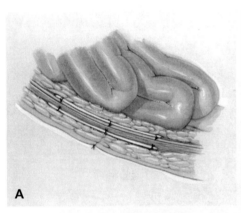

A

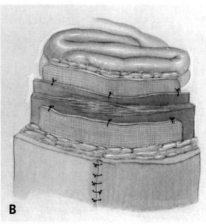

B

Figure 63.8 The sandwich technique after interposition of the big omentum: application of a synthetic net intraperitoneally and for fascia reinforcement. (A) Cross-section; and (B) view from outside.

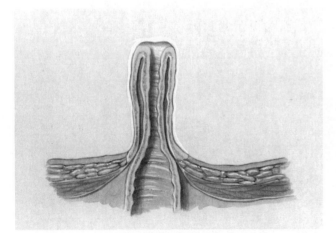

Figure 63.9 A trunk-like stoma prolapse.

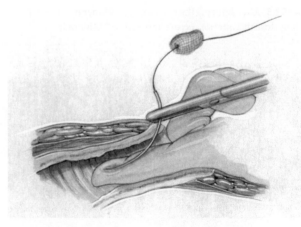

Figure 63.10 In repositioning keep the needle tip under digital control and use a double-armored 1/0 Vicryl rapid stitch.

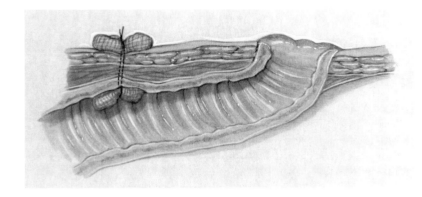

Figure 63.11 Fixation of the conduit over a swab with repeated stitches.

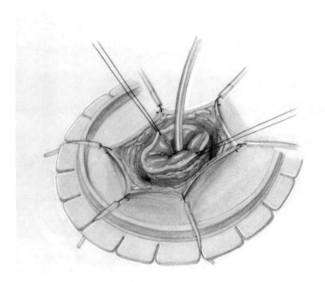

Figure 63.12 For open correction of the prolapse make a circular incision after repositioning, and insert a 20 Fr Foley catheter using a Scott retractor.

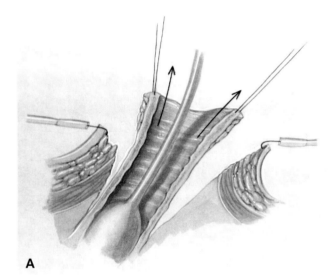

A

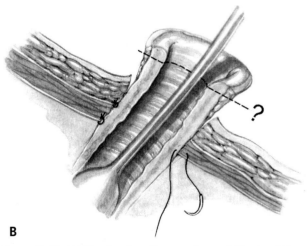

B

Figure 63.14 (A) The situation after complete mobilization. (B) Shortening of the trunk-like prolapse and fixation on the anterior and posterior layer of the rectus sheath.

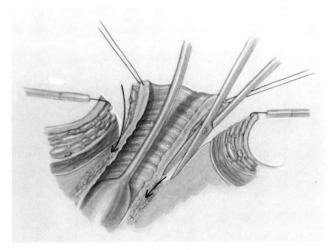

Figure 63.13 Mobilization of the conduit.

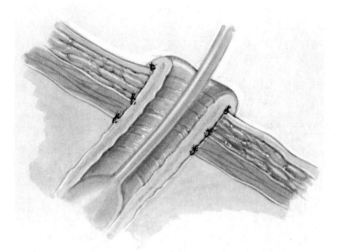

Figure 63.15 Inner fixation of the peritoneum, posterior rectus sheath, and seromuscular layer with 3/0 Maxon, and of the anterior rectus sheath and fascia with 3/0 Ethibond.

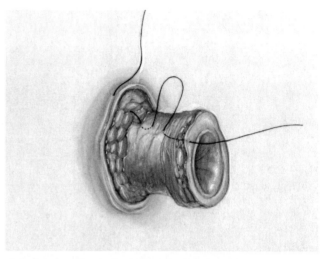

Figure 63.16 After the final resection of the bowel loops, create a slightly prominent stoma.

Section 9
Special Techniques

Chapter 64
Splenectomy for Iatrogenic Splenic Injury

U. Humke, T. Lindenmeir, and M. Ziegler

Introduction

Intraoperative, iatrogenic splenic injury accounts for about 10–24% of all splenectomies worldwide [1,2]. Left-sided transperitoneal nephrectomy in particular is associated with an increased risk for iatrogenic splenic injury (reported incidence 5–21%). Reliable data are missing in the literature for retroperitoneal access to the left kidney, but a certain risk for retractor-induced splenic injury has been postulated.

In general there are two mechanisms that can affect the spleen:
- Direct, sharp preparation of the colonic ligaments with accidental incisional injury of the splenic parenchyma.
- Indirect, blunt tension on the splenic capsule from badly placed retractors may damage the splenic parenchyma and cause significant bleeding.

Sudden intraoperative signs of hemorrhage and destabilization of circulatory parameters should always lead to immediate exploration of the spleen to exclude or consequently treat iatrogenic injury.

Patient counseling and consent

The risk of iatrogenic splenic injury should be explained to the patient before all (open and laparoscopic) transperitoneal operations for left renal tumors, left adrenal tumors, and urinary diversion procedures with the use of transverse or descending colon.

Indications

This procedure is indicated in intraoperative injury of the spleen with local and circulatory signs of hemorrhage. Management follows the classification of splenic injury by Roth *et al.* [4] (Fig. 64.1):
- Stages I and II: conservative management with organ preservation if possible.
- Stages III and IV: in most cases splenectomy is necessary.

Limitations and risks

Organ-preserving surgery carries the risk of recurrent bleeding and should be absolutely avoided for uncomplicated postoperative recovery if the patient is at high risk. If there is a doubt, decide on splenectomy.

After conservative management of a stage I injury, monitor for possible delayed rupture of the splenic parenchyma 10–20 days after the primary injury. In overwhelming postsplenectomy infection (OPSI) syndrome there is fulminant postsplenectomy sepsis with disseminated intravasal coagulation. Mortality rises to 45% [5], caused by splenectomy-related immunologic defects (decreased IgM) combined with infection through either *Streptococcus* pneumonia, *Haemophilus* influenza, or *Neisseria* meningitis—which are most prevalent in children and older adults [3].

Contraindications

There are no contraindications as bleeding from splenic injury can be life-threatening making surgical treatment mandatory.

Preoperative management

Use routine bowel preparation for transperitoneal surgery.

Anesthesia

General anesthesia.

Special instruments/suture material

For splenectomy there are no special instruments needed. Spleen-sparing surgery needs the following:
- Absorbable atraumatic 2/0 and 0/0 sutures.
- Fibrin glue.
- Collagen pads.
- Infrared coagulator or argon beam laser.
- Polyglycolic acid knitted mesh.

Anatomical considerations

Due to embryological development there is a double blood supply to the spleen:

- Blood from the main vessels from the celiac trunk (splenic artery) and to the portal vein (splenic vein), both running close alongside the pancreatic tail, which often reaches the splenic hilum (Fig. 64.2C, D).
- Blood from the short gastric vessels, coming from the great curvature of the stomach, which can fully compensate complete ligature of the main vessels (Fig. 64.2a).

Splenic ligaments fix the spleen (splenocolic and splenorenal ligaments, which are vulnerable to splenic injury) and contain the vessels (splenogastric and splenodiaphragmatic ligaments) (Fig. 64.2A–C).

Operative technique

- First of all, the splenic injury needs to be staged (Fig. 64.1).
- Place the retractors carefully to make the spleen visible.
- Remove blood, with manual compression of the hilar splenic vessels or compression of the injured parenchyma with hot towels to stop the bleeding; get control and an overview.
- Make a decision for repair of the injury or splenectomy.

Splenectomy

- A normal-sized spleen should be dorsally excised.
- Follow the steps detailed in Fig. 64.2.
- Remove the organ, and oversew any small bleeders.
- Oversew the greater curvature of the stomach with single sutures.
- Close the retroperitoneum.
- Place drainage if necessary.

Repair of splenic injury

- For small parenchymal injuries, use single parenchymal sutures, only slightly tightened (Fig. 64.3B).
- For deep parenchymal injuries, use coagulation of the parenchyma with an argon beam laser or infrared coagulator. Digital compression of the parenchyma stops bleeding while coagulating. Alternatively, or in addition, apply a polyglycolic acid knitted mesh for permanent compression.
- Injuries of the lower or upper pole of the spleen are suitable for partial resection (Fig. 64.4).
- Placement of drainage after reconstructive surgery is strongly recommended.
- Autotransplantation of splenic tissue is rarely used to maintain immunologic function after splenectomy—mostly in children—although its efficacy is not proven. The splenic parenchyma is sharply cut into pieces of 60–80 g. The pieces are wrapped in an omentum flap and are fixed with sutures in the former position of the spleen.

Tips

- It is most important to manually compress the parenchyma or hilar vessels to stop bleeding, to remove blood, and to clearly expose and stage the splenic injury.
- Place a nasogastric tube for easier definition of the greater curvature of the stomach.
- Use small step dissection of the smaller gastric vessels alongside the greater curvature to avoid the risk of clamping and/or ligating part of the stomach wall (fistula formation!).
- Do not use blind clamping of the hilar splenic vessels as there is a risk of a clamp injury of the pancreatic tail and adrenal injury with consecutive bleeding, pancreatitis, and the formation of pancreatic pseudocysts.
- Always ligate the splenic artery and vein close to the splenic hilum; there is a risk of pancreatic ischemia if the ligation is too close to the celiac trunk.

Postoperative care

- Perform ultrasonography on day 2 and 5.
- Remove drainage on day 2.
- Start oral feeding on day 2.
- After a splenectomy, give antibiotic prophylaxis with penicillin and the administration of pneumococcal polysaccharide vaccine [1].

Complications

- *Recurrent bleeding* (2%): this is the most important complication. It occurs with subphrenic hematoma or abscess formation with lower pulmonary atelectasis.
- *Intraoperative gastric, pancreatic, or adrenal injury*: repair with atraumatic sutures immediately. There is a risk of fistula formation.
- *Thrombocytosis*: use routine thrombosis prophylaxis (stockings, mobilization) and heparin. If the thrombocytes exceed 800,000–1,000,000/mm^3 some authors recommend aggregation inhibitors or cumarine until there is normalization of the thrombocyte count.
- *OPSI syndrome*: strictly follow the protocol for fever and leucocytosis, with antibiotic treatment.

Troubleshooting

In cases of significant persistent or recurrent bleeding after reconstruction of the spleen, perform an immediate or secondary splenectomy, whenever symptoms occur. Do not risk excessive blood loss and coagulopathy.

To do

- Think of the spleen while operating in the left upper abdomen or close to the left kidney.

- Remind your assistant of the spleen while handling retractors in this area.
- Avoid retractors in this area whenever possible.
- Carefully inspect the spleen if injury is supposed.
- Always place an intraperitoneal drainage tube after reconstruction of the spleen; after splenectomy it is optional.
- Be aware of possible postoperative clinical signs due to complications of the pancreas or stomach.

Not to do

- Do not ignore even slight, permanent bleeding of unclear origin in the left upper abdomen.
- Avoid blind positioning of retractors in the left upper abdomen.
- Do not leave behind reconstructed spleen if it is obviously still bleeding.

References

1 Cooper CS, Cohen MB, Donovan JF. Splenectomy complicating left nephrectomy. J Urol 1996;155:30–6.
2 Da SE, Pereiro AM, Pereiro AB, Ferreira CC, Pesqueira SD, Zungri TE. Iatrogenic splenectomy in surgery of renal tumours. Actas Urol Esp 1997;21:476–9
3 Meekes I, van der Staak F, van Oostrom C. Results of splenectomy performed on a group of 91 children. Eur J Pediatr Surg 1995;5:19–22.
4 Roth H, Daum R, Benz G. Stadieneinteilung der Milzruptur — chirurgische Konsequenzen im Kindesalter. Chirurg 1986;57: 194–7.
5 Waghorn DJ, Mayon WR. A study of 42 episodes of overwhelming post-splenectomy infection: is current guidance for asplenic individuals being followed? J Infect 1997;35:289–9

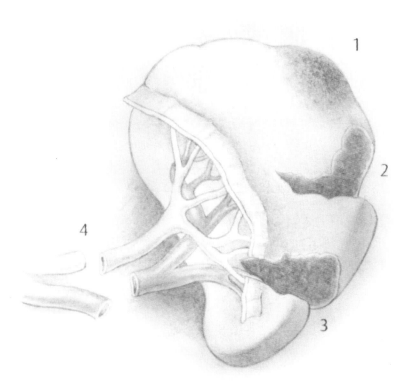

Figure 64.1 Classification of splenic injury (Roth *et al.* 1986 [4]): 1, stage I: subcapsular hematoma; 2, stage II: extrahilar parenchymal rupture; 3, stage III: intrahilar transparenchymal rupture; 4, stage IV: complete disruption of the hilar vessels.

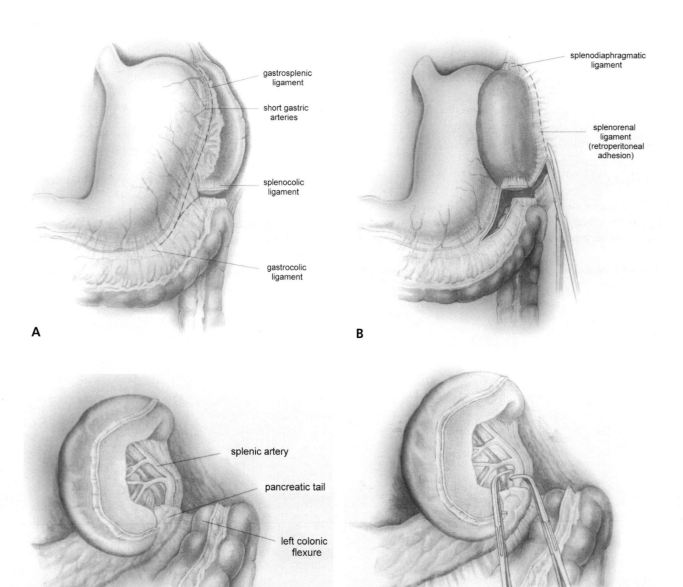

A

- gastrosplenic ligament
- short gastric arteries
- splenocolic ligament
- gastrocolic ligament

B

- splenodiaphragmatic ligament
- splenorenal ligament (retroperitoneal adhesion)

C

- splenic artery
- pancreatic tail
- left colonic flexure

D

Figure 64.2 The technique of splenectomy. (A) Dissection of the splenocolic and gastrocolic (in part) ligaments to detach the colonic flexure, and dissection of the gastrosplenic ligament with careful stepwise ligation of the short gastric arteries. (B) Retraction of the spleen medially and incision of the retroperitoneal fold 1–2 cm lateral to the splenic parenchyma alongside the splenorenal ligament. (C) Further luxation of the spleen medially and exposition of the splenic artery and vein dorsally in the splenodiaphragmatic ligament. Note identification of the pancreatic tail. (D) Separate clamping, dissection, and ligation of the splenic artery and vein distally to the pancreatic tail, with further dissection of the splenodiaphragmatic ligament.

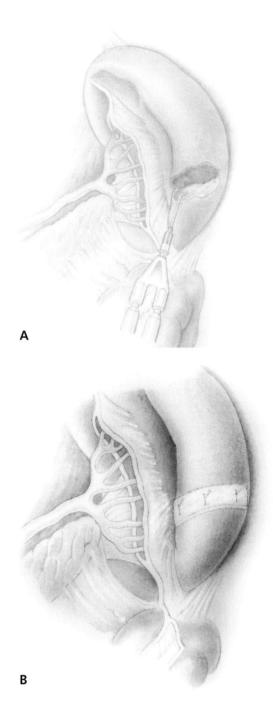

A

B

Figure 64.3 Management of stage II splenic injury. (A) Application of fibrin glue on the ruptured parenchyma (with or without preceeding coagulation). (B) Compression of the ruptured parenchyma, application of a collagen pad covering the ruptured capsule, and fixation with single parenchymal sutures.

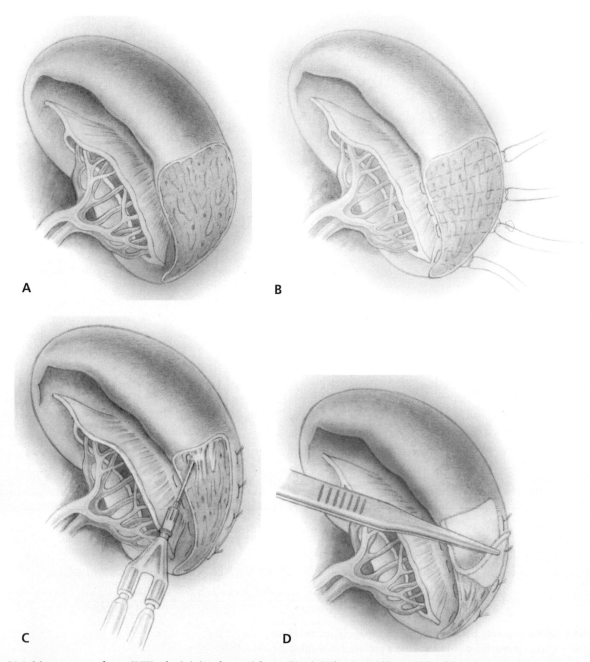

Figure 64.4 Management of stage II/III splenic injury by partial resection. (A) The resected lower pole of the spleen after coagulation (argon beam laser or infrared). (B) Placement of U-shaped single parenchymal sutures passing the splenic capsule. (C) Tying the parenchymal sutures with slight tissue compression and application of fibrin glue. (D) Application of a collagen pad.

Chapter 65
Mobilization of the Liver

C. G. Stief and W. F. A. Hiller

Introduction

Mobilization of the liver is used to adequately expose large right-sided adrenal tumors or extensive cranial recurrent renal cell carcinoma. It is also used in extirpation of renal tumors with intravenous extension ('tumor thrombus') cranial to the (right) renal vein.

Patient counseling and consent

Patients should be warned of the risk of lesions of the liver with possible severe bleeding and/or bile fistula. There is also a risk of excessive blood loss in cases of intravenous neoplastic extension infiltrating the vena cava.

Indications

• Large adrenal tumors.
• Cranial recurrent renal cell carcinoma.
• Renal tumors with infradiaphragmatic, intravenous neoplastic extension into the caval vein cranial to the (right) renal vein.

Anesthesia

General anesthesia.

Special instruments/suture material

A laparotomy set and large frames (Sieber frame or similar) are needed.

Operative technique

• Cut the round ligament of the liver.
• Cut the ligamentum falciforme hepatis.

Mobilization of the right liver lobe

• Dissect the adhesions at the lower margin of the liver between the liver and Gerota's fascia.
• Cut the right triangular and falciform ligaments of the liver and perform step-by-step mobilization of the right liver lobe while the assistant carefully retracts the liver ventrally to the left.
• Dislocate the right liver lobe, if necessary severing the ligamentum venae cavae immediately caudal to the entry of the right hepatic vein and demonstration of the retrohepatic inferior caval vein, while taking care to protect the smaller accessory hepatic veins supplying the caval vein.

Mobilization of the left liver lobe

• Dissect the hepatogastric ligament.
• Sever the left triangular ligament of the liver and mobilize segments II and III.

Tips

• Place the patient in the hyperlordosis position.
• Perform a transverse upper abdominal laparotomy plus a median extension cranially ('Mercedes star').

Postoperative care

No specific drains or blood tests are necessary for liver mobilization. If the pancreas was involved, check the serum for amylase and lipase (reactive pancreatitis).

Complications

• During mobilization of the liver, parenchymal lacerations may occur. These are due particularly to inadequate freeing of adhesions at the lower liver margin as well as excessive pull.
• Smaller superficial lesions can be controlled with bipolar electrocoagulation.
• More extensive and deeper hepatic lesions require a specific

suture ligation of the vessel involved (4/0 Prolene). Nonspecific, penetrating sutures are to be avoided.

To do

- Place the patient in the hyperlordosis position.
- Use a self-retracting system.
- Operate with two assistants.
- Use bipolar scissors for dissection.
- Be prepared for a total vascular occlusion of the liver in large tumors by exposing and securing the suprahepatic and infrahepatic caval veins and the liver hilum.

Not to do

- Do not put too much traction on the liver when mobilizing it.
- If clamping of the liver hilum is required (Pringle's maneuver) due to excessive bleeding from injuries to the liver or from the liver veins, in cases where a cavotomy has been done and vascular clamping is insufficient, ischemia should not exceed 30–40 min in a healthy liver.
- Avoid Pringle's maneuver in cases of liver cirrhosis.

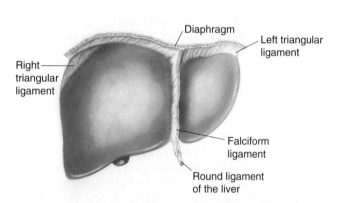

Figure 65.1 Ventral view of the liver

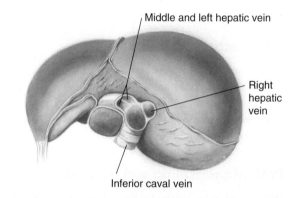

Figure 65.3 Cranial view of the liver.

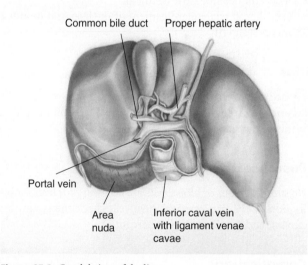

Figure 65.2 Caudal view of the liver.

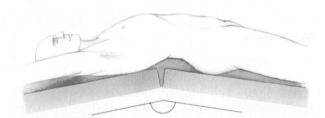

Figure 65.4 Position the patient in hyperlordosis.

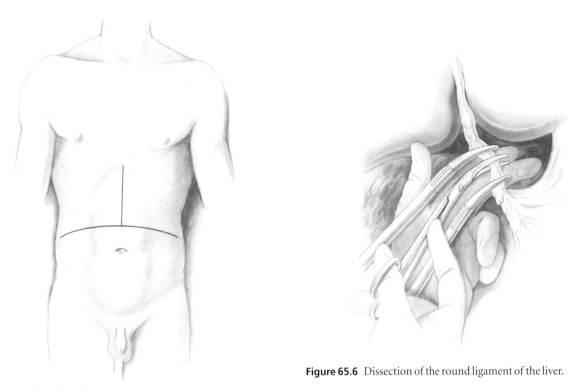

Figure 65.6 Dissection of the round ligament of the liver.

Figure 65.5 Line of incision.

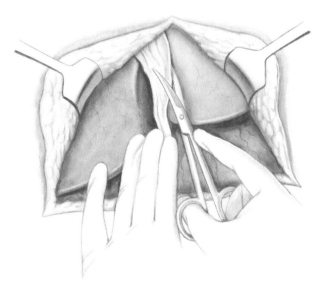

Figure 65.7 Dissection of the falciform ligament.

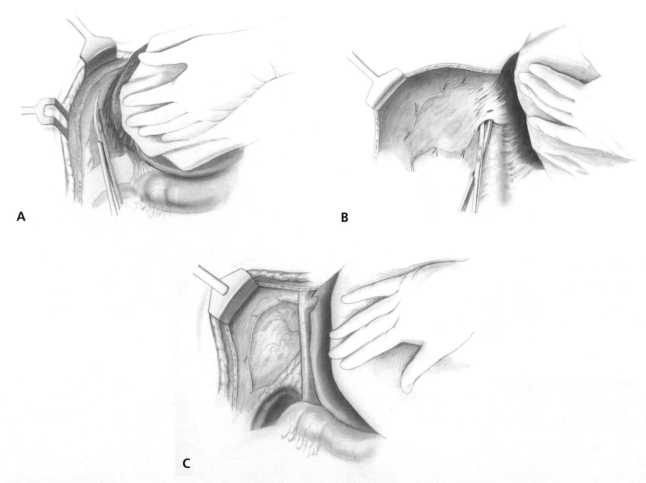

Figure 65.8 (A) Retraction of liver to the left ventral, (B) severance of the right triangular ligament, and (C) step-by-step mobilization of the right liver lobe.

Chapter 66

Surgical Repair of Large Vessel Injuries during Retroperitoneal Surgery

W. Schmiedt, M. Fisch, and R. Wammack

Introduction

The accidental injury of large vessels during surgical interventions is not rare and its incidence is about 7% during radical gynecological interventions (Wertheim Meigs) or in retroperitoneal lymphadenectomy (testicular cancer) [1]. Most of these are minor injuries that can be sutured without increased blood loss or postoperative morbidity. However, there is an increased incidence of major injuries in retroperitoneal tumor surgery (Wilms' tumor, neuroblastoma), in patients who have had previous irradiation, and in 'bulky disease' [2–4].

After chemotherapy the dissection plane between the tumor and the vessel wall is missing, thus leading to 'dissection underneath the adventitia'. Postoperative ruptures of the aorta due to lesions of the adventitia have been described [4]. In a series of 710 patients who had previously had chemotherapy, and were now undergoing retroperitoneal lymphadenectomy, 10 patients (1.4%) needed replacement of the aorta (seven intraoperatively, three postoperatively) [4]. The incidence of major injuries in clinical stages B2 and C of testicular cancer is even higher (6.2%) [5]. In another series of retroperitoneal lymphadenectomy procedures, the complication rate was 100% ($n = 103$) [6].

An aortoenteric fistula represents another severe complication leading to death [4].

The repair of vessel injuries encompasses primary control of the bleeding (done by the surgeon of primary intervention) and vascular surgery (done by the vascular surgeon).

Temporary control of bleeding (Figs 66.1–66.13)

- In arterial bleeding, use digital compression and tangential placement of a Satinsky clamp under vision.
- The 'blind' placement of clamps is risky (injury to the surrounding tissue or the vascular wall).
- Complete clamping of the aorta is only done in major longitudinal, horizontal, or complete ruptures (often after chemotherapy/irradiation). The level of complete clamping is proximal and distal to the injury (there may be remaining minor bleeding from the lumbar arteries).
- In difficult anatomical situations, insufficient access, or bad exposure, insert a balloon catheter for temporary closure of the vessel (Fig. 66.6).
- In cases with insufficient control of bleeding, use subdiaphragmal clamping of the aorta (perform an access anteriolateral thoracotomy: excellent exposure, fast, and simple approach to the aorta).
- Venous lesions are more difficult to repair despite the lower intravascular pressure. Control the bleeding with manual compression proximal and distal to the lesion (Fig. 66.3).

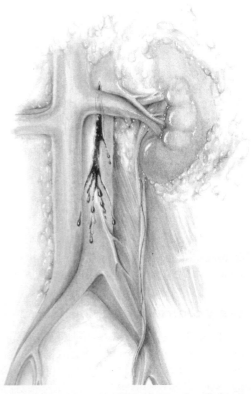

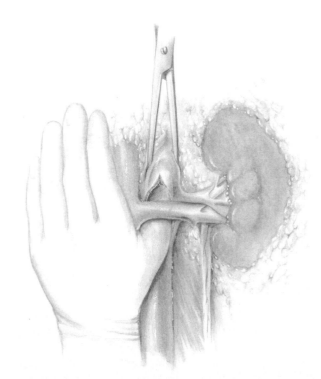

Figure 66.3 If exposure is bad due to severe bleeding, the surgeon's thumb occludes the aortic lumen until a straight vascular clamp is positioned at the suprarenal aorta.

Figures 66.1–66.13 Repair of injuries to the abdominal aorta.

Figure 66.1 Irregular rupture of the anterior aortic wall up to the level of the left renal vein.

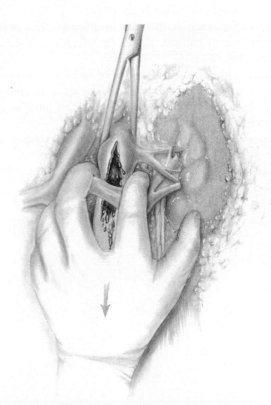

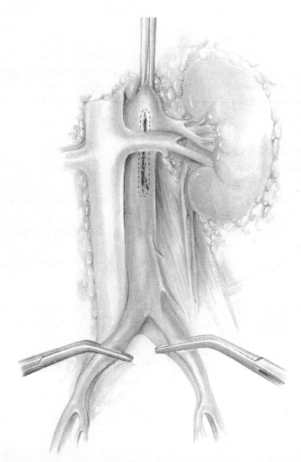

Figure 66.2 In direct clamping of the suprarenal aorta, the surgeon's hand is keeping the renal vein downwards and the vena cava laterally.

Figure 66.4 Additional clamping of the aorta is needed distal to the injury.

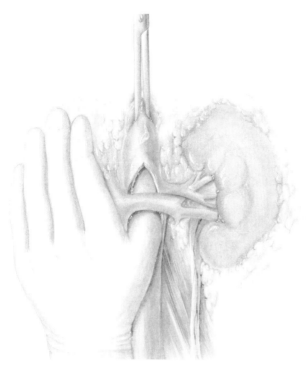

Figure 66.5 If the rupture extends cranial to the branch of the renal artery, then clamping of the aorta above the branch of the superior mesenteric artery may be possible in selected cases.

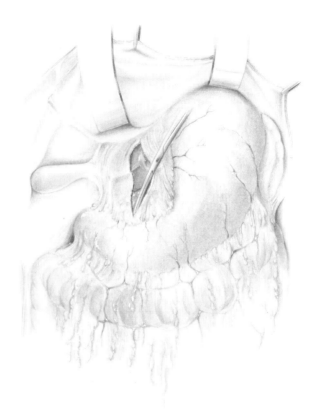

Figure 66.7 When clamping the aorta distal to the diaphragm, retract the left liver lobe.

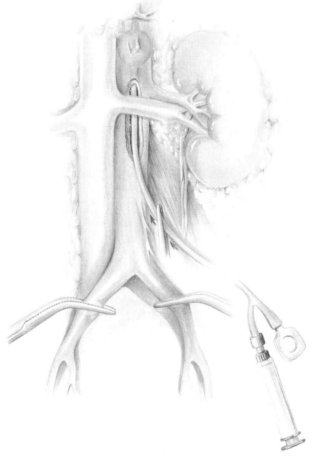

Figure 66.6 If a vascular clamp cannot be placed, bleeding is controlled by the insertion of a balloon catheter; in an emergency situation even a bladder catheter can be used.

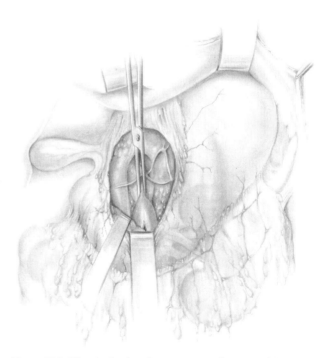

Figure 66.8 Then incise the minor omentum, being careful to avoid injuring the esophagus.

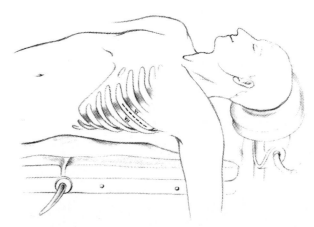

Figure 66.9 When clamping the intrathoracic aorta, perform a left-sided anterolateral thoracotomy between the sixth and seventh rib.

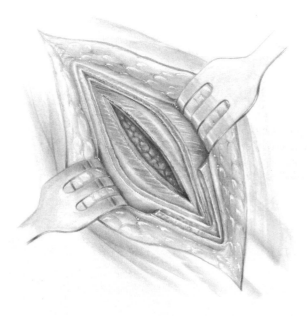

Figure 66.11 Distraction of the anterior serratus muscle along its fibers and incision of the intercostal musculature close to the upper border of the rib.

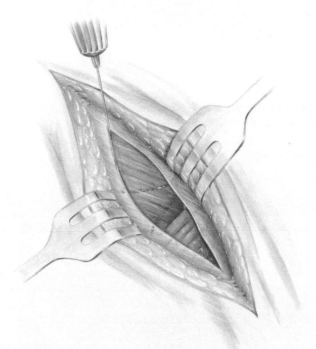

Figure 66.10 Incision of the subcutaneous tissue and the thoracic fascia.

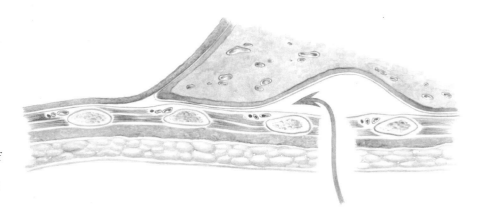

Figure 66.12 During blind dissection of the layer between the thoracic wall and the lung, the lung is moved cranially and medially, and a rib retractor is inserted.

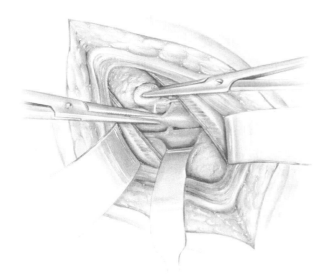

Figure 66.13 Incision of the parietal pleura above the aorta and clamping of the aorta cranial to the diaphragm, respecting the vagal nerve.

Vascular surgery (Figs 66.14–66.17)

- Options include:
  - direct vascular sutures;
  - reconstruction with a 'patch' plasty;
  - replacement by transplants (interposition of vascular prosthesis).
- Method of choice: direct sutures (best postoperative results) [7].
- Transplantation of a patch (Dacron): this approach is used if vascular sutures lead to a narrowing of the lumen.
- Vascular prosthesis: used for major wall injuries or defects [7].

Special instruments/suture material

- Atraumatic vascular clamps of different sizes and angulations (Pean, Roberts, and Satinsky clamps with De Bakey teeth).
- Vascular clips (Mueller and bulldog clamps).
- Retractors (rib retractor such as the Finochietto or Mercedes thoracic retractor).
- Direct vascular sutures: resorbable monofilament suture material (e.g. polydioxanone, polyglycaprone).
- Ligation of vessels: polyglycolic acid, polyglyconate, or polyglactin.
- Alloplastic replacement: nonabsorbable suture material such as polypropylene.

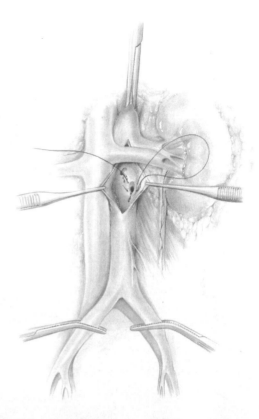

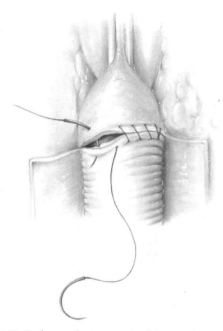

Figure 66.16 End-to-end anastomosis of the anterior aortic wall is performed with the Dacron prosthesis.

Figures 66.14–66.17 Surgical repair of vessel injuries.
Figure 66.14 The branches of the lumbar arteries are sutured.

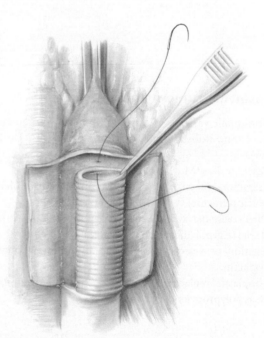

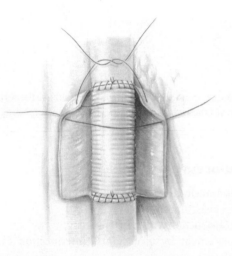

Figure 66.17 The original vascular wall is closed in front of the prosthesis. Additional coverage with tissue (fat, peritoneum) as interposition between the duodenum and the prosthesis is advantageous.

Figure 66.15 The aorta is replaced with a Dacron prosthesis. Anastomosis of the posterior aortic wall with the posterior wall of the prosthesis is done using a nonabsorbable double-armed suture (e.g. Prolene). To avoid loosening of the intima plaques, the stitch is placed in-to-out.

Operative technique

See Figs 66.18–66.23.

Tips

To avoid aortoenteric fistulas, tissue (greater omentum, retroperitoneal fat, or peritoneum) should be interposed between the aorta and duodenum, especially in simultaneous lesions of the vascular adventitia and seromuscularis of the bowel.

To do

• First control the bleeding, then repair the injury.
• If after aortic injury exposure is bad, then clamp the aorta at a higher level (inferior to the diaphragm or cranial (thoracotomy)).

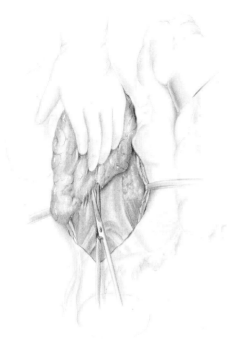

Figure 66.19 After previous chemotherapy, a dissection plane between the tumor and the vascular wall is lacking.

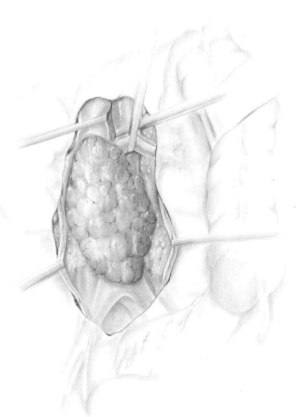

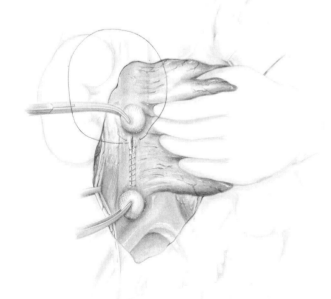

Figures 66.18–66.23 Surgical repair of injuries to the vena cava.
Figure 66.18 'Bulky disease' in a patient with testicular cancer: a large retroperitoneal tumor is attached to the major vessels; vessel loops are placed around the proximal and distal vena cava and aorta, as well as the renal vessels.

Figure 66.20 For rupture of the vena cava and to achieve good exposure, compress the vena cava distally and proximally to the injury and use a continuous suture.

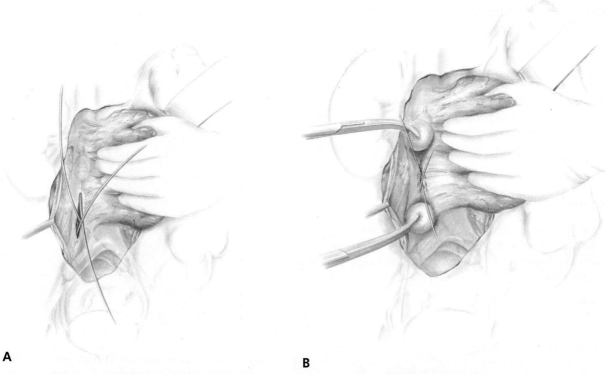

A

B

Figure 66.21 Access to the vena cava is limited by the tumor and further mobilization of the tumor may enlarge the venous injury. (A) Primary control of the bleeding is done by compression of the vena cava. (B) Insertion of an occlusive catheter, which is deflated and removed immediately before the suture is accomplished.

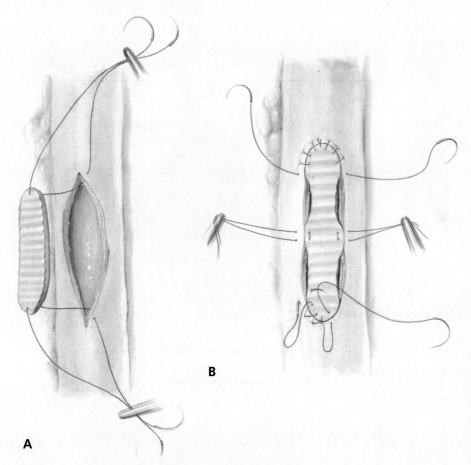

B

A

Figure 66.22 A Dacron or autologous venous patch is used when the defect is so large that simple suturing will lead to narrowing of the lumen. Nonabsorbable suture material (4/0 or 5/0 Prolene, double-armed) is used, with the direction of the stitch in-to-out.

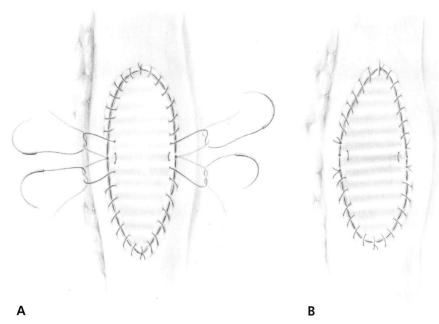

A   **B**

Figure 66.23 Flush the vessel with heparin solution before anastomosis with the patch is accomplished; minor bleeding through the stitch canals stops after compression for several minutes.

Not to do

- Do not suture or place the clamps blindly.
- In venous injuries do not use a narrowing suture (risk of postoperative thrombosis); instead use patching.

References

1 Palfalvi L, Bosze P, Ungar L. Vascular injuries in the surgical management of gynaecological malignancies. Eur J Surg Oncol 1993;19:601–3.

2 Donohue JP, Thornhill JA, Foster RS, Bihrle R. Vascular considerations in postchemotherapy retroperitoneal lymph-node dissection: part I — vena cava. World J Urol 1994;12:182–6.

3 Baniel J, Foster RS, Rowland RG, Bihrle R, Donohue JP. Complications of postchemotherapy retroperitoneal lymph node dissection. J Urol 1995;153:976–80.

4 Donohue JP, Thornhill JA, Foster RS, Bihrle R. Vascular considerations in postchemotherapy retroperitoneal lymph-node dissection: part II. World J Urol 1994;12:187–9.

5 Kelly R, Skinner D, Yellin AE, Weaver FA. En bloc aortic resection for bulky metastatic germ cell tumors. J Urol 1995;153:1849–51.

6 Christmas TJ, Smith GL, Kooner R. Vascular interventions during postchemotherapy retroperitoneal lymph-node dissection for metastatic testis cancer. Eur J Surg Oncol 1998;24:292–7.

7 Gefäßverletzungen. In: vom Vorstand der Deutschen Gesellschaft für Gefäßchirurgie, Herausgeber: Leitlinien zu Diagnostik und Therapie in de Gefäßchirurgie. Dt ÄrzteVerl, Köln, 1998;123–7.

Chapter 67
Chronic Sacral Neuromodulation

C. Seif, K.-P. Jünemann, and P.-M. Braun

Introduction

This chapter describes the authors' method of choice. High patient compliance is absolutely mandatory. It is important to exclude patients with urinary bladder tumors, stress incontinence, or complete para- or tetraplegia.

Indications

The procedure is indicated in anticholinergic therapy-refractory overactive bladder (motor and sensory urge syndrome with or without incontinence), idiopathic retention in chronic pelvic pain when combined with urge symptoms, and in detrusor–sphincter dyssynergia.

Limitations/risks

• Planned MRI investigations.
• The patient must be mentally capable of managing the stimulator.
• Electrode- or impulse generator (IPG)-related infections.
• Cable damage or cable breaking.

Contraindications

• Malignancy with a life expectancy < 3 years.
• Grade II or higher cystocele.
• Vertical or rotatory descensus.
• Stress incontinence.
• Anatomical subvesical obstruction.

Preoperative management

• A positive bilateral PNE (peripheral nerve evaluation) test is mandatory (more than 50% improvement of symptoms during a 5-day (minimum) test period).
• X-ray the os sacrum to rule out any malformations.
• Start 30 min preoperatively with antibiotics (third-generation cephalosporin) and continue with ciprofloxacin for 3–5 days.

Anesthesia

Local anesthesia is possible, but the authors prefer general anesthesia.

Special instruments/suture material

All required instruments are delivered with the electrode/IPG kit.

Operative technique

• Place the patient in a prone position with a 30–45° flexion of the hip and knee joints. Place a ground electrode on the shoulder and connect to the external stimulator (stimulation parameters: amplitude 8 V; impulse widths 210 μs; rate 20 Hz).
• Use a sterile wrapping.
• Puncture both sacral foramina at the S3 level (sometimes S4).
• Stimulate the PNE needle to identify the correct location until you observe anal sphincter contraction and/or flexion of the ipsilateral big toe.
• Withdraw the PNE needle mandrin.
• Insert the guidewire.
• Insert the dilatator, and remove the guidewire and dilatator mandrin.
• Insert the electrode and perform the test stimulation to see if the electrode is in the correct position.
• If all four electrode rings show positive responses, retract the dilatator totally.
• Perform a skin incision two finger breadths below the iliac crest on the side that the patient wishes to have the IPG (this depends on whether the patient is right- or left-handed).
• Tunnel through the subcutaneous tissue by means of the tunneling device. Start from the site of the electrode exit up to

the skin incision, where the subcutaneous bag for the IPG is created.
- Withdraw the tunneling device, leaving the plastic tube in place.
- Guide the electrode through the plastic tube.
- Repeat the steps on the other side.
- Connect the electrodes via extension cables with the IPG. Place two fixation ligatures at the gluteal fascia. Insert the IPG and tie the IPG ligatures. Close the subcutis and cutis.
- Start stimulation on the first or second postoperative day.

Tips

When puncturing the S3 foramen, you will notice resistance on passing through the sacral fascia. When the electrode is inserted, the proximal electrode rings can be covered by the dilatator; then retract the dilatator until the second mark on the electrode can be seen and redo the test stimulation.

Open the electrode or IPG kit shortly before it is needed and have a bowl with nebacetine (1 g in 300 mL 0.9% NaCl) ready to wash and rinse the electrodes and IPG before their final implantation.

Postoperative care

- Inspect the wound carefully and start stimulation only if the wound is normal.
- Perform an X-ray for correct electrode placement documentation.
- Perform a blood test on the first and fifth postoperative days to rule out infection.

Troubleshooting

Perform control stimulation by looking at anal sphincter contraction and/or flexion of the ipsilateral big toe after each of the following steps:
- PNE needle punction.
- Withdrawal of the PNE mandarin.
- Guidewire insertion.

- Dilatator insertion.
- Electrode implantation and dilatator withdrawal.
- After guiding the electrode through the plastic tube.
- Before connecting to the IPG.

In cases of uncertainty about whether a patient should receive a neuromodulator or not, because the PNE test was not totally convincing, the final stimulation electrodes may be implanted as described above and then connected to an external stimulation device (Fig. 67.10). In this case the test period can be extended — if the patient responds to this therapy, the electrodes can remain in place and only the IPG is then implanted in a second step.

References

1 Braun PM, Seif C, Scheepe JR *et al.* Chronic sacral bilateral neuromodulation. Using a minimal invasive implantation technique in patients with disorders of bladder function. Urologe A 2002; 41(1):44–7.
2 Seif C, Eckermann J, Bross S, Martinez Portillo FJ, Jünemann KP, Braun PM. Findings with bilateral sacral neurostimulation: 62 PNE-tests in patients with neurogenic and idiopathic bladder dysfunctions. Neuromodulation 2004;7(2):141–5.
3 Spinelli M, Giardiello G, Gerber M, Arduini A, van den Hombergh U, Malaguti S. New sacral neuromodulation lead for percutaneous implantation using local anesthesia: description and first experience. J Urol 2003;170(5):1905–7.

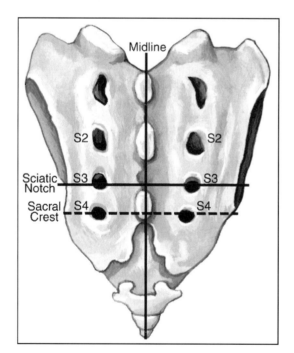

Figure 67.2 Locate the S3 foramina four finger-breadths caudal of a line between the spina iliaca posterior and superior and one finger-breadth to the side.

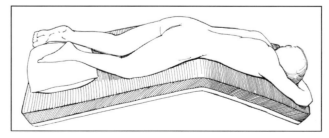

Figure 67.1 Position of patient placement.

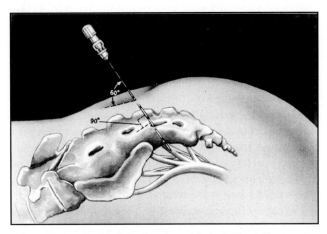

Figure 67.3 Puncture the S3 foramen with the PNE needle at a 60° angle to the skin to follow the physiologic path of the spinal nerve.

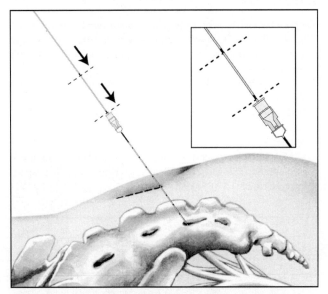

Figure 67.4 After withdrawal of the PNE mandrin, insert the guidewire until the first mark can be seen at the upper end of the PNE needle.

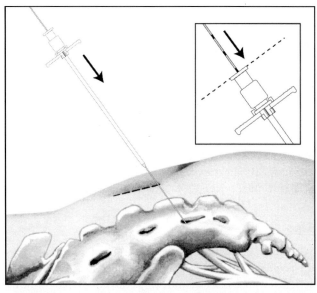

Figure 67.5 Withdraw the PNE needle and insert the dilatator up to the same mark on the guidewire as illustrated in Fig. 67.4.

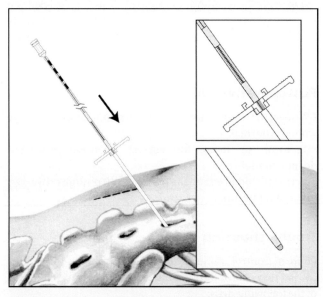

Figure 67.6 Withdraw the dilator mandarin and insert the electrode after withdrawing the guidewire and dilatator mandrin.

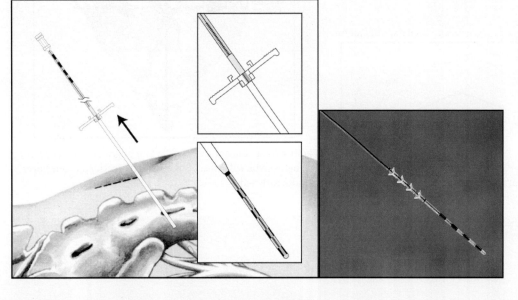

Figure 67.7 Start to perform test stimulation via a distal ring electrode to check whether the positioning is still correct and withdraw the dilatator up to a second mark on the electrode and perform a test stimulation at the remaining three electrode rings. When all four electrodes show positive stimulation responses, the dilatator can be removed carefully while holding the electrodes in place. Little anchors on the electrode surface fix the electrodes permanently.

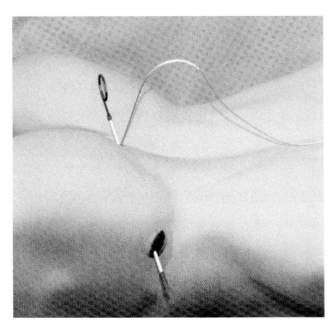

Figure 67.8 Tunneling to the subcutaneous pocket.

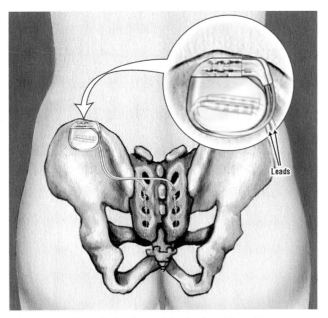

Figure 67.9 Electrode fixation and the final position of the electrodes and the IPG (this shows a final version with bilateral electrodes).

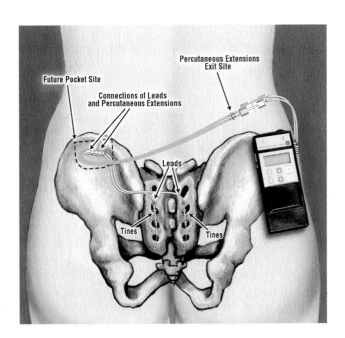

Figure 67.10 Two-stage implantation with an external stimulator for extended subchronic testing.

Chapter 68

GMF Procedure for Complex Pelvic Reconstruction in Bladder Exstrophy: the Giessen–Mainz–Frankfurt Multidisciplinary Approach

R. Stein, T. H. Jünger, F. Kerschbaumer, H.-P. Howaldt, and R. Hohenfellner

Introduction

In bladder exstrophy, primary bladder closure is the gold standard worldwide and treatment of pubic diastasis is a key step in the reconstructive surgery. To treat pubic diastasis, different types of osteotomies are often used in primary as well as in secondary bladder closure [19]. However, in patients with wide pubic diastasis, permanent closure of the pelvic arch remains a challenge.

Penile deformity in bladder exstrophy is part of this complex anomaly. The phallus is foreshortened in male patients in large part due to the wide separation of the corpora cavernosa secondary to pubic diastasis. Mitchell's technique of penile disassembling facilitated penile reconstruction in a cosmetic as well as functional way [1]. Despite the progress in genital reconstruction made with this technique, the improvements in the appearance of the penis are limited by the treatment of the underlying deformity of the pelvic bones. Due to the anatomical relationship between the corpora cavernosa and the distance between the pubic rami, reconstruction of the pelvic arch is a prerequisite to success in phallic reconstruction. Gaining adequate penile length remains an unresolved problem in this group of patients [2–7,12].

The technique of callus distraction was originally described by Ilizarov for lengthening of underdeveloped limbs and treatment of infected bone fractures in 1968. It is now widely used also in orthopedic and maxillofacial surgery [13,15,17]. We performed gradual callus distraction prior to genital reconstruction in a boy with bladder exstrophy in the expectation that the approximation and upward rotation of the bony insertions of the corpora cavernosa would result in lengthening of the penis [20].

Indications

This procedure is indicated in genital reconstruction in male patients with exstrophy/epispadias with a wide diastasis of the symphysis. It is also indicated in approximation of the os pubis during primary or secondary bladder closure.

Limitations

Its use is limited in small children and in patients with a thin os pubis (fixation of the pins must be possible).

Contraindications

The technique is contraindicated in small diastasis of the symphysis and in infection of the skin.

Anesthesia

General anesthesia.

Preoperative management

Three-dimensional imaging of the pelvis is needed to plan the operative procedure using, for example, a stereolithography model for mock surgery. Imaging of the upper urinary tract (sonography) should also be done.

Special instruments/suture material

- Multidirectional device routinely used for mandibular lengthening (Normed®, Tuttlingen, Germany).
- Raspatory.
- Oscillating saw.
- Bone pins for the multidirectional device system.

Operative technique

- Place the patient in a lithotomy position.
- Use careful disinfection and mark the three incision lines on both sites (spina iliaca anterior superior, ramus superior ossis pubis, and ramus inferior ossis pubis).
- Explore the crista iliaca anterior superior. After making a 2–3 cm long skin incision, the periost is opened with the scalpel in a longitudinal direction.
- The periost is pushed away from the bone by the raspatory. Make two parallel burr holes (2 mm) within the distance of 1 cm and drill in the Schanz screws (3.0–3.5 mm diameter).
- The second skin incision is performed over the ramus superior ossis pubis (3–4 cm). During exploration of the bone, care should be taken not to compromise the vena artery or femoral nerve. They are usually lateral of the incision.
- Partially sever the base of the pectineus muscle, as much as necessary (2–3 cm). Make a longitudinal incision and detach the periost from the bone.
- The inferior pins are placed close to the strong intersymphysal ligament at the ramus superior ossis pubis.
- Bilateral osteotomies of the rami superior are made with the oscillating saw, 1–2 cm proximal to the two holes of the pins, with preservation of the periosteum. The 50–60 mm pins are drilled in.
- The third skin incision is carried out at the junction of the ramus inferior ossis pubis to the os ischii and exposes the cartilaginous junction. A longitudinal incision of the perichondrium is made. In small infants transect the junction using the scalpel, in older children use the oscillating saw.
- A flexible distractor is fixed at the Schanz screws on both sites and both distractors are fixed in the midline.
- Close the wounds.

Postoperative care

- Start the distracting phase at day 5 (when antibiotics are given) [11].
- The correct positions of the pins are checked radiographically. The distraction rate of 1–2 mm per day is checked every second day by ultrasound [9] and sometimes, if necessary, radiographically.
- Monitor bone growth, possible complications — such as infections, premature ossification, and mineralization — and the timing of the distraction phase.
- Distraction is limited by the soft tissue between the os pubis.
- The direction of the distraction is medial and cranial to rotate the ramus inferior ossis pubis upward. This maneuver achieves approximation of both corpora cavernosa.
- Immobilization for 4–6 weeks is sufficient.
- The final stability is achieved after the functional exercises.

References

1 Aadalen RJ, O'Phelan EH, Chisholm TC, McParland FA, Jr. Sweetser TH, Jr. Exstrophy of the bladder: long-term results of bilateral posterior iliac osteotomies and two-stage anatomic repair. Clin Orthop 1980;151:193–200.

2 Cook FE, Leslie JT, Brannon EW. Preliminary report: a new concept of abdominal closure in infants with exstrophy of the bladder. J Urol 1962;87:823–4.

3 Edgerton MT, Gillenwater JY. A new surgical technique for phalloplasty in patients with exstrophy of the bladder. Plast Reconstr Surg 1986;78(3):399–410.

4 Frey P. Anterior pelvic osteotomy of the superior pubic ramus to facilitate bladder exstrophy repair. Dialog Ped Urol 1993; 16(1):4–5.

5 Frey P, Cohen SJ. Bladder exstrophy — anterior osteotomy of the pelvis — a new surgical technic for facilitating stabilization of the pelvis and abdominal closure [in German]. Z Kinderchir 1988;43(3):171–3.

6 Gearhart JP, Forschner DC, Jeffs RD, Ben-Chaim J, Sponseller PD. A combined vertical and horizontal pelvic osteotomy approach for primary and secondary repair of bladder exstrophy. J Urol 1996;155(2):689–93.

7 Gokcora IH, Yazar T. Bilateral transverse iliac osteotomy in the correction of neonatal bladder extrophies. Int Surg 1989;74(2): 123–5.

8 Ilizarov GA. General principles of transosteal compression and distraction osteosynthesis. In: Proceedings of the Scientific Session of Institutes of Traumatology and Orthopedics. Leningrad, USSR, 1968:35–9.

9 Jünger TH, Klingmüller V, Howaldt HP. Application of ultrasound in callus distraction of the hypoplastic mandible: an additional method for the follow-up. J Craniomaxillofac Surg 1999;27(3):160–7.

10 Kerschbaumer F. Operative approaches to the pelvis. In: Operative Approaches in Orthopedic Surgery and Traumatology (Bauer R, Kerschbaumer F, Poisel S, eds). Thieme, New York, 1987:103–9.

11 Klein C, Howaldt H-P. Lengthening of the hypoplastic mandible by gradual distraction in childhood — a preliminary report. J Craniomaxillofac Surg 1995;23:68–74.

12 McKenna PH, Khoury AE, McLorie GA, Churchill BM, Babyn PB, Wedge JH. Iliac osteotomy: a model to compare the options in bladder and cloacal exstrophy reconstruction. J Urol 1994; 151(1):182–6; discussion 6–7.

13 McLorie GA, Bellemore MC, Salter RB. Penile deformity in bladder exstrophy: correlation with closure of pelvic defect [see comments]. J Pediatr Surg 1991;26(2):201–3.

14 Mitchell ME, Bagli DJ. Complete penile disassembly for epispadias repair: the Mitchell technique. J Urol 1996;155(1):300–4.

15 Perovic S, Brdar R, Scepanovic D. Bladder exstrophy and anterior pelvic osteotomy. Br J Urol 1992;70(6):678–82.

16 Schmidt AH, Keenen TL, Tank ES, Bird CB, Beals RK. Pelvic osteotomy for bladder exstrophy. J Pediatr Orthop 1993; 13(2):214–19.

17 Shultz WG. Plastic repair of exstrophy of the bladder combined with bilateral osteotomy of the ilia. J Urol 1958;79:453–8.

18 Sponseller PD, Gearhart JP, Jeffs RD. Anterior innominate os-

teotomies for failure or late closure of bladder exstrophy. J Urol 1991;146(1):137–40.

19 Sponseller PD, Jani MM, Jeffs RD, Gearhart JP. Anterior innominate osteotomy in repair of bladder exstrophy. J Bone Joint Surg Am 2001;83A(2):184–93.

20 Stein R, Junger TH, Anders M *et al*. The Giessen–Mainz–

Frankfurt procedure: a new method for complex pelvic reconstruction for bladder exstrophy. J Urol 2001;165(4): 1235–9.

21 Woodhouse CR, Kellett MJ. Anatomy of the penis and its deformities in exstrophy and epispadias. J Urol 1984;132(6): 1122–4.

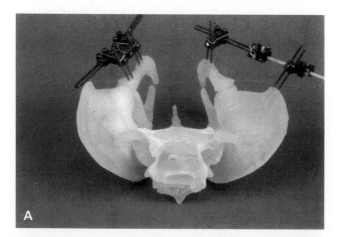

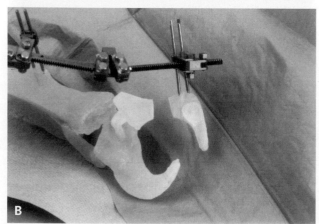

Figure 68.1 Stereolithography model with the attached multidirectional device: (A) cranial view, and (B) a detail.

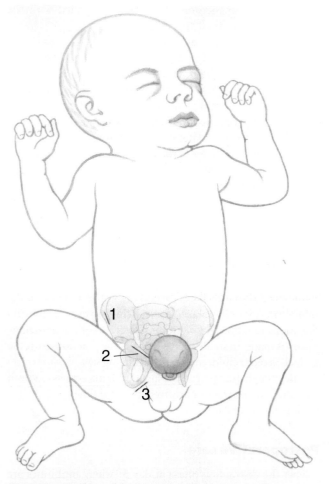

Figure 68.2 Marking of the three skin incision (1, spina iliaca anterior superior; 2, ramus superior ossis pubis; 3, the junction of the ramus inferior ossis pubis and os ischii).

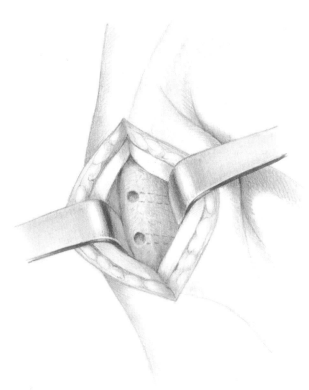

Figure 68.3 Exposure of the spina iliaca anterior superior, transection of the cartilage, and drilling two burr holes.

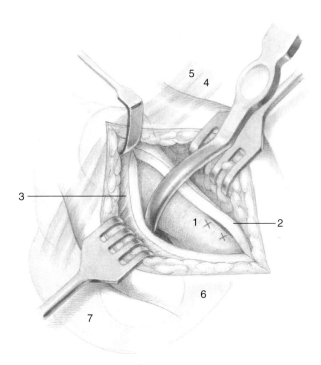

Figure 68.4 Exploration of the ramus superior ossis pubis. After severance of the pectineus muscle and incision of the periost, two burr holes are drilled in the crista pubica. 1, ramus superior ossis pubis; 2, cartilage; 3, pectineus muscle; 4, femoral vein; 5, femoral artery; 6, ramus inferior ossis pubis; 7, os ischii.

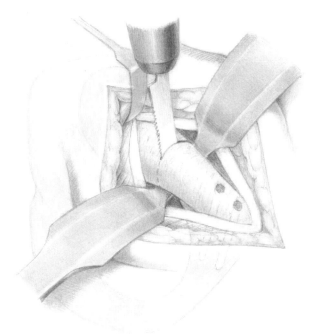

Figure 68.5 Transection of the ramus superior ossis pubis with the oscillating saw.

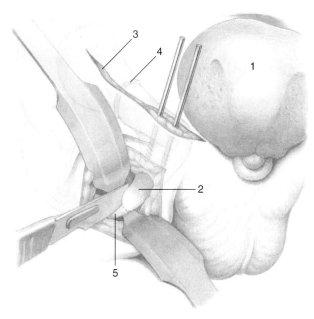

Figure 68.6 Exposure of the junction of the ramus inferior ossis pubis and the os ischii. The cartilaginous junction is transected with the scalpel. 1, bladder exstrophy; 2, ramus inferior ossis pubis; 3, skin incision; 4, osteotomy; 5, os ischii.

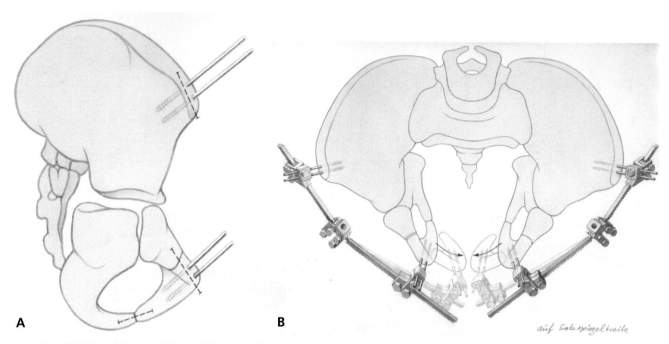

A   **B**

Figure 68.7 (A) Bilateral fixation of the multidirectional device at the pins. (B) The direction of the distraction is marked with the arrow.

Chapter 69
Primary Reconstruction of Cloacal Exstrophy

P. C. Black, R. W. Grady, and M. E. Mitchell

Introduction

Reconstruction of cloacal exstrophy poses one of the most significant surgical challenges in pediatrics. These infants may present with neurologic, pulmonary, cardiac, and limb anomalies in addition to abnormalities of the genitourinary and gastrointestinal tracts. The physical appearance at birth (Fig. 69.1) underscores the enormity of the challenge to reconstruct these children satisfactorily, giving them safe and continent bladder function as well as acceptable sexual and bowel function.

In primary repair, the bladder, bladder neck, and urethra form a single unit, which is closed and placed deep into the pelvis. As most of these patients have a rudimentary hindgut, an imperforate anus, and poor pelvic floor support, a rectal reservoir is usually not advised. Further, because of lower CNS abnormalities and a high potential for aberrant innervation of the sphincteric mechanism, rectal pull-through is not possible in many patients. The already short length of the bowel limits its use in reconstruction.

Patient counseling and consent

Single-stage reconstruction may be safely performed only in select circumstances—usually in patients with small omphaloceles and without significant pelvic diastasis. More often, the presence of a large omphalocele, wide pubic diastasis, or compromised pulmonary function makes an early, staged repair necessary; in this case, the principles of complete primary repair are applied in a sequential fashion.

Gender assignment in male patients has been controversial in the past, but recent data suggests that these children should not be routinely designated female for reasons of prenatal imprinting with testosterone [2]. Wide symphyseal diastasis and small phallus size pose special challenges for satisfactory reconstruction of the external genitalia.

Indications

This procedure is indicated in cloacal exstrophy.

Limitations and risks

- Perform within 24–48h of birth, when possible, to take advantage of the pliability of the pelvis.
- Reconstruction should be carried out in a tertiary center with urologic and surgical specialists experienced with cloacal exstrophy.
- Airway pressure monitoring after closure of the omphalocele is used as a parameter for intra-abdominal pressure; use single-stage closure only if the pressure remains low and there is no undue risk from prolongation of the anesthetic.
- Aggressive closure of a large abdominal defect may result in increased abdominal pressure with anuria secondary to decreased renal vascular perfusion.
- Staged repair involves the following steps:
  - Omphalocele closure with removal of the hindgut plate from cloacal exstrophy, tubularization of the hindgut, and creation of a colostomy.
  - This is followed, after convalescence of the child (2–6 weeks), with bladder closure.
  - An interval of several weeks to months poses minimal risk to the bladder as long as it is protected from desiccation.
  - In the most severe cases with a large omphalocele that contains the liver, it is necessary to treat this defect on its own as a first stage.

Contraindications

- Cardiopulmonary complications should be stabilized preoperatively.
- A large omphalocele (especially with inclusion of the liver) requires repair prior to exstrophy reconstruction.

Preoperative management

• Cover the bladder and hindgut after delivery with a hydrophilic dressing (e.g. Vigilon®, Bard Medical, Covington, GA).
• Ligate the umbilicus with a silk suture rather than a plastic clamp in order to protect the bladder from superficial trauma.
• Give prophylactic broad-spectrum antibiotics (e.g. second generation cephalosporin).
• Check the karyotype preoperatively.
• Perform renal ultrasonography and an echocardiogram.
• Perform a plain X-ray of the abdomen and pelvis.

Anesthesia

General anesthesia with caudal injection.

Special instruments/suture material

• Small tray with fine instruments.
• Surgical loupes (2–4× magnification).
• Tungsten electrocautery (Colorado tip®, Biomed Inc., Evergreen, CO).
• Two 3.5 Fr umbilical artery catheters.
• Sutures: 4/0 to 7/0 PDS®, Maxon®, Monocryl®, and Vicryl®; 5/0 chromic catgut.
• 6 Fr modified Malecot catheter for suprapubic tube (Cook Inc., Bloomington, IN).
• Dressings: Telfa® (The Kendall Company Ltd, Mansfield, MA), Duoderm® (ConvaTec Ltd, Princeton, NJ), and Tegaderm® (3M Health Care Ltd, St Paul, MN).

Operative technique

The procedure described here is for a male patient.
• Give a preoperative single injection of caudal anesthetic.
• Place 5/0 Monocryl® stay sutures transversely in each hemiglans (these will become sagittal with rotation of the corpora).
• Insert 3.5 Fr umbilical artery catheters in the ureters and fix with 6/0 chromic sutures.
• Initiate the dissection superiorly.
• Close the omphalocele.
• Ligate the umbilical vessels only if necessary.
• Separate the lateral bladder plates from the surrounding skin with tungsten electrocautery, proceeding from superior to inferior.
• Separate the centrally located hindgut from the two halves of the bladder plate.
• Reduce the intussusception of the terminal ileum in the hindgut and tabularize the hindgut; the distal end is used later for the colostomy.
• Reapproximate the two halves of the bladder in the midline (this is the stopping point for a staged procedure).

• Penile degloving: start with a ventral penile circumcising incision; dissect between Buck's fascia and the dartos on the ventral and lateral aspects of the corpora, taking care not to injure the neurovascular bundles (located laterally). Make a medial dissection on the tunica albuginea of the corpora cavernosa (Buck's fascia is absent medially).
• Dissect a wedge of the urethra with its underlying spongiosa; this is critical to preserve the urethral blood supply and to maintain maximal urethral width for later tubularization.
• Separate the two hemiglans and corpora cavernosa in the midline (in severe cloacal exstrophy the two halves of the penis may already be totally separate).
• Make bilateral deep incisions into the intersymphyseal band lateral and posterior to the distal prostatic urethra and bladder neck; this allows the bladder, bladder neck, and urethra to move posteriorly into the pelvis (key maneuver).
• Insert a suprapubic catheter (modified 6 Fr Malecot) through the umbilicus, which is moved superiorly to a more anatomically normal position.
• Close the bladder in two layers with absorbable monofilament sutures (running 4/0 Monocryl® and interrupted 4/0 PDS®).
• Tubularize the urethra in two layers with 5/0 Maxon® and 4/0 Vicryl® over the previously placed ureteral catheters. If the penile halves are totally separate, then the urethral plate may also be separate, making posterior (dorsal) and anterior (ventral) closure necessary.
• Place two symphyseal sutures (0/0 PDS® in a figure-of-eight) through firm symphyseal tissue, and knot anteriorly.
• Carefully inspect the corpora and lower extremities for impaired vascular perfusion following closure of the symphysis; consider pelvic osteotomies if the vasculature appears compromised.
• Perform a running fascial closure with 2/0 PDS®.
• Reapproximate the corpora cavernosa in the midline with interrupted 6/0 PDS® sutures.
• Glanular reconstruction is done with 5/0 or 6/0 PDS® for shaping and 6/0 or 7/0 Vicryl® for reapproximation of the epithelial edges.
• Construct the neomeatus with 6/0 or 7/0 Vicryl® using standard hypospadias techniques, after bringing the tubularized urethra up towards the glans ventrally (it is not usually possible to reach the glans).
• Close the penile skin, with reverse Byars' flaps as necessary, using 6/0 chromic or 6/0 Vicryl®.
• Colostomy formation is performed using the distal end of the tubularized hindgut brought out to the left lower quadrant and matured in standard fashion.
• Close the abdominal incision in two layers with running 5/0 and 6/0 Monocryl® sutures.
• Reconstruct the umbilicus at the time of closure of the incision.
• Apply a three-layer dressing to the penis—Telfa®, Duoderm®, and Tegaderm®—with fixation to the abdomen.

Tips

• Conserve the appendix for possible future Mitrofanoff appendicovesicostomy (often not possible).
• Conserve the hindgut for optimal nutrition, fluid absorption, and possible future bladder and/or vaginal reconstruction.
• Optimal symphyseal apposition improves fascial competence after closure; pelvic osteotomies are required more frequently than for classic exstrophy and are almost always necessary for reconstruction done more than 48 h after birth, especially if vascular compromise is apparent in the corpora cavernosa and lower extremities after closure of the symphyseal diastasis.
• When there is inadequate urethral length, the neomeatus is established on the proximal penile shaft and hypospadias repair can be performed later; redundant ventral foreskin should be left in place for urethroplasty.

Postoperative care

• Use immobilization in a spica cast (pelvis and lower extremities) with external fixator or Bryant's traction.
• Give prophylactic antibiotics: ampicillin and gentamicin (if there is no renal impairment) until they can be taken by mouth, then trimethoprim/sulfamethoxazole until the tubes are taken out.
• Provide acute pain service consultation and continuous morphine infusion.

• Perform intravenous hyperalimentation (usually necessary).
• Provide decubitus prophylaxis, especially if there is concomitant neurologic disease.
• Spontaneous dislodgement of the ureteral catheters occurs after 7–10 days.
• The spica cast is taken off after 3 weeks.
• Perform a voiding trial after 4 weeks, and then remove the suprapubic tube if there is adequate bladder emptying.

Results

Of six patients with single-stage reconstruction:
• two had normal voiding and no incontinence;
• two had dry intervals;
• two had complete incontinence, pending further reconstruction.

References

1 Grady RW, Mitchell ME. Complete primary repair of exstrophy [comments]. J Urol 1999;162:1415.
2 Mathews RI, Perlman E, Marsh DW, Gearhart JP. Gonadal morphology in cloacal exstrophy: implications in gender assignment. Br J Urol Int 1999;84:99–100.
3 Mitchell ME, Carr MC. Epispadiekorrektur nach Mitchell [complete penile disassembly]. Akt Urol 1999;30:269–74.
4 Plaire J, Mitchell ME. Single stage reconstruction of cloacal exstrophy. In: Dialogues in Pediatric Urology (Weiner J, ed.). W.J. Miller, New York, 2000:6.

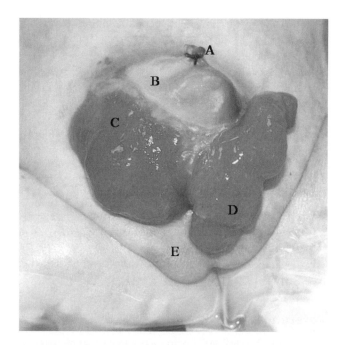

Figure 69.1 Preoperative appearance of a newborn male with cloacal exstrophy. (For color, see Plate 69.1, between pp. 112 and 113.)

Key for Figs 69.1–69.13: A, umbilical cord; B, omphalocele; C, bladder plate; D, intussuscepted terminal ileum; E, scrotum; F, penis (right and left); G, urethral plate; H, glans penis; I, appendix (right and left); J, small bowel; K, hindgut; L, ileocecal valve; M, colostomy; N, ureteral orifices; O, corpus cavernosum (right and left); P, ureteral stent; Q, penile skin (internal aspect); R, sutures through the urethral plate and corpus spongiosum; S, deep paravesical dissection (right and left); T, reapproximation of the dorsal urethra and corpus spongiosum; U, suprapubic catheter.

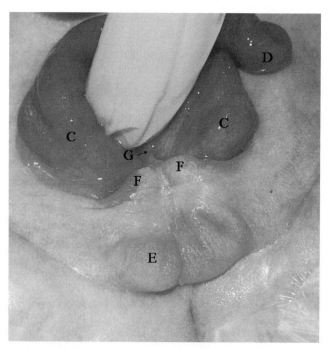

Figure 69.2 Preoperative appearance of the external genitalia in a male newborn with cloacal exstrophy when the intussuscepted bowel (D) is retracted. (For color, see Plate 69.2.)

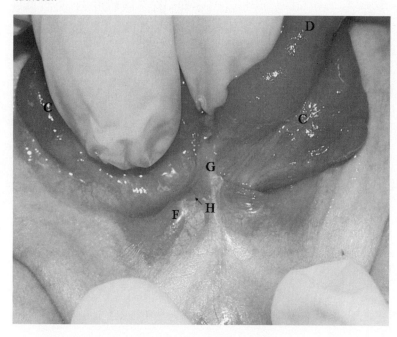

Figure 69.3 Close up of genitalia including a hemi-penis (F), glans penis (H), and urethral plate (G). (For color, see Plate 69.3.)

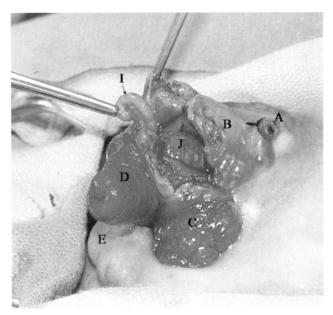

Figure 69.4 The dissection is started below the omphalocele. (For color, see Plate 69.4, between pp. 112 and 113.)

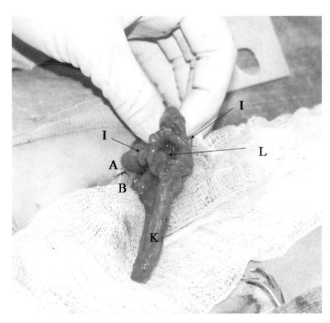

Figure 69.6 Complete release of the hindgut (K), showing the ileocecal valve (L) and split appendix (I). (For color, see Plate 69.6.)

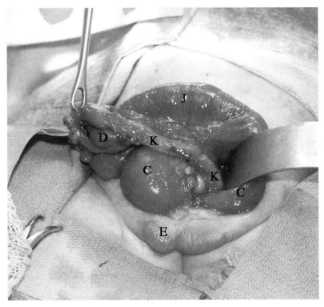

Figure 69.5 Dissection of the hindgut (K) and small gut (J). (For color, see Plate 69.5.)

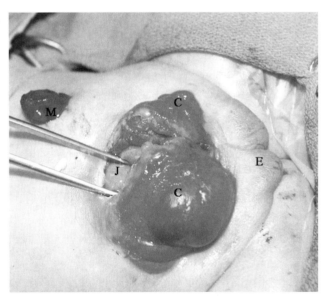

Figure 69.7 The surgical field after construction of the colostomy (M). (For color, see Plate 69.7.)

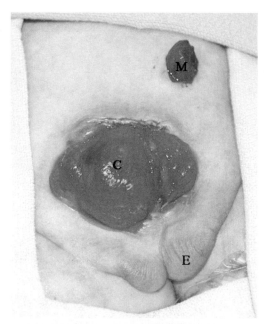

Figure 69.8 Surgical field after closure at the end of the first stage. (For color, see Plate 69.8, between pp. 112 and 113.)

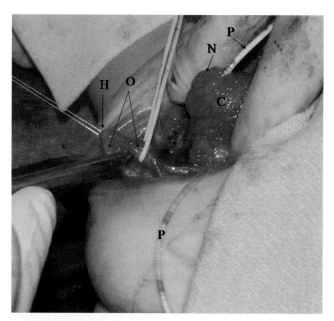

Figure 69.10 Dissection of the corpora cavernosa. (For color, see Plate 69.10.)

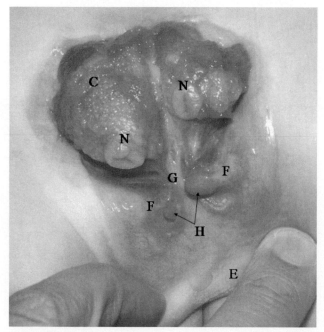

Figure 69.9 Appearance before the second-stage surgery. (For color, see Plate 69.9.)

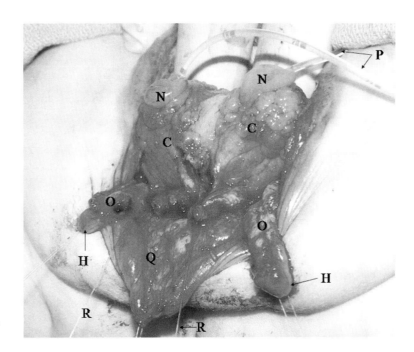

Figure 69.11 Complete penile disassembly. (For color, see Plate 69.11, between pp. 112 and 113.)

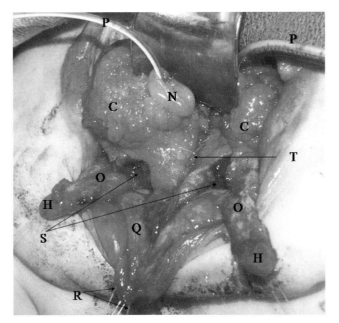

Figure 69.12 Deep dissection lateral to the urethra and bladder neck. (For color, see Plate 69.12.)

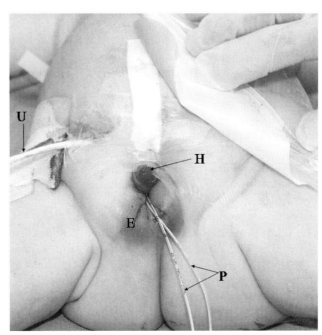

Figure 69.13 Appearance after bladder closure.

Chapter 70
Surgical Treatment of Prune Belly Syndrome

F. T. Dénes

Introduction

Prune belly syndrome (PBS) is characterized by abdominal flacidity, cryptorchism, and variable degrees of bilateral ureterohydronephrosis associated with renal dysplasia (Fig. 70.1). It occurs in 1:30,000 to 1:50,000 births. The clinical presentation varies from severe cases, that are stillborn or die prematurely due to renal and pulmonary insufficiency, to cases that present only mild abdominal flaccidity and urinary tract dilatation, with normal renal function. The patients that present at least one good functioning kidney generally survive the neonatal period, but depending on the degree of renal dysplasia, ureterohydronephrosis, and vesicoureteral reflux, may present further renal impairment, associated to secondary obstruction or pyelonephritis.

Based on the presumption of spontaneous improvement of the urinary tract abnormalities, clinical treatment with antibiotic prophylaxis has been recommended in mild and intermediate forms of the disease. Surgical treatment was exceptional, performed in most cases late in childhood, when the urinary tract had already suffered additional injuries. The procedures were performed, in general, to remove non-functioning renal units or to perform urinary diversion. Orchiopexy was performed late, in children who survived early childhood.

The concept of early comprehensive surgical treatment of PBS patients is based on the fact that most associated urinary tract abnormalities (such as vesicoureteral reflux, ureteral obstruction due to megaureter with excessive kinking, increased vesical residue due to enlarged, hypotonic bladders, and urachal diverticuli), as well as abdominal flaccidity, can be adequately corrected by reconstructive surgery, preventing further damage. Urinary tract reconstruction includes nephroureterectomy of nonfunctioning units, unilateral or bilateral reductive ureteroplasty with ureterovesical reimplantation, and reductive cystoplasty—according to individual needs. Abdominoplasty is also adapted to each patient's anatomical features. Furthermore, since orchiopexy is necessary in all cases and has better results when performed during the first year of life, it is done simultaneously with early urinary tract reconstruction and abdominoplasty.

There are no age limits to this comprehensive procedure, and all patients that survive the first weeks of life are potential candidates. The best results are obtained in very young children, if adequate anesthesiologic and postoperative care can be ensured.

Indications

All children with PBS, who present adequate or potentially normal renal function, are candiates for this procedure.

Contraindications

The technique is contraindicated in active urinary tract infection, pulmonary insufficiency, and impaired renal function.

Preoperative management

• Careful morphological and functional evaluation of the urinary tract is crucial in the planning of the reconstruction of the urinary tract.
• Renal function must be evaluated in both kidneys. Severely obstructed units must be drained preoperatively, in order to evaluate unilateral function and to treat infection.
• Urinary tract infection must be effectively eliminated before surgery.
• In selected cases with deteriorating renal function due to ureteral obstruction, but no infection, emergency reconstruction can be an alternative to primary diversion.
• Previous pyelostomy, ureterostomy, or vesicostomy are not contraindications for the procedure.

Anesthesia

General anesthesia should be performed by experienced pediatric anesthesiologists. Adequate fluid administration must be ensured to prevent dehydration due to prolonged procedures (that may take up to 240–300 min of operating time) and peritoneal exposition.

Operative technique

• After anesthesia, the child is raised from the table, and the thorax, abdomen, dorsum, and genitals are completely prepared, and the patient is laid supine. The dressing is fixed in order to allow complete access to the abdomen, both lumbar regions, and the scrotum during surgery.

• The abdominal wall is palpated and grasped to re-evaluate flaccidity and redundancy (Fig. 70.2). An ellipsoid figure is demarcated according to the redundant skin area, not necessarily equivalent in both sides. The umbilicus is also demarcated with a small circle, in order to be preserved (Fig. 70.3).

• Incise and remove the skin and subcutaneous tissue within the outer demarcation line, preserving the aponeurotic fascia and the umbilicus (Fig. 70.4).

• The aponeurotic fascia, with its residual muscle, is incised along an elliptical paramedian line on the most redundant side, which extends to the upper and lower extremities of the skin incision (Fig. 70.5).

• The bladder, together with the urachal diverticulum (or urachal fistula), is detached from the anterior abdominal wall. An eventual vesicostomy is undone. This maneuver exposes the peritoneal contents, and the lack of colonic and splenic fixation allows easy inspection of the retroperitoneal structures, including the dilated ureters and kidneys. The testes are identified as intraperitoneal structures, lying close to the common iliac vessels, with a mesenterium-like structure that contains its vessels and the deferens.

• The testes are liberated initially, preserving the deferens with its perideferential vessels, and the spermatic pedicle, which lies upon the dilated ureteral folds.

• Urinary tract reconstruction is planned as described by Woodard (Fig. 70.6) [6]. Previous dissection of the spermatic vessels enables radical liberation of the ureters, with removal of the eventual ureterostomies or pyelostomies. In the case of a nonfunctioning kidney, nephroureterectomy must be performed. Otherwise, care must be taken not to skeletonize the ureter completely, particularly its proximal segments. If an evident pyeloureteral obstruction is still present after adequate dissection, a nondismembered pyeloureteral anastomosis can be performed. The distal and redundant ureteral segments are removed, and the proximal segments are straightened without skeletonization (Figs 70.7 and 70.8).

• The noncontractile bladder dome with the urachal diverticulum is excised, care being taken to avoid overresection of the bladder (Fig. 70.9).

• The ureters are reimplanted in the the bladder either with the Politano–Leadbetter (bilateral reimplantation) or Paquin psoas hitch (unilateral reimplantation) techniques (Fig. 70.10), employing ureteral stents exteriorized transvesically. Eventual tailoring or infolding of the proximal ureteral seg-ments can be performed judiciously, preserving the ureteral vasculature.

• Before closure, the bladder is drained with an urethral catheter or a cystostomy.

• Orchiopexy is performed, making an orifice in the inguinal aponeurotic fascia and extending a tunnel in the inguinal subcutaneous fat to the ipsilateral hemiscrotum. Through this tunnel the testis is brought down to the scrotum, and is positioned in a previously prepared subdartus pouch. While in infants the testes easily reach the scrotum, section of the spermatic vessels is sometimes necessary in older children to perform a successful orchiopexy.

• The aponeurosis is closed in a vest-over fashion, the larger leaf with the umbilicus placed below, and the smaller above. They are thus sutured to each other, with the umbilicus exposed through a 'buttonhole' in the upper leaf, where it is sutured (Fig. 70.11). No abdominal drains are left.

• The skin edges, already approximated by the previous maneuver, are sutured according to the initial demarcation (Fig. 70.12).

• Circumcision is performed at the end of the procedure.

Tips

• Precise estimation of the redundant cutaneous surface is made by careful preoperative evaluation of the abdominal wall, with the child in upright and supine positions.

• Judicious use of the electric scalpel and forceful traction of the skin and subcutaneous fat enable the quick removal of the patch with preservation of the aponeurotic fascia.

• Bowel manipulation must be minimal and careful, to avoid postoperative ileus. Due to lack of fixation, replacement in the peritoneal cavity before closure must respect anatomy, to avoid obstruction and volvus.

• In order to optimize orchiopexy, it must be performed after ureterovesical reimplantation. The spermatic vessels must be left below the ureters.

Postoperative care

• Ventilatory assistance and physiotherapy is mandatory due to decreased abdominal support for ventilation.

• Urinary drainage must be ensured with adequately fixated splints. Residual abdominal flaccidity may predispose to dislodgement.

• Manipulation of the splints must be minimal to avoid retrograde contamination of the residually dilated urinary tract.

• There should be stepwise removal of the splints, ensuring that the bladder empties itself adequately.

Results

Table 70.1 shows the surgical results for 32 patients.

Table 70.1 Surgical results (32 patients in 18 years, with no intraoperative complications and no postoperative deaths).

	Preoperative status	Postoperative status	Postoperative complications (early and late)
Abdomen			Inguinal hernia (unilateral), 1
Flaccidity	32	2 (late reoccurrence)	
Urinary tract			Vesicoureteral obstruction, 3:
			transient (bilateral), 1
			definitive (unilateral), 2
			Acute tubular necrosis, 1
			Severe urinary infection, 3
			(Reoperations: 6 in 4 patients)
Pyelocaliceal dilatation	15	4	
Ureteral dilatation	24	4*	
Vesicoureteric reflux (unilateral)	10	0	
Vesicoureteric reflux (bilateral)	11	0	
Hypotonic bladder	••	Mild, 9; Severe, 3	
Recurrent urinary tract infection	19	4	
Impaired renal function	7	2	
Testes			
Intra-abdominal	64		
Scrotal/normal		54	
Scrotal/atrophic		5	
Inguinal		5	
Respiratory tract			Transient postoperative respiratory distress, 2

References

1 Arap S, Dénes FT, Silva FAQ, Góes GM. Le syndrome d'aplasie des muscles de la paroi abdominale antérieure. J Urol Nephrol 1978;3:161–71.
2 Coplen DE, Snow BW, Duckett JW. Prune belly syndrome. In: Adult and Pediatric Urology, 3rd edn (Gillenwater JY, Grayhack JT, Howards SS, Duckett JW, eds). Mosby-Year Book, St Louis, 1996:2297–316.
3 Greskovich FJ, Nyberg LM. The prune belly syndrome: a review of its etiology, defects, treatment and prognosis. J Urol 1998; 140:707–12.
4 Randolph J. Total surgical reconstruction for patients with abdominal muscular deficiency ('prune-belly') syndrome. J Pediatr Surg 1977;12:1033–43.
5 Reinberg Y, Manivel JC, Pettinato G, Gonzalez R. Development of renal failure in children with the prune belly syndrome. J Urol 1991;145:1017–19.
6 Smith EA, Woodard JR. Prune-belly syndrome. In: Campbell's Urology, 8th edn (Walsh PC, Retik AB, Vaughan ED, Jr, Wein AJ, eds). W.B. Saunders, Philadelphia, 2002:2117–35.

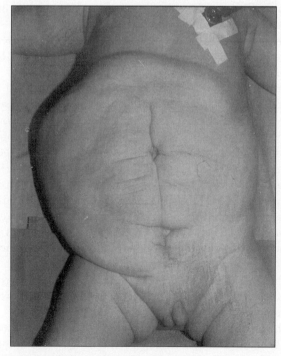

Figure 70.1 Characteristic abdominal flaccidity with cutaneous wrinkles and empty scrotum.

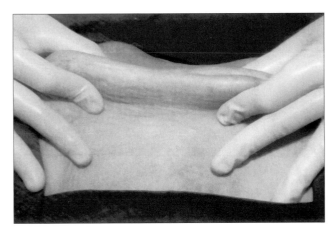

Figure 70.2 Abdominal palpation to evaluate cutaneous redundancy.

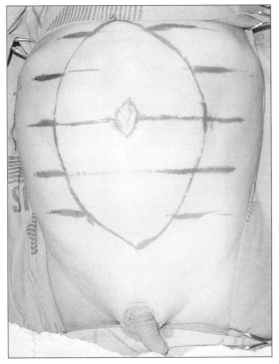

Figure 70.3 Demarcation of excessive skin to be removed.

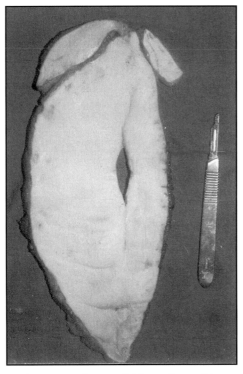

Figure 70.4 Fragments of removed skin patch: one side may be larger than the other, according to differences in abdominal flaccidity.

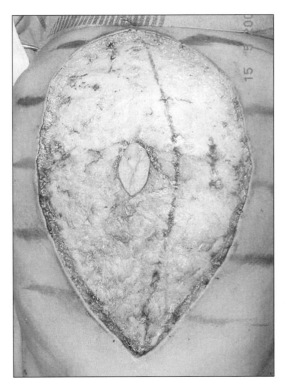

Figure 70.5 Musculoaponeurotic fascia exposed after removal of the skin patch, with the lines of aponeurotic incision and 'buttonhole' drawn.

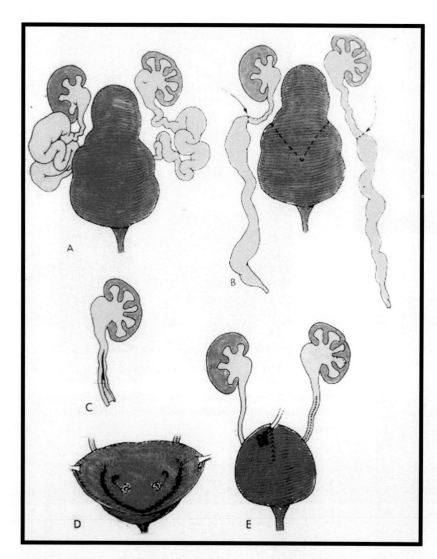

Figure 70.6 Steps of urinary tract reconstruction: A, initial finding of dilated and redundant distal ureteral segments; B, removal of these segments after judicious dissection; C, ureteral tailoring or infolding, performed in the proximal segment, when necessary; D, ureteral reimplantation in the bladder after removal of its dome; E, closure of the bladder.

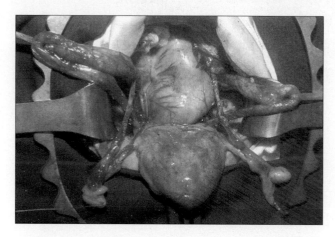

Figure 70.7 Complete the ureteral and testicular dissection, the latter with preservation of the gonadal vessels and vas deferens. Mobilization of the bladder dome is also observed.

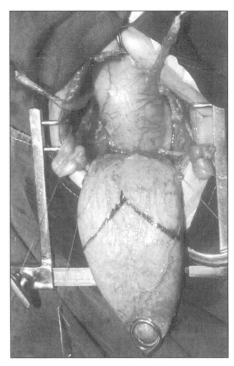

Figure 70.8 After removal of the dilated distal ureteral segments, the proximal ureters are straightened for reimplantation. The testes are repaired. The bladder is delineated for removal of its hypocontractile dome with the urachal diverticulum.

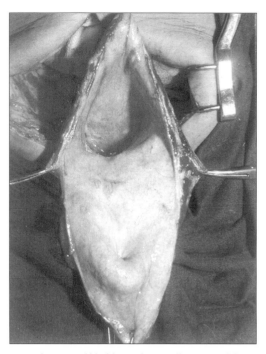

Figure 70.9 The opened bladder with partially removed dome (including urachal fistula).

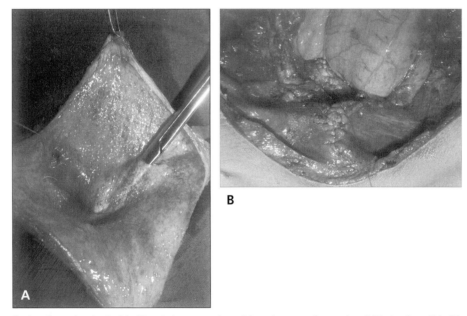

Figure 70.10 Ureteral reimplantation in the bladder: (A) preparation of the submucosal tunnel and (B) the closed bladder after the bilateral Politano–Leadbetter procedure.

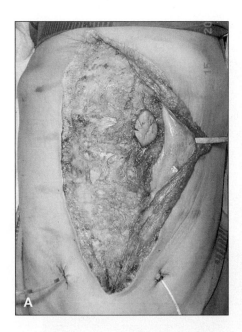
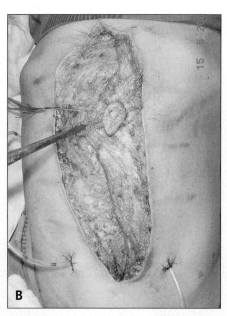

Figure 70.11 Closure of the abdominal wall: (A) overlap suture of the musculoaponeurotic fascial leafs and (B) exteriorization of the umbilicus through the 'buttonhole' in the outer fascia.

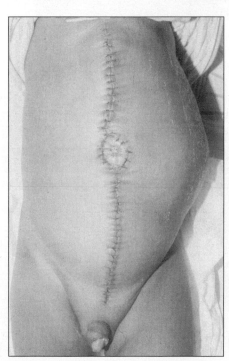

Figure 70.12 Early postoperative abdominal view: partial flaccidity may remain after extensive reconstruction, but further spontaneous improvement with growth is not precluded. The circumcised penis is also seen.

Chapter 71
Anterior Transanorectal Approach for the Repair of Urethrovaginal Fistulas

J. Franc-Guimond and R. González

Introduction

The anterior transanorectal approach to the vagina is a derivation of the transanorectal approach described by Kilpatrick and Mason [2]. In patients with normal rectal anatomy, it is not necessary to incise the posterior rectal wall in order to gain excellent access to the vagina and uterus when the vaginal route is insufficient [4]. The approach is also useful in males to repair urethrorectal fistulas and to remove large prostatic utricles. Rectal function and continence are not affected by this approach. With a good mechanical bowel preparation, a protective colostomy is not necessary. Here we illustrate its application in a girl with a twice-recurrent urethrovaginal fistula and urinary incontinence resulting from a perineal injury from a landmine [3]. Either as a result of the injury or the previous surgical procedures, the vagina had a complete transverse cicatricial septum. The urethral fistula, adjacent to the bladder neck, communicated with the cephalad vaginal chamber (Fig. 71.1). This type of post-traumatic fistula and resulting vaginal anatomy have been previously described [1]. This anatomy and the early pubertal development precluded the more conventional transvaginal approach.

Indications

This approach is useful for complex vaginal reconstruction in prepubertal females and in those with vaginal stenosis or atresia precluding a transvaginal approach. It is particularly useful for constructing an intestinal neovagina when the uterus is present.

Preoperative management

Mechanical bowel cleansing is needed using polyethylene glycol, and the patient is given perioperative antibiotics to cover Gram-negative and -positive bacteria as well as anaerobes.

Anesthesia

General anesthesia with endotracheal intubation. Some prefer nasal intubation to have a more secure fixation of the tube in the prone position. An epidural block is useful in older patients for postoperative pain control.

Special instruments/suture material

- Standard instrumentation.
- Lone Star retractor system (Lone Star Medical Products Inc., Houston, TX).
- Optical magnification with coaxial illumination.
- Fine tip electrode for monopolar diathermy (Colorado tip) and bipolar coagulator.

Surgical approach

The patient should be prone on the operating table with the buttocks elevated. Small children are best placed in the middle of the table and operated on from the side. Adults can be placed at the end of the table with the legs supported in stirrups if the surgeon prefers to operate from the midline.

Operative technique

- The perineum is shaved and the rectum and vagina are washed with Povidone; skin antisepsis is also with Povidone.
- Define the anatomy endoscopically (this can be done in advance in the dorsal lithotomy position or in the prone position).
- Make an incision with fine needle cautery (pure cutting) from the anal verge to the posterior vaginal fourchet.
- Open the anterior rectal wall in the midline for an extension of 5 cm or more (but not above the peritoneal reflection) according to the exposure needed.
- Place a gauze pack in the rectum to prevent the spillage of intestinal contents during the procedure.
- Thus the posterior vaginal wall is exposed and is opened in

the midline from the introitus to the level of the transverse cicatricial septum.

- Identify the cervix and cephalad vaginal compartment by palpation and opening of the cephalad vaginal chamber in the posterior midline.
- Expose the fistula located on anterior vagina wall. The introduction of a sound or lachrymal duct probe through the urethral meatus helps identification of the fistula.
- The edges of the fistula are dissected, elevating the anterior vaginal wall from the underlying urethra and bladder neck circumferentially.
- A Foley catheter of appropriate size is inserted in the urethra and is directed towards the bladder.
- The edges of the fistula are freshened and it is closed with interrupted Vicryl sutures in a longitudinal fashion.
- An incision is made along the inner aspect of the left labium major and a generous posteriorly based subcutaneous tissue flap is prepared (Martius).
- A tunnel is prepared between the anterior vagina wall and the pubis and urethra to allow passing the Martius flap to cover the urethral repair. The flap is secured in place with fine Vicryl sutures.
- The transverse vaginal scar is excised and the anterior vaginal wall is repaired in a transverse direction with interrupted Vicryl sutures.
- The posterior vaginal wall is closed longitudinally with a PDS running suture. A second interrupted layer can be applied.
- The anterior rectal wall is closed in two running layers with PDS.
- The anal sphincter and anal verge are close with interrupted PDS sutures.
- The perineal body is reapproximated with two or three interrupted PDS sutures.
- The rectum and vagina are calibrated with Hegar dilators to ensure an adequate circumference.
- The skin is closed with fine Monocryl sutures.
- A soft rectal tube and light vaginal packing are left in place.
- The patient is turned to the supine position and a percutaneous cystostomy tube is placed.

Postoperative care

- Continue the perioperative antibiotic regime.
- The rectal tube and vaginal packing are removed after 48 h.
- The patient can ambulate on the third postoperative day.
- Remove the urethral catheter after 1 week.
- After 30 days clamp the cystostomy tube and remove it when the patient is voiding well.
- A postoperative cystogram is optional.

Tips

- In infants and small children prepare the field circumferen-

tially below the rib cage and drape to allow turning the patient prone and supine without having to redrape. An extremity sheet is useful for this purpose.
- Operate from the side of the patient. This allows better lighting and positioning of the assistants.
- Use colored solutions such as methylene blue or indigo carmine to identify the fistulas and verify that closures are watertight.
- In prolonged procedures, avoid nerve injury by careful padding of pressure points.

To do

- Perform a preoperative urine culture, and operate with sterile urine.
- Wait many months after the trauma to avoid operating on inflamed tissues.
- Interpose well-vascularized tissue between the structures involved in the fistula such as omental or Martius flap.

References

1 Didusch W. A collection of urogenital drawings. American Cystoscope Makers Inc., New York, 1952: 167.
2 Kilpatrick FR, Mason AY. Post-operative recto-prostatic fistula. Br J Urol 1969;41:649–54.
3 Mauermann J, González R, Franc-Guimond J, Filipas D. The anterior sagittal transrectal approach (ASTRA) for traumatic urethrovaginal fistula closure. J Urol 2004;171:1650–1.
4 Rosi F, De Castro R, Ceccarelli PI. Anterior transanorectal approach to the posterior urethra in the pediatric age group. J Urol 1998;160:1173–7.

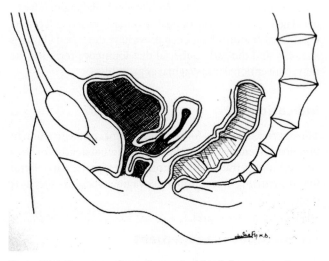

Figure 71.1 Anatomy of a urethrovaginal fistula in cross-section. The vagina is divided transversally by a cicatricial septum making the transvaginal approach impossible.

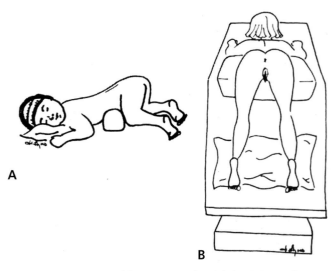

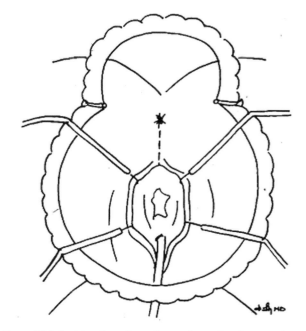

Figure 71.2 Position of the patient on the table for: (A) an infant or (B) an older child or adult.

Figure 71.3 Incision from the anal verge (upper) to the posterior fourchet using a self-retaining retractor.

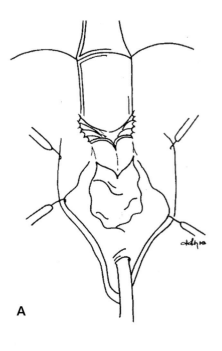

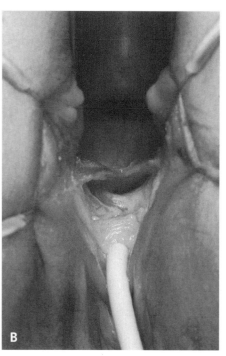

Figure 71.4 Midline opening of the anterior rectal and posterior vaginal walls.

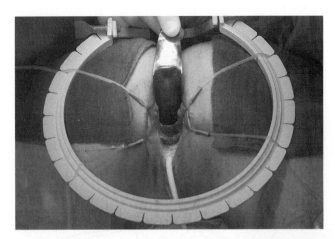

Figure 71.5 Use of the self-retaining retractor.

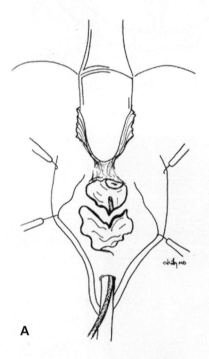

A

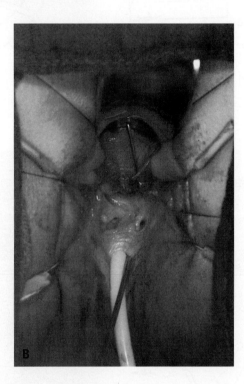

B

Figure 71.6 Midline opening on the cephalad part of the vagina demonstrating the cervix. The metal probe introduced in the urethral meatus leads to the fistula in the anterior wall of the cephalad portion of the vagina.

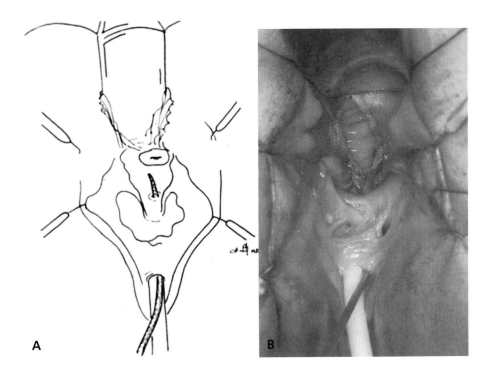

Figure 71.7 The septum separating the upper and lower vaginal chambers has been divided providing better exposure to the fistula.

A

B

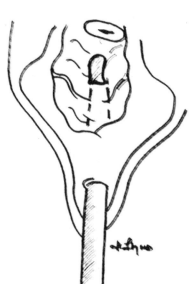

Figure 71.8 The urethral catheter, which goes preferentially to the cephalad portion of the vagina, is guided into the bladder.

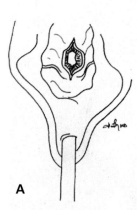

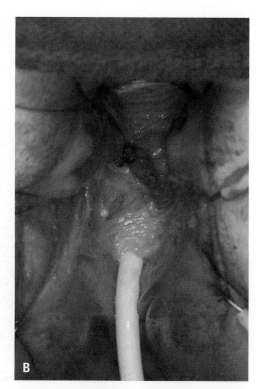

Figure 71.9 Mobilization of the edges of the fistula.

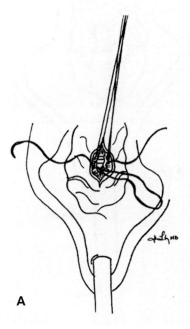

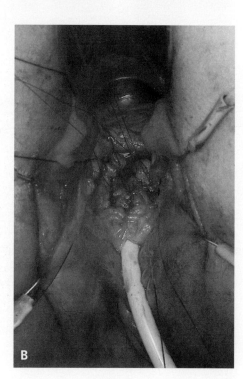

Figure 71.10 Closure of the fistula with interrupted sutures over the catheter.

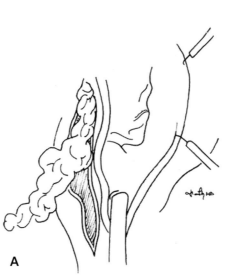
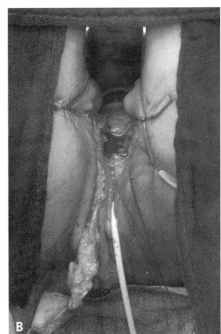

Figure 71.11 Incision on the left labium major; a posteriorly based subcutaneous tissue flap (Martius) is mobilized.

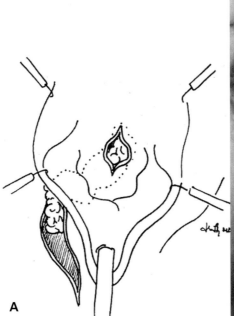
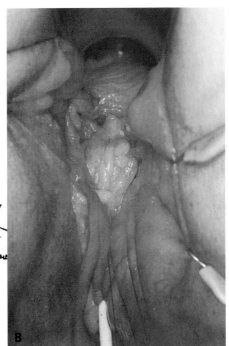

Figure 71.12 Creation of a tunnel ventral to the vagina to rotate the Martius flap and interpose it between the urethra and the vagina.

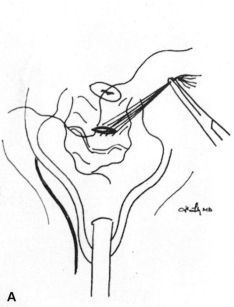

A

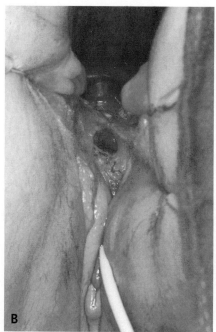

B

Figure 71.13 Tranversal closure of the anterior vaginal wall at the level of the fistula.

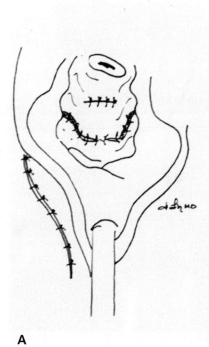

A

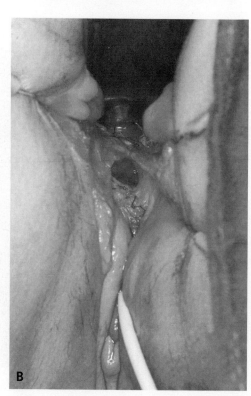

B

Figure 71.14 Completed repair of the anterior vaginal wall joining the upper and lower portions previously separated by the cicatricial septum.

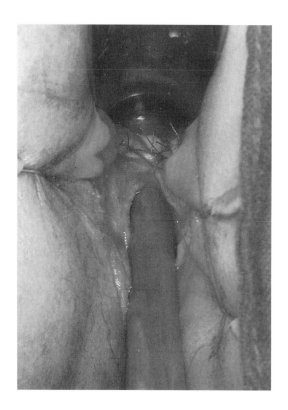

Figure 71.15 The posterior vaginal wall has been closed and the vagina is calibrated with a Hegar dilator.

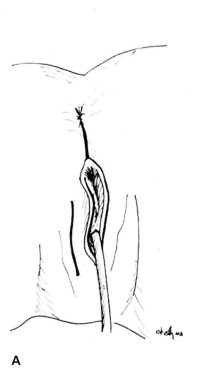

A

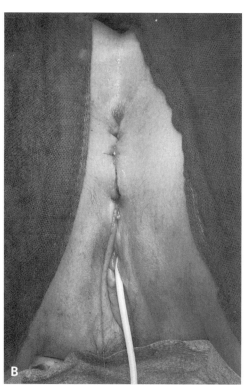

B

Figure 71.16 Completed closure.

Chapter 72
Totally Extraperitoneal Endoscopic Hernia Repair with Synthetic Mesh

J.-U. Stolzenburg

Introduction

Inguinal hernia repair by means of laparoscopic placement of synthetic mesh is an accepted and very successful treatment modality. There are two main surgical access techniques to reach the preperitoneal space and place the synthetic mesh. The transabdominal (transabdominal preperitoneal technique or TAPP) or the extraperitoneal (totally extraperitoneal technique or TEP) route. Both of these laparoscopic techniques use the principle of tension-free hernia repair, covering the entire myopectineal area with a large piece of mesh. This results in covering the hernial defect and potential sites for recurrences.

The preperitoneal mesh technique (TEP) is favored for the repair of inguinal hernias because of the clear visibility of all possible hernial defects and its direct access to the posterior inguinal anatomy. The trend in laparoscopic/endoscopic surgery toward the TEP repair has shown it to be equally effective but with fewer complications [1,2]. The extraperitoneal endoscopic hernia repair can also be safely performed concurrently with endoscopic extraperitoneal lymph node dissection or radical prostatectomy [3,4].

Indications

This procedure is indicated in all inguinal hernias and recurrent hernias.

Contraindications

Incarcerated hernias contradict the use of this approach.

Preoperative management

Single-shot broad-spectrum antibiotics; ensure the bladder is empty.

Special instruments/suture material

- Standard laparoscopic tower: high flow (CO_2) insufflator, monitor, camera (Olympus Visera camera OTV-S7), light source CLV-S40, and video laparoscope (Endo-Eye) 0° optic 10 mm for the Visera control unit 'OTV-S7V-B' set.
- Trocars: 1 × Ballontrokar PDB 1000 (Tyco) trocar, 1 × Hassan-type optical trocar, 2 × 5.5 mm trocars insulated with thread.
- Instruments (5 mm): 2 × atraumatic forceps, 1 × Metzenbaum scissors, 1 × Hook scissors.
- Synthetic mesh (e.g. Prolene).

Advantages of preperitoneal hernia repair

The technique completely avoids intraperitoneal entry and, therefore, its complications. Staples or stitches are not necessary for fixation of the mesh.

Operative technique (left inguinal hernia repair)

- The patient is placed in a dorsal supine position with a 10° Trendelenburg tilt.
- A 15 mm left infraumbilical incision is performed.
- Balloon trocar dissection of the preperitoneal space is performed, with placement of the optical trocar (Hassan type) and CO_2 insufflation (pressure 12 mmHg) (see Chapter 29).
- A 5 mm trocar is placed right of the paramedian and as cranial as possible.
- The key to a safe dissection of the extraperitoneum is the creation of a space directly underneath and lateral to the epigastric vessels. At this level visualization of the transversus abdominis muscle needs to be obtained. The dissection is continued laterally in a cranial direction.
- Placement of the second 5 mm trocar is two fingers medial to the anterior superior iliac spine.
- Loose areolar tissue is dissected away from the lateral ab-

dominal wall. The spermatic cord structures are carefully identified, and the transverse fascia, the rectus muscle, and the pubic arch are exposed.

- In direct hernias, the hernial sac is found medial to the epigastric vessels; traction and countertraction maneuvers are used to reduce the hernial sac.
- In indirect hernias, the peritoneal sac will travel on the anteromedial aspect of the spermatic cord as it enters the internal ring. The hernial sac is carefully dissected free from the cord.
- A large indirect hernia (e.g. inguinal scrotal hernia) can be divided at the internal ring.
- Closure of the peritoneal defect is essential (suture or loop ligation).
- The spermatic cord is elevated and an opening is created posteriorly for the mesh.
- Extracorporeal preparation of the Prolene mesh ($8–10 \times 13–15$ cm).
- A 6 cm incision is made in the middle of the mesh, and a 0.5 cm hole is cut out for the spermatic cord.
- The incision in the mesh is covered by a further 4×6 cm Prolene mesh, secured with 3/0 Prolene. This flap is temporarily fixed at the medial aspect of the main mesh by a stay suture. The mesh is rolled up and fixed by two stay sutures.
- The mesh is placed through the 12 mm Hassan trocar into the preperitoneal space underneath the spermatic cord.
- The stay sutures are cut in sequence (first the lateral, then the medial, and third the flap stay suture) and the mesh is subsequently unfolded around the spermatic cord to cover the hernial defect and the entire myopectineal area. No staples or sutures are necessary for mesh fixation.
- Insert the wound drain via the lateral trocar site if necessary.
- Observe the mesh position whilst slowly evacuating the CO_2 insufflation.
- Close the trocar sites in layers.

Tips

- *Bilateral hernia repair*: place the first 5 mm trocar as cranial and lateral as possible (on the side of the paraumbilical incision). Free the preperitoneal space along the pubic arch across to the other side. Two pieces of mesh need to be used.
- *Unable to free the hernial sac*: this may occur with large inguinal scrotal hernias. Divide the hernial sac at the external inguinal ring and dissect it free of the spermatic cord. Close the peritoneal opening. A third 5 mm working trocar in the mid-line may be necessary to assist with larger hernias.
- *Large direct hernial defect*: cut and place the mesh in an asymmetric fashion underneath the cord. The medial aspect of the mesh should be larger.
- *Rolled-up mesh*: mark the lateral aspect of the mesh with a long suture. This enables easy recognition and placement *in situ*.

Postoperative care

Remove the drain on the first postoperative day (if present). The patient can resume normal activities in 7 days.

References

1 Kraehenbuehl L, Schaefer M, Feodorovici MA, Buechler MW. Laparoscopic hernia surgery: an overview. Dig Surg 1998;15:158–66.
2 Ramshaw BJ, Tucker JG, Duncan TD *et al*. Technical considerations of the different approaches to laparoscopic herniorrhaphy: analysis of 500 cases. Am Surg 1996;62:69–72.
3 Stolzenburg JU, Pfeiffer H, Nehaus JM, Sommerfeld M, Dorschner W. Repair of inguinal hernias using the mesh technique during extraperitoneal pelvic lymph node dissection. Urol Int 2001;67: 19–23.
4 Stolzenburg JU, Rabenalt R, Dietel A, Do M, Pfeiffer H, Doschner W. Hernia repair during endoscopic (laparoscopic) radical prostatectomy. J Laparoendosc Adv Surg Tech 2003;13:27–31.

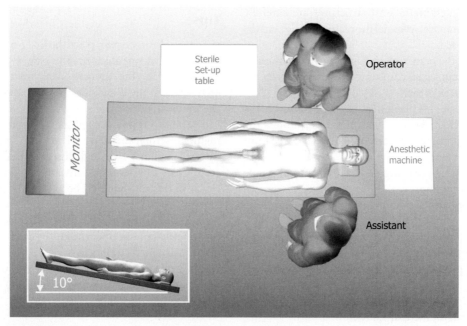

Figure 72.1 Patient positioning and operative set-up. The surgeon stands on the right side for a left hernia repair.

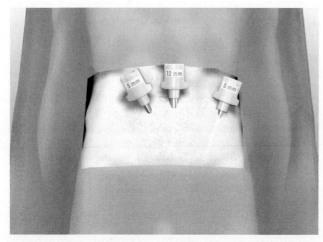

Figure 72.2 Trocar placement for a left hernia repair. The assistant holds the left working trocar and the camera.

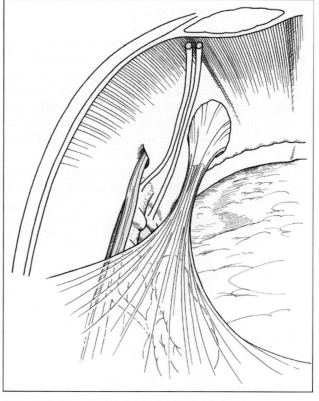

Figure 72.3 Direct hernia. The defect lies medial to the epigastric vessels. The hernial sac is easily freed with blunt traction and countertraction maneuvers.

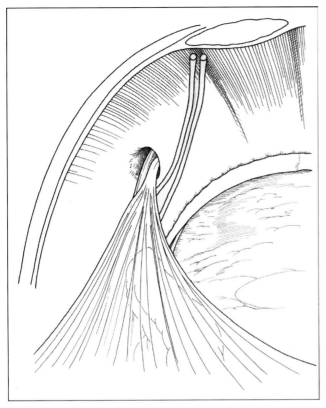

Figure 72.4 Indirect hernia. The hernial sac enters the internal inguinal canal along the spermatic cord, lateral to the inferior epigastric vessels.

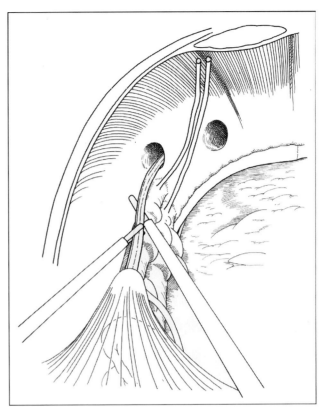

Figure 72.6 Preparation for mesh placement. The spermatic cord is dissected free up to the internal inguinal canal.

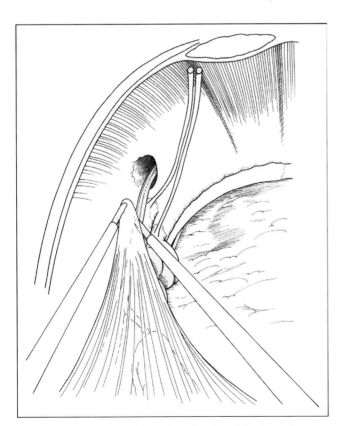

Figure 72.5 Dissection of the indirect hernia. Whilst the assistant places cranial traction on the peritoneum, the hernia can be separated with blunt dissection. Sharp dissection may be required in rare circumstances.

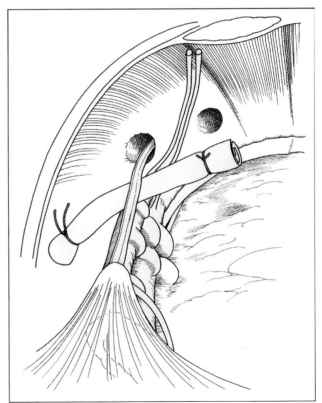

Figure 72.7 The extracorporeal prepared mesh is placed into the extraperitoneal space via the Hassan trocar underneath the spermatic cord.

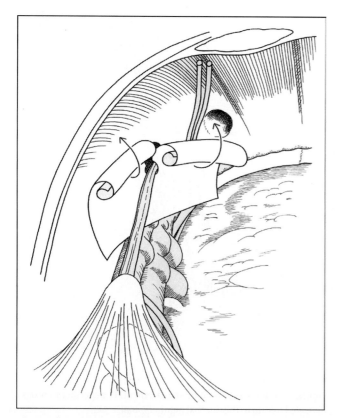

Figure 72.8 The mesh is unfolded in sequence: first the lateral half and then the medial half. Finally, the flap is released and placed over laterally.

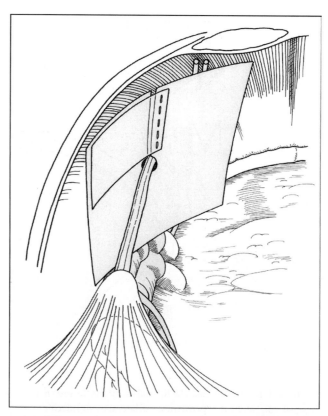

Figure 72.9 Correct positioning of the mesh and disufflation of CO_2 under vision.

Section 10
Miscellaneous

Chapter 73

Secondary Malignancies following Intestinal Urinary Diversion

T. Kälble and M. Austen

Tumor development following ureterosigmoidostomy is a worldwide accepted late complication, the risk being up to 477-fold increased compared to the general population. For benign disease the mean latency period from the operation to the tumor diagnosis is 20 years (range 2–48 years) for adenomas and 26 (6–54) years for adenocarcinomas. The mean latency period for malignant primary disease is about 50% shorter with 10 (1–21) years for adenomas and 13 (6–27) years for adenocarcinomas [22,23].

Although own animal experiments [22–24,26] showed a similar tumor risk in rectal bladders with and without the separation of feces and urine in a rat model, the assessment of tumor risk in urinary diversions via isolated intestinal segments without urine/feces mixture is controversial.

Up to now, 81 benign and malignant tumors in conduits (*n* = 18) [3,9,11,27–29,39,40,42,46,49,52,55], cystoplasties (*n* = 45) [3–8,10,11,14–17,19,20,21,30,32,35,36,38,43,47,50, 51,56,57], rectal bladders (*n* = 5) [11,31,37,45,47], neobladders (*n* = 3) [12,41,48], colonic pouches (*n* = 6) [1,2,13,33,34,53], and ileal ureter replacements (*n* = 4)[3,47; R. Hohenfeller, pers. comm., 2000] have been published, 47 in ileum and 34 in colon segments (Table 73.1). The median latency period for developing malignant tumors in urinary diversion using ileum is 21 (2–40) years and using colon is 12 (1–28) years. In 48 patients with benign primary disease after a median latency period of 21.5 (2–40) years, malignant tumors occurred; in 18 patients with malignant primary disease the median latency period was shortened to 8 (1–22) years. These facts suggest a similar tumor risk in all urinary diversions using small or large bowel — malignant diseases predisposing for a shorter induction period.

Fifty-five of 67 (82.1%) of the malignant tumors occurred in cystoplasties, colonic pouches (Indiana or Florida pouch), rectal bladders, colonic/ileal neobladders, or ureter replacements suggesting an increased tumor risk in continent urinary diversions. This statement, however, is speculation due to the unknown figures of unreported tumors and of the different operations performed in the world. Apart from that, cystoplasties are mainly operated in younger patients for be-

nign disease with longer survival times than conduits, which are operated mainly in elder patients for malignant disease with survival times being possibly too short for tumor induction.

Comparing the tumor risk following ureterosigmoidostomy and cystoplasty, the data can be interpreted in different ways. There were 45 tumors following cystoplasty and more than 200 following ureterosigmoidostomy [22,25], which suggests an increased risk following ureterosigmoidostomy. On the other hand ureterosigmoidostomies have been performed from 1911 until the end of the 1980s in large numbers worldwide; in less developed countries this approach is still the urinary diversion of first choice. The indication for cystoplasty, however, is much less common. Taking into account this fact the 45 tumors might well correspond to the more than 200 cases of carcinomas and adenomas following ureterosigmoidostomy. There are nine case reports published so far following orthotopic bladder substitution or catheterizable pouches — five of them being published in the last 4 years — that suggest that the tumor risk is similar following neobladders or pouches as well, but that most patients with neobladders or pouches have not reached the latency period yet.

Strikingly, the tumor spectrum is different between ureterosigmoidostomies and urinary diversions via isolated intestinal segments. Following ureterosigmoidostomy the most common diagnoses are adenoma and adenocarcinoma. Following urinary diversions using isolated intestinal segments, carcinoids, transitional cell carcinomas, squamous cell carcinomas, signet ring cell carcinomas, oat cell carcinoma, and leiomyosarcomas occurred as well as adenomas and adenocarcinomas.

Interestingly, in three patients following cystoplasty, transitional cell carcinoma and adenocarcinoma occurred simultaneously [10,17,43]. These clinical data are confirmed by our own animal experiments with the observation of transitional cell carcinoma and adenocarcinoma in the same rat following urinary diversion via the rectal bladder [22–24,26].

The location of tumors following ureterosigmoidostomy

Table 73.1 Case reports in the world literature of tumors following urinary diversion via isolated intestinal segments.

	Colon	Ileum	Total
Conduit	6	12	18
Cystoplasty	15	30	45
Rectal bladder	5	–	5
Neobladder	2	1	3
Colonic pouch	6	–	6
Ureter replacement	–	4	4
Total	34	47	81

and diversion using isolated gut segments is different as well. Twenty-four of 43 (55.8%) tumors in urinary diversions using ileum and in 17/30 (56.7%) tumors using colonic segments without feces/urine mixture grew directly at or near to the urointestinal anastomosis. The other tumors occurred in the intestinal and/or the vesical part of the urinary diversion or near the stoma in conduits. Following ureterosigmoidostomy, however, the tumors grew only at the urocolonic borderline.

In this review we have only considered patients where there was no relationship between the secondary tumor and the original disease resulting in the urinary diversion.

In summary there is an increased tumor risk in all urinary diversions via isolated intestinal segments compared to the general population. Regular endoscopic controls are mandatory. The German Urological Association guidelines recommend annual endoscopic controls [18]. Our data show that 11.9% (8/67) of malignancies following urinary diversion using isolated gut segments occurred within the first 5 years postoperatively. Annual endoscopic controls beginning from the third postoperative year would therefore be a good compromise and should be recommended. In conduits regular inspection of the stoma is necessary as well. Apart from that, urinary diversions have to be completely removed in cases of conversion because of the fact that tumors have been detected at ureteral implant sites after undiversion too [4,37,44,54].

So far, based on the literature, the tumor risk seems to be similarly increased in all forms of urinary diversion although this estimation can be criticized due to the unknown number of unpublished tumors and the unknown figure of operated urinary diversions worldwide. Whether patients with ureterosigmoidostomies have an even higher risk than those with orthotopic bladder substitutes, pouches, or cystoplasties cannot yet be answered.

References

1 Ahlstrand C, Herder A. Primary adenocarcinoma of distal ileum used as outlet from right colonic urinary reservoir. Scand J Urol Nephrol 1998;32:70.

2 Albertini JJ, Sujka SK, Helal MA, Seigne JD, Lockhart JL. Adenocarcinoma in a continent colonic urinary reservoir. Urology 1998;84:499.

3 Ali-El-Dein B, El-Tabey N, Abdel-Latif M, Abdel-Rahim M, El-Bahnasawy MS. Late uro-ileal cancer after incorporation of ileum into the urinary tract. J Urol 2002;167:84.

4 Austen M. Karzinominzidenz und Karzinomprophylaxe sekundärer Tumoren in verschiedenen Formen der Harnableitung. PhD dissertation, Marburg, 2003.

5 Barrington JW, Fulford S, Griffiths D, Stephenson TP. Tumors in bladder remnant after augmentation enterocystoplasty. J Urol 1997;157:482.

6 Bono Ariño A, Sanz Vélez JI, Esclarin Duny MA, Berné Manero JM, Vera álvarez J. Adenocarcinoma de células en anillo de sello en colocistoplastia. Actas Urol Esp 2001;17:31.

7 Carr LK, Herschorn S. Early development of adenocarcinoma in a young woman following augmentation cystoplasty for undiversion. J Urol 1997;157:2255.

8 El Otmany A, Hamada H, Al Bouzidi A, Oukheira H, Boujida M, Souadka A. Carcinome malpighien sur iléocystoplastie d'agrandissement pour vessie tuberculeuse. Prog Urol 1999;9:534.

9 Erb RE, Kaufman AJ, Koch MO, Dutt KS. Adenocarcinoma in a sigmoid conduit: case report. Urol Radiol 1999;12:115.

10 Fernandez-Arjona M, Herrero L, Romero JC, Nieto S, Martin R, Pereira I. Synchronous signet ring cell carcinoma and squamous cell carcinoma arising in an augmented ileocystoplasty. Eur Urol 1996;29:125.

11 Filmer RB, Spencer JR. Malignancies in bladder augmentations and intestinal conduits. J Urol 1990;143:671.

12 Frese R, Doehn C, Baumgärtel M, Holl-Ulrich K, Jocham D. Carcinoid tumor in an ileal neobladder. J Urol 2001;165:522.

13 Gazzaniga MS, Turbow B, Ahlering TE, Shanberg AM. Adenocarcinoma in an Indiana pouch urinary diversion. J Urol 2000;163:900.

14 Gepi-Attee S, Ganabathi K, Abrams PH, MacIver AG. Villous adenoma in augmentation colocystoplasty: a case report and discussion of the pathogenesis. J Urol 1992;147:128.

15 Goldman HB, Dmochowski RR, Noe HN. Nephrogenic adenoma occurring in an augmented bladder. J Urol 1996;155:1410.

16 Grainger R, Kenny A, Walsh A. Adenocarcinoma of the caecum occurring in a caecocystoplasty. Br J Urol 1988;61:164.

17 Gregoire M, Kantoff P, de Wolf WC. Synchronous adenocarcinoma and transitional cell carcinoma of the bladder associated with augmentation: case report and review of the literature. J Urol 1993;149:115.

18 Guidelines of the DGU. Leitlinie zur Nachsorge von Patienten mit Harnableitung unter Verwendung von Darmsegmenten. Urologe A 2000;39:483.

19 Ishida T, Koizumi H. A case of adenocarcinoma of the reconstructed bladder following ileocystoplasty. Nippon Hinyokika Gakkai Zasshi 1997;88:439.

20 Jung JL, Abouelfadel Z, Dettloff H. Adénocarcinome développé sur une anse iléale après cystoplastie d'agrandissement. Ann Urol (Paris) 1996;30:69.

21 Kadow C, Heaton ND, Paes T, Yates-Bell AJ, Packham DA. Adenocarcinoma in a substitution caecocystoplasty. Br J Urol 1989;63:649.

22 Kälble T. Karzinogenese nach Ureterosigmoideostomie im Vergleich zu anderen ureterointestinalen Harnableitungen—

Klinische und tierexperimentelle Untersuchung–Habilitationsschrift. Heidelberg, 1991.

23 Kälble T. Ätiologie, Inzidenz und Prophylaxe von Tumoren in verschiedenen Formen der intestinalen Harnableitung. Akt Urol 1996;27:166–74.

24 Kälble T, Busse K, Amelung F, Waldherr R, Berger MR, Edler L. Tumor induction and prophylaxis following different forms of intestinal urinary diversion in a rat model. Urol Res 1995;23:365.

25 Kälble T, Schreiber W, Berger MR *et al.* Karzinomrisiko in verschiedenen Formen der Harnableitung unter Verwendung von Darm. Akt Urol 1993;24:1–7.

26 Kälble T, Tricker AR, Berger MR *et al.* Tumor induction in a rat model for ureterosigmoidostomy without evidence of nitrosamine formation. J Urol 1991;146:862–6.

27 Kedar R, Arger PH, Rovner ES, Nisenbaum HL. Colonic polyp in a urinary diversion causing hematuria: diagnosis on ultrasonography. J Ultrasound Med 2000;19:797.

28 Kerfoot BP, Steele GS, Datta MW, Richie JP. Carcinoid tumor in an ileum conduit diversion. J Urol 1999;162:1685.

29 Kochevar J. Adenocarcinoid tumor, goblet cell type, arising in a ureteroileal conduit: a case report. J Urol 1984;131:957.

30 Koizumi S, Johnin K, Kataoka A, Nakai M, Tomoyoshi T. Adenocarcinoma occuring 37 years after augmentation ileocystoplasty for tuberculous bladder atrophy: report of a case. Hinyokika Kiyo 1997;43:743.

31 Kotanagi H, Ito M, Koyama K, Sato K, Kato T. Colon cancer in rectal bladder. J Gastroenterol 2001;36:718.

32 Lane T, Shah J. Carcinoma following augmentation ileocystoplasty. Urol Int 2000;64:31.

33 L'Esperance JO, Lakshmanan Y, Trainer AF, Jiang Z, Blute RD, Ayvazian PA. Adenocarcinoma in an Indiana pouch after cystectomy for transitional cell carcinoma. J Urol 2001;165:901.

34 Lisle D, Cataldo P, Bibawi SE, Wood M. Colonic adenocarcinoma occurring in an Indiana pouch. Dis Colon Rectum 2000;43:864.

35 Llarena Ibarguren R, Pertusa Peña CP, Zabala Egurrola JA, Olaizola Furtes G. Adenocarcinoma de colon. Desarrolo sobre colocistoplastia. Arch Esp Urol 1989;42:459.

36 Louis L, Vanegas JP, Schulman CC, Simon J. Carcinome des dérivations urinaires une observation et revue de la littérature. Acta Urol Belg 1997;65:81.

37 Metzger PP. Adenocarcinoma developing in a rectosigmoid conduit used for urinary diversion — report of a case. Dis Colon Rectum 1989;32:247.

38 Nahas WC, Iizuka FH, Mazzucchi E, Antonopoulos IM, Lucon AM, Arab S. Adenocarcinoma of an augmented bladder 25 years after ileocystoplasty and 6 years after renal transplantation. J Urol 1999;162:490.

39 Ng FC, Woodhouse CRJ, Parkinson MC. Adenocarcinoma in an ileal conduit. Br J Urol 1996;77:314.

40 Pelaez C, Leslie JA, Thompson IM. Adenocarcinoma in a colon conduit. J Urol 2002;167:1780.

41 Redondo Martínez E, Rey López A. Adenoma nefrogénico en mucosa intestinal. Un caso en una anastomosis uretro-sigmoidea. J Arch Esp Urol 1998;51:284.

42 Sakano S, Yoshihiro S, Joko K, Kawano H, Naito K. Adenocarcinoma developing in an ileal conduit. J Urol 1995;153:146.

43 Sato M, Fukui S, Fujita I, Kawakita M, Sakaida N, Okamura M. Adenocarcinoma of the ileal segment with transitional cell carcinoma of the bladder following ileocystoplasty: a case report. Hinyokika Kiyo 2000;46:33.

44 Schipper H, Decter A. Carcinoma of the colon arising at ureteral implant sites despite early external diversion: pathogenetic and clinical implications. Cancer 1981;47:2062.

45 Shaaban AH, Sheir KZ, El-Baz MA. Adenocarcinoma in an isolated rectosigmoid bladder: case report. J Urol 1992;147:457.

46 Shishido T, Itou T, Ono Y, Arai Y, Miki M. Adenocarcinoma of the renal pelvis and transitional cell carcinoma of the ureter occurring 11 years after radical cystectomy for bladder cancer: a case report. Hinyokika Kiyo 2001;47:187.

47 Shokeir AA, Shamaa M, El-Mekresh MM, El-Baz M, Ghonheim A. Late malignancy in bowel segments exposed to urine without fecal stream. Urology 1995;46:657.

48 Stillwell TJ, Myers RP. Adenomatous polyp in defunctionalized colonic segment used as a urinary bladder. Urology 1988;32:538.

49 Strand WR, Alfert HJ. Nephrogenic adenoma occurring in an ileal conduit. J Urol 1987;137:491.

50 Takahashi A, Tsukamoto T, Kumamoto Y, Sato Y, Shibuya A. Adenocarcinoma arising in the ileal segment of a defunctionalized ileocystoplasty. Acta Urol Jpn 1993;39:753.

51 Téllez Martínez-Fornes M, Burgos Revilla FJ, Del Hoyo Campos J, Rivas Escudero JA, Navio Niño S, Allona Almagro A. Adenocarcinoma de colon metastasico en paciente portador de cecocistoplastia de ampliacion. Actas Urol Esp 1993;17:80.

52 Tsuboniwa N, Miki T, Kuroda M, Maeda O, Saiki S, Kinouchi T. Primary adenocarcinoma in an ileal conduit. Int J Urol 1996;3:64.

53 Uesugi T, Uno S, Hayashi K. Colonic adenocarcinoma associated with dysplastic lesions in an Indiana pouch. J Urol 2002;168:2117.

54 Weinstein T, Zevin D, Kyzer S, Korzets A, Halperin M, Luria B. Adenocarcinoma at ureterosigmoidostomy junction in a renal transplant recipient 15 years after conversion to ileal conduit. Clin Nephrol 1995;44:125.

55 Yamada Y, Fujisawa M, Nakagawa H, Tanaka H, Gotoh A, Gohji K. Squamous cell carcinoma in an ileal conduit. Int J Urol 1998;5:613.

56 Yip SKH, Wong MP, Cheung MC, Li JHC. Mucinous adenocarcinoma of renal pelvis and villous adenoma of bladder after caecal augmentation of bladder. Aust NZ J Surg 1999;69:247.

57 Yoshida T, Kim CJ, Konishi T, Yoshiki T, Park KI, Tomoyoshi T. Adenocarcinoma of the bladder 19 years after the augmentation ileocystoplasty: report of a case. Nippon Hinyokika Gakkai Zasshi 1998;89:54.

Chapter 74
Abdominal Compartment Syndrome: Urologic Aspects

Raanan Tal

Introduction

The term abdominal compartment syndrome (ACS) describes the effects of elevated intra-abdominal pressure (IAP) on multiple organ systems. The deleterious effects of increased IAP have been known since the 19th century but our understanding of their pathogenesis is still evolving. A high index of suspicion among critically ill patients, monitoring of IAP among patients at risk, and prompt treatment are the cornerstones of successful management of this disorder. This chapter reviews the latest information about the effects of elevated IAP on different organs and systems and the pathogenesis, diagnosis, and treatment of ACS with an emphasis on renal dysfunction and other urologic aspects.

History

Although the term ACS was first used by Kron *et al.* [18] only in the early 1980s, the disorder has been recognized since 1863, when Marey and Burt described the respiratory effects of elevated IAP. In 1876, Wendt reported an association of elevated IAP with renal dysfunction; in 1890, Heinricius demonstrated that in animal models an elevation in IAP led to death presumably from respiratory failure; and in 1911 Emerson described the cardiovascular derangements due to elevated IAP in animals. Early in World War II, Ogilvie detailed the surgical management of the 'burst abdomen' and in 1940 Gross identified the clinical triad that could be anticipated when the abdominal cavity is overstuffed: respiratory failure (due to upward displacement of the diaphragm), impaired venous return (from pressure on the inferior vena cava), and intestinal obstruction (from compression of the viscera).

Definition and etiology

ACS is defined as the cardiovascular, pulmonary, renal, splanchnic, gastrointestinal, abdominal wall/wound, and intracranial disturbances resulting from an acute and rapid increase in IAP [23]. Normal IAP is atmospheric (zero) or subatmospheric (negative) when measured in spontaneously breathing animals [23]. Mechanical ventilation produces a positive IAP close to the end-expiratory pressure with values of up to 10 mmHg, which are considered normal. Following abdominal surgery, pressures are typically in the range of 3–15 mmHg [19]. The diagnosis of ACS is made when IAP exceeds 25 mmHg in the presence of one of the following signs of clinical deterioration: oliguria, raised pulmonary pressure, hypoxia, decreased cardiac output, hypotension, or acidosis. The diagnosis is confirmed when abdominal decompression results in clinical improvement [20]. In the current literature, different definitions for ACS are used. Meldrum *et al.* [21] defined ACS as an IAP of >20 mmHg complicated by one of the following: peak airway pressure (PAP) >40 cmH$_2$O, oxygen delivery index (DO$_2$I) <600 mL O$_2$/min/m^2, or urine output (UO) < 0.5 mL/kg/h; while Ertel *et al.* [11] defined ACS as the development of significant respiratory compromise, including an elevated inspiratory pressure of >35 mbar, a decreased Horowitz quotient (<150 torr (<20 kPa)), renal dysfunction (urine output <30 mL/h), hemodynamic instability necessitating catecholamines, and a rigid or tense abdomen.

ACS and resultant renal dysfunction have been described in many diverse clinical scenarios [19,23], in trauma patients with intraperitoneal, extraperitoneal, or pelvic injuries, and in nontraumatic conditions. The most common cause is increased IAP due to intraperitoneal conditions, such as hemorrhage, edema, bowel distension, mesenteric venous obstruction, abdominal packs, tense ascites, peritonitis, and tumors. Pneumoperitoneum induction, widely used for laparoscopic procedures, has been shown to cause elevated IAP with adverse effects on the cardiovascular system and renal function, including decreased aortic and inferior vena cava bloodflow and oliguria [3,16]. Unilateral pneumoretroperitoneum, however, causes lesser systemic and renal hemodynamic alterations [7]. The effects produced by the gas insufflation are reversible, with complete resolution between 2 and 24 h after decompression [7,16]. ACS has also been described after ureteral perforation, leading to intraperitoneal urine leakage and as a consequence of increased retroperitoneal volume secondary to pancreatitis, hemorrhage, or edema after pelvic trauma or abdominal aortic surgery [14,23]. Extrinsic abdominal compression can also lead to ACS: IAP may rise in burn patients with abdominal eschars or after a tight surgical abdominal closure.

In most critically ill patients, the development of ACS is multifactorial. Massive fluid resuscitation, combined with capillary leak (e.g. in shock, sepsis, burns, or reperfusion injury), leads to visceral edema, an increase in visceral volume, and IAP. Poor pulmonary compliance due to acute lung dysfunction requires high positive pressure ventilation. This pressure is transmitted to the abdominal cavity exacerbating the existing elevation of IAP. The circulatory effects of elevated IAP further compromise abdominal wall and visceral perfusion, leading to a vicious cycle of increased edema, decreased abdominal wall compliance, and in turn elevation of IAP [23]. The diagnosis of ACS should be considered in any trauma or critically ill patient in the setting of abdominal distension and deteriorating cardiac, pulmonary, or renal function [17]. The incidence of elevated IAP in surgical patients admitted to an intensive care unit has been reported to be as high as 33%. Among patients with renal function impairment, 69% had increased IAP [24].

Measurement of IAP

Several methods of measuring IAP have been described in the literature. Kron et al. used intravesical pressure to reflect IAP [18]. They measured the intravesical pressure with a manometer attached to a Foley catheter placed in the bladder. Cheatham et al. revised Kron's technique and described a closed system device that enabled repeated measurements of the intravesical pressure and, thereby, close, convenient, and safe monitoring of the IAP [4]. Fusco et al. showed that intravesical pressure closely approximates IAP and that the instillation of 50 mL of liquid into the bladder improves the accuracy of the IAP measurement [12]. Other techniques include intragastric pressure measurement obtained by a nasogastric tube and intrarectal pressure measurement obtained by the introduction of a 12 Fr balloon-tipped catheter into the rectum 8–10 cm above the anal verge, but these methods seem to be technically less reliable [22]. The measurement of IAP is essential, as the clinical examination cannot reliably identify patients with elevated IAP. Kirkpatrick et al. found that the sensitivity of the clinical examination was only 40% for an IAP higher than 10 mmHg, and 56% for an IAP higher than 15 mmHg [15].

ACS and its pathophysiologic derangements appear above a critical IAP value that varies from patient to patient and even within a given patient. Burch et al. [2] described a grading system for IAP as follows: grade I, 10–15 cmH_2O; grade II, 16–25 cmH_2O; grade III, 26–35 cmH_2O; and grade IV, >35 cmH_2O. Although physiologic changes could be found already in association with grade I elevations, decompression was clinically insignificant and unwarranted. These authors recommended that at higher pressures, treatment should be determined on the basis of the patient's physiologic responses. Meldrom et al. [2,21], on the basis of their finding that renal dysfunction, defined as urine output less than 0.5 mL/kg/h, was absent in patients with grades I and II ACS but was present in 65% and 100% of patients with grades III and IV, respectively, concluded that most grade III and all grade IV elevations require operative intervention and decompression. Cheatham et al. [5] proposed a new parameter in the assessment of elevated IAP named 'abdominal perfusion pressure'; defined as the mean arterial pressure minus the IAP. These authors showed that the abdominal perfusion pressure was superior to the IAP in predicting survival and served as a clinically useful resuscitation endpoint in patients with ACS.

Pathogenesis and treatment

The deleterious consequences of elevated IAP on the abdominal viscera, abdominal wall, respiratory system, cardiovascular system, central nervous system, and urinary system are well described in the literature [19,23]. The cause of the urinary system dysfunction is probably multifactorial. The renal dysfunction of ACS is characterized by oliguria progressing to anuria and unresponsiveness to volume expansion [23]. Oliguria can be seen at an IAP of 15–20 mmHg, and anuria at 30 mmHg or greater. Biancofiore et al. showed that an abdominal pressure of 25 mmHg had the best sensitivity/specificity ratio for renal failure [1]. Indeed, at an IAP greater than 20 mmHg, all intraperitoneal and retroperitoneal viscera demonstrate a marked reduction in bloodflow. The one exception is the adrenal gland, for which measurements of perfusion clearly indicate a paradoxical increase in bloodflow even at IAPs as high as 40 mmHg [19]. Harman et al. studied the hemodynamic effects of elevated IAP on renal function and cardiac output in dogs [13]. At a pressure of 20 mmHg, renal bloodflow and glomerular filtration rate (GFR) were 25% lower than the values measured at a pressure of 0 mmHg and renal vascular resistance was 15-fold higher than systemic vascular resistance. At 40 mmHg, the dogs became anuric and the renal bloodflow and glomerular filtration rates were 7% of the baseline with a cardiac output of 37% of the baseline. Volume expansion corrected the deficit in cardiac output but renal bloodflow and GFR remained less than 25% of the normal value. These findings suggest that renal dysfunction secondary to elevated IAP is not related only to reduced cardiac output.

The pathogenesis of these renal derangements is probably multifactorial: a combination of reduced cardiac output, elevated renal venous pressure, increased renal parenchymal pressure, and direct compression of the renal vein. Elevated IAP compresses the resistance vessels, increasing afterload, and compresses the inferior vena cava decreasing preload. These processes result in decreased cardiac output and reduced renal bloodflow with activation of the rennin–

angiotensin–aldosterone system. The combination of decreased renal bloodflow, increased renal parenchymal pressure, and direct renal vein compression reduces the pressure gradient across the glomerular membrane and, thereby, the GFR, leading to changes in intrarenal bloodflow and corticomedullary blood shunting. These hemodynamic alterations promote the release of rennin, with the formation of angiotensin II, a potent vasoconstrictor, further reducing renal bloodflow and GFR. With reduced GFR, there is a reduction of sodium delivery to the macula densa and further release of renin from the juxtaglomerular cells, leading to a vicious cycle [10]. Aldosterone secretion mediates sodium and water retention contributing to oliguria [23]. The reduction in GFR in ACS is refractory to volume loading suggesting that the renal vein hypertension may play a greater role than the reduction in renal bloodflow [19]. This assumption is also supported by the general ineffectiveness of treatment with dopaminergic agonists and loop diuretics [23]. Doty *et al.* showed that high renal parenchymal pressure alone does not lead to renal dysfunction, whereas renal vein compression alone does create the pathophysiologic derangements seen in ACS, suggesting that renal vein compression is the single most important factor [9,10]. Ureteric compression has also been implicated as a contributory factor in the development of oliguria and urinary system dysfunction but the insertion of ureteral catheters has no favorable effect [19,23].

The cornerstones of ACS management are prevention, a high index of suspicion, early recognition, and prompt decompressive laparotomy to reverse the urinary system dysfunction. Prolonged fluid resuscitation to maintain intravascular volume and cardiac output may aggravate bowel edema and ascites, resulting in a vicious cycle with aggravation of the ACS [17]. Prevention can be achieved by awareness of the high prevalence of ACS, reported to be 5–15% among severe abdominal trauma victims, and knowing the risk factors associated with ACS [11]. Ertel *et al.* [11] found that risk factors associated with ACS are active bleeding requiring damage control laparotomy and packing, combined abdominal and pelvic injuries, primary abdominal fascial closure (in contrast to mesh closure), massive bowel distension secondary to reperfusion injury after fluid resuscitation, and resolution of shock and uncontrolled intra-abdominal bleeding, not uncommonly due to coagulopathy, necessitating re-exploration. Early diagnosis of ACS mandates close monitoring of IAP in every patient at risk since it may occur within a few hours. In certain circumstances the development of ACS can be prevented by simple measures such as the avoidance of tense abdominal closure, but the presence of active bleeding poses a real treatment challenge owing to the conflict between the need to achieve pressure to tamponade the bleeding and the avoidance of increased IAP. The treatment of ACS is prompt surgical decompressive laparotomy and temporary abdominal wall closure using a mesh or a 'Bogota bag'. Minimally invasive decompression techniques, namely laparoscopic and percutaneous procedures, for selected indications have been described but they are not widely used [6,8]. Kopelman *et al.* [17] noted that survivors of ACS underwent surgical decompression earlier than nonsurvivors and suggested that the length of time a patient remains intra-abdominally hypertensive is more significant than the absolute increase in abdominal pressure. Early recognition of predictive variables and identification of patients at risk will hopefully lead to early treatment and avoidance of the morbidity and mortality associated with ACS.

Summary

ACS is prevalent in various surgical conditions and in a large percentage of critically ill patients. The measurement of IAP is an important tool in early diagnosis of ACS and can be performed easily by measuring the intravesical pressure. ACS adversely affects multiple organ systems; the pathogenesis of the renal dysfunction is probably multifactorial: a combination of reduced cardiac output, reduced GFR mediated by secretion of renin and angiotensin, aldosterone-mediated water reabsorption, increased renal parenchymal pressure, and direct compression of the renal vein. Successful treatment requires a high index of suspicion, prompt recognition, and early surgical abdominal decompression.

References

1 Biancofiore G, Bindi L, Romanelli AM *et al.* Renal failure and abdominal hypertension after liver transplantation: determination of critical intra-abdominal pressure. Liver Transpl 2002;8: 1175–81.

2 Burch JM, Moore EE, Moore FA *et al.* The abdominal compartment syndrome. Surg Clin North Am 1996;76:833–42.

3 Chang DT, Kirsch AJ, Sawczuk IS. Oliguria during laparoscopic surgery. J Endourol 1994;8:349–52.

4 Cheatham ML, Safcsak K. Intraabdominal pressure: a revised method for measurement. J Am Coll Surg 1998;186:594–5.

5 Cheatham ML, White MW, Sagraves SG *et al.* Abdominal perfusion pressure: a superior parameter in the assessment of intra-abdominal hypertension. J Trauma 2000;49:621–7.

6 Chen RJ, Fang JF, Lin BC *et al.* Laparoscopic decompression of abdominal compartment syndrome after blunt hepatic trauma. Surg Endosc 2000;14:966.

7 Chiu AW, Chang LS, Birkett DH *et al.* The impact of pneumoperitoneum, pneumoretroperitoneum, and gasless laparoscopy on the systemic and renal hemodynamics. J Am Coll Surg 1995; 181:397–406.

8 Corcos AC, Sherman HF. Percutaneous treatment of secondary abdominal compartment syndrome. J Trauma 2001;51:1062.

9 Doty JM, Saggi BH, Blocher CR *et al.* Effects of increased renal parenchymal pressure on renal function. J Trauma 2000;48: 874–7.

10 Doty JM, Saggi BH, Sugerman HJ *et al.* Effect of increased renal venous pressure on renal function. J Trauma 1999;47:1000–3.

11 Ertel W, Oberholzer A, Platz A *et al.* Incidence and clinical pattern

of the abdominal compartment syndrome after 'damage-control' laparotomy in 311 patients with severe abdominal and/or pelvic trauma. Crit Care Med 2000;28:1747–53.

12 Fusco MA, Martin RS, Chang MC. Estimation of intra-abdominal pressure by bladder pressure measurement: validity and methodology. J Trauma 2001;50:297–302.

13 Harman PK, Kron IL, McLachlan HD *et al.* Elevated intra-abdominal pressure and renal function. Ann Surg 1982; 196:594–7.

14 Katz R, Meretyk S, Gimmon Z. Abdominal compartment syndrome due to delayed identification of a ureteral perforation following abdomino-perineal resection for rectal carcinoma. Int J Urol 1997;4:615–17.

15 Kirkpatrick AW, Brenneman FD, McLean RF *et al.* Is clinical examination an accurate indicator of raised intra-abdominal pressure in critically injured patients? Can J Surg 2000;43: 207–11.

16 Kirsch AJ, Hensle TW, Chang DT *et al.* Renal effects of CO_2 insufflation: oliguria and acute renal dysfunction in a rat pneumoperitoneum model. Urology 1994;43:453–9.

17 Kopelman T, Harris C, Miller R *et al.* Abdominal compartment syndrome in patients with isolated extraperitoneal injuries. J Trauma 2000;49:744–9.

18 Kron IL, Harman PK, Nolan SP. The measurement of intra-abdominal pressure as a criterion for abdominal re-exploration. Ann Surg 1984;199:28–30.

19 Nathens AB, Brenneman FD, Boulanger BR. The abdominal compartment syndrome. Can J Surg 1997;40:254–8.

20 Mayberry JC. Prevention of the abdominal compartment syndrome. Lancet 1999;354:1749–50.

21 Meldrum DR, Moore FA, Moore EE *et al.* Prospective characterization and selective management of the abdominal compartment syndrome. Am J Surg 1997;174:667–73.

22 Obeid F, Saba A, Fath J *et al.* Increases in intra-abdominal pressure affect pulmonary compliance. Arch Surg 1995;130:544–8.

23 Saggi BH, Sugerman HJ, Ivatury RR *et al.* Abdominal compartment syndrome. J Trauma 1998;45:597–609.

24 Sugrue M, Buist MD, Hourihan F *et al.* Prospective study of intra-abdominal hypertension and renal function after laparotomy. Br J Surg 1995;82:235–8.

Chapter 75
Nerve Injuries in Urologic Surgery

M. Eicke, R. Hohenfellner, and J. Leissner

Classification [1]

• *Neurapraxia*: this is the temporary blockade of signal transmission without a structural axon lesion. The functional deficits persist for hours to weeks. Electrophysiologically, it can be diagnosed by transmission blockade at the trauma site with persisting motor or sensory potentials when stimulated distally.
• *Axonotmesis*: this is defined by axon transection with intact nerve sheets. Post-traumatically, a degeneration is observed of the nerves distal to the lesion site. It has a good prognosis, although regeneration time varies. At the site of the injury, nerve growth is 0.25 mm/day, and distal to the injury it is approximately 3–4 mm/day. The rule of thumb is that the length of the nerve structures to be regenerated in millimeters approximately equals the time in days until the beginning of functional recovery.
• *Neurotmesis*: this is the complete transection of the nerve including its sheets. Due to the elasticity of the nerves, a dehiscence of several centimeters of the proximal and distal nerve endings can be observed. Spontaneous regeneration cannot be expected. In addition, neuroma can occur later on.

Pain syndromes

• *Causalgia*: this is characterized by burning pain, triggered by tactile stimuli, with a waveform character. It is associated with vegetative symptoms. It reaches its maximum after weeks, and improves after months to years.
• *Post-traumatic neuralgia*: this is characterized by flash-like, dull and drilling pain, starting in the first few hours after the trauma. The intensity increases with cold temperatures.
• *Neuroma pain*: this follows a complete lesion with or without nerve suture or nerve interposition, and is extremely painful. Revision becomes necessary.

Anatomy

Remember that six important nerves arising from T12–L5 enter the paravertebral structures (plexus lumbosacralis) through the psoas muscle (Fig. 75.1): the iliohypogastric nerve, ilioinguinal nerve, genitofemoral nerve, femoral nerve, cutaneous femoral lateral nerve, and obturatoric nerve. These nerves are located in the retroperitoneum, and travel later on in a lateral and anterior direction on the surface of the abdominal wall. (Lesions of the ischiadic nerve are extremely rare.)

The closer the lesions are to the point where the nerves arise (as in kidney surgery or lymphadenectomy), the higher the risk of complete deficiency later on. Notice also that double innervations of muscles, such as the ilioinguinal/iliohypogastric or obturatoric/femoral nerves, as well as a double sensory innervation of some regions may compensate for deficiency symptoms (again the ilioinguinal/iliohypogastric and genitofemoral nerves).

For lesions of the pelvic plexus, see Chapter 76.

Nerve injuries from pelvic surgery

Obturatoric nerve (L2–L4) (Fig. 75.2)
Location of nerve injury
• Point of exit from the psoas muscle at its medial rim: reported in extended lymphadenectomy and radical pelvic surgery.
• At the fossa obturator and Cooper's ligament: reported in laparoscopy.

Remarks
Indirect lesions are also observed after radical transurethral resection (TUR) of the prostate. Prostatitis may lead to capsule perforation and cause ostitis ossis pubis with spasm of the adductor muscle and hip contraction. Intraoperative spasm of the adductor muscle in transurethral resection of prostate and bladder tumors may even cause bladder destruction. Local anesthesia of the nerve in addition to regional anesthesia may reduce this risk.

Function
• Motor: hip adduction (musculus adductor magnus et

Table 75.1 Functional tests for different muscles.

Muscle	Functional test
M. pectineus	Thigh adduction in the hip
M. sartorius	Thigh abduction, flexion, and outside rotation
M. quadriceps femoris	Knee extension and thigh elevation
M. vastus medius, lateralis, intermedius	Knee extension and heel elevation with extended knee
M. rectus femoris	Hip extension with extended knee
M. iliopsoas	Hip flexion with knee flexed by 90°

longus) and outside rotation (musculi gracilis, pectineus, obturatorius externus, adductor brevis).
• Sensory: medial part of the distal thigh.

Femoral nerve (L1–L4)
Location of nerve injury
• Between the psoas and iliacus muscles: reported in psoas hitch (rare) and hernia repairs.
• Lateral and dorsal femoral artery and vein: reported in extreme abduction and self-retractor compression of the inguinal ligament.

Remarks
Sometimes a deep suture inside the psoas muscle may cause the lesion. Also, rare cases are reported of lesions due to hernia fixation. There is severe motor dysfunction.

Function
• Motor: Table 75.1 lists the functional tests for different muscles.
• Sensory: ventral part of the thigh and the medial side of the lower leg (saphenous nerve).

Genitofemoral nerve (L1–L2)
Location of nerve injury
• Genital branch of the genitofemoral nerve (penetrates the abdominal wall 1–3 cm lateral of the deep inguinal ring): reported in psoas hitch operations, hernia repair, and neurinoma near the ureter stump in kidney transplants.
• Femoral branch of the genitofemoral nerve (below the inguinal ligament): reported as a rare lesion in urologic surgery.

Remarks
Remember that there is double sensory innervation by the ilioinguinal nerve of the scrotum, labium, and penis.

Function
• Motor: contraction of the labia majora and cremaster.
• Sensory: labia majora, scrotum penis (genital branch), skin at the inguinal ligament (trigonum femorale scarpae), and spermatic neuralgia with flash-like intense pain (femoral branch).

Cutaneous nerves of the thigh (L2–L3)
Location of nerve injury
• Between the fascia of the iliacus muscle and the crista iliaca (usually 1–4 cm medial of the spina iliaca anterior superior): reported in lithotomy and laparoscopic hernia surgery.

Remarks
There is dysesthesia and a severe burning pain on the lateral side of the thigh (meralgia paraesthetica). The region lateral to the deep inguinal ring is referred to as the 'triangle of pain' or the 'trapezoid of disaster'. Neurolysis may become necessary.

Function
• Motor: no function.
• Sensory: lateral thigh.

Pudendal nerve
Location of nerve injury
• Above and below the sacrotuberous ligament, through Alcock's canal and the transversus perinei muscles: reported in induratio penis plastica operations causing loss of sensation of the glans penis and coldness.

Remarks
Pudendus anesthesia is used in pelvic pain.

Function
• Motor: perineal nerve: bulbospongiosis muscle (ejaculation, bladder control) and the sphincter anus externus muscle.
• Sensory:
  • perineal nerve: perineal region and skin of the scrotum;
  • dorsal nerve of the penis: the penis.

Intercostal nerve (T11–T12) (Fig. 75.3)
Location of nerve injury
• Lower rim of the 11th or 12th ribs: reported in colostomies and paraventral incisions.

Remarks
Paresthesia of the skin nerves is reversible within 3–6 months.

Iliohypogastric nerve (T12–L1) (Figs 75.4, 75.5)
Location of nerve injury
• Between the transverses and internal obliquus muscles: reported in colostomies located laterally in the abdominal wall.

Function
• Motor: paralysis of the abdominal wall muscles (musculi transversus abdominis, obliquus internus abdominis; torsional elevation of the trunk) in combined injuries with the ilioinguinal nerve.
• Sensory: lateral inguinal region.

Ilioinguinal nerve (T12–L1) (Fig. 75.4)
Location of nerve injury
• Distal from the iliohypogastric nerve and below the fascia of the oblique muscles: reported in colostomies.

Function
• Motor: deficits only in combined lesions with the iliohypogastric nerve (abdominal wall).
• Sensory: dorsum penis, and the proximal section of the labia majora and scrotum.

Nerve injuries from kidney exploration
(Fig. 75.6)

Iliohypogastric nerve (T12–L1)
Location of nerve injury
• First, this muscle perforates the psoas muscle. Then, it is located on top of the quadratus lumbar muscle; further distally the nerve is embedded between the transverse abdominal and oblique internal muscles. Damage is reported in secondary operations, with scar tissue between the fatty capsule and the kidney causing dislocation of the nerve.

Ilioinguinal nerve (T12–L1)
Location of nerve injury
• This nerve perforates the psoas muscle together with the iliohypogastric nerve, which is located below it. As the iliohypogastric nerve it runs on top of the quadratus lumbar muscle. Nephrectomy, surgery on retroperitoneal tumors, or hematoma may cause a lesion. Damage results in paresis of the abdominal wall and sensory deficits at the dorsum penis and the proximal section of the labia majora/scrotum.

Reference

1 Seddon HJ. Three types of nerve injury. Brain 1943;66:238–88.

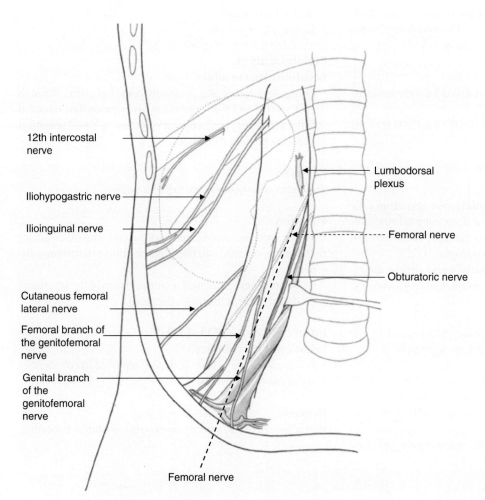

Figure 75.1 Topography of the most relevant retroperitoneal and inguinal nerves.

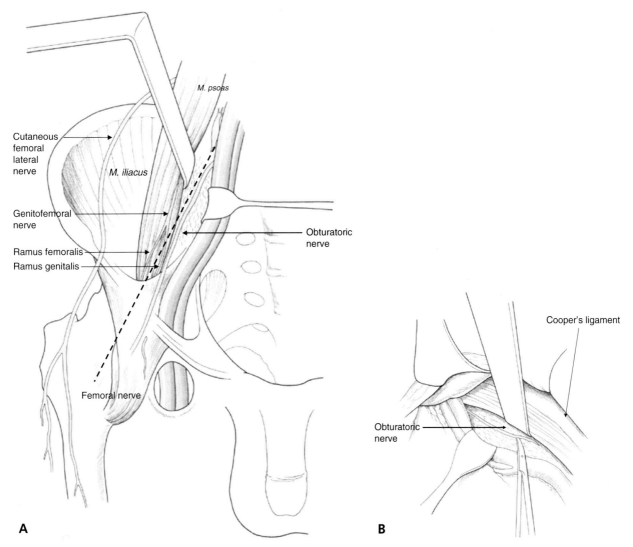

Figure 75.2 The obturatoric nerve is at high risk during extended lymph node resection.

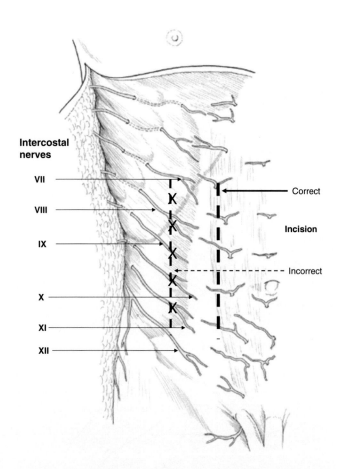

Intercostal nerves

VII

VIII

IX

X

XI

XII

Correct

Incision

Incorrect

Figure 75.3 The lower six intercostal nerves between the oblique transverse and internal abdominal muscles provide motor innervation of the abdominal wall (a lesion may cause abdominal wall relaxation or hernia formation). The cutaneous branches VII, VIII, and IX innervate the supraumbilical region, while branches X, XI, and XII innervate the infraumbilical region.

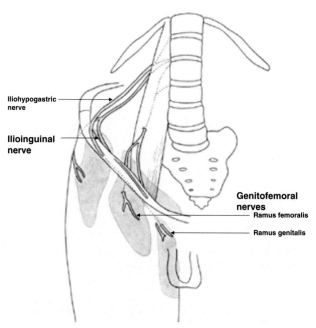

Iliohypogastric nerve

Ilioinguinal nerve

Genitofemoral nerves
— Ramus femoralis
— Ramus genitalis

Figure 75.4 The topography and sensory areas of the ilioinguinal, iliohypogastric (these nerves perforate the psoas, located on the quadratus lumbar muscle), and genitofemoral nerves. Risks are posed by the scar tissue from renal 'redo' operations on the backside of the kidney.

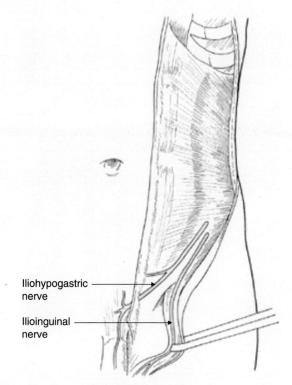

Iliohypogastric nerve

Ilioinguinal nerve

Figure 75.5 The topography of the parainguinal incision, which could damage the iliohypogastric nerve. Remember the double (or triple) genital skin innervation by the ilioinguinal nerve and the genital branch of the genitofemoral nerve.

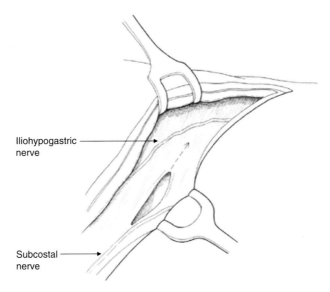

Figure 75.6 Kidney exploration poses a risk for iliohypogastric and intercostal (T12) nerve lesions.

Chapter 76
Pelvic Plexus: Topographical Considerations and Clinical Consequences

J. Leissner

Introduction

An exact knowledge of anatomical structures is mandatory for every surgeon. Usually, vessels, large nerves, and organs are recognized very early on by the individual surgeon because violating these structures has direct and often severe consequences. Precise knowledge about minor structures comes later, when the long-term effects of surgery also become obvious. This is especially true for the nerve fibers of the autonomic nerve system in the small pelvis, where a number of organs, including their blood supply and innervation, are located within a very small space. Surgery in the pelvis is complex and dangerous, and is often complicated by severe bleeding.

The autonomic nerve system in the pelvis has been neglected for a long time. A new interest has arisen in the last few years from different points of view: pediatric surgeons learned its significance for antireflux surgery, oncologists found its importance during radical prostatectomy, and for every form of bladder substitution the preservation of the autonomic nerves is of interest.

This chapter discusses the topography of the pelvic plexus and assesses injuries to the plexus incurred by antireflux surgery.

Functional anatomy

The pelvic plexus is an association of sympathetic and parasympathetic neurons near the bladder, and is involved in eliminative and reproductive functions. The sympathetic part comes from two main lumbar splanchnic nerves arising from L2 and L3 levels. The parasympathetic part is formed by three pelvic splanchnic nerves. The efferent nerve fibers run from the plexus to the genitourinary system and the rectum (Fig. 76.1). In addition to the innervation of the bladder, the plexus is responsible for sexual and reproductive functions and for defecation.

Study: materials, methods, and results

Human cadavers, fixed with Thiel's solution, were used for the dissection [11]. The nerves were visualized with methylene blue staining [7]. The superior hypogastric plexus and the hypogastric nerves were identified as the pathway to the pelvic plexus (Fig. 76.2). Following dissection of the surrounding fatty tissue, the afferent and efferent nerve bundles from the pelvic plexus were identified (Fig. 76.3).

The plexus itself is located between the dorsal wall of the bladder and the anterior surface of the rectum, embedded in fatty tissue. The main portion is found about 1.5 cm dorsal and medial to the ureterovesical junction. The bundles of the pelvic plexus end at the distal ureter, the trigone, the rectum, and in the female, the uterus and vagina.

The adventitia of the ureter is surrounded immediately by a network of small vessels. The next layer surrounding the ureter is a plane formed by thin tissue fibers, which were dissected without compromising the longitudinal blood vessels of the ureter. Analogous to the rectum, this layer was named the mesoureter (Fig. 76.4).

For evaluating critical nerve pathways that may be damaged during antireflux surgery, the ureter was dissected using Overholt clamps (Fig. 76.5). The terminal branches of the pelvic plexus running to the ureter were immediately destroyed when dissection was performed outside the plane of the mesoureter. When dissection was continued dorsal and medial to the ureterovesical hiatus, the branches running through the trigone, as well as the main bulk of the pelvic plexus, were also damaged.

Clinical consequences

Voiding dysfunction and urinary retention are rare complications of antireflux surgery. However, long-term effects such as renal insufficiency or urinary diversion can be fatal for patients. As mainly reported for bilateral antireflux surgery with extravesical techniques, bladder insufficiency has been suspected to be caused by intraoperative damage to the neural structures [2].

Intravesical techniques

If ureteral dissection is performed only in the intramural part, as described by Cohen [1], the risk of destroying nerve fibers of the pelvic plexus is minimal (Fig. 76.6). In contrast, the risk is higher when performing a more extensive dissection of the ureter. When ureteral dissection is continued extravesically, as often performed for the Politano–Leadbetter technique (Fig. 76.7), the preparation should be close to the ureter in the layer of the mesoureter to avoid damage to the efferent nerve fibers [8].

Extravesical techniques

In the original Lich–Gregoir technique [3], myotomy is performed starting from the ventral aspect of the ureterovesical hiatus and ending at the top of the bladder (Fig. 76.8). The distal ureter should therefore be mobile, but extensive dissection—particularly dorsal and caudal to the ureterovesical hiatus—is unnecessary (Fig. 76.9). In contrast, the horizontal incision described by Hendren [4] has a higher risk of destroying the neural structures of the pelvic plexus. In the detrusorraphy technique, the circumferential myotomy around the ureterovesical hiatus and the vest-type sutures to anchor the ureter onto the trigone are the steps during which nerve structures are damaged [12].

Critical points during dissection also include unexpected bleeding from the uterine vessels or branches of the paravesical or paravaginal venous plexus. Because the nerve fibers cannot be identified intraoperatively, clamping or deep stitches may compromise the branches of the pelvic plexus.

Ureterocystoneostomy

When the ureter is dissected and a terminal segment approximately 1–1.5 cm is left above the bladder entrance to perform the psoas hitch procedure, there is no risk of damaging the pelvic plexus, even when it is performed bilaterally [9].

Conclusions

In order to avoid damaging the structures of the pelvic plexus, attention should be drawn to the following aspects:
- Dissect the ureter close to the adventitia in the layer of the mesoureter, where no bleeding appears.
- Avoid preparation dorsal and medial to the ureterovesical hiatus, and subtrigonal preparation.

- If bleeding occurs during dissection of the distal ureter, avoid deep stitches or clamping that includes the structures dorsal and medial to the distal ureter.

Since bilateral extravesical antireflux procedures cause a higher risk of postoperative voiding dysfunction, reflux correction should be performed over two sessions [10]. In gynecological and rectal surgery, nerve-sparing techniques of the pelvic plexus based on anatomical studies have already been successfully developed to decrease postoperative voiding dysfunction [5,10]. In urologic surgery attention should be given to the pelvic plexus and its terminal branches in all reconstructive procedures of the bladder and distal ureter.

References

1 Cohen SJ. Ureterozystoneostomie: eine neue Antireflux Technik. Akt Urol 1975;6:1–7.
2 Fung LCT, McLorie GA, Jain U, Khoury AE, Churchill BM. Voiding dysfunction after ureteral reimplantation: a comparison of extravesical and intravesical techniques. J Urol 1995;153:1972–5.
3 Gregoir W. Lich–Gregoir operation. In: Surgical Pediatric Urology (Epstein HB, Hohenfellner R, Williams DI, Herausgeber, eds). Thieme, Stuttgart, 1977:265–72.
4 Hendren WH. Reoperation for the failed ureteral implantation. J Urol 1974;111:403.
5 Höckel M, Konerding MA, Heussel CP. Liposuction-assisted nerve-sparing extended radical hysterectomy: oncologic rationale, surgical anatomy, and feasibility study. Am J Obstet Gynecol 1998;178:971.
6 Leissner J, Allhoff EP, Wolff W et al. The pelvic plexus and antireflux surgery—topographical considerations and clinical consequences. J Urol 2001;165:1652–5.
7 Nahlieli O, Levy Y. Intravital staining with methylene blue as an aid to facial nerve identification in parotid gland surgery. J Oral Maxillofac Surg 2001;59:355–6.
8 Politano VA, Leadbetter F. An operative technique for the correction of vesico-ureteric reflux. J Urol 1958;79:932–6.
9 Riedmiller H, Becht E, Hertle L. Psoas-hitch ureteroneocystostomy: experience with 181 cases. Eur Urol 1984;10:145.
10 Sugihara K, Moriya Y, Akasu T et al. Pelvic autonomic nerve preservation for patients with rectal carcinoma. Oncologic and functional outcome. Cancer 1996;78:1871.
11 Thiel W. Die Konservierung ganzer Leichen in natürlichen Farben. Ann Anat 1992;174:185–95.
12 Zaontz MR, Maizels M, Sugar EC, Firlit CF. Detrusorraphy: extravesical ureteral advancement to correct vesicoureteral reflux in children. J Urol 1987;138:947–9.

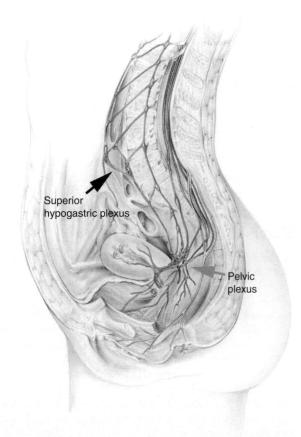

Figure 76.1 Pelvic plexus and innervation of the bladder showing the sympathetic nerves, parasympathetic nerves, and pudendal nerve. (For color, see Plate 76.1, between pp. 112 and 113.)

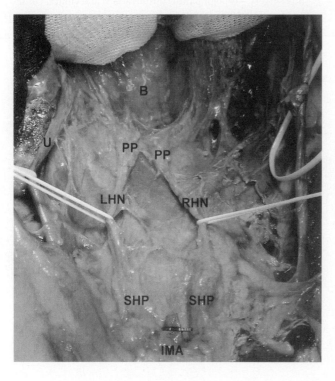

Figure 76.2 Dissection of the superior hypogastric plexus, the hypogastric nerves, and the two main portions of the pelvic plexus in a male cadaver. B, bladder; IMA, inferior mesenteric artery; LHN, left hypogastric nerve; PP, pelvic plexus; RHN, right hypogastric nerve; SHP, superior hypogastric plexus; U, ureter.

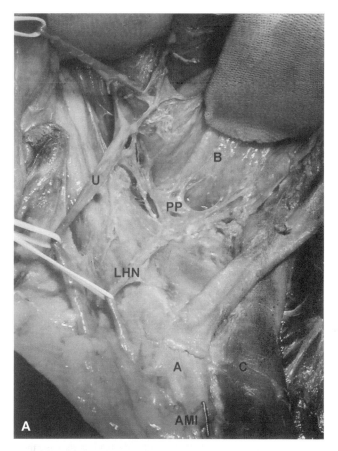

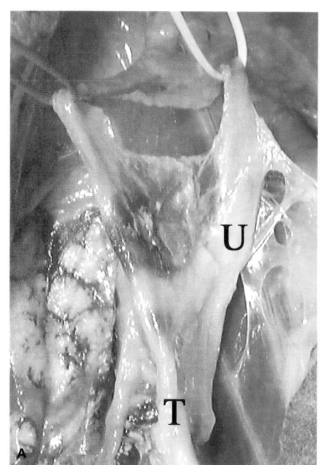

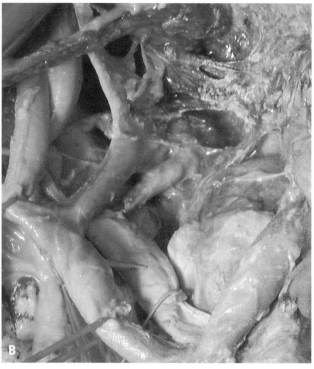

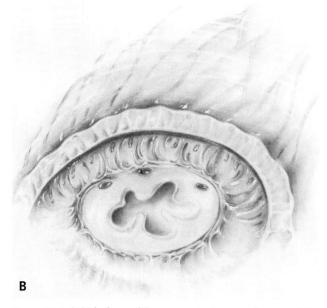

Figure 76.3 (A) The left hypogastric nerve with a network of pelvic plexus nerve bundles. Branches run to the distal ureter (U) and bladder (B) trigones. A, aorta; AMI, inferior mesenteric artery; C, inverior vena cava; LHN, left hypogastric nerve; PP, pelvic plexus. (B) Nerve bundles of the left hypogastric nerve and pelvic plexus are visualized with methylene blue staining. (For color, see Plate 76.3, between pp. 112 and 113.)

Figure 76.4 (A) The layer of the mesoureter between the ureter (U) and the testicular vessels (T). In this layer the ureter can be dissected without compromising the blood supply and without damaging the nerve structures. (B) Layers of the ureter beginning from the center: lumen, lamina muscularis, adventitia with blood vessels, mesoureter, and nerve structures. (For color, see Plate 76.4.)

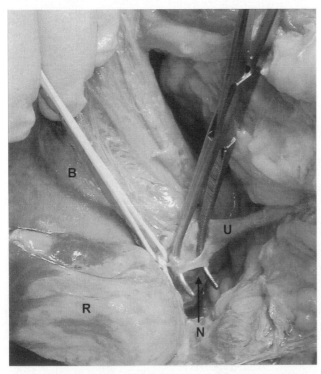

Figure 76.5 Dissection of the distal ureter (U). An Overholt clamp is used to dissect the nerve bundles of the pelvic plexus. B, bladder; N, pelvic plexus nerve fibers; R, rectum.

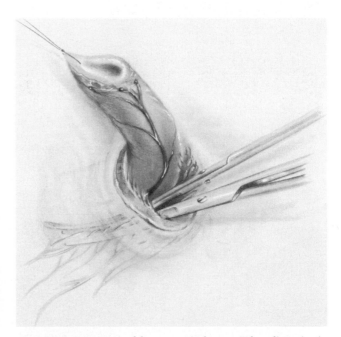

Figure 76.7 Dissection of the extravesical ureter. When dissection is performed outside the layer of the mesoureter, the nerve structures (grey) are easily damaged.

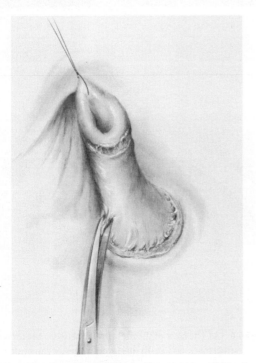

Figure 76.6 For the Cohen technique the ureter is mobilized intramurally only, with no risk of damaging the nerve structures.

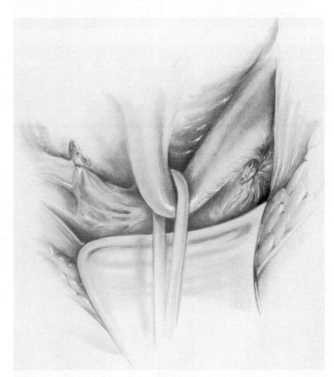

Figure 76.8 For the Lich–Gregoir procedure myotomy is performed starting at the ureterovesical hiatus and ending at the top of the bladder. Nerve bundles are located dorsal and medial to the ureterovesical hiatus.

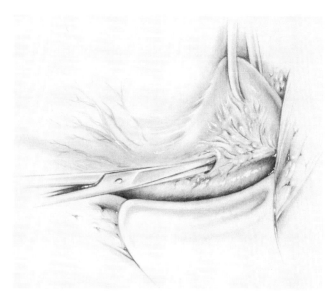

Figure 76.9 Extravesical identification of the ureter. Note the location of the neural bundles and the risk of damage when the dissection is far away from the ureter.

Index

Note: page numbers in *italics* refer to figures, those in **bold** refer to tables. 'Plate' refers to the color plate section